Handbook of Experimental Pharmacology

Volume 130

Springer
Berlin
Heidelberg
New York
Barcelona
Budapest
Hong Kong
London
Milan
Paris
Santa Clara
Singapore
Tokyo

The Pharmacology of Pain

Contributors

I. Appleton, D.L.H. Bennett, J.-M. Besson, P.J. Birch,
V. Chapman, M. Devor, A. Dickenson, A. Dray,
H.L. Fields, M. Fitzgerald, D.L. Hammond, K. Hole,
B.L. Kieffer, M. Koltzenburg, J. Lai, T.O. Malan,
S.B. McMahon, H.J. McQuay, M.J. Millan, R.A. Moore,
M.H. Ossipov, F. Porreca, M.C. Rowbotham, A. Tjølsen,
S. Wiesenfeld-Hallin, X.-J. Xu

Editors
A. Dickenson and J.-M. Besson

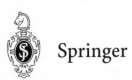 Springer

Professor A. Dickenson
University College London
Department of Pharmacology
Gower Street
London WC1E 6BT
UNITED KINGDOM

Dr. J.-M. Besson
INSERM, U.161
Physiopharmacologie du Système Nerveux
et Laboratoire de Physiopharmacologie
de la Douleur (EPHE)
2, rue d'Alésia
F-75014 Paris
FRANCE

With 41 Figures and 21 Tables

ISBN 3-540-62785-5 Springer-Verlag Berlin Heidelberg New York

Library of Congress Cataloging-in-Publication Data
The pharmacology of pain / editors, A. Dickenson and J.-M. Besson: contributors, I. Appieton . . . [et al.].
p. cm. — (Handbook of experimental pharmacology; v. 130)
Includes bibliographical references and index.
ISBN 3-540-62785-5 (alk. paper)
1. Pain. 2. Analgesia. I. Dickenson, A.H. II. Besson, Jean-Marie R. III. Appleton, I. (Ian)
IV. Series.
[DNLM: 1. Pain—drug therapy. 2. Nociceptors—drug effects. 3. Receptors, Neurotransmitter—
drug effects. 4. Analgesics—pharmacology. 5. Anesthetics—pharmacology.
W1 HA51L v. 130 1997 / WL 704 P536 1997]
QP905.H3 vol. 130
[RB127] 615'. 1s—dc21 [615'.783]
DNLM/DLC
for Library of Congress
97-23531
CIP

Cover design: *design & production* GmbH, Heidelberg

Typesetting: Best-set Typesetter Ltd., Hong Kong

SPIN: 10503571   27/3020 – 5 4 3 2 1 0 – Printed on acid-free paper

Preface

Pain is a symptom of many clinical disorders, afflicts a large proportion of the population and is largely treated by pharmacological means. However, the two main classes of drugs used are the opioids and the non-steroidal anti-inflammatory drugs, drugs that have a long history. The last decade has seen remarkable advances in our understanding of some of the pharmacological bases of pain and analgesia and this book aims to reflect these rapid changes in our understanding of pain mechanisms. One impetus to these scientific advances has been dialogue and interactions between scientists and clinicians; as a result we now has a number of animal models of clinical pain states, to mimic certain aspects of clinical pathophysiological pain states. Molecular aspects of receptors and the synthesis of tools for probing receptor function have also been rapid growth areas. A number of controlled clinical studies using novel licensed drugs have also resulted from recent research, offering hope to certain patients with severe intractable pain. However, we desperately need the pharmaceutical industry to develop new drugs based on these novel targets for analgesic therapy. This book attempts to provide an overview of the important areas of the pharmacology of pain.

This book, although providing an account of the pharmacology of pain transmission and its control based on the underlying anatomical organization and physiological responses, does not attempt to cover these latter two areas. Neither does it provide details of all aspects of opioid function since the *Handbook of Experimental Pharmacology*, volume 104, covered this area in great detail in 1993. Those readers who wish to have a better understanding of the anatomy and physiology of pain and analgesia are referred to several recent reviews, listed at the end of this preface, which amplify some of the details given in this book.

The study of the receptor systems involved in the transmission of pain and its modulation involves the investigation of processes occurring at the peripheral endings of sensory neurones as well as central events. Whereas acute pain rarely presents as a clinical problem, pain caused by inflammation and tissue damage can be produced by operative procedures, trauma, childbirth, cancer etc. In addition, pain from nerve damage, neuropathic pain, can be produced by trauma and tumours invading nervous tissue. The mechanisms of inflammatory and neuropathic pain are very different from acute pain, and there is considerable plasticity in both the transmission and modulating systems in these prolonged pain states. Due to state- and time-dependent plasticity a full range of models spanning the short and longer term inflammatory and neuropathic states is a prerequisite for characterization of all potential receptor systems involved in pain and analgesia.

Models for studying pain have to take into account these different mechanisms and the plasticity inherent in the pharmacology. Simple models of acute pain will not reveal many of the receptors and channels important in the more persistent pain states. Some of the animal models of pain are discussed by KJELL HOLE and colleagues in Chap. 1.

Peripheral Events

The transmission of acute pain involves activation of sensory receptors on peripheral C-fibres, the nociceptors. However, once tissue damage and inflammation occurs, the actions of prostanoids, bradykinin, 5HT etc. on their excitatory receptors plays a major role in sensitization and activation of C-fibres. ANDY DRAY discusses new aspects of excitatory events in the periphery (Chap. 2), PHIL BIRCH covers the roles of the tachykinins at both the peripheral and central levels (Chap. 6) and IAN APPLETON provides a basis for the production of new and more benign NSAIDs based on different forms of the cycloxygenase enzyme (Chap. 3). Other factors such as NGF and cytokines are also important at the peripheral level, and resultant changes in the phenotype of the sensory neurones are considered by MCMAHON and BENNETT (Chap. 7).

Neuropathic pain states are generated in the peripheral sensory neurones by events that are independent of nociceptors. Clustering of sodium channels around areas of nerve damage set up ectopic activity that can spread to the ganglion cells. Sympathetic activity can facilitate these events. Thus membrane stabilizers and agents acting on the sympathetic nervous system have a place in the control of neuropathic pain, and this is covered by HOWARD FIELDS, MARSHALL DEVOR and MICHAEL ROWBOTHAM (Chap. 5).

MARTIN KOLTZENBURG reviews the evidence for an involvement of the sympathetic nervous system in nerve damage related pains (Chap. 4).

Central Excitatory Systems

The arrival of sensory information from nociceptors in the dorsal horn of the spinal cord adds considerable complexity to study of pain and analgesia due to the fact that most of the receptors found in the CNS are also present in the areas where the C-fibres terminate. The density of neurones in these areas is equal to or exceeds that seen elsewhere in the CNS.

Interactions between peptides and excitatory amino acids (EAA) are critical for setting the level of pain transmission from the spinal cord to the brain and motoneurones.

The AMPA receptor for the EAA, the release of substance P and its actions on the neurokinin-1 receptor removes the Mg^{2+} block of the NMDA receptor. Other peptides may also contribute. Activation of the NMDA receptor underlies *wind-up*, and this increased responsivity of dorsal horn neurones is probably the basis for *central hypersensitivity*. The NMDA receptor does not participate in responses to acute stimuli but is involved in persistent inflammatory and neuropathic pains. Adenosine appears to be released in response to NMDA receptor activation and then, by actions on the A1 receptor, acts as a negative feedback system. TONY DICKENSON reviews the roles of these systems (Chap. 8).

Nitric oxide is generated in the spinal cord and periphery and this gas, together with other chemical transmitters such as the peptide cholecystokinin, are discussed by X.-J. XU and ZSUSANNA WIESENFELD-HALLIN (Chap. 9).

Induction of the immediate early gene, *c-fos*, in spinal neurones is rapid and, since it relates to the intensity of stimulus, can be used as a marker of activity and a powerful tool for the study of modulatory effects. VICTORIA CHAPMAN and JEAN-MARIE BESSON review this area (Chap. 10).

Central Inhibitory Systems

Excitatory transmission can be controlled by simply blocking the effects of excitatory transmitters but can also be controlled by the augmentation of inhibitory controls. The roles of the mu, delta and kappa opioid receptors have been established, and despite the long history of the use of opium there are still opportunities for the development of better opioid analgesics. Most clinically used drugs act on the mu receptor, and the delta receptor may provide a target for opioids with fewer side-effects than with morphine. The endogenous opioid peptides have controlling influences on the spinal transmission of pain whereas the dynorphins have complex actions.

BRIGITTE KIEFFER covers the cloning of the opioid receptors and molecular aspects of the receptors (Chap. 11), whereas FRANK PORRECA et al. reviews the functional aspects of the multiple opioid receptors in different pain models (Chap. 12). HENRY McQUAY and ANDREW MOORE point out the key influence of metabolism and tolerance to opioids with the presently available drugs (Chap. 13). Tonic $GABA_A$ and $GABA_B$ receptor controls are important in controlling acute, inflammatory and neuropathic pain states. The former receptor appears to prevent low-threshold inputs from triggering nociception, and DONNA HAMMOND provides a review of the roles of this inhibitory amino acid (Chap. 14).

Monoamine systems originating in the midbrain and brainstem act on the spinal transmission of pain. $Alpha_2$ adrenoceptors appear to be important in the roles of noradrenaline. There is still great confusion regarding the relative roles of the multiple 5HT receptors. MARK MILLAN reviews this field (Chap. 15).

A decade ago it was held that infants did not feel pain – this view has radically changed but there is little basis for a rational approach to analgesia in young children. There are dramatic alterations in receptor ontogeny, location and function during development. The pharmacology of pain in immature is very different form the adult, and MARIA FITZGERALD discusses this area (Chap. 16).

We would like to thank all our contributors to this book for their enthusiasm and, in many cases, for their promptness in providing their chapters. We are also grateful to our colleagues in London and Paris for their assistance and wish to thank DORIS WALKER at Springer-Verlag for her guidance in the project.

Additional Reading

Besson JM, Chaouch A (1987) Peripheral and spinal mechanisms of pain. Physiol Rev 67:67–186
Belmonte C, Cervero F (1996) Neurobiology of nociceptors. Oxford University Press, Oxford, p 531
Pain 1996 – an overview. IASP, Seattle
Postgraduate Educational Issue (1995) Inflammatory and neurogenic pain; new molecules, new mechanisms. Br J Anaesthesia 75:123–227
Willis WD, Coggeshall RE (1991) Sensory mechanisms of the spinal cord. Plenum, New York

List of Contributors

APPLETON, I., School of Biological Sciences, The Stopford Building,
The University of Manchester, Oxford Road, Manchester,
M13 9PT, United Kingdom

BENNETT, D.L.H., Department of Physiology,
St. Thomas Hospital Medical School, Lambeth Palace Road,
London SE1 7EH, United Kingdom

BESSON, J.-M., Physiopharmacologie du Système Nerveux, INSERM U.161
and Laboratoire de Physiopharmacologie de la Douleur (EPHE),
2 rue d'Alésia, F-75014 Paris, France

BIRCH, P.J., Astra Research Centre Montreal, 7171 Frederick Banting,
St. Laurent, Quebec, Canada H4S 1Z9

CHAPMAN, V., Physiopharmacologie du Système Nerveux, INSERM U.161
and Laboratoire de Physiopharmacologie de la Douleur (EPHE),
2 rue d'Alésia, F-75014 Paris, France

DEVOR, M., Department of Cell and Animal Biology, Life Sciences Institute,
Hebrew University of Jerusalem, Jerusalem 91904, Israel

DICKENSON, A., Department of Pharmacology, University College London,
Gower Street, London WC1E 6BT, United Kingdom

DRAY, A., Astra Research Centre Montreal 7171 Frédérick-Banting,
St-Laurent, Québec, Canada H4S 1Z9

FIELDS, H.L., Department of Neurology,
University of California San Francisco, 505 Parnassus Avenue, M-794,
San Francisco, CA 94143-0114, USA

FITZGERALD, M., Department of Anatomy and Developmental Biology,
University College London, Gower Street, London WC1 6BT,
United Kingdom

HAMMOND, D.L., Department of Anesthesia and Critical Care,
University of Chicago, 5841 South Maryland Ave., M/C 4028, Chicago,
IL 60637, USA

HOLE, K., Department of Physiology, University of Bergen, Arstadveien 19, N-5009 Bergen, Norway

KIEFFER, B.L., CNRS UPR 9050 ESBS, Parc d'Innovation, Boulevard S. Brandt, F-67400 Illkirch, France

KOLTZENBURG, M., Department of Neurology, University of Würzburg, Josef-Schneider-Str. 11, D-97080 Würzburg, Germany

LAI, J., Department of Pharmacology, The University of Arizona Pain Institute, Health Sciences Center, Tucson, AZ 85724, USA

MALAN, T.O., Department of Anesthesiology, University of Arizona, Health Sciences Center, Tucson, AZ 85724, USA

McMAHON, S.B., Department of Physiology, St. Thomas Hospital Medical School, Lambeth Palace Road, London SE1 7EH, United Kingdom

McQUAY, H.J., Pain Research and Nuffield Department of Anesthetics, University of Oxford, Oxford OX3 7LJ, United Kingdom

MILLAN, M.J., Institut de Recherches Servier, Centre de Recherches de Croissy, Psychopharmacology Department, 125, Chemin de Ronde, F-78290 Croissy-sur-Seine (Paris), France

MOORE, R.A., Pain Research and Nuffield Department of Anesthetics, University of Oxford, Oxford OX3 7LJ, United Kingdom

OSSIPOV, M.H., Department of Pharmacology, The University of Arizona Pain Institute, Health Sciences Center, Tucson, AZ 85724, USA

PORRECA, F., Department of Pharmacology, The University of Arizona Pain Institute, Health Sciences Center, Tucson, AZ 85724, USA

ROWBOTHAM, M.C., Department of Neurology, University of California San Francisco, 505 Parnassus Avenue, M-794, San Francisco, CA 94143-0114, USA

TJØLSEN, A., Department of Physiology, University of Bergen, Arstadveien 19, N-5009 Bergen, Norway

WIESENFELD-HALLIN, S., Karolinska Institute, Department of Medical Laboratory Sciences and Technology, Section of Clinical Neurophysiology, Huddinge University Hospital, S-141 86 Huddinge, Sweden

XU, X.-J., Karolinska Institute, Department of Medical Laboratory Sciences and Technology, Section of Clinical Neurophysiology, Huddinge University Hospital, S. 141 86 Huddinge, Sweden

Contents

CHAPTER 3

Non-steroidal Anti-inflammatory Drugs and Pain

CHAPTER 4

The Sympathetic Nervous System and Pain

CHAPTER 5

**Excitability Blockers: Anticonvulsants and Low Concentration
Local Anesthetics in the Treatment of Chronic Pain**
H.L. FLELDS, M.C. ROWBOTHAM, and M. DEVOR. With 1 Figure   93

CHAPTER 8

Mechanisms of Central Hypersensitivity: Excitatory Amino Acid Mechanisms and Their Control

CHAPTER 9

Novel Modulators in Nociception
X.-J. Xu and Z. Wiesenfeld-Hallin

CHAPTER 10

Pharmacological Studies of Nociceptive Systems Using the C-Fos Immunohistochemical Technique: An Indicator of Noxiously Activated Spinal Neurones
V. CHAPMAN and J.-M. BESSON. With 13 Figures 235

CHAPTER 11

Molecular Aspect of Opioid Receptors

CHAPTER 14

**Inhibitory Neurotransmitters and Nociception: Role of GABA
and Glycine**
D.L. HAMMOND 361

CHAPTER 16

Neonatal Pharmacology of Pain
M. FITZGERALD. With 4 Figures 447

CHAPTER 1
Animal Models of Analgesia

A. Tjølsen and K. Hole

A. Introduction

Measurement of pain and analgesia in animals poses a variety of problems. In addition to the fact that pain itself constitutes a multiplicity of sensory entities, the term pain is poorly defined in relationship to animals and animal behaviour.

Pain is defined by the International Association for the Study of Pain as "an unpleasant sensory and emotional experience associated with actual or potential tissue damage, or described in terms of such damage" (MERSKEY 1984). A noxious stimulus is one which is damaging to normal tissue, and a nociceptor is a receptor that is preferentially sensitive to a noxious stimulus or to a stimulus which would become noxious if prolonged (SHERRINGTON 1947). Activity in the nociceptor and nociceptive pathways and other neurophysiological processes induced by a noxious stimulus is called nociception. Analgesia is the absence of pain in response to stimulation which would normally be painful, while hypoalgesia is diminished pain. An increased response to a stimulus which is normally painful is called hyperalgesia, the basic concept of inflammatory pain.

According to the above definitions, the term pain is often avoided when describing animal models of nociception. In general, pain tests in animals are in fact tests of nociception. Pain is a subjective and personal psychological experience that at best can be measured only indirectly in animals. Animal models of analgesia must hence be animal models of nociception and antinociception.

B. Animal Models and Ethics

Over the years many tests of nociception and pain in animals have been developed, and the species most frequently used in pain research are rats and mice. We describe some of the most commonly used methods, which may illustrate important aspects of investigations on pain in animals. Special emphasis is put on methodological problems in the tests.

While the use of anaesthetics and analgesics is standard in invasive biomedical research involving intact animals, analgesics cannot be used in models for studying behavioural responses to nociceptive stimulation. Therefore special considerations must be given to the approval of models and protocols for pain research in animals. The type and intensity of noxious stimulation and the duration of the stimulus should be examined thoughtfully. In addition, the ability of the animal to terminate or limit the noxious stimulus may be an important factor in evaluating models for acute pain.

The Committee for Research and Ethical Issues of the International Association for the Study of Pain has published the following guidelines for investigations of experimental pain in conscious animals:

- Experiments must be reviewed by scientists and laypersons, and the potential benefit must be made clear.
- If possible, the investigator should try the pain stimulus on himself.
- A careful assessment of the animal's deviation from normal behaviour should be given.
- A minimal pain stimulus necessary for the purposes of the experiment should be used.
- Pain-relieving agents or procedures should be used, as long as this does not interfere with the aim of the investigation.
- The duration must be as short as possible, and the number of animals kept to a minimum.

Several tests of nociception measuring acute pain at or close to the pain threshold do not pose problems with respect to these guidelines, while there may be difficulties in applying the present guidelines to chronic pain models. It is not always possible to try the pain stimulus on the experimenter himself, and pain-relieving agents generally interfere with the purpose of the experiments. Adequate evaluations of the intensity and duration of pain necessary to achieve the experimental objective are also difficult (Roberts 1989). For these reasons improved guidelines are needed for use in models of chronic pain.

C. Factors Affecting Measurements of Nociception

When an animal model of nociception or pain has been chosen, many factors affect the outcome of the measurements. Conflicting results in various studies may be explained by differences in nociceptive model or study design that are not necessarily obvious. Because of this one should be aware that the animal model used must be characterized as well as possible, and results should be evaluated critically with regard to the exact conditions under which testing has been performed.

The choice of species and strain of animals is among the more obvious factors that influence the results of tests. The time of day when testing is performed is another factor, there being considerable diurnal variation in nociceptive sensitivity. Factors concerning the nociceptive stimulus used may be important for the test result. It is of importance which area on the body is used for the test, as nociceptive thresholds vary from one area to another. The size of the stimulated area is also crucial for the threshold and response to stimulation. A multitude of mechanisms affect the sensitivity for pain and the response to noxious stimulation, and the interval between consecutive stimuli may therefore be important for the responses. When a heat stimulus is used, the temperature of the stimulated area of skin is an important factor in determining the response. In certain tests, such as the tail-flick test, the effect of variation in skin temperature may seriously confound the results.

D. Tests of Nociception and Analgesia

When investigating the supposed analgesic effect of drugs, it is essential to be aware that the measured analgesic effects may vary considerably between different models. This is because nociceptive tests may differ with regard to whether the stimulus threshold or the response is measured. Furthermore, different types of stimuli are used. There are two main types of tests. In the first the response to the stimulation is fixed, i.e. a standard response is defined. Here what is measured is the strength or duration of the stimulus when the response occurs, and the test measures mainly the threshold of the stimulus required to elicit a certain response. Examples include the tail-flick and hot-plate tests. In the second type the stimulus is standardized, and the strength or duration of the response is measured. Rather than determining a threshold for the response, this type of test measures the gain of the response. Examples include the formalin and writhing tests.

Animal models of nociception include highly variable types of stimulation, with regard to both modality and duration. Stimuli may be mechanical, using von Frey hairs for stimulation, as in a test of allodynia, or pressure or pinch, as in the paw pressure test. Thermal stimulation may be applied using thermodes, laser beams, or focused heat lamps, as in the tail-flick test. Chemical agents may also be used for stimulation, as in the writhing and formalin tests.

This section describes a number of tests for nociception and analgesia. Tests that are more important or are used more widely are described in more detail.

I. Direct Measurements of Pain, Behavioural Responses

1. Acute Stimulation of Nociceptors

a) Reflex Response Measurements

Tail-Flick and Tail Immersion Tests. The tail-flick test was first described more than 50 years ago (D'AMOUR and SMITH 1941) and is still an extensively used test of nociception in rats and mice. Radiant heat is focused on the tail, and the time is measured until the animal flicks the tail away from the beam. This tail-flick latency is a measure of the nociceptive sensitivity of the animals and is prolonged, for instance, by opioid analgesics. A spinal transection above the lumbar level does not block the tail-flick response. This test thus determines a spinal nociceptive reflex rather than measuring pain directly. Nevertheless it is considered very useful both in basic pain research and in pharmacological investigations of analgesic drugs.

This is a useful test of nociception only if it is carefully performed, and if possible sources of error are taken into account. A particular problem with tests that use thermal stimulation is the possible effect of skin temperature. The tail flick occurs when the temperature at the level of the nociceptors in the skin reaches a critical value. Obviously the time required for heating the skin to this critical temperature depends on the initial temperature of the skin, a parameter determined by local blood flow within the limits given by deep body and ambient temperatures. As a consequence the tail-flick latency is negatively correlated to the ambient temperature (BERGE et al. 1988). This may be a source of variation in the test results, even within a single laboratory. More important is the fact that many experimental treatments affect blood flow and thereby tail skin temperature. A reduction in tail skin temperature may be interpreted as analgesia, and an increase in temperature as hyperalgesia (TJØLSEN et al. 1989). The reduced tail-flick latency observed after transection of the spinal cord, selective lesions of raphe-spinal serotonergic systems, and systemic and intrathecal administration of serotonin receptor blocking drugs can be accounted for completely by increased skin temperature due to functional impairment of these systems.

The conclusion is that tail skin temperature is of great importance for the results of the tail-flick test. The problem may be solved by recording the tail skin temperature and correcting the tail-flick latency data for changes in the temperature. For this purpose a regression analysis or an analysis of covariance may be performed (TJØLSEN et al. 1989).

The tail immersion test is very similar to the tail-flick test. Here the tail is heated, and the time is measured that elapses before the response, a flick of the tail. In this variety of the test the tail is heated by immersion in hot water kept at a constant temperature.

Paw Pressure and Tail Pinch Tests. These nociceptive tests employ mechanical stimuli and taking the threshold for response as outcome. In both tests an increasing pressure is applied, to a paw or to the tail, respectively, and the force is recorded when withdrawal response or vocalization occurs (RANDALL and SELITTO 1957). Mechanical threshold tests of nociception may be used in models without long-term changes in nociceptive sensitivity, such as a test of drug effect on acute pain stimuli (MALCANGIO et al. 1992) and in models of chronic pain, neuropathy or long-term inflammation to quantify the hyperalgesia observed in many of these models (RANDALL and SELITTO 1957; AHLGREN and LEVINE 1993).

Shock Titration. The response to electric shocks to the feet has been used as a measure of pain sensitivity in rats (CARR et al. 1984; MINOR et al. 1986).

However, an electric shock is a very complex stimulus, pain probably being only a minor component. This test should therefore be used with caution, and only for special purposes.

b) Behaviour Coordinated at Higher Levels

Hot-Plate Test. The hot-plate test was described in 1944 (WOOLFE and MACDONALD 1944) and is one of the most commonly used tests of nociception and analgesia in rodents. Originally the test measured nociceptive responses of mice placed on the hot-plate at temperatures varying from 55° to 70°C, but the test has since been modified, and most researchers use a constant temperature of about 55°C (for description of the method see HUNSKAAR et al. 1985). Despite the extensive literature of studies using the hot-plate test there is a paucity of work on the methodological aspects of the test. The latency to various behavioural responses, including jumping, kicking and dancing, shaking of a foot, holding the foot tightly against the body and licking the forepaw, the hindpaw or both, has been used as a measure of pain sensitivity in mice and rats. In recent years most investigators have employed either forepaw or hindpaw lick as the end-point. These responses occur in nearly all animals, licking the forepaw usually preceding the hindpaw lick.

At a temperature of 55°C the analgesic effects of morphine and other opiate analgesics are easily identified and quantified in the hot-plate test. However, at this temperature non-narcotic analgesics have no or only weak antinociceptive effects. Various modifications have been made to detect the activities of such drugs. When the temperature is reduced to 50°C or lower, the analgesic effects may be detectable, but the variability increased, making statistical analysis difficult (TABER 1974). In addition to sensitivity problems, the variability of the results is a major difficulty with the hot-plate test. The response latencies of control animals vary considerably between different research reports, even from the same laboratory.

Increasing Temperature Hot-Plate Test. This test (HUNSKAAR et al. 1986; TJØLSEN et al. 1991b) has several advantages over the conventional hot-plate test. Here the temperature of the plate is set below pain threshold, and the temperature is gradually increased until a response is observed. The temperature of the plate when the response occurs is recorded as the nociceptive end-point. The licking of a hindpaw may be used as the response recorded. To avoid the scoring of mere grooming behaviour, it may be an advantage to score the second hindpaw lick. Forepaw lick may be a part of heat-dissipating mechanisms and should not be used as an end-point.

The increasing temperature hot-plate test may be performed using a conventional hot-plate that is turned on at a plate temperature of 42°–43°C, the temperature increasing gradually until the nociceptive response is observed, or a cut-off temperature (50°–52°C) is reached. The hot-plate test also involves a thermal stimulus, and the constant temperature hot-plate test may have similar problems as the tail-flick test. In the increasing temperature hot-plate test this problem is reduced, since the end-point is the plate temperature when a hindpaw lick occurs, regardless of the time it takes before the response occurs. This test is therefore less, if at all, influenced by the pretest skin temperature. The test has been shown to be more sensitive than the traditional hot-plate test, for instance, when studying the analgesic effect of mild analgesics (Hunskaar et al. 1986). The nociceptive threshold in this test is similar to that found using other methods.

Formalin Test. Here diluted formalin is injected subcutaneously into a paw, and nociceptive behaviour is measured (in mice and rats, for instance, licking and biting of the injected paw; Tjølsen et al. 1992). Two phases of the response are observed: an early phase starting immediately after injection and lasting for 5–10 min and a late phase 15–60 min after injection (Dubuisson and Dennis 1977). While the stimulus for the early phase is a direct chemical stimulation of the nociceptors, that for the late phase involves inflammation. In addition, the response in the late phase depends on changes in processing of the information in the spinal cord due to the afferent barrage during the early phase (Coderre et al. 1990). It is an interesting aspect of this test that two different types of stimulus are employed in the same test to study possibly varying analgesic effects of a drug in the two phases of the test. It may also be claimed that this test is a better model of clinical pain than the hot-plate and tail-flick tests.

It has recently been shown that in mice the late phase is very sensitive both to changes in ambient temperature and to drugs and lesions that affect peripheral blood flow and skin temperature (Rosland 1991). Hence changes in blood flow and skin temperature may also be interpreted in terms of analgesia or hyperalgesia. Drugs may influence blood flow as a 'side effect', and CNS lesions and stress may also affect peripheral blood flow.

For studies of the late phase, which is the more commonly studied, it is recommended to use ambient temperatures that are not too low (above 23°C) and formalin concentrations of 1%–5% (0.4%–2% formaldehyde). The early phase does not seem to be sensitive to moderate changes in ambient temperature, and in this phase the use of lower concentrations of formalin (0.02%–0.1% formaldehyde) may increase the possibility of observing either an increase or an attenuation of the response (Rosland et al. 1990). These recommendations are clearly valid for mice, and although the role of skin temperature in the formalin test has not been investigated in rats, it is likely that similar mechanisms may apply in this species.

Rats show a more complex behavioural response than mice in this test. The method of scoring the behavioural response in rats is usually an adaptation of the method originally described by Dubuisson and Dennis (1977). A rating scale is used for different behaviours, and a total pain rating is calculated with the ratings weighted according to the time spent in each rating category. The main assumption is that the animal has a one-dimensional nociceptive experience, and that each behavioural category adds to this experience. However, pain in both animals and in humans may in fact be multi-dimensional. Different behaviours displayed by the animal may express different aspects of nociception and not necessarily merely varying intensities of a single nociceptive modality. The importance of observing the integrated motor performance when evaluating the complex perception of pain in animals has been emphasized (CHAPMAN et al. 1985). For this type of data the adequate treatment may be a multivariate statistical analysis (TJØLSEN et al. 1991a). This type of analysis may also make it possible to distinguish nociceptive from non-nociceptive (for instance motor) behavioural changes, improving both the amount and the relevance of the information obtained from the data in future studies.

Chemically Induced Writhing: The Abdominal Stretch Assay. In this widely used test the intraperitoneal injection of an irritant induces a syndrome called 'writhing', which consists of contractions of the abdomen, twisting and turning of the trunk, and extension of the hind limbs. Several compounds have been shown to elicit this syndrome, such as phenylquinone (SIEGMUND et al. 1957), acetic acid (KOSTER et al. 1959), bradykinin and acetylcholine. In recent years acetic acid and phenylquinone have been used most frequently (for an example of the method see GOETTL and LARSON 1994). Administration of relatively small doses of non-narcotic drugs, especially non-steroid anti-inflammatory drugs, abolishes the writhing syndrome in a dose-dependent manner. The test is commonly employed as a screening method because of its simplicity and sensitivity.

The main disadvantage of this method is its lack of specificity, as many drugs without certain analgesic effects in humans can effectively inhibit the writhing response (CHERNOV et al. 1967). In addition, there is wide variation in the response between mouse strains; ED_{50} values for acetylsalicylic acid have been found to vary from 50 to 200 mg/kg (BROWN and HUGHES 1962).

The mechanism of the syndrome is not known, but many mediators have been proposed. No significant differences are detected in histamine, serotonin and prostaglandin content of peritoneal fluid from writhing (using phenylquinone) and control mice, while other reports indicate involvement of the prostaglandin system in writhing induced by at least some irritants. It has been claimed that various irritants may be considered as models of different pain reactions, for example distinguishing between inflammatory and non-inflammatory pain.

The writhing test is most widely used in mice (GOETTL and LARSON 1994), but it has also been used in a few studies in rats. The test is simple to perform and sensitive and is therefore preferred in many laboratories. However, because of the poor specificity the results of this test should be interpreted with caution.

Colonic Distension. The central mechanisms of visceral and other deep tissue pains are not as well understood as those of cutaneous, superficial pain. For this reason a number of tests have been described in which more adequate physiological visceral stimuli are used. One test that includes the administration of a visceral stimulus is the colonic distension test (GEBHART and NESS 1991). Here the rectum and distal colon are distended with constant pressure by means of a balloon. Distension of a section of gut mimics a natural, painful stimulus, and the test is used in awake, unanaesthetized animals. It is also minimally invasive.

Quantification of responses may be complicated in nociceptive testing. In this model it has been suggested to use a passive avoidance paradigm to evaluate the nociceptive-aversive character of the stimulus. Rats placed on a platform in an open field naturally step down from the platform to explore the environment. If, when both forepaws are placed on the floor of the field, the colon/rectum is distended, the rat quickly learns passively to avoid the stimulus in subsequent trials by remaining on the platform for the duration of a trial. Hence the mean latency for stepping down increases with the strength of the distension stimulus used in the conditioning trials, and this may be used as an indication of the pain experienced by the animal (GEBHART and NESS 1991).

2. Intrathecal Injection of Nociceptive Neurotransmitters

The excitatory amino acid glutamate and the neuropeptide substance P are important neurotransmitters in primary sensory nociceptive neurones. When these substances are injected intrathecally into the lumbar region in rats or mice, biting and scratching directed towards the caudal part of the body occur (HYLDEN and WILCOX 1983; AANONSEN and WILCOX 1987; WILCOX 1988). Other substances that may be administered to the spinal cord include capsaicin, which causes the release of substance P from primary afferent terminals, and several amino acid agonists, such as N-methyl-D-aspartate and α-amino-3-hydroxy-5-methyl-isoxazole (MJELLEM-JOLY et al. 1991). A state of pain is thus induced without peripheral stimulation of nociceptors, and it is possible, for instance, to investigate central as opposed to peripheral effects of analgesic drugs.

This test has mostly been performed with percutaneous injections in awake mice, or through preimplanted catheters in rats. Recently an improved method for intrathecal catheterization of rats has been described in which the morbidity associated with the implantation is much lower than in the classical method (STØRKSON et al. 1996). A percutaneous catheter-through-needle approach is used in the lumbar region in halothane anaesthesia, in contrast to the insertion of a long catheter through a slit in the exposed atlanto-occipital membrane in the neck.

3. Long-Term Peripheral Stimulation

a) Skin

Injection of Irritants. In rats the injection of carrageenan or yeast sub-cutaneously in a paw causes localized inflammation. This inflammatory process causes nociceptive behaviour, with focused behaviour such as licking of the injected site, and lifting and protection of the paw (KAYSER and GUILBAUD 1987). The local inflammation caused by injected irritants also induces a state of hyperalgesia. To test mechanical hyperalgesia pressure is applied to the inflamed area by means of a metal cylinder, and the force at which the animals begin to vocalize or struggle is recorded. Several modifications of the test have been described (RANDALL and SELITTO 1957; VINEGAR et al. 1976). Hyperalgesia for thermal stimuli may be tested in a similar way, applying a heat stimulus (REN et al. 1992).

Drugs can be administered before, at the time of, or after the injection of the inducing agent. Oedema and hyperalgesia do not seem to be correlated in this model. The contralateral, non-injected paw may be used as a control. Therefore the test has been used to distinguish between drugs acting in the CNS and locally at the site of inflammation. The test is sensitive to the non-narcotic analgesics and is relatively simple to perform.

Irradiation. Exposure to ultraviolet light induces a condition of localized inflammation of the skin with hyperalgesia in the exposed area. Such a cutaneous inflammation may be induced on the plantar surface of a hindpaw of rats (PERKINS et al. 1993). The hyperalgesia to a heat stimulus may then be measured, for example, by recording the latency to withdrawal to a focused beam of radiant heat. This may be considered a model of persistent cutaneous inflammatory hyperalgesia.

b) Joint Inflammation

Monoarthritis. Carrageenan or uric acid injected intra-articularly into the knee or ankle joint of rats induces a monoarthritis, with dysfunction that lasts 2–3 days. This dysfunction, protective ("nocifensive") behaviour and hyperalgesia may be used as models of joint pain (OKUDA et al. 1984; CODERRE and WALL 1987; TONUSSI and FERREIRA 1992). A limited monoarthritis may be obtained by injection of complete adjuvant in the tibio-tarsal joint of rats (BUTLER et al. 1992; BESSE et al. 1992). This arthritis seems to be pronounced, limited to a single joint and stable over 6 weeks. It is reported that animals in this model gain weight and remain active as control rats (BUTLER et al. 1992), indicating little systemic disturbance. It seems that the model is useful for assessing treatments for prolonged joint pain.

General Adjuvant-Induced Arthritis. Intradermal injection of heat-killed *Mycobacterium tuberculosis* in Freund's complete adjuvant into the tail of rats induces polyarthritis (Costa et al. 1981, for review: Besson and Guilbaud 1988). The arthritic condition develops over weeks and lasts for several months. This disease in rats shows many similarities to various human arthritic conditions, and most anti-inflammatory drugs are effective in adjuvant arthritis. The drugs have the same rank order of potency as in humans (Pircio et al. 1975), and results from the test are predictive for the effect of such agents in man.

In this chronic model of adjuvant arthritis, the nociceptive stimulation is tonic rather than phasic in nature. Thus the model may elucidate possible changes in neurochemistry, metabolism and drug tolerance in test animals compared to normal animals. However, the animals suffer from an immunological disease and may not be a model for all chronic pain conditions. Drug effects are often measured as the influence on foot swelling, and this may not be indicative of nociception. The vocalization response induced by manipulation of the tarso-tibial joint has been used to measure nociception. Simultaneous measurement of oedema (paw volume) and recording of vocalizations have also been claimed to separate anti-inflammatory from antinociceptive activity of drugs.

c) Muscle

Several methods of stimulation of muscle nociceptors have been used to model muscle pain. Experimental myositis may be induced by intramuscular injection of a solution containing carrageenan (Hoheisel et al. 1994). Nociceptive stimulation of muscular tissue is obtained with injection of a variety of compounds, among others bradykinin (Hoheisel et al. 1993). In these models nociception has been assessed mainly by means of electrophysiological methods in anaesthetized animals.

d) Surgical Trauma

Surgically induced trauma to a joint has also been used as a model of joint pain. Section of a cruciate ligament has been used as a model of osteoarthritis in dogs (Brandt et al. 1991). Nociceptive behaviour and the effect of analgesics may be investigated in a model of post-operative pain. One of the issues that has been studied is the effect of pre-emptive analgesia or analgesics given before or during surgery on the pain experienced post-operatively. Experimental surgical injuries may be used to model post-operative pain in animals. A recent study has used ovariohysterectomy as model surgery (Lascelles et al. 1995).

4. Models of Neuropathic Pain

a) Nerve Damage

Neuroma Model. The first animal model of painful neuropathy was reported by WALL and colleagues in 1979. They sectioned the rat's sciatic nerve and either tied the proximal stump tightly or implanted it in a polyethylene tube sealed at its far end. The saphenous nerve was also cut, such that the hindpaw was completely denervated. It has been suggested that this procedure, known as the neuroma model, replicates the human syndromes seen after an amputation (phantom pain) or after nerve transection in an intact limb (anaesthesia dolorosa). Within several days rats (and mice) with this condition begin to self-mutilate the hindpaw on the side of the nerve transection: a behaviour named 'autotomy'. This behaviour has been proposed to be the animal's response to spontaneous pain or dysesthesia (WALL et al. 1979; WIESENFELD and LINDBLOM 1980). This model has been very successful in identifying pathophysiological mechanisms that are likely to contribute to human painful peripheral neuropathies. The usefulness of the autotomy model and the extent to which autotomy reflects a sensation of pain have been discussed. Experiments with long-term lidocaine anaesthesia of a limb do not, however, induce autotomy, indicating that the autotomy syndrome is not induced merely by the loss of sensation (BLUMENKOPF and LIPMAN 1991). These results support the contention that autotomy is a behavioural response to pain and therefore a valid measure of nociception in animals.

Chronic Constriction Injury. A peripheral mononeuropathy may be produced in rats by placing four loosely constrictive ligatures around the common sciatic nerve (BENNETT and XIE 1988; BENNETT 1993). This constitutes a widely used model of neuropathy, known as the Bennett or Bennett and Xie model. In this chronic constriction model hyperalgesia is found to noxious heat stimuli and to mustard oil (BENNETT and XIE 1988) and to mechanical stimuli (ATTAL et al. 1990). There are indications that older rats fail to develop allodynia after sciatic nerve ligation (TANCK et al. 1992); this study noted that rats 107 days of age failed to develop allodynia to cold and developed less mechanical allodynia. Studies designed to investigate therapies for neuropathic allodynic syndromes should probably use younger animals.

Tight Ligatures. Partial nerve injury may cause conditions of neuropathic pain in humans. An animal model has been developed that involves unilateral ligation of about half of the sciatic nerve in the thigh (SELTZER et al. 1990; SHIR and SELTZER 1990). An attempt has been made to compare the Bennett and Xie and Seltzer models with regard to time course and magnitude of hyperalgesia (DOUGHERTY et al. 1992). To evaluate the hypothesis that neuropathic pain develops as a result of injury-associated discharges, in addition, the effect of anaesthesia of the sciatic nerve during injury were investigated. It seemed that the neuropathy develops somewhat faster in the

Bennett and Xie model than in the Seltzer model. There were also indications that local anaesthesia during the nerve damage reduced the extent and duration of the neuropathy in the Bennett and Xie model, suggesting that injury-related discharge is an important factor in the development of hyperalgesia in this model. A model somewhat similar to the partial ligation of the sciatic nerve has been described. This model involves tight ligation of spinal nerves, in rats either L5 or L5 and L6 (Kim and Chung 1992; Sheen and Chung 1993; Kim et al. 1993). This model induces symptoms of neuropathy much as the sciatic ligation model does but is suggested to be more constant and yields a complete separation between injured and intact segments. This model has also been used in primates, on spinal nerve L7 (Carlton et al. 1994).

Cryogenic Nerve Lesion. Lesions of peripheral nerves by freezing may also induce a syndrome of neuropathic pain. Cryogenic nerve lesion (DeLeo and Coombs 1991; DeLeo et al. 1994; Willenbring et al. 1994) seems to be a valid mononeuropathy animal model. This involves freezing of the proximal sciatic nerve (sciatic cryoneurolysis), using a cryoprobe cooled to $-60°C$ in a 30/5/30s freeze-thaw-freeze sequence. After this treatment all animals demonstrated some degree of autotomy.

   Although the technique used to produce each of these model neuropathic conditions is slightly different, the post-surgical sensory aberrations are similar to those in human neuropathic disorders. The phenomena of heat hyperalgesia, mechanical allodynia, cold allodynia and spontaneous pain are characteristic of these animal models. It has also been found that the sensory abnormalities are sympathetically maintained (Kim and Chung 1992; Shir and Seltzer 1991; Kim et al. 1993).

   Measurements of sensitivity to heat in neuropathic areas should be made with caution. Skin blood flow and skin temperature in such areas are prone to be abnormal, and it is known from a number of studies that the response latency to a nociceptive heat stimulus is inversely correlated to the temperature of the skin (Tjølsen et al. 1989; Lascelles et al. 1995). Hence increased skin temperature would cause shortened response latencies, and this could easily be interpreted as an increased sensitivity for heat (Luukko et al. 1994).

   Models of neuropathy are interesting and important because of the potential for testing the effect of treatments of neuropathic conditions and hypotheses concerning the pathophysiology of such conditions. Neuropathic disorders are among the most difficult to treat by pharmacological means.

b) Diabetic Animals

Altered pain sensations, including hyperalgesia and spontaneous pain, can exist without inflammation or traumatic injury. For example, many patients with diabetes mellitus complain of mechanical hyperalgesia and pain. Rats with streptozotocin-induced diabetes as well as strains of rats that spontaneously develop diabetes have been used as models to study the complications of diabetes mellitus, including altered pain sensation (AHLGREN and LEVINE 1993, 1994; AHLGREN et al. 1992; COURTEIX et al. 1993). Results suggest that increased C fibre excitability is an important cause of hyperalgesia in diabetic neuropathy. Streptozotocin-induced diabetes has been used to assess the pharmacological activity of several analgesic drugs known to be more or less (or not) effective in human painful diabetic neuropathy (COURTEIX et al. 1994). Interestingly, the findings correspond very well with the experience from patients with diabetic neuropathy and hence indicate a high pharmacological predictivity of the model.

5. Models of Central Pain

a) Spinal Cord Injury

A model of spinal cord injury with a chronic pain-related syndrome has been developed by WIESENFELD-HALLIN and collaborators (XU et al. 1992). This model involves an ischemic spinal cord injury induced photochemically by laser irradiation for 5–20 min. The procedure results in an acute allodynia-like phenomenon which lasts for several days and is possibly related to dysfunction of the $GABA_B$ system in the spinal cord. In some rats this is followed by a chronic allodynia-like symptom, with an onset varying between 1 week and 1.5 months after injury, expressed as a painful reaction to light pressure to the skin at or near the corresponding dermatome. The chronic allodynia-like phenomenon is being used as a model for studying the mechanisms of chronic central pain.

II. Physiological Correlates of Pain or Nociception

Although the concept of pain can be studied only by means of behavioural measures in awake, intact animals, important elements of the nociceptive systems may be studied in preparations where the animals cannot experience pain. The response of neurones to noxious stimulation of peripheral tissues has been studied in several areas of the CNS: in the spinal cord, the brainstem, the thalamus and the cerebral cortex. Electrical recordings can be made from neurones in all these areas in intact, anaesthetized animals, and their response to noxious stimulation and pharmacological treatment investigated. Tissue slices from the spinal cord can be prepared with intact dorsal roots in such a way that allows study of the response of neurones in the dorsal horn to stimulation of the root.

1. Electrophysiological Methods

a) Microneurography

To evaluate the role of tissue factors in peripheral mechanisms of nociception primary afferents may be studied in either animals or humans. Recordings can be made from single fibres in peripheral nerves, reflecting the activity in single primary afferents. The afferents can be classified into the different classes of receptors, including the different classes of nociceptors. In rats recordings from primary afferents may be carried out either in vitro or in vivo. In in vitro preparations, consisting of a nerve with a skin flap, the receptive fields are superfused at the highly permeable corium side with controlled solutions (KRESS et al. 1992).

b) Dorsal Horn Recording

The dorsal horn of the spinal cord plays a key role in modulation and transmission of nociceptive information from the peripheral tissues to the supraspinal areas. By recording action potentials from single cells in the dorsal horn with extracellular electrodes it is possible to investigate the spontaneous and evoked activity in nociceptive systems on this level (DICKENSON and SULLIVAN 1987, 1990). By pharmacological manipulations both the effects and mechanisms of action of analgesics and the physiological mechanisms of nociceptive regulation may be studied. Peripheral electrical stimulation constitutes in this model a well-defined stimulus that enables the quantitation of the response of dorsal horn neurones separately to the different classes of peripheral fibres ($A\beta$, $A\delta$, C fibres). With this acute model analgetic and hyperalgesic effects of drugs may be studied directly.

The same method of recording may be used to evaluate the changes in nociceptive transmission in models of long-lasting pain, for example, after subcutaneous injection of carrageenan (STANFA et al. 1992). It is also possible directly to study the firing pattern of single neurones after injection of formalin in the receptive field, obtaining a response pattern mirroring the behavioural response to formalin in awake animals (see "Formalin Test"; HALEY et al. 1990).

By methods of intracellular recording it is furthermore possible to study modulation of the membrane potential of nociceptive neurones below the threshold for eliciting action potentials (KING et al. 1988; WOOLF and KING 1990; WOOLF and THOMPSON 1991). With such methods studies may be performed of the relative importance of inhibitory and excitatory mechanisms in the fine regulation of nociceptive sensitivity in the dorsal horn.

2. Biochemical and Histochemical Methods

The concentration of neurotransmitters involved in nociception may be used as an indication of the activity in nociceptive systems. For example, the concentration of excitatory amino acids in the dorsal horn has been found to increase as a response to noxious stimulation (SKILLING et al. 1988).

The expression of immediate-early genes (c-*fos*, c-*jun* and others) in the spinal cord is affected by nociceptive stimulation, showing a stimulus-response relationship (HUNT et al. 1987). This may indicate that induction of immediate-early genes is correlated to the central changes that occur as a response to painful stimuli. It has also been shown that the induction of genes of this class by noxious stimuli may be inhibited by morphine (PRESLEY et al. 1990). On this basis it seems that studies of gene induction, transcription and peptide synthesis is a valuable supplement to other tests of nociception in the study of pain and analgesia. Supporting this, measurement of specific mRNA for several neuropeptides including dynorphin (IADOROLA et al. 1988) has shown changes in transcription during noxious stimulation.

E. Comparative Aspects

Detecting and avoiding noxious stimuli are fundamental functions of the nervous system of animals. It is therefore not surprising that similar regulatory systems for nociception are found over a wide range of animal species. The vast majority of studies of nociception have been performed in rodents, and hence the knowledge of systems involved in nociception and nociceptive signal processing is based on these species. Other species have occasionally been used; the formalin test was originally described, for instance, in cats and rats, and it has been also adapted for monkeys.

Some focus has been put on the advantages of utilizing non-mammalian species, in that these are lower on the phylogenetic spectrum (e.g. STEVENS 1992). It has been assumed that reptiles and amphibia have less capacity to experience pain or distress than mammals. In the crocodile, however, both the hot-plate and the formalin tests have been shown to be useful tests of nociception, and in these tests crocodiles are also very sensitive to the analgesic effect of morphine (KANUI et al. 1990). Crocodiles also show a marked nociceptive response to instillations into the eye of diluted capsaicin, unlike birds and amphibians.

Several amphibian models of nociception have been described, and it has generally been difficult to show antinociceptive effects of reasonable doses of opioids. However, a model using cutaneous application of various concentrations of acetic acid in frogs has been developed (STEVENS 1992), and in this model opioid analgesia is most conveniently studied. The model involves the application of progressively higher concentrations of acetic acid on the hindlimb, and the end-point is defined as the concentration which elicits a characteristic wiping response.

F. Conclusion

By definition, pain is a psychological experience (MERSKEY 1984). In animals pain can at best be assessed indirectly, by behavioural measures. Investigation of behavioural responses in animals is an important and necessary part of the study of pain, and this type of research necessitates the use of intact, unanesthetized animals. There is a great need for more, thorough, methodological studies of such tests of nociception. Animal models of pain pose ethical problems, and ethical guidelines have been recommended by the International Association for the Study of Pain. Parts of the nociceptive systems may also be studied in animal preparations, both in anaesthetized animals and in in vitro preparations.

References

Aanonsen LM, Wilcox GL (1987) Nociceptive action of excitatory amino acids in the mouse: effects of spinally administered opioids, phencyclidine and sigma-agonists. J Pharmacol Exp Ther 243:9–19

Ahlgren SC, Levine JD (1994) Protein kinase C inhibitors decrease hyperalgesia and C-fiber hyperexcitability in the streptozotocin-diabetic rat. J Neurophysiol 72:684–692

Ahlgren SC, Levine JD (1993) Mechanical hyperalgesia in streptozotocin-diabetic rats. Neuroscience 52:1049–1055

Ahlgren SC, White DM, Levine JD (1992) Increased responsiveness of sensory neurons in the saphenous nerve of the streptozotocin-diabetic rat. J Neurophysiol 68:2077–2085

Attal N, Jazat F, Kayser V, Guilbaud G (1990) Further evidence for "pain-related" behaviours in a model of unilateral peripheral mononeuropathy. Pain 41:235–251

Bennett GJ (1993) An animal model of neuropathic pain: a review. Muscle Nerve 16:1040–1048

Bennett GJ, Xie YK (1988) A peripheral mononeuropathy in rat that produces disorders of pain sensation like those seen in man. Pain 33:87–107

Berge OG, Garcia-Cabrera I, Hole K (1988) Response latencies in the tail-flick test depend on tail skin temperature. Neurosci Lett 86:284–288

Besse D, Weil-Fugazza J, Lombard MC, Butler SH, Besson JM (1992) Monoarthritis induces complex changes in mu-opioid, delta-opioid and kappa-opioid binding sites in the superficial dorsal horn of the rat spinal cord. Eur J Pharmacol 223:123–131

Besson JM, Guilbaud G (1988) The arthritic rat as a model of clinical pain? Excerpta Medica, Amsterdam

Blumenkopf B, Lipman JJ (1991) Studies in autotomy: its pathophysiology and usefulness as a model of chronic pain. Pain 45:203–209

Brandt KD, Braunstein EM, Visco DM, O'Connor B, Heck D, Albrecht M (1991) Anterior (cranial) cruciate ligament transection in the dog: a bona fide model of osteoarthritis, not merely of cartilage injury and repair. J Rheumatol 18:436–446

Brown DM, Hughes BO (1962) Practical aspects of strain variation in relation to pharmacological testing. Pharmacol Pharmacol 14:399–405

Butler SH, Godefroy F, Besson J, Weil-Fugazza J (1992) A limited arthritic model for chronic pain studies in the rat. Pain 48:73–81

Carlton SM, Lekan HA, Kim SH, Chung JM (1994) Behavioral manifestations of an experimental model for peripheral neuropathy produced by spinal nerve ligation in the primate. Pain 56:155–166

Carr KD, Aleman DO, Holland MJ, Simon EJ (1984) Analgesic effects of ethylketocyclazocine and morphine in rat and toad. Life Sci 35:997–1003

Chapman CR, Casey KL, Dubner R, Foley KM, Gracely, Reading AE (1985) Pain measurement: an overview. Pain 22:1–31

Chernov HI, Wilson DE, Fowler F, Plummer AJ (1967) Non-specificity of the mouse writhing test. Arch Int Pharmacodyn 167:171–178

Coderre TJ, Wall PD (1987) Ankle joint urate arthritis (AJUA) in rats: an alternative model of arthritis to that produced by Freund's adjuvant. Pain 28:379

Coderre TJ, Vaccarino TJ, Melzack R (1990) Central nervous system plasticity in the tonic pain response to subcutaneous formalin injection. Brain Res 535:155–158

Costa M, Sutter P, Gybels J, Hees J (1981) Adjuvant-induced arthritis in rats: a possible animal model of chronic pain. Pain 10:173–185

Courteix C, Eschalier A, Lavarenne J (1993) Streptozocin-induced diabetic rats: behavioural evidence for a model of chronic pain. Pain 53:81–88

Courteix C, Bradin M, Chantelauze C, Lavarenne J, Eschalier A (1994) Study of the sensitivity of the diabetes induced pain model in rats to a range of analgesics. Pain 57:153–160

D'Amour FE, Smith DL (1941) A method for determing loss of pain sensation. J Pharmacol 72:74–79

DeLeo JA, Coombs DW (1991) Autotomy and decreased spinal substance P following peripheral cryogenic nerve lesion. Cryobiology 28:460–466

DeLeo JA, Coombs DW, Willenbring S, Colburn RW, Fromm C, Wagner R, Twitchell BB (1994) Characterization of a neuropathic pain model: sciatic cryoneurolysis in the rat. Pain 56:9–16

Dickenson AH, Sullivan AF (1987) Evidence for a role of the NMDA receptor in the frequency dependent potentiation of deep rat dorsal horn nociceptive neurons following C-fiber stimulation. Neuropharmacology 26:1235–1238

Dickenson AH, Sullivan AF (1990) Differential effects of excitatory amino acid antagonists on dorsal nociceptive neurones in the rat. Brain Res 506:31–39

Dougherty PM, Garrison CJ, Carlton SM (1992) Differential influence of local anesthetic upon two models of experimentally induced peripheral mononeuropathy in the rat. Brain Res 570:109–115

Dubuisson D, Dennis SG (1977) The formalin test: a quantitative study of the analgesic effects of morphine, meperidine, and brain stem stimulation in rats and cats. Pain 4:161–174

Gebhart GF, Ness TJ (1991) Central mechanisms of visceral pain. Can J Physiol Pharmacol 69:627–634

Goettl VM, Larson AA (1994) Activity at phencyclidine and mu opioid sites mediates the hyperalgesic and antinociceptive properties of the N-terminus of substance P in a model of visceral pain. Neuroscience 60:375–382

Haley JE, Sullivan AF, Dickenson AH (1990) Evidence for spinal N-methyl-D-aspartate receptor involvement in prolonged chemical nociception in the rat. Brain Res 518:218

Hoheisel U, Mense S, Simons DG, Yu XM (1993) Appearance of new receptive fields in rat dorsal horn neurons following noxious stimulation of skeletal muscle – a model for referral of muscle pain. Neurosci Lett 153:9–12

Hoheisel U, Koch K, Mense S (1994) Functional reorganization in the rat dorsal horn during an experimental myositis. Pain 59:111–118

Hunskaar S, Berge OG, Hole K (1985) Antinociceptive effets of orphenadrine citrate in mice. Eur J Pharmacol 111:221–226

Hunskaar S, Berge OG, Hole K (1986) A modified hot-plate test sensitive to mild analgesics. Behav Brain Res 21:101–108

Hunt SP, Pini A, Evan G (1987) Induction of c-fos-like protein in spinal cord neurons following sensory stimulation. Nature 328:632–634

Hylden JLK, Wilcox GL (1983) Pharmacological characterization of substance P-induced nociception in mice: modulation by opioid and noradrenergic agonists at the spinal level. J Pharmacol Exp Ther 226:398–404

Iadorola MJ, Douglass J, Civelli O, Naranjo JR (1988) Differential activation of spinal cord dynorphin and enkephalin neurons during hyperalgesia: evidence using cDNA hybridization. Brain Res 455:205–212

Kanui TI, Hole K, Miaron JO (1990) Nociception in crocodiles – capsaicin installation, formalin and hot plate test. Zool Sci 7:537–540

Kayser V, Guilbaud G (1987) Local and remote modifications of nociceptive sensitivity during carrageenan-induced inflammation in the rat. Pain 28:99–107

Kim SH, Chung JM (1992) An experimental model for peripheral neuropathy produced by segmental spinal nerve ligation in the rat. Pain 50:355–363

Kim SH, Na HS, Sheen K, Chung JM (1993) Effects of sympathectomy on a rat model of peripheral neuropathy. Pain 55:85–92

King AE, Thompson SWN, Urban L, Woolf CJ (1988) An intracellular analysis of amino acid induced excitation of deep dorsal horn neurons in the rat spinal cord slice. Neurosci Lett 89:286–292

Koster R, Anderson M, deBeer EJ (1959) Acetic acid for analgesic screening. Fed Proc 18:412

Kress M, Koltzenburg M, Reeh PW, Handwerker HO (1992) Responsiveness and functional attributes of electrically localized terminals of cutaneous C-fibers in vivo and in vitro. J Neurophysiol 68:581–595

Lascelles BDX, Waterman AE, Cripps PJ, Livingston A, Henderson G (1995) Central sensitization as a result of surgical pain: investigation of the pre-emptive value of pethidine for ovariohysterectomy in the rat. Pain 62:201–212

Luukko M, Konttinen Y, Kemppinen P, Pertovaara A (1994) Influence of various experimental parameters on the incidence of thermal and mechanical hyperalgesia induced by a constriction mononeuropathy of the sciatic nerve in lightly anesthetized rats. Exp Neurol 128:143–154

Malcangio M, Malmberg-Aiello P, Giotti A, Ghelardini C, Bartolini A (1992) Desensitization of GABA-B receptors and antagonism by CGP 35348, prevent bicuculline- and picrotoxin-induced antinociception. Neuropharmacology 31:783–791

Merskey M (1984) Pain terms: a list with definitions and notes on usage. Recommended by the International Association for the Study of Pain Subcommittee on Taxomony. Pain 18:287–297

Minor BG, Archer T, Post C, Jonsson G, Mohammed AK (1986) 5-HT agonist induced analgesia modulated by central but not peripheral noradrenaline depletion in rats. J Neural Transm 66:243–259

Mjellem-Joly N, Lund A, Berge OG, Hole K (1991) Potentiation of a behavioural response in mice by spinal coadministration of substance P and excitatory amino acid agonists. Neurosci Lett 133:121–124

Okuda K, Nakahama H, Miyakawa H, Shima K (1984) Arthritis induced in cat by sodium urate; a possible animal model for tonic pain. Pain 18:287–297

Perkins MN, Campbell E, Dray A (1993) Antinociceptive activity of the bradykinin B1 and B2 receptor antagonists, des-Arg9, (Leu8)-BK and HOE 140, in two models of persistent hyperalgesia in the rat. Pain 53:191–197

Pircio A, Fedele C, Bierwagen M (1975) A new method for the evaluation of analgesic activity using adjuvant-induced arthritis in the rat. Eur J Pharmacol 31:207–215

Presley RW, Menétrey D, Levine JD, Basbaum AI (1990) Systemic morphine suppresses noxious stimulus-evoked Fos protein-like immunoreactivity in the rat spinal cord. J Neurosci 10:323–335

Randall LO, Selitto JJ (1957) A method for measurement of analgesic activity on inflamed tissue. Arch Int Pharmacodyn Ther 111:409–418

Ren K, Hylden JL, Williams GM, Ruda MA, Dubner R (1992) The effects of a noncompetitive NMDA receptor antagonist, MK-801, on behavioural hyperalgesia and dorsal horn neuronal activity in rats with unilateral inflammation. Pain 50:331–344

Roberts VJ (1989) Ethical issues in the use of animals for pain research. In: Chapman CR, Loeser JD (eds) Advances in pain research and therapy, vol 12. Raven, New York, pp 169–174

Rosland JH (1991) The formalin test in mice: the influence of ambient temperature. Pain 45:211–216

Rosland JH, Tjølsen A, Mæhle B, Hole K (1990) The formalin test in mice: effect of formalin concentration. Pain 42:235–242

Seltzer Z, Dubner R, Shir Y (1990) A novel behavioral model of neuropathic pain disorders produced in rats by partial sciatic nerve injury. Pain 43:205–218

Sheen K, Chung JM (1993) Signs of neuropathic pain depend on signals from injured nerve fibers in a rat model. Brain Res 610:62–68

Sherrington C (1947) The integrative action of the nervous system, 2nd edn. Yale University Press, New Haven

Shir Y, Seltzer Z (1990) A-fibers mediate mechanical hyperesthesia and allodynia and C-fibers mediate thermal hyperalgesia in a new model of causalgiform pain disorders in rats. Neurosci Lett 115:62–67

Shir Y, Seltzer Z (1991) Effects of sympathectomy in a model of causalgiform pain produced by partial sciatic nerve injury in rats. Pain 45:309–320

Siegmund E, Cadmus R, Lu G (1957) A method for evaluating both non-narcotic and narcotic analgesics. Proc Soc Exp Biol Med 95:729

Skilling SR, Smullin DH, Beitz AJ, Larson AA (1988) Extracellular amino acid concentrations in the dorsal spinal cord of freely moving rats following veratridine and nociceptive stimulation. J Neurochem 51:127–132

Stanfa LC, Sullivan AF, Dickenson AH (1992) Alterations in neuronal excitability and the potency of spinal mu, delta and kappa opioids after carrageenan-induced inflammation. Pain 50:345–354

Stevens CW (1992) Alternatives to the use of mammals for pain research. Life Sci 50:901–912

Størkson R, Kjørsvik A, Tjølsen A, Hole K (1996) Lumbar catheterization of the spinal subarachnoid space in the rat. J Neurosci Methods 65:167–172

Taber RI (1974) Predictive value of analgesic assays in mice and rats. In: Braude MC, Harris LS, May EL, Smith JP, Villarreal JE (eds) Narcotic antagonists. Raven, New York, pp 191–211 (Advances in biochemical psychopharmacology, vol 8)

Tanck EN, Kroin JS, McCarthy RJ, Penn RD, Ivankovich AD (1992) Effects of age and size on developement of allodynia in a chronic pain model produced by a sciatic nerve ligation in rats. Pain 51:313–316

Tjølsen A, Lund A, Berge OG, Hole K (1989) An improved method for tail flick testing with adjustment for tail skin temperature. J Neurosci Methods 33:259–265

Tjølsen A, Berge OG, Hole K (1991a) Lesion of bulbo-spinal serotonergic or noradrenergic pathways reduce nociception as measured by the formalin test. Acta Physiol Scand 142:229–236

Tjølsen A, Rosland JH, Berge OG, Hole K (1991b) The increasing temperature hot plate test: an improved test of nociception in mice and rats. J Pharmacol Methods 25:241–250

Tjølsen A, Berge OG, Hunskaar S, Rosland JH, Hole K (1992) The formalin test: an evaluation of the method. Pain 51:5–17

Tonussi CR, Ferreira SH (1992) Rat knee-joint carrageenin incapacitation test: an objective screen for central and peripheral analgesics. Pain 48:421–427

Vinegar R, Truax JF, Selph JL (1976) Quantitative comparison of the analgesic and antiinflammatory activities of aspirin, phenacetin and acetaminophen in rodents. Eur J Pharmacol 37:23–30

Wall PD, Devor M, Inbal R, Scadding JW, Schonfeld D, Seltzer Z, Tomkiewicz MM (1979) Autotomy following peripheral nerve lesions: experimental anesthesia dolorosa. Pain 7:103–113

Wiesenfeld Z, Lindblom U (1980) Behavioural and electrophysiological effects of various types of peripheral nerve lesions in the rat: a comparison of possible models of chronic pain. Pain 8:285–298

Wilcox GL (1988) Pharmacological studies of grooming and scratching behaviour elicted by spinal substance P and excitatory amino acids. Ann NY Acad Sci 525:228–236

Willenbring S, Deleo JA, Coombs DW (1994) Differential behavioral outcomes in the sciatic cryoneurolysis model of neuropathic pain in rats. Pain 58:135–140

Woolf CJ, King AE (1990) Dynamic alterations in the cutaneous mechanoreceptive fields of dorsal horn neurons in the rat spinal cord. J Neurosci 10(8):2717–2726

Woolf CJ, Thompson SWN (1991) The induction and maintenance of central sensitization is dependent on N-methyl-D-aspartic acid receptor activation; implications for the treatment of post-injury pain hypersensitivity states. Pain 44:293–299

Woolfe G, MacDonald AD (1944) The evaluation of the analgesic action of pethidine
    hydrocholoride (demerol). J Pharmacol Exp Ther 80:300–307
Xu XJ, Hao JX, Aldskogius H, Seiger Å, Wiesenfeld-Hallin Z (1992) Chronic pain
    related syndrome in rats after ischemic spinal cord lesion: a possible animal model
    for pain in patients with spinal cord injury. Pain 48:279–290
Zimmermann M (1983) Ethical guidlines for investigations of experimental pain in
    conscious animals. Pain 16:109–110

CHAPTER 2

Peripheral Mediators of Pain

A. DRAY

A. Introduction

Pain is a cardinal feature of normal physiological protective mechanisms to avoid tissue damage. In the periphery pain is signalled by fine C and Aδ afferent nerve fibres which respond to noxious stimuli (mechanical, heat, cold and chemical). Indeed all tissues, with the exception of the neuropil of the CNS, are innervated by such afferent fibres. However, pain is not a uniform sensation, and both the quality of pain and the initiation of protective responses are determined by many factors within the spinal cord and in higher brain structures involved in the integration and modification of nociceptive signals.

When significant tissue damage occurs, pain is often more persistent and is associated with inflammation. In these circumstances hyperalgesia and tenderness around the inflamed region occurs. Activation and sensitisation of peripheral nociceptors, by chemical mediators produced by tissue injury and inflammation, partially account for this. In hyperalgesia however, there is also an important contribution from changes in the central processing of pain signals which allows signals generated by normally innocuous stimuli, such as gentle stroking, to be perceived as painful. Activity in peripheral fibres is essential for the initiation and maintenance of these central changes.

Inflammation is a common and complex feature of clinical pain. The action of chemical mediators produced during inflammation is responsible for the multiplicity of events that occur, including hyperalgesia, alterations in cell phenotype and the expression of new molecules (neurotransmitters, enzymes, ion channels and receptors) in the peripheral and central nervous system (LEVINE et al. 1993; DRAY 1994). In addition, a number of exogenous irritants, directly or indirectly, cause activation of peripheral fibres inducing pain and hyperalgesia. This discussion addresses the actions of these substances on sensory neurones and the way in which they are involved in pain signalling and in the functional remodelling of peripheral afferent fibres.

B. Chemical Signalling in Fine Afferent Neurones

The majority of nociceptors, the polymodal nociceptors, respond to thermal and mechanical stimulation, but chemical signalling is likely to be the most common and diverse form of signal generation in all types of fine afferent fibres. These stimuli can directly active peripheral fibres to induce pain or, more importantly, induce sensitisation to a range of exogenous stimuli occurs.

A small proportion of afferent fibres, the "silent or "sleeping" nociceptors are found in the skin, joints and viceral organs which are normally unresponsive to intense stimuli. However, when influenced by inflammatory mediators or following the administration of irritants these fibres exhibit spontaneous activity or become sensitised and responsive to sensory stimuli (SCHEIBLE and SCHMIDT 1988; SCHMELZ et al. 1994). Indeed, afferent fibres may be affected by chemical stimuli without producing specific sensations. This depends on the generation and propagation of nerve impulses to the spinal dorsal horn and on synaptic interactions in spinal cord. Some chemicals, however, may induce little obvious excitability change but rather have a trophic influences on afferent fibre function, thereby altering neuronal phenotype and cellular neurochemistry (DRAY 1992; RANG et al. 1994; AKOPIAN et al. 1996a).

There are several important sources from which pathophysiological mediators are generated: damaged tissues, the vasculature, immune cells and surrounding tissues, sensory and sympathetic nerves. They act via a multiplicity of receptors coupled for the most part, with a limited repertoire of cellular regulatory intermediates (G proteins, second messengers) to regulate permeability and cellular ion concentration. In reality the afferent nerve terminal may be exposed to a great many substances, but there is little information about the composition or concentrations of various components in different conditions. Thus the net effect on peripheral neurones is difficult to predict.

C. Mediators Generated by Tissue Damage and Inflammation

A common cause of muscle ache and discomfort due to the hypoxia/anoxia of muscle exercise is the generation of protons (lactic acid). In addition, proton production is increased in inflammation and is likely to be involved in inflammatory hyperalgesia. Indeed, protons induce a direct activation of nociceptors which accounts for the sharp stinging pain produced by intradermal injections of acidic solutions, and low extracellular pH enhances the effects of other inflammatory mediators (BEVAN and GEPPETTI 1994).

Acidic solutions produce a rapid, transient increase in the membrane cation permeability of sensory neurones as well as a more prolonged ion permeability increase. This produces both a sustained nerve activation and an enhancement of sensitivity to mechanical stimuli (STEEN et al. 1992). The mechanism of proton-induced activation of sensory neurones is similar to that induced by the selective sensory neuronal stimulant capsaicin and neural sensitivity to both agents is regulated by nerve growth factor (NGF; BEVAN and YEATS 1991; DRAY 1992; BEVAN and GEPPETTI 1994). Indeed capsaicin, an exogenous irritant obtained from chilli peppers, activates nociceptors via a specific membrane receptor (DRAY 1992). Thus proton-induced activation may be an endogenous mechanism for activation of the capsaicin receptor. However, data obtained using the selective capsaicin antagonist capsazepine have been inconclusive. While capsazepine is ineffective against proton-induced activation of somatic sensory neurones (DRAY 1992), it attenuates proton-induced membrane changes and proton-induced neuropeptide release (heart, trachea) in visceral sensory systems. It is possible that protons induce the release of capsaicin-like molecules, or that visceral and somatic fibres differ in their mechanism of activation by protons. In support of these suggestions capsazepine was shown to block the release of calcitonin gene related peptide (CGRP) induced by proton activation of prostacyclin production (LOU and LUNDBERG 1992; SANTICIOLI et al. 1992). In addition, proton-induced activation of tracheal afferent fibres was also antagonised by capsazepine (Fox et al. 1995).

Sensory neurone activation may also lead to the generation of nitric oxide (NO) through NOS catalysis of L-arginine. Small and medium-sized sensory neurones contain constitutive nitric oxide synthase (NOS) and can thus make NO when activated by the increased intracellular calcium produced following nerve stimulation. Although intradermal injection of NO induces a delayed burning pain in humans (HOLTHUSEN and ARNDT 1994), there is little evidence for direct activation of sensory neurones by NO (McGEHEE et al. 1992). However, NO donors such as sodium nitroprusside may activate cerebral sensory fibres directly, causing release of the vasodilator CGRP (WEI et al. 1992). Because of this, NO has been suggested to contribute to migraine and other types of head pain (OLESEN et al. 1994).

Interestingly, NO has also been shown to change neural responsiveness to bradykinin. Thus the attenuation of neural responsiveness to repeated administrations of bradykinin, attributed to receptor desensitisation, is promoted by guanylate cyclase or cGMP, which have been considered to mediate the effects of NO. Conversely, desensitisation is reduced by NOS-inhibitors (N^w-nitro-L-arginine methyl ester and 7-nitroindazole; McGEHEE et al. 1992; BRADLEY and BURGESS 1993; RUEFF et al. 1994). The molecular details of these interactions are not known but may involve the regulation of the bradykinin B_2 receptor-effector coupling mechanism.

It may be of greater significance that NO production is enhanced following injury and inflammation by the activity of inducible NOS. NO may consequently contribute to the ectopic discharges induced by peripheral nerve lesions as the increased sensory neuronal excitability is reduced by NOS inhibitors (VERGE et al. 1992).

Intradermal administration of ATP produces a sharp, transient pain due to direct activation of sensory neurones resulting from increased cation permeability (BLEEHAN and KEELE 1977). Recently a number of purinergic receptors have been identified on sensory neurones through which ATP causes these effects. In particular the identification and characterisation of the $P2X_2$

and P2X$_3$ receptor (CHEN et al. 1995; LEWIS et al. 1995) which are specifically localised on small sensory neurones may provide a clearer understanding of the pharmacological action of ATP. Moreover, the selection of one or other of these receptors may be unique targets against which new analgesic can be developed, although it has been suggested that ATP-gated channels are heteropolymerised P2X receptor subunits (LEWIS et al. 1995).

The rapid hydrolysis of ATP generates adenosine, which also provokes pain and hyperalgesia when administered intradermally, intravenously or onto a blister base (BLEEHAN and KEELE 1977). This is likely to be due to the activation of adenosine A$_2$ receptors which are coupled with adenylate cyclase (TAIWO and LEVINE 1990). The production of cAMP and a reduction of potassium ion permeability accounts for afferent fibres hyperexcitability. On the other hand, adenosine may also activate A1 receptors which are negatively coupled to cAMP activation to cause a reduced afferent excitability by blocking Ca2$^+$ conductance or increasing K$^+$ permeability. This may cause antinociception, as demonstrated with adenosine ligands (TAIWO and LEVINE 1990; KARLSTEN et al. 1992). These findings suggest that selective A1 receptor agonists would be useful analgesic agents provided that systemic side effect problems (motor impairment or cardiovascular effects) can be overcome. An alternatively approach to producing an adenosine-mediated analgesia is to inhibit the degradation of endogenous adenosine with an adenosine kinase inhibitor such as 5'amino-5'deoxyadenosine (KEIL and LEANDER 1992).

Kinins are also potent algogenic and proinflammatory peptides produced by two major biochemical pathways. Bradykinin is the major product of kininase catalysis of high molecular weight kininogen in the blood, while cleaved of low molecular weight kininogen in other tissues by proteolytic enzymes, produces lysyl-bradykinin (kallidin). Kinins are also produced during acute inflammation following the release of cellular proteases from immune cells (mast cells, basophils; see BHOOLA et al. 1992). Rapid degradation of bradykinin and kallidin occurs through kininases activity to yield the major active metabolites des-Arg-9 bradykinin and des-Arg-10 kallidin, respectively, and a number of inactive metabolites.

Bradykinin and kallidin mediate pain and hyperalgesia via the activation of G protein coupled kinin receptors, B$_1$ and B$_2$. The preferred agonist for the B$_2$ receptor is bradykinin but kallidin also acts via the B$_2$ receptor both by direct interaction and, potentially, via conversion to bradykinin by aminopeptidases. Thus far this receptor has accounted for the majority of the pharmacological effects attributed to kinins. A number of selective peptidic and non-peptidic B$_2$ antagonists have been developed and have been critical for receptor characterisation and for evaluating the function role of kinins (DRAY and URBAN 1996).

The B$_1$ receptor is not normally abundant but appears to be overexpressed under the influence of inflammatory mediators and growth promoters (reviewed by MARCEAU 1995). The B$_1$ receptor also appears to have a prominent role in inflammatory hyperalgesia (DRAY and PERKINS 1993). Interestingly, the B_1 receptor has little homology with the B_2 receptor (MENKE et al. 1994) and is likely to be pharmacological distinct from the B_2 receptor. The major metabolites of bradykinin and kallidin, des-Arg-9 bradykinin and des-Arg-10 kallidin, respectively, have greater affinity for the B1 receptor than the parent peptides (see HALL 1992). However, it is worth noting that the major active metabolite of kallidin, des-Arg-10 kallidin, has much greater affinity for the B1 receptor than des-Arg-9 bradykinin. The implications of this for hyperalgesia are unclear, but these data suggest different roles for the B_1 receptor in vascular tissues than in other tissues.

Bradykinin induces pain by direct stimulation of B_2 receptors which occur on nociceptors (C and $A\delta$ fibres) in most tissues (skin, joint, muscle, tooth pulp, viscera). A variety of studies using receptor selective antagonists have confirmed that this receptor is important in producing pain in pathological conditions as a number of B2 receptors antagonists reduce nociceptor activation and the pain produced by irritants or inflammatory mediators (STERANKA et al. 1988; PERKINS et al. 1993; HEAPY et al. 1993).

However, of greater significance in the pathophysiology of pain is the sensitisation of sensory fibres to physical (heat, mechanical) and chemical stimuli (MELLER and GEBHART 1992; MENSE 1993; SCHEIBLE and GRUBB 1993). Sensitisation of sensory fibres occurs through lowering of the activation threshold to exogenous stimuli or by prolonging the discharges following fibre activation. Bradykinin may sensitise fibres by synergistic interactions with other inflammatory algogens such as prostaglandins (PGs), serotonin (5HT) and cytokines or by the release of histamine from mast cells.

B2 receptor signal transduction occurs via the activation of phospholipase C and cleavage of membrane phospholipids. Membrane depolarisation arises from an increase in sodium ion permeability production by the activation of protein kinase C and the phosphorylation of membrane proteins (BURGESS et al. 1989a; DRAY et al. 1992b; SCHEPELMANN et al. 1993). Depolarisation also induces a secondary increase calcium permeability which causes sensory neuropeptide release, activation of NOS and the generation of cGMP (BURGESS et al. 1989b). Bradykinin-induced activation of sensory nerves can be attenuated by indomethacin supporting a role for prostanoids generated via activation of phospholipase C (GAMMON et al. 1989; DRAY et al. 1992). Indeed, PGE_2 has been shown to directly increase sodium ion permeability in sensory neurones thus causing neural excitation (SCHEIBLE and SCHMIDT 1988; BIRRELL et al. 1991) and the secondary release of substance P (NICOL and CUI 1992). Prostanoids may also contribute to sensory neuronal activation by enhancing and prolonging ionic conductance through tetrodotoxin (TTX) resistant sodium channels found only in small sensory neurones (GOLD et al. 1996; AKOPIAN et al. 1996b).

Although B_1 receptors are constitutively expressed in some tissues, they are not present in abundance under normal conditions. Cytokines, particularly interleukin (IL) 1β, increase B_1 receptor expression (MARCEAU 1995) and may trigger the synthesis of new receptor, unmask existing receptors or facilitate B_1

receptor-effector coupling. B_1 receptor activation is important in inflammatory hyperalgesia induced by a number of different agents including Freund's complete adjuvant, carrageenan or UV irradiation as well as following the systemic administration of IL-1β (DRAY and PERKINS 1993).

The contribution of B_1 receptors can be measured by the increased effectiveness of B_1 agonists in exacerbating hyperalgesia and by the fact that B_1 receptor antagonists produce analgesia (DAVIS and PERKINS 1994; CRUWYS et al. 1994; KHASAR et al. 1995). In keeping with this, des-Arg-9 bradykinin, which selectively activates B_1 receptors, is present in greater abundance than bradykinin during inflammation (BURCH and DEHAAS 1988).

Sensory neurones are not directly activated by des-Arg-9 bradykinin (DRAY et al. 1992; NAGY et al. 1993) and thus do not contribute significantly to B1 receptor-induced hyperalgesia. However, hyperalgesia is mediated indirectly via the release of other mediators such tumor necrosis factor-α (TNFα) and IL-1β from immune cells (macrophages and leucocytes; TIFFANY and BURCH 1989) or by PG release (DAVIS and PERKINS 1994). These agents are discussed below.

Prostanoids (PGs, leukotrienes, hydroxy-acids) are generated from archidonic acid by cyclo-oxygenase (COX) and lipoxygenase enzyme and are also important mediators of inflammatory hyperalgesia. Normally PG synthesis is regulated by COX-1 activity, but during inflammation larger amounts of prostanoids are synthesised due to the induction of another synthetic enzyme COX-2. Since the properties of COX-1 and COX-2 differ, it is possible to inhibit COX-2 differentially with newer types of non-steroidal anti-inflammatory drugs (MITCHELL et al. 1993; BOYCE et al. 1994; SEIBERT et al. 1994; DRAY and URBAN 1996).

Normally PG do not evoke pain when injected intradermally into human skin (CRUNKHORN and WILLIS 1971), but PGE_1 and prostacyclin have been reported to increase the activity of nociceptors directly (BIRRELL et al. 1991; SCHEIBLE and SCHMIDT 1988), and PGE_2 stimulates the release of substance P from sensory neurones in culture. These depolarising effects may be due to increased membrane sodium ion conductance. More usually PGs sensitise sensory neurones, reducing their activation threshold and enhancing their responses to other stimuli (LEVINE et al. 1993; DRAY 1994). PGE_2 and prostacyclin in particular cause the sensitisation of sensory neurones to exogenous stimuli. These PGs act upon EP and IP receptors, respectively (COLEMAN et al. 1994). An EP3 receptor subtype has recently been identified in the majority of small sensory neurones and may be important for initiating sensitisation. A number of mechanisms have been proposed to account for this. In visceral sensory neurones (nodose ganglion cells) and to some extent in somatic afferent neurones, increased excitability is associated with the inhibition of a long-lasting spike after-hyperpolarisation (slow-AHP). The slow-AHP is regulated by a cAMP-dependent, calcium-activated potassium conductance mechanism (WEINREICH and WONDERLIN 1987). Thus the slow-AHP, following a single action potential, normally produces a state of reduced excitability which limits the number of evoked action potentials. PGs and bradykinin (through prostanoid formation) inhibit the slow-AHP by stimulating cAMP formation (UNDEM and WEINREICH 1993). This sensitising mechanism accounts for the actions of a number of pro-algesic substances which activate G protein coupled receptors.

Prostanoids, particularly PGE_2, may also contribute to sensory neuronal activation by enhancing and prolonging ionic conductance through TTX-resistant sodium channels (GOLD et al. 1996). Both the magnitude and the rate of sodium channel inactivation are increased, suggesting a likely mechanism for increased cell firing. In addition, the delay to the increase of the sodium current produced by PGE2 and the prolonged duration of this effect suggest that a secondary diffusable intracellular messenger is involved (GOLD et al. 1996).

5HT excites sensory neurones direct by increasing their sodium permeability, and this may accounts for mild and transient pain produced when 5HT is applied to a blister base (RICHARDSON et al. 1985). A similar effect may occur when 5HT is released from platelets and mast cells during injury or inflammation. Since 5HT-induced neural activation is blocked by the 5HT3/4 antagonist ICS 205.930 (tropisetron), interactions with a 5-HT3 receptor are considered to be involved (RICHARDSON et al. 1985). However, it is possible that ICS 205.930 also produces some effects via Na^+ channel blockade since the 5-HT3 receptor binding site is part of a cation (Na^+) selective ion channel.

5-HT also activates sensory neurones via G protein coupled 5HT-1 and 5-HT2 receptors (TAIWO et al. 1992; RUEFF and DRAY 1992). This induces a decrease in potassium ion permeability causing membrane depolarisation and repetitive neuronal firing following neural stimulation. In keeping with this a lowered threshold to heat and pressure stimuli and hyperalgesia have been measured in behavioural experiments (BECK and HANDWERKER 1974). Activation of cAMP-dependent processes occurs during 5HT-induced sensitisation since hyperalgesia can be blocked by an inhibitor of cAMP and augmented by inhibition of phosphodiesterase (TAIWO and LEVINE 1991b). As described above, the cAMP-mediated reduction of K^+ permeability has also been proposed to be the mechanism that attenuates the slow-post spike AHP which increases sensory neural excitability and provokes repetitive firing (TODOROVIC and ANDERSON 1990).

$5HT_{1D}$ like receptors have also been postulated to be present on fine afferent fibres which innervate the dura mater of the brain. Stimulation of these nociceptors may induce pain, release sensory neuropeptides and initiate a number of pro-inflammatory effects (DAVIS and DOSTROVSKY 1988; JANIG and KOTZENBURG 1991). Indeed, neuropeptide-containing C fibres arise mainly from the trigeminal nerve and supply blood vessels, brain parenchyma and the dura mater. Activation of pial sensory fibres induces the release of substance P and CGRP (MOSKOWITZ et al. 1983; KUROSAWA et al. 1995) while electrical stimulation of the trigeminal ganglion or infusion of substance P or neurokinin A produce vasodilatation and plasma extravasation in the dura mater but not in brain (Markowitz et al. 1987). Activation of 5HT1D receptors may reduce afferent excitability, plasma extravasation and the vasodilatation brought about by sensory neuropeptide release. A number of anti-migraine agents including sumatriptan are thought to act on these receptors (Humphrey and Feniuk 1991; Buzzi and Moskowitz 1990).

Histamine can be released following mast cell degranulation by a number of inflammatory mediators including substance P, IL-1 and NGF. It can then act on sensory neurones to produce itching at low concentrations and pain at higher concentrations (Simone et al. 1991). Indeed, sensory neurones express histamine H_1 receptors, and H_1 receptor activation increases membrane calcium permeability in a variety of sensory neurones. This is likely to evoke the release of sensory neuropeptides as well as the release of PGs and monohydroxyeicosatetraenoic acids from endothelial cells, leading to hyperalgesia and other pro-inflammatory effects (Rang et al. 1994).

D. Mediators Released from Neurones

A number of sensory neuropeptides, particularly the neurokinins (substance P and neurokinin A) and CGRP, are released from sensory nerve endings to affect the viability and activity of target tissues (Dray 1994). During inflammation, however, the neurokinins substance P and neurokinin A contribute in a number of ways to neurogenic inflammation, to the associated hyperalgesia in the periphery and to the excitability changes that occur in the spinal dorsal horn.

The effects of neurokinins are mediated through the activation of one or other specific neurokinin receptors NK1, NK2 and NK3 (Maggi et al. 1992). To date NK1 and NK2 receptors have been shown to be involved in the pro-inflammatory and hyperalgesic effects of neurokinins. During inflammation the neuropeptide content of sensory nerves is increased by the actions of neurotrophins such as NGF (Donnerer et al. 1992) so that the effects of substance P and neurokinin A to cause vasodilation, plasma extravasation, mast cell degranulation and immune cell stimulation are more pronounced. CGRP is also released from sensory nerve endings, but rather than producing plasma extravasation directly it induces a powerful arteriolar vasodilation, thereby increasing blood flow into venules and thus acts synergistically with substance P to enhance plasma extravasation. Other sensory neuropeptides such as galanin and somatostatin, although less abundant than the neurokinins, may reduce neurogenic inflammation since they decrease afferent excitability and reduce neuropeptide release from sensory fibres. Plasma extravasation induced by NK1 receptors seems to be of special significance in dural blood vessels and thus may be important in relation to vascular headache. Indeed, NK1 receptor antagonists potently attenuate the plasma extravasation induced by sensory nerve stimulation (Moussaoui et al. 1993) and are predicted to have clinical anti-migraine activity.

Neurokinins may also directly depolarise sensory neurones by reducing membrane potassium ion permeability (DRAY and PINNOCK 1982). This suggests that under appropriate conditions neurokinins may induce pain by stimulating afferent nerve endings in the periphery. Other studies have postulated that the presence of NK1 receptors on primary afferent nerve terminals regulates afferent excitability in the spinal cord (MALCANGIO and BOWERY 1994). Thus neurokinins may be important for direct regulation of nociception at several stages, although it is not clear whether this is an auto-regulatory mechanisms, via peptide release from afferent fibres themselves or release from other tissues such as sympathetic fibres.

In support of the involvement of NK1 receptors in nociception several NK1 antagonists produce analgesia. Thus the non-peptide antagonist RP67580 reduced mechanical hyperalgesia in rats with streptozotocin-induced diabetic neuropathy but not in normal animals. A similar antagonist CP 96345 abolishes carrageenan- and formalin-induced inflammatory hyperalgesia (BIRCH et al. 1992). However, it is not clear whether these antagonists induce their effects by block of peptidergic transmission in the spinal cord or act at peripheral NK1 sites as well.

Interactions of sympathetic neurones and nociceptive afferents have been postulated during inflammation. However, direct interactions of sympathetic nerves or sympathetic transmitters with afferent fibres have been demonstrated only after peripheral nerve damage or inflammation (MCMAHON 1991; TREEDE et al. 1992). Thus afferent fibre can be sensitised during inflammation by the release of prostanoids from activated sympathetic fibres (LEVINE et al. 1993). In addition, sympathetic nerve stimulation, or the direct administration of noradrenaline, is able to excite fine afferent fibres after injury to a sensory nerve trunk (SATO and PERL 1991; DEVOR et al. 1994). This can be attenuated by a number of α-adrenergic receptor blocking drugs, suggesting that α-adrenergic receptors are expressed on fine afferent fibres (SATO and PERL 1991; DEVOR et al. 1994). It is important to note however that following peripheral nerve injury, activity in large A fibre afferents can also sustain the spinal hyperexcitability necessary for maintaining hyperalgesia and allodynia (THOMPSON et al. 1995). Postganglion sympathetic nerves play a prominant role in regulating large Aβ fibres activity via the ingrowth of sympathetic fibres to innervate dorsal root ganglion (DRG) neurones and the expression of adrenergic α-receptors on sensory ganglion cells (MCLACHLAN et al. 1993; DEVOR et al. 1994).

Although neuropeptide Y (NPY) receptors 1 and 2 have also been found on sensory neurones, it is unclear what function they serve although they are likely to be involved in regulating nociception. Thus NPY can be released from sympathetic fibres in which it is co-localised with sympathetic transmitter or from large afferent fibres in the spinal cord in which it is expressed following nerve injury (MANTYH et al. 1994). Indeed, Y_1 receptors activation increases DRG excitability and neuropeptide release through increased calcium permeability, but Y_2 receptor activation inhibits calcium conductance and sensory

transmitter release (COLMERS and BLEAKMAN 1994), thereby reducing neurogenic inflammation (LEVINE et al. 1993). Presently it is not clear what the net
effect of NPY is on nociception although it is believed that Y_2 receptors
predominate on sensory neurones (ZHANG et al. 1995). Whether a selective
agonist or antagonist of NPY receptors would be of greatest benefit for analgesia may be determined soon as a non-peptide NPY1 receptor antagonist,
BIBP 3226 has been reported (WIELAND et al. 1995).

E. Inflammatory Mediators from Immune Cells

A number of cytokines (IL-1β, IL-6, IL-8, TNFα) are released from a variety
of immune cells and can induce powerful hyperalgesia. This is mediated indirectly via several mechanisms including (a) the release of prostanoids from
several tissues, (b) increasing the expression of NGF or kinin receptors, and
(c) by affecting the neurochemistry of sympathetic fibres (JONAKAIT 1993;
CUNHA et al. 1991, 1992). So far there is no evidence that cytokines can directly
affect the excitability of sensory fibres although they may be produced by
damaged sensory neurones (R.A. Murphy, personal communication, 1995)
and possibly be released by them onto innervated tissues.

Various cytokines (IL-1β, IL-6, IL-8 and TNFα), particularly IL-1β show
potent pro-inflammatory and hyperalgesic actions (FERREIRA et al. 1988; DAVIS
and PERKINS 1994) by stimulating the synthesis and release of pro-hyperalgesic
mediators (peptides, NGF) or the expression of receptors (kinin B_1 receptors)
on sensory and sympathetic neurones as well as on immune cells (DAVIS and
PERKINS 1994; SEABROOK et al. 1995). A number of new strategies have been
adopted to reduce cytokine activity and hopefully reducing inflammatory
hyperalgesia, including blockade of IL-1β activity with tri-peptides related to
Lys-D-Pro-Thr (FERREIRA et al. 1988), inhibition of cytokine synthesis using IL-
1β converting enzyme inhibitors or by interfering with cytokine-mediated
gene transcription and translation (LEE et al. 1993; ELFORD et al. 1995).

The neurotrophin NGF is normally produced by the peripheral target
tissues of afferent fibres and by supporting cells including fibroblasts, Schwann
cells and keratinocytes. It is essential for the survival and development of
sensory neurones and for maintaining their phenotype (LEWIN and MENDELL
1993) acting via a specific tyrosine kinase receptor (trkA) to regulate specific
gene transcription processes. During inflammation, however, NGF production
is stimulated (DONNERER et al. 1992) by other inflammatory mediators such as
cytokines (IL-1β and TNFa; SAFIEH-GARABEDIAN et al. 1995). NGF appears to
induce a rapid but indirect sensitisation of nociceptors, particularly to thermal
stimuli, via mast cell degranulation and the release of other mediators and
through the expression of kinin B_1 receptors. In the longer term NGF induces
phenotypic changes in small sensory neurones via an alteration in gene regulation. This leads to the increased synthesis of several neuropeptides including
neurokinins and CGRP and upregulates a number of other proteins such as

vanilloid receptors, membrane sodium channels and proton-activated ion channels (AGUAYO and WHITE 1992; WINTER et al. 1988, 1993). Related to these changes is increased sensitivity to mechanical and exogenous chemical stimuli and the production of hyperalgesia. In keeping with this, anti-NGF antibodies reduce the hyperalgesia and neurochemical changes induced by NGF and inflammation (LEWIN and MENDELL 1993; WOOLF et al. 1994).

A number of studies have shown that during inflammation opioid peptide production and release is induced from immune cells (SCHÄFFER et al. 1994). This is coupled with the expression of opioid receptors on sensory and sympathetic neurones. Thus a number of studies confirm that opioids produce analgesic activity (STEIN 1993; CZLONKOWSKI et al. 1993) through μ-, δ-, or k-opioid receptors on primary afferent nerve terminals (ANDREEV et al. 1994) and sympathetic fibres (TAIWO and LEVINE 1991) Indeed, ongoing activity in C fibres following injury to peripheral nerve terminals is inhibited by μ and κ receptor agonists (ANDREEV et al. 1994).

Depression of neural excitability is mediated by μ, δ and κ receptors via receptor-coupled activation of a G protein and inhibition of adenylate cyclase. This reduces membrane excitability by reducing calcium permeability and/or by increasing potassium ion conductance (SHEN and CRAIN 1990; CRAIN and SHEN 1990). These data suggest that both primary afferents and sympathetic fibres can be targets for peripherally acting opiates which would lack the sedative and psychotropic effects of existing, centrally acting compounds.

There has also been much interest recently in the discovery of opioid-like receptors (orphan receptors) in the nervous system which differ from μ, δ and κ receptors. A recently isolated receptor, ORL1, is similar in sequence to other G protein coupled opioid receptors but does not bind opioid peptides or ligands. The natural ligand may be a pro-algesic peptide which resembles dynorphin A and has been named nociceptin (MEUNIER et al. 1995) or ophanin FQ (REINSCHEID et al. 1995) by the groups that have characterised it. Thus far there is little information about the occurrence of this receptor or the action of the peptide in peripheral neurones.

F. Exogenous Modulators of Sensory Fibre Activity: Vanilloids (Capsaicin Analogues)

Capsaicin, the pungent principle in hot chili peppers, produces a burning pain by selective activation of nociceptors (references in DRAY 1992; SZALLASI 1994). This appears to require precise chemical structural requirements (WALPOLE and WRIGGLESWORTH 1993) and is mediated by a specific membrane receptor, known as the vanilloid receptor. Thus capsaicin recognition sites on sensory neurones have been proposed from structure-activity studies using capsaicin-like ligands, particularly the naturally occurring analogue resiniferatoxin (SZOLSCÁNYI 1994; SZALASI 1994). In addition, the capsaicin antagonist capsazepine has provided direct pharmacological evidence that resiniferatoxin binding and capsaicin-induced activation of sensory neurones was mediated by specific receptor interactions (Bevan et al. 1992; Dickenson and Dray 1991; James et al. 1993) Indeed, there may be multiple capsaicin binding sites, indicating that subtypes of vanilloid receptor exist both on sensory neurones and on other tissues (Ninkina et al. 1994; Szallasi 1994; Dray et al. 1992). In support of this, capsaicin-evoked depolarisation of sensory neurones has been shown to be mutiphasic and only partially susceptible to capsazepine (Dray et al. 1992; Petersen et al. 1995). These findings raise questions about the relative functions of various capsaicin receptors and their natural ligand as well as how these might be further exploited to produce analgesics.

Nociceptor activation accounts for the burning pain sensation that capsaicin induces upon intradermal injection or after topical application to the skin and mucous membranes (Bevan and Szolcanyi 1990; Dray 1992). In addition, capsaicin given locally or systemically induces sensory neuropeptide release and thus triggers a number of proinflammatory effects and local reflexes. However, following neural activation capsaicin rapidly induces sensory neurones to become inexcitable, and consequently noxious stimuli are no longer effective. In addition, the release of sensory neuropeptides from these peptide-containing afferents is prevented, thus contributing to an attenuation of neurogenic inflammation. Capsaicin has therefore been used topically in the treatment of several painful conditions such as cluster headache, reflex sympathetic dystrophy, post-mastectomy pain, post-herpetic neuralgia and diabetic neuropathy which are often resistant to conventional analgesic therapies. The major drawback to capsaicin therapy has been the irritant and burning sensation that it evokes upon initial application. Unfortunately, the non-irritant antagonist capsazepine does not appear to be analgesic (Perkins and Campbell 1992), and thus capsaicin analogues must be agonists to induce fibre inactivation and analgesia. Other capsaicin analogues such NE19550 (olvanil) and NE21610 (nuvanil) are analgesic and anti-inflammatory while NE21610 given intradermally is analgesic against heat but not mechanical pain in humans (Brand et al. 1987; Davis et al. 1995). However, these analogues still retain significant pungency.

G. Ion Channels Activity and Chronic Pain

The over-expression of membrane ion channels during inflammation and nerve injury increases membrane excitability, creates abnormal nerve activity and can initiate spontaneous ectopic activity in peripheral neurones (neuroma tissue and DRG; Devor 1994; Matzner and Devor 1994; Waxman et al. 1994).

These changes may account for some aspects of inflammatory and neuropathy pain. In particular TTX-sensitive sodium channels are over-expressed in large axons following nerve injury while TTX-resistant channels, found in many small nociceptive neurones, may be upregulated by the increases in NGF production seen in inflammation (AGUAYO and WHITE 1992). It is particularly significant that the nociceptor sensitisation induced by prostanoids may occur through the enhancement and prolongation of TTX-resistant sodium channel activity (GOLD et al. 1996). Other types of sodium channel are also increased such as the type III sodium channels in nerve injury and PN1 sodium channels by NGF (WAXMAN et al. 1994; TOLEDO-ARAL et al. 1995). The over expression of sodium channels has been viewed as attractive targets for novel analgesics which may be designed to block the active conformation of the channel which would be associated with nerve activation and nociception, thus leaving normal physiological pain transmission intact.

A variety of anticonvulsant drugs (cabamazepine, phenytoin), local anaesthetics (lidocaine, tocainide) and antiarrythmic drugs (mexilitene) have been used with varying degrees of success in the treatment of chronic pain associated with neuropathy and sympathetic dystrophy (MARCHETTINI et al. 1992; TANELIAN and BROSE 1991), conditions which are poorly controlled by conventional opioid analgesics. Their efficacy may be related to the fact that they block sodium channels, having a higher affinity for the open or activated conformation of the channel (RAGSDALE et al. 1991; SCHWARZ and GRIGAT 1989). However, their site and exact mechanism of action as analgesic is still unclear. For example, in experimental models of neuropathic pain, lidocaine selectively blocks ectopic discharges originating from the DRG or from the neuroma without affecting axonal conduction (DEVOR et al. 1992). This selectivity may be explained by a block of active Na^+ channels below the threshold needed for generating spontaneous activity or, as indicated above, a use-dependent block of open sodium channels resulting in the inhibition of tonic ongoing discharge (RAGSDALE et al. 1991). Since activity in postganglionic sympathetic fibres may also contribute significantly to neuropathic pain (DEVOR et al. 1994; KIM and CHUNG 1991), blockade of abnormal activity in these fibres may be an alternative target for novel channel blocking drugs.

Voltage-dependent T-, N- and L-calcium channels also contribute significantly to the excitability of sensory neurones, but N-channels are particularly important as they control the release of neurochemicals from peripheral and central terminals. N- and L-channels can be blocked by endogenous chemical transmitters (opioids, γ-aminobutyric acid, NPY) but also by a number of selective drugs (dihydropyridines) to prevent nociceptive signalling. Unfortunately, present drugs which block voltage-activated channels are not selective for sensory neurones, and side effects may therefore be anticipated. However, abnormal calcium channel activity in small sensory neurones has been implicated in diabetic neuropathy (KOSTYUK et al. 1995) and in the generation of ectopic discharges in sensory ganglia after peripheral nerve injury. Thus the spontaneous discharges of experimental nerve injury can be blocked by verapamil and a number of N- channel, ω-conotoxin derivatives (XIAO and BENNETT 1995; ZHANG et al. 1994). Clearly calcium channel activity in chronic pain conditions needs molecular characterisation to reveal whether novel channels may account for abnormalities in excitability. If so, the blocking of this may offer new directions for the control of neuropathic pain. A similar strategy can be adopted to characterise potassium channels in sensory neurones in chronic pain conditions. Indeed, drug-induced opening of potassium channels would result in membrane hyperpolarisation and inhibition of membrane excitability. Although a number of new K channel stimulants are available, none has been targeted directly for analgesia (references in Dray and Urban 1996).

H. Summary

Fine peripheral sensory fibres are sensitive to a range of chemical stimuli. Their activity and metabolism is powerfully regulated by the products of tissue injury and inflammation as well as by a number of exogenous irritant chemicals. For the most part these interactions are produced by specific receptors coupled with second messenger cascades and membrane ion channels. These processes affect membrane excitability but also have the potential to alter gene transcription, thereby inducing long-term alterations in the biochemistry of sensory neurones with consequences up- or downregulation of neurochemicals, expression of novel ion channels (Na^+ channels) and receptors (capsaicin, NPY) as well as the induction of novel enzymes (inducible NOS). Many substances produce direct activation of nociceptors (bradykinin, ATP, capsaicin), thereby causing acute pain. More importantly, however, inflammatory mediators induce hyperalgesia through nociceptor sensitisation. This results from direct activation of cellular kinases and altered membrane excitability or indirectly via the synthesis and release of other cellular regulators (prostanoids, cytokines, NGF). Selective modification of these processes would give rise to novel analgesic and anti-inflammatory agents (Dray et al. 1994). In addition, abnormal excitability arising from inflammation and nerve injury may involve the over-expression or appearance of new ion channels and receptors. Greater knowledge of these events as well as ways of selective inactivation of nociceptors (e.g. capsaicin analogues) will also be required to produce new analgesics.

References

Aguayo LG, White G (1992) Effects of nerve growth factor on TTX- and capsaicin-sensitivity in adult rat sensory neurones. Brain Res 570:61–67

Akopian AN, Abson NC, Wood JN (1996a) Molecular genetic approach to nociceptor development and function. Trends Neurosci 19:240–246

Akopian AN, Sivoletti L, Wood JN (1996b) A tetrodotoxin-resistant voltage-gated sodium channel expressed by sensory neurons. Nature 379:257–262

Andreev N, Urban L, Dray A (1994) Opioids suppress spontaneous activity of polymodal nociceptors in rat paw skin induced by ultraviolet irradiation. Neuroscience 58:793–798

Bevan SJ, Geppetti P (1994) Protons: small stimulants of capsaicin-sensitive sensory nerves. Trends Neurosci 17:509–512

Beck PW, Handwerker HO (1974) Bradykinin and serotonin effects on various types of cutaneous nerve fibres. Pflugers Arch 347:209–222

Bevan S, Yeats J (1991) Protons activate a cation conductance in a sub-population of rat dorsal root ganglion neurons. J Physiol (Lond) 433:145–161

Bevan S, Szolcsanyi J (1990) Sensory neuron-specific actions of capsaicin: mechanisms and applications. Trends Pharmacol Sci 11:330–333

Bevan S, Hothi S, Hughes G, James IF, Rang HP, Shah K, Walpole CSJ, Yeats JC (1992) Capsazepine: a competitive antagonist of the sensory neurone excitant capsaicin. Br J Pharmacol 197:44–552

Bhoola KD, Figueroa CD, Worthy K (1992) Bioregulation of kinins: kallikreins, kininogens, and kininases. Pharmacol Rev 44:1–80

Birch PJ, Harrison SM, Hayes AG, Rogers H, Tyers MB (1992) The non-peptide NK1 receptor anatgonist, (±)–CP-96,345, produces antinociception and anti-oedema effects in the rat. Br J Pharmacol 105:508–510

Birrell GJ, McQueen DS, Iggo A, Coleman RA, Grubb BD (1991) PGI2-induced activation and sensitization of articular mechanonociceptors. Neurosci Lett 124:5–8

Bleehan T, Keele CA (1977) Observations on the algogenic actions of adenosine compounds on the human blister base preparation. Pain 3:367–377

Boyce S, Chan C, Gordon R, Li C, Rodger IW, Webb KJ, Rupniak NMJ, Hill RG (1994) A selective inhibitor of cyclooxygenase-2 elicits antinociception but not gastric ulceration in rats. Neuropharmacology 33:1609–1611

Bradley C, Burgess G (1993) A nitric oxide synthase inhibitor reduces desensitisation of bradykinin-induced activation of phospholipase C in sensory neurones. Trans Biochem Soc 21:43–53

Brand LL, Berman E, Schwen R, Loomans M, Janusz J, Bohne R, Maddin C, Gardner J, LaHann T, Farmer R, Jones L, Chiabrando C, Fanelli R (1987) NE-19550: a novel, orally active anti-inflammatory analgesic. Drugs Exp Clin Res 13:259–265

Burch, RM, DeHaas C (1988) A bradykinin antagonist inhibits carageenin oedema in the rat. Naunyn Schmiedebergs Arch Pharmacol 342:189–193

Burgess GM, Mullaney J, McNeil M, Dunn P, Rang HP (1989a) Second messengers involved in the action of bradykinin on cultured sensory neurones. J Neurosci 9:3314–3325

Burgess GM, Mullaney I, McNeill M, Coote PR, Minhas A, Wood JN (1989b) Activation of guanylate cyclase by bradykinin in rat sensory neurones is mediated by calcium influx: possible role of the increase in cyclic GMP. J Neurochem 53:1212–1218

Buzzi M G, Moskowitz MA (1990) The antimigraine drug sumatriptan (GR43175), selectively blocks neurogenic plasma extravasation from blood vessels in dura mater. Br J Pharmacol 99:202–206

Chen C-C, Akopian AN, Sivilotti L, Colquhoun D, Burnstock G, Wood J (1995) A P2X purinoceptor expressed by a subset of sensory neurons. Nature 377:428–431

Coleman RA, Smith WL, Narumiya S (1994) Classification of prostanoid receptors: properties, distribution and structure of the receptors and their subtypes. Pharmacol Rev 46:205–229

Colmers WF, Bleakman D (1994) Effects of neuropeptide Y on the electrical properties of neurons. Trends Neurosci 17:373–379

Crain MC, Shen K-F (1990) Opinoids can evoke direct receptor-mediated excitatory effects on sensory neurons. Trend Pharmacol Sci 11:77–81

Crunkhorn P, Willis AL (1971) Cutaneous reaction to intradermal prostaglandins. Br J Pharmacol 41:49–56

Cruwys SC, Garrett NE, Perkins MN, Blake DR, Kidd BL (1994) The role of bradykinin B1 receptors in the maintenance of intra-articular plasma extravasation in chronic antigen-induced arthritis. Br J Pharmacol 113:940–944

Cunha FQ, Lorenzetti BB, Poole S, Ferreira SH (1991) Interleukin-8 as a mediator of sympathetic pain. Br J Pharmacol 104:765–767

Cunha FQ, Poole S, Lorenzetti BB, Ferreira SH (1992) The pivotal role of tumor necrosis factor a in the development of inflammatory hyperalgesia. Br J Pharmacol 107:660–664

Czlonkowski A, Stein C, Herz A (1993) Peripheral mechanisms of opioid antinociception in inflammation: involvement of cytokines. Eur J Pharmacol 242:229–235

Davis KD, Dostrovsky JO (1988) Cerebrovascular application of bradykinin excites central sensory neurons. Brain Res 446:401–406

Davis KD, Meyer RA, Turnquist JL, Filloon TG, Pappagallo M, Campbell JN (1995) Cutaneous injection of the capsaicin analogue, NE-21610 produces analgesia to heat but not to mechanical stimuli in man. Pain 61:17–26

Davis AJ, Perkins MN (1994) The involvement of bradykinin B1 and B2 receptor mechanisms in cytokine-induced mechanical hyperalgesia in the rat. Br J Pharmacol 113:63–68

Devor M (1994) The pathophysiology of damaged peripheral nerves. In: Wall PD, Melzack R (eds) Textbook of pain, 3rd edn. Churchill-Livingstone, Edinburgh, pp 79–100

Devor M, Wall PD, Catalan N (1992) Systemic lidocaine silences ectopic neuroma and DRG discharge without blocking nerve conduction. Pain 48:261–268

Devor M, Jänig W, Michaelis M (1994) Modulation of activity in dorsal root ganglion neurons by sympathetic activation in nerve-injured rats. J Neurophysiol 71:38–47

Dickenson AH, Dray A (1991) Selective antagonism of capsaicin by capsazepine: evidence for a spinal receptor site in capsaicin-induced antinociception. Br J Pharmacol 104:1045–1049

Donnerer J, Schuligoi R, Stein C (1992) Increased content and transport of substance P and calcitonin gene-related peptide in sensory nerves innervating inflamed tissue: evidence for a regulatory function of nerve growth factor in vivo. Neuroscience 49:693–698

Dray A (1992) Neuropharmacological mechanisms of capsaicin and related substances. Biochem Pharmacol 44:611–615

Dray A (1994) Tasting the inflammatory soup: role of peripheral neurones. Pain Rev 1:153–171

Dray A, Perkins M (1993) Bradykinin and inflammatory pain. Trends Neurosci 16:99–104

Dray A, Pinnock RD (1982) Effects of Substance P on adult rat sensory ganglion neurones in vitro. Neurosci Lett 33:61–66

Dray A, Urban L (1996) New pharmacological strategies for pain relief. Annu Rev Pharmacol Toxicol 36:253–280

Dray A, Patel I, Naeem S, Rueff A, Urban L (1992a) Studies with capsazepine on peripheral nociceptor activition by capsaicin and low pH: evidence for a duel effect of capsaicin. Br J Pharmacol 107:236P

Dray A, Patel IA, Perkins MN Rueff A (1992b) Bradykinin-induced activation of nociceptors: receptor and mechanistic studies on the neonatal rat spinal cord-tail preparation in vitro. Br J Pharmacol 107:1129–1134

Dray A, Urban L Dickenson A (1994) Pharmacology of chronic pain. Trends Pharmacol Sci 15:190–197

Elford PR, Heng R, Revesz L, MacKenzie AR (1995) Reduction of inflammation and pyrexia in the rat by oral administration of SDZ 224-015, an inhibitor of the interleukin-1β converting enzyme. Br J Pharmacol 115:601–606

Ferreira SH, Lorenzetti BB, Bristow AF, Poole S (1988) Interleukin-1 beta as a potent hyperalgesic agent antagonized by a tripeptide analogue. Nature 334:698–700

Fox AJ, Urban L, Barnes PJ, Dray A (1995) Effects of capsazepine against capsaicin- and proton-evoked excitation of single airway C-fibres and vagus nerve from the guinea pig. Neuroscience 67:741–752

Gammon CM, Allen AC, Morell P (1989) Bradykinin stimulates phosphoinositide hydrolysis and mobilisation of arachidonic acid in dorsal root ganglion neurons. J Neurochem 53:95–101

Gold MS, Reichling DB, Shuster MJ, Levine JD (1996) Hyperalgesic agents increase a tetrodotoxin-resistant Na^+ current in nociceptors. Proc Natl Acad Sci USA 93: 1108–1112

Hall JM (1992) Bradykinin receptors: pharmacological properties and biological roles. Pharmacol Ther 56:131–190

Heapy CG, Shaw JS, Farmer SC (1993) Differential sensitivity of antinociceptive assays to the bradykinin antagonist Hoe 140. Br J Pharmacol 108:209–213

Holthusen H, Arndt JO (1994) Nitric oxide evokes pain in humans on intracutaneous injection. Neurosci Lett 165:71–74

Humphrey PPA, Feniuk W (1991) Mode of action of the anti-migraine drug sumatriptan. Trends Pharmacol Sci 12:444–446

James IF, Ninkina N, Wood JN (1993) The capsaicin receptor. In: Wood J (ed) Capsaicin in the study of pain. Academic, London, pp 83–104

Janig W, Kolzenburg M (1991) Receptive properties of pial afferents. Pain 45:77–85

Jonakait GM (1993) Neural-immune interactions in sympathetic ganglia. Trends Neurosci 10:419–423

Karlsten R, Gordh T, Post C (1992) Local antinociceptive and hyperalgesic effects in the formalin test after peripheral administration of adenosine analogues in mice. Pharmacol Toxicol 70:434–438

Keil GJ, Lander GE (1992) Spinally-mediated antinociception is induced in mice by an adenosine kinase-, but not by an adenosine deaminase-inhibitor. Life Sci 51:PL171–176

Khasar SG, Miao FJ-P, Levine JD (1995) Inflammation modulates the contribution of receptor-subtypes to bradykinin-induced hyperalgesia. Neuroscience 69:685–690

Kim SH, Chung JM (1991) Sympathectomy alleviates mechanical allodynia in an experimental animal model for neuropathy in the rat. Neurosci Lett 134:131–134

Kostyuk E, Pronchuk N, Shmigoi A (1995) Calcium signal prolongation in sensory neurons of mice with experimental diabetes. Neuroreport 6:1010–1012

Kurosawa M, Messlinger K, Pawlak M, Schmidt RF (1995) Increases of meningeal blood flow after electrical stimulation of rat dura mater encephali: mediation by calcitonin-gene related peptide. Br J Pharamacol 114:1397–1402

Lee JC, Badger AM, Griswold DE, Dunnington D, Truneh A, Votta B, White JR, Young PR, Bender PE (1993) Bicyclic imidazolines as a novel class of cytokine biosynthesis inhibitors. Ann N Y Acad Sci 696:149–170

Levine JD, Fields HL, Basbaum AI (1993) Peptides and the primary afferent nociceptor. J Neurosci 13:2273–2286

Lewin GR, Mendell LM (1993) Nerve growth factor and nociception. Trends Neurosci 16:353–358

Lewis C, Noldhart S, Holy C, North RA, Buell G, Supranant A (1995) Coexpression of P2X2 and P2X3 receptor subunits can account for ATP-gated currents in sensory neurons. Nature 377:432–435

Lou Y-P, Lundberg JM (1992) Inhibition of low pH evoked activation of airway sensory nerves by capsazepine, a novel capsaicin-receptor antagonist. Biochem Biophys Res Commun 189:537–544

Maggi CA, Patacchini R, Rovero P, Giachetti A (1992) Tachykinin receptors and tachykinin receptor antagonists. J Autonom Pharmacol 13:23–29

Malcangio M, Bowery NG (1994) Effect of tachykinin NK1 receptor antagonist, RP 67580 and SR 140333, on electrically-evoked subtance P release from rat spinal cord. Br J Pharmacol 113:635–641

Mantyh PW, Allen CJ, Rogers S, DeMaster E, Ghilard JR, Mosconi T, Kruger L, Mannon PJ, Taylor IL, Vigna SR (1994) Some sensory neurones express neuropeptide Y receptors: potential paracrine inhibition of primary afferent nociceptors following peripheral nerve injury. J Neurosci 14:3958–3968

Marceau F (1995) Kinin B1 receptors: a review. Immunology 30:1–26

Marchettini P, Lacerenza M, Marangoni C, Pellegata G, Sotgiu ML, Smirne S (1992) Lidocaine test in neuralgia. Pain 48:377–382

Matzner O, Devor M (1994) Hyperexcitability at sites of nerve injury depends on voltage-sensitive Na⁺ channels. J Neurophysiol 72:349–359

Markowitz S, Saito K Moskowitz MA (1987) Neurogenically mediated leakage of plasma protein occurs from blood vessels in dura mater but not brain. J Neurosci 7:4129–4136

McGehee DS, Goy MF Oxford GS (1992) Involvement of the nitric oxide-cyclic GMP pathway in the desensitization of bradykinin responses of cultured rat sensory neurons. Neuron 9:315–324

McLachlan EM, Janig W, Devor M, Michaelis M (1993) Peripheral nerve injuries triggers noradrenergic sprouting within dorsal root ganglia. Nature 363:543–546

McMahon SB (1991) Mechanisms of sympathetic pain. Br Med Bull 47:584–600

Meller ST, Gebhart GF (1992) A critical review of the afferent pathways and the potential chemical mediators involved in cardiac pain. Neuroscience 48:501–524

Mense S (1993) Nociception from skeletal muscle in relation to clinical muscle pain. Pain 54:241–289

Menke JG, Borkowski JA, Bierilo K, MacNeil T, Derrick AW, Schneck KA, Ransom RW, Strader KD, Linemeyer DL, Hess JF (1994) Expression cloning of a human B1 bradykinin receptor. J Biol Chem 269:21583–21586

Meunier J-C, Mollereau C, Toll L, Suaudeau C, Molsand C, Alvinerle P, Butour J-L, Guillemot J-C, Ferrara P, Monsarrat B, Mazargull H, Vassart G, Parmentier M, Costentin J (1995) Isolation and structure of the endogenous agonist of opioid receptor-like ORL1 receptor. Nature 377:532–535

Mitchell A, Akarasereenont P, Thiemermann C, Flower RJ, Vane JR (1993) Selectivity of nonsteroidal antiinflammatory drugs as inhibitors of constitutive and inducible cyclooxygenase. Proc Natl Acad Sci USA 90:11693–11697

Moskowitz MA, Brody M, Liu-Chen LY (1983) In vitro release of immunoreactive substance P from putative afferent nerve endings in bovine pia arachnoid. Neuroscience 9:809–814

Moussaoui SM, Phillipe L, Le Prado N, Garret C (1993) Inhibition of neurogenic inflammation in the meninges by a non-peptide NK-1 receptor antagonists RP 67580. Eur J Pharmacol 238:421–424

Nagy I, Pabla R, Matesz, Dray A, Woolf CJ, Urban L (1993) Cobalt uptake enables identification of capsaicin and bradykinin sensitive sub-populations of rat dorsal root ganglion cells in vitro. Neuroscience 56:167–172

Nicol GD, Cui M (1994) Enhancement by prostaglandin E2 of bradykinin activation of embryonic rat sensory neurones. J Physiol (Lond) 480:485–492

Ninkina NN, Willoughby JJ Beech MM, Coote PR, Wood JN (1994) Molecular cloning of a resiniferatoxin-binding protein. Mol Brain Res 22:39–48

Olesen J, Thomsen LL, Iversen H (1994) Nitric oxide is a key molecule in migraine and other vascular headaches. Trends Pharmacol Sci 15:149–153

Perkins MN, Campbell EA (1992) Capsazepine reversal of the analgesic action of capsaicin in vivo. Br J Pharmacol 107:329–333

Perkins MN, Campbell E, Dray A (1993) Anti-nociceptive activity of the B1 and B2 receptor antagonists desArg9Leu8Bk and HOE 140, in two models of persistent hyperalgesia in the rat. Pain 53:191–197

Petersen M, LaMotte RH, Klusch A Kniffki K-D (1995) capsaicin ilicits inward current with two components differing in time course and response to pH in adult rat sensory neurons. Soc Neurosci 21:648

Ragsdale DS, Scheuer T, Catterall WA (1991) Frequency and voltage-dependent inhibition of type IIA Na⁺ channels, expressed in a mammalian cell line, by local anesthetic, antiarrhythmic, and anticonvulsant drugs. Mol Pharmacol 40:756–765

Rang HP, Bevan SJ, Dray A (1994) Nociceptive peripheral neurones: cellular properties. In: Wall PD, Melzack R (eds) Textbook of pain. Churchill Livingstone, Edinburgh, pp 57–78

Reinscheid RK, Nothacker H-P, Bourson A, Ardati A, Henningsen RA, Bunzow JR, Grandy DK, Langen H, Monsma Jr FJ, Civelli O (1995) Orphanin FQ: a neuropeptide that activates an opioid like G protein-coupled receptor. Science 270:792–794

Richardson BP, Engel G, Donatsch P, Stadler PA (1985) Identification of serotonin M-receptor subtypes and their specific blockade by a new class of drugs. Nature 316:126–131

Rueff A, Dray A (1992) 5-Hydroxytryptamine-induced sensitization and activation of peripheral fibres in the neonatal rat are mediated via different 5-hydroxytryptamine-receptors. Neuroscience 50:899–905

Rueff A, Patel IA, Urban L, Dray A (1994) Regulation of bradykinin sensitivity in peripheral sensory fibres of the neonatal rat by nitric oxide and cyclic GMP. Neuropharmacology 33:1139–1145

Safieh-Garabedian B, Poole S, Allchorne A, Winter J, Woolf CJ (1995) Contribution of interleukin-1 beta to the inflammation-induced increase in nerve growth factor levels and inflammatory hyperalgesia. Br J Pharmacol 115:1265–1275

Santicioli P, Del Bianco E, Giachetti AM Maggi CA (1992) Capsazepine inhibits low pH- and capsaicin-induced release of calcitonin gene-related peptide (CGRP) from rat soleus muscle. Br J Pharmacol 107:464P

Sato J, Perl ER (1991) Adrenergic excitation of cutaneous pain receptors induced by peripheral nerve injury. Science 251:1608–1610

Scheible H-G, Grubb BD (1993) Afferent and spinal mechanisms of joint pain. Pain 55:5–54

Scheible H-G, Schmidt RF (1988) Excitation and sensitization of fine articular afferents from cat's knee joint by prostaglandin E2. J Physiol (Lond) 403:91–104

Schäfer M, Carter L, Stein C (1994) Interleukin 1 beta and corticotropin-releasing factor inhibit pain by releasing opioids from immune cells in inflamed tissue. Proc Natl Acad Sci USA 91:4219–4223

Schepelmann K, Messlinger K, Schmidt RF (1993) The effect of phorbol ester on slowly conducting afferents of the catts knee joint. Exp Brain Res 92:391–398

Schmelz M, Schmidt R, Ringkamp M, Handwerker HO, Torebjork HE (1994) Sensitization of insensitive branches of C nociceptors in human skin. J Physiol (Lond) 480:389–394

Schwarz JR, Grigat G (1989) Phenytoin and carbamazepine: potential- and frequency-dependent block of Na currents in mammalian myelinated nerve fibers. Epilepsia 30:286–294

Seabrook GR, Bowery BJ, Hill RG (1995) Bradykinin receptors in mouse and rat isolated suprior cervical ganglia. Br J. Pharmacol 115:368–372

Seibert K, Zhinag Y, Leahy K, Hauser S, Masferrer J, Perkins W, Isakson P (1994) Pharmacological and biochemical demonstration of the role of cyclooxygenase 2 in inflammation and pain. Proc Natl Acad Sci USA 91:12013–12017

Shen K-F, Crain SM (1990) Dynorphin prolongs the action potential of mouse sensory ganglion neurons by decreasing a potassium conductance whereas another specific kappa opioid does so by increasing a calcium conductance. Neuropharmacology 29:343–349

Simone DA, Alrejom M, LaMotte RH (1991) Psychophysical studies of the itch sensation and itchy skin ("allokenis") produced by intracutaneous injection of histamine. Somatosens Motor Res 8:271–279

Steen KH, Reeh PW, Anton F, Handwerker HO (1992) Protons selectively induce lasting excitation and sensitization to mechanical stimuli of nociceptors in rat skin, in vitro. J Neurosci 12:86–95

Stein C (1993) Peripheral mechanisms of opioid analgesia. Anesth Analg 76:182–191

Steranka RR, Manning D, DeHass CJ, Ferkany JW, Borosky SA, Connor JR, Vavrek RJ, Stewart JM, Snyder SH (1988) Bradykinin as a pain mediator: receptors are localized to sensory neurons, and antagonists have analgesic actions. Proc Natl Acad Sci USA 85:324–3249

Szallasi A (1994) The vanilloid (capsaicin) receptor: receptor types and species differences. Gen Pharmacol 25:223–243

Szolcsányi J (1993) Actions of capsaicin on sensory neurones. In: Wood JN (ed) Capsaicin in the study of pain. Academic, London, pp 1–26

Taiwo YO, Levine JD (1990) Direct cutaneous hyperalgesia induced by adenosine. Neuroscience 38:757–762

Taiwo YO, Levine JD (1991a) Kappa- and delta-opioids block sympathetically dependent hyperalgesia. J Neurosci 11:928–932

Taiwo YO, Levine JD (1991b) Further confirmation of the role of adenyl cyclase and of cAMP-dependent protein kinase in primary afferent hyperalgesia. Neuroscience 44:131–135

Taiwo YO, Heller PH, Levine JD (1992) Mediation of serotonin hyperalgesia by the cAMP second messenger system. Neuroscience 48:479–483

Tanelian DL, Brose WG (1991) Neuropathic pain can be relieved by drugs that are use-dependent sodium channel blockers: lidocaine, carbamazepine, and mexiletine. Anesthesiology 74:949–951

Thompson SWN, Dray A, Urban L (1995) Nerve Growth factor induces mechanical allodynia associated with neurokinin-1 receptor activation and novel A fibre-evoked reflex activity in the rat. Pain 62:219–231

Tiffany CW, Burch RM (1989) Bradykinin stimulates tumor necrosis factor and interleukin-1 release from macrophages. FEBS 247:189–192

Todorovic S, Anderson EG (1990) 5-HT2 and 5-HT3 receptors mediate two distinct depolarizing responses in rat dorsal root ganglion neurons. Brain Res 511:71–79

Toledo-Aral JJ, Brehms P, Halegoua S, Mandel G (1995) A single pulse of nerve growth factor triggers long-term neuronal excitability through sodium channel gene induction. Neuron 14:607–611

Treede R-D, Meyer RA, Raja SN, Campbell JN (1992) Peripheral and central mechanisms of cutaneous hyperalgesia. Prog Neurobiol 38:397–421

Undem BJ, Weinreich D (1993) Electrophysiological properties and chemosensitivity of guinea pig nodose ganglion neurons in vitro. J Autonom Nerv Syst 44:17–34

Verge VMK, Xu Z, Xu X-J, Wiesenfelt-Hallin Z, Hokfelt T (1992) Marked increase in nitric oxide synthase mRNA in rat dorsal root ganglia after peripheral axotomy: in situ hybridization and functional studies. Proc Natl Acad Sci USA 89:11617–11621

Walpole CSJ, Wrigglesworth R (1993) Structural requirements for capsaicin agonists and antagonists. In: Wood J (ed) Capsaicin in the study of pain. Academic, London, pp 63–81

Waxman SG, Kocsis JD, Black JA (1994) Type III sodium channel mRNA is expressed in embryonic but not adult spinal sensory neurons, and is reexpressed following axotomy. J Neurophysiol 72:466–470

Wei P, Moskowitz MA, Boccalini P, Kontos HA (1992) Calcitonin gene-related peptide mediates nitroglycerin and sodium nitroprusside-induced vasodilatation in feline cerebral arterioles. Circ Res 70:1313–1319

Weinreich D, Wonderlin WF (1987) Inhibition of calcium-dependent spike after-hyperpolarization increases excitability of rabbit visceral sensory neurons. J Physiol (Lond) 394:415–427

Wieland HA, William KD, Entzeroth M, Weinen W, Rudolf K, Eberlein W, Doods HN (1995) Subtype selectivity and antagonistic profile of the nonpeptide Y1 receptor antagonist BIBP 3226. J Pharmacol Exp Ther 275:143–149

Winter J, Forbes CA, Sternberg J, Lindsay JM (1988) Nerve growth factor (NGF) regulates adult rat cultured dorsal root ganglion neuron responses to capsaicin. Neuron 1:973–981

Winter J, Walpole CSJ, Bevan S, James IF (1993) Characterization of resiniferatoxin binding sites on sensory neurons: coregulation of resiniferatoxin binding and capsaicin sensitivity in adult rat dorsal root ganglia. Neuroscience 57:747–757

Woolf CJ, Safieh-Garabedian B, Ma Q-P, Crilly P, Winter J (1994) Nerve Growth factor contributes to the generation of inflammatory sensory hypersensitivity. Neuroscience 62:327–331

Xiao W-H, Bennett GJ (1995) Synthetic omega-conopeptides applied to the site of nerve injury suppress neuropathic pain in rats. J Pharmacol Exp Ther 274:666–672

Zhang JM, Kitabata LM, LaMotte RH (1994) Verapamil inhibits the spontaneous activities originating in dorsal root ganglion cells after chronic nerve constriction in rats. Soc Neurosci 20:760

Zhang X, Ji RR, Nilssen S, Villar M, Ubink R, Ju G, Wiesenfeld-Hallin Z, Hokfelt T (1995) Neuropeptide Y and galanin binding sites in rat and monkey lumbar dorsal root ganglia and spinal cord and effect of peripheral axotomy. Eur J Neurosci 7:367–380

CHAPTER 3

Non-steroidal Anti-inflammatory Drugs and Pain

I. APPLETON

A. Inflammatory Pain and NSAIDs

During inflammation numerous events occur resulting in nociception of peripheral stimuli. Inflammatory cells and peripheral nerves release a variety of mediators including prostaglandins (PGs). This results in a change of high-threshold mechanoceptors into nociceptors. Changes in the central nervous system (CNS) also occur. This is particularly evident in the dorsal horn of the spinal cord where reflex and metabolic activity of neuronal cells is increased. Collectively these events result in hyperalgesia. Traditionally it was believed that non-steroidal anti-inflammatory drugs (NSAIDs) reduce the enhanced nociceptor activity in the periphery by inhibition of the sensitising effects of PGs. This is based on the finding that all of the hyperalgesic eicosanoids induce cyclic adenosine monophosphate, which in turn mediates the peripheral hyperalgesia of primary afferent nociceptors (TAIWO et al. 1989). However, as is discussed below, numerous other analgesic mechanisms of action separate from inhibition of PG formation are now attributed to NSAIDs.

Aspirin, the most common NSAID, has been widely used for pain relief for decades, but it was not until 1971 that its possible mode of action was first demonstrated (VANE 1971). Here it was shown that NSAIDs inhibit the enzyme cyclo-oxygenase (COX) thus resulting in a decrease in the pain-sensitising effects of PGs. However, despite intense research discrepancies between their analgesic, antipyretic and anti-inflammatory activity have occurred.

The major advantage of NSAIDs for the control of pain is that, unlike opiates, chronic usage does not lead to tolerance or addiction. However, serious side effects are associated with their use, including haemorrhage, gastric ulceration, renal and hepatic failure, skin reactions and asthma. As NSAIDs are used on such vast scales, the development of NSAIDs with analgesic properties free from these effects would be highly beneficial. Within the past 3 years such drugs have been developed; their possible clinical usage in inflammation and analgesia is discussed below.

B. Cyclo-oxygenase

Arachidonic acid is an integral part of cell membrane phospholipids. Free arachidonic acid is released via the rate-limiting action of phospholipase A_2 on phosphatidylcholine or phospholipase C on phosphatidylinositol. Once generated, arachidonic acid is converted to PGG_2 followed by PGH_2. The PGH_2 is subsequently converted to PGs and thromboxanes by the COX pathway, leukotrienes and hydroxyeicosatetraenoic acids by the lypoxygenase pathway or lipid epoxides and diols through the epoxygenase pathway (for review see Smith et al. 1991).

I. Isoforms of Cyclo-oxygenase

Different NSAIDs have varying inhibitory effects on PG formation depending on the source of COX (Flower and Vane 1974). It has been suggested that different intracellular pools of COX may exist. More recent work has identified a second mitogen-inducible isoform of COX, COX-2 (Xie et al. 1991; Kujubu et al. 1991), the intracellular location of COX-1 (the original target of NSAIDs) and COX-2 being distinct (see Sect. B.I.1).

1. Cyclo-oxygenase 1

COX-1 is a constitutive isoform found in virtually all cell types. It is a homodimeric enzyme with a subunit molecular weight of 72 kDa. The gene for COX-1 contains multiple transcription start sites (Wang et al. 1993), and its DNA has now been identified in numerous sources (Funk et al. 1991; DeWitt and Smith 1988; DeWitt et al. 1990). It encodes a 600 amino acid protein with four glycosylation sites. The site for aspirin acetylation (Ser-530) lies close to the carboxyl terminus. The COX-1 mRNA is found constitutively in numerous tissues and is approximately 2.8 kb in length. Recently Picot et al. (1994) determined the X-ray crystallography structure of COX-1 protein.

2. Cyclo-oxygenase 2

The major differences between COX-1 and COX-2 lie in the presence of a TATA box and regulatory sites for glucocorticoids and cytokines in the COX-2 gene (Xu et al. 1995). In addition, COX-2 protein has a unique 18 amino acid insert near the carboxyl terminal. Similar to COX-1, the COX-2 protein has a serine site for aspirin acetylation and five possible glycosylation sites. The COX-2 enzyme is able to utilise a larger number of substrates than COX-1 (Smith et al. 1994). The COX-2 mRNA is approximately 4 kb and is usually expressed in low amounts. However, constitutive expression of COX-2 is found in the testis, brain and lung (Simmons et al. 1991). The distribution of COX mRNA in human tissues has been mapped by O'Neill and Ford-Hutchinson (1993).

The original hypothesis of Flower and Vane (1974) that different intracellular pools of COX exist has now received credence through molecular biology. The activity of COX-1 is mainly in the endoplasmic reticulum, whereas COX-2 is predominantly around the nucleus, with trace amounts in the cytoplasm (Smith et al. 1994). It is not intended here to detail the regulation of COX-1 and COX-2; rather the reader is referred to APPLETON et al. (1996). However, an important point to note is that glucocorticoids such as dexamethasone selectively inhibit COX-2 (MASFERRER et al. 1992; DE WITT and MEADE 1993; EVETT et al. 1993) whereas COX-1 is unaffected (DE WITT and MEADE 1993).

II. Cyclo-oxygenase Isoforms and Inflammation

The rapid increase in PG levels in inflammation in conjunction with the rapid induction of COX-2 may implicate this isoform in acute inflammation. In the rat carrageenan-induced pleurisy, it has been demonstrated that COX activity corresponds to COX-2 protein (TOMLINSON et al. 1994). Furthermore, dexamethasone suppresses the induction of COX-2 and PG release in this model (KATORI et al. 1995). Similarly in the Arthus reaction and pertussis pleurisy COX-2 is the predominant isoform with COX-1 protein remaining constant (MOORE et al. 1995).

In the murine air pouch model of chronic granulomatous inflammation COX activity profiled the levels of COX-2 protein with COX-1 levels remaining constant (VANE et al. 1994). The major source of COX-2 immunoreactivity being the macrophage (APPLETON et al. 1995). However, the finding that COX-2 is the predominant isoform in inflammation does not dictate that it is the isoform responsible for the elaboration of PGs. Recent work in our Department using the murine air pouch model has shown that nimesulide, a selective COX-2 inhibitor (GROSSMAN et al. 1995), rather than inhibiting COX activity causes a significant increase in PG levels and has little effect on granuloma dry weight (Gilroy 1995, personal communication). Furthermore, WILBORN et al. (1995) have demonstrated that in alveolar and peritoneal macrophages COX-1 alone accounts for the elaboration of PGs, with COX-2 being to a certain extent redundant.

In rheumatoid arthritis synovial fluids contain elevated levels of PGE2. Under basal conditions synovial explants express COX-1 and COX-2 protein. However, following stimulation with interleukin (IL) 1β or phorbol myristate acetate, COX-2 protein and mRNA is markedly increased whilst COX-1 levels show slight alterations. Furthermore, this induction of COX-2 mRNA is blocked by dexamethasone, with COX-1 levels unchanged (CROFFORD et al. 1994). Therefore in a number of acute and chronic models of inflammation and in rheumatoid arthritis COX-2 is the predominant isoform of COX.

1. Selective Inhibitors of Cyclo-oxygenase Isoforms and Inflammation

The information concerning the selectivity of NSAIDs for COX-1 and COX-2 is primarily from in vitro cell systems and isolated enzyme preparations. It is not intended to detail here the selectivity of NSAIDs; rather the reader is referred to APPLETON et al. (1995). Most of the clinically available NSAIDs are equipotent inhibitors of COX-1 and COX-2. However, it is generally accepted that aspirin is more selective for COX-1. The fact that there is a dissociation between the analgesic effects and anti-inflammatory effects of aspirin raises the question of whether COX-2 inhibitors would be of greater analgesic efficacy.

At present there are no COX-2 specific inhibitors in clinical usage for pain or inflammation. However, several experimental compounds are available. NS-398 (N-[2-cyclohexyloxy-4-nitrophenyl] methanesulfonamide]) selectively blocks COX-2 in vitro (Futaki et al. 1994) and in vivo in the rat carrageenan–air pouch model of inflammation (Futaki et al. 1993a; Masferrer et al. 1994) whilst sparing COX-1 and thus gastric side effects (Futaki et al. 1993b; Masferrer et al. 1994). Similar gastric sparing and anti-inflammatory effects are reported with the selective COX-2 inhibitors L-745|337 and SC-58125 (1-[(4-methyl sulfonyl) phenyl]-3-triflouromethyl-5-(4-flourophenyl) pyrazole) in rat carrageenan-induced paw oedema (Chan et al. 1994; Seibert et al. 1994).

III. Side Effects of NSAID Therapy

The most common side effects of NSAID usage are gastric and renal. COX-1 is constitutively expressed in the stomach. In models of gastric ulcers PGE1, PGE2 and PGI$_2$ have a protective effect against gastric erosions induced by a number of agents (Ferguson et al. 1973; Lee et al. 1973; Whittle 1976). Removal of these cytoprotective effects may account for the gastric and renal side effects associated with the use of aspirin and indeed other NSAIDs.

A recent development for reducing the gastrointestinal effects of NSAIDs is the linkage with a nitric oxide (NO) donor. NO maintains gastric blood flow and inhibits leucocyte adherence (Kubes et al. 1991) and therefore counteracts the effects of NSAIDs. Examples of NSAID-NO compounds include diclofenac nitroxybutylester and ketoprofen nitroxybutylester. In models of acute and chronic inflammation these agents suppress inflammation whilst sparing the gastric mucosa (Reuter et al. 1994; Cuzzolin et al. 1994). Other strategies for preventing the gastric side effects of NSAIDs based on NO include the use of transdermal nitroglycerin patches, which have recently been demonstrated to dose-dependently protect the gastric mucosal damaged induced by indomethacin (Barrachina et al. 1995). Other possible side effects of NSAID therapy are dependent on isoform selectivity. Thus whilst COX-1 inhibition results in gastric and renal side effects, COX-2 inhibition may have effects on the brain and female reproductive system, organs which constitutively express COX-2 (see Sect. C.II.1). An example of this can be seen in COX-2 knock out mice which are infertile (Herschmann et al. 1994)

C. Prostaglandins and Inflammatory Pain

It was first demonstrated by Ferreira 1972 that PGs alone do not produce pain but rather sensitise afferent nociceptors to the effects of other pain-producing substances such as bradykinin and histamine. The hyperalgesic effects of bradykinin are not only potentiated by PGs but may also involve induction of PGs. This is based on the observation that the effects of bradykinin can be blocked by pretreatment with indomethacin, suggesting that activation of bradykinin receptors causes the release of PGs from sympathetic nerves. The major PGs involved in hyperalgesia are PGE_2 and PGI_2. The resultant hyperalgesia and duration of these two mediators are different. Injection of PGE_2 results in a delayed onset but long-lasting hyperalgesic state (FERREIRA 1972; MONCADA et al. 1975), whereas PGI_2 effects are more rapid and quickly decline. Furthermore, PGI_2 is a more potent hyperalgesic agent than PGE_2 (FERREIRA et al. 1978). Differences in the effects of these two PGs may account for the efficacy of NSAIDs in different pathophysiological pain. For example, certain types of headache (where PGI2 has been implicated) respond rapidly to NSAID therapy. Sunburn and back pain which are to a certain extent resistant to NSAID therapy may be due to the involvement of PGE_2.

I. Non-steroidal Anti-inflammatory Drugs and Inflammatory Pain

Inhibition of peripherally formed PGs has been ascribed as the mechanism of action for the analgesic effects of NSAIDs (WILLIS 1969; JUHLIN and MICHAELSON 1969; FERREIRA 1972). However, in numerous models of pain this mechanism alone does not account for the analgesic properties of NSAIDs (McCORMACK and BRUNE 1991; WEISSMAN 1992; BRUNE et al. 1991). For example, dipyrone, paracetamol and phenazone have little effect on PG biosynthesis but are potent analgesics (BRUNE and APLERMANN 1983; BRUNE et al. 1981, 1991; HIGGS et al. 1987). Similarly, aspirin at analgesic and antipyretic doses has little anti-inflammatory activity (ABRAMSON and WEISSMANN 1989; WEISSMANN 1991). In addition, diflunisal, naproxen, azapropazone, tolmetin and oxaprozin are weak inhibitors of PG production but are more potent analgesics than aspirin in dental pain (McCORMACK and BRUNE 1991).

1. Selective Inhibition of COX-2 and Inflammatory Pain

There is relatively little information concerning the isoform of COX responsible for the production of the PGs involved in pain, much of which is based on work using COX isoform selective inhibitors. For example, the selective COX-2 inhibitors, SC-58125 and L745337 [5-methanesulfonamido-6-(2,4-diflourothiophenyl)-1-indanone] have analgesic effects on thermal injury and the carrageenan-induced rat paw hyperalgesia assay, respectively (SEIBERT et al. 1994; CHAN et al. 1994). The selective COX-2 inhibitor NS-398 has also been shown to be effective in models of pain. In rat adjuvant arthritic pain NS-398 was up to five times more effective than diclofenac and loxoprofen and equipotent to indomethacin. In acetic acid–induced writhing in mice it was found to be as potent as indomethacin and diclofenac. NS-398 has also been demonstrated to be effective in models of pyrexia. In lipopolysaccharide (LPS) induced fever it is upto 4.5 times more potent than indomethacin and loxoprofen. As with the other COX-2 inhibitors, little effect on the gastric mucosa is found (FUTAKI et al. 1993c). These studies suggest that selective inhibition of COX-2 would provide equal or greater relief of pain than existing NSAID therapy without the associated side effects of traditional analgesics.

II. Prostaglandins and Central Nociceptive Processing

In addition to direct hyperalgesic action of PGs (see Sect. C), PGs are also involved in the processing of nociceptive signals induced by other agents. Activation of excitatory amino acid receptors (EAAs) such as N-methyl-D-aspartate (NMDA) receptors and metabotropic EAA receptors results in an influx of extracellular Ca^{2+} and intracellular mobilisation of Ca^{2+}, respectively. This stimulates the metabolism of arachidonic acid by phospholipase A_2 (DUMUIS et al. 1990). Metabotropic EAA receptor activation also stimulates phospholipase C which metabolises diacyglycerol, resulting in a further increase in arachidonic acid (GAMMON et al. 1989). This arachidonic acid is then further metabolised by COX to the PGs.

Intrathecal administration of NSAIDs blocks the tail-flick response induced by substance P or NMDA (MALMBERG and YAKSH 1992). In contrast, intrathecal treatment with arachidonic acid potentiates the nociceptive response to formalin (YASHPAL and CODERRE 1993). It has therefore been postulated that the role of PGs is in the development of persistent pain.

1. COX-2 in the Central Nervous System

PGs as well as being involved in central nociceptive processing also have numerous physiological roles. PGD2 and PGE_2 are involved in the sleep-wake cycle (UENO et al. 1983; MATSUMURA et al. 1989). PGs are also involved in the control of luteinising hormone-releasing hormone production and thermoregulation and may have anti-convulsant properties (see VANE and BOTTING 1994).

It has recently been shown that COX-2 is constitutively present in the brain where it is the predominant COX isoform (YAMAGATA et al. 1993). Similar to COX-2 in other organs, it is upregulated by stress, and its effects can be blocked by dexamethasone. In the unstimulated brain it is found in the granule and pyramidal cells of the hippocampus, pyramidal cells of the pyriform cortex, neurones of neocortical layers II and III with lower levels being expressed in the striatum, thalamus and hypothalamus. No COX-2 is present in the white matter. These findings therefore suggest a role of COX-2 in both physiological and pathophysiological neuronal function.

In preovulatory rats the release of luteinising hormone-releasing hormone is preceded by an increase in COX activity in the hypothalamus (OJEDA and CAMPBELL 1982). This raises the possibility that a COX-2 inhibitor capable of penetrating the blood brain barrier, whilst having analgesic properties, could affect the normal reproductive cycle. This may help to explain the observation that COX-2 knock out mice are infertile (HERSCHMANN et al. 1994). Other possible side effects of COX-2 inhibition may be the induction of seizures in epileptics. This is based on the finding that glucocorticoids such as dexamethasone (which specifically inhibits COX-2) induce seizures (MCEWAN et al. 1986).

III. Analgesic and Anti-inflammatory Effects of NSAIDs Separate from Inhibition of Peripheral PG Formation

The dissociation between the anti-inflammatory and analgesic properties of NSAIDs is best exemplified by work using NSAID enantiomers. The S form of flurbiprofen, a 2-arylpropionic acid derivative, has anti-inflammatory and analgesic properties whereas the R form has little effect on PG formation and inflammation but blocks nociception. Additionally, whilst the S form is ulcerogenic, the R form has negligible effects. This work suggests that NSAID-induced analgesia can be independent of PG synthesis inhibition (BRUNE et al. 1991).

Inflammation-induced hyperalgesia obviously depends not only on PGs. Recent work has shown that IL-1β upregulates nerve growth factor which in turn has a major role in the production of hyperalgesia in rats given an intraplantar injection of Freund's complete adjuvant. Furthermore, dexamethasone (selective COX-2 inhibitor) and indomethacin are able to reduce the levels of both mediators as well as substance P levels (SAFIEH-GARABEDIAN et al. 1995). This work again exemplifies the other, in this instance peripheral, effects of COX inhibitors.

It is now emerging that NSAIDs in addition to peripheral effects on nociception can also have central effects (reviewed by URQUHART 1993; McCORMACK and BRUNE 1991; McCORMACK 1994). For example, ibuprofen has been shown to have central analgesic effects in humans (SANDRINI et al. 1992). However, not all the NSAIDs may have central effects. In the formalin test in mice nociception occurs in two phases, the first due to an effect on nociceptors and the second due to inflammation (DUBUISSON and DENNIS 1977). Aspirin and paracetamol are antinociceptive in both phases whereas indomethacin is active only in the late inflammatory phase (HUNSKAAR and HOLE 1987). However, it should be noted that in this model the late phase is not exclusively PG dependent, and that NO is also involved (see Sect. C.II). Given the interaction of PGs and NO and the direct and indirect effects that NSAID manipulation of PG and NO levels can have (see Sect. D.IV), interpretation of these results may not be as conclusive as first thought.

In general the central nociceptive effects of NSAIDs are due to opiod, serotonergic and NO mechanisms. It is not intended to elucidate all of these pathways here; rather the reader is referred to an extensive review of the topic by BJORKMAN (1995).

1. NSAIDs and Substance P

Diclofenac can block the effects of substance P by binding to substance P receptors (quoted in BJORKMAN 1995). Similarly, ketoprofen can significantly reduce the amount of substance P in the hypothalamus and spinal cord (DUBOURDIEU and DRAY 1989). The role of substance P in inflammatory pain is well established. For example, sensory denervation of substance P with capsaicin treatment significantly reduces inflammation and nociception in a rat model of polyarthritis (CRUWYS et al. 1995). Administration of aspirin or paracetamol can also attenuate nociceptive processes induced by substance P. For example, they attenuate pain related behaviour induced by the intrathecal injection of substance P and by intrathecal administration of capsaicin (HUNSKAAR et al. 1985). Thus NSAIDs may not only decrease the amount of substance P at sites of inflammation and in the CNS but may in addition block its nociceptive effects.

2. NSAIDs and Immediate-Early Genes

Other central effects of NSAIDs may be via regulation of immediate-early genes, which are upregulated in nociception. Intraplantar injection of carrageenan results in peripheral oedema and upregulation of c-FOS in the dorsal horn of rats. Treatment with piroxicam dose-dependently reduces the appearance of c-FOS. This effect directly correlated with its anti-inflammatory effects on foot swelling (BURITOVA et al. 1995)

The anomalies between anti-inflammatory, analgesic and antipyretic effects of NSAIDs may be further explained by recent studies. Aspirin and sodium salicylate can inhibit NF-κB (KOPP and GHOSH 1994), a transcription factor involved in the activation of the inflammatory cytokines IL-1, IL-6, IL-8, tumour necrosis factor-α and interferon-β (GRILLI et al. 1993). Previous work has demonstrated the pivotal role of tumour necrosis factor-α in the development of inflammatory hyperalgesia, an effect which can be blocked by steroidal anti-inflammatory drugs (CUNHA et al. 1992). The finding that the non-steroidal aspirin can block the transcription of tumour necrosis factor-α could provide a mechanism to explain these observations. Large doses of aspirin also acetylate Ser 516 on ovine COX-2, resulting in the production of 15-hydroxyeicosatetreanoic acid, an effect not observed with COX-1 (HOLTZMAN et al. 1991). 15-Hydroxyeicosatetreanoic acid has potent anti-inflammatory properties including inhibition of LTB4 formation and carrageenan-induced arthritis (FOGH et al. 1989).

3. NSAIDs and Apoptosis

An intriguing possible mode of action of NSAIDs has recently been proposed by LU et al. (1995). They demonstrated that a number of NSAIDs are capable of inducing apoptosis or programmed cell death in v-*src* transformed chicken embryo fibroblasts. In addition, it was shown that rather than inhibiting COX-

1 and COX-2 NSAID treatment results in induction of their mRNA and protein. It was suggested that COXs and their products prevent apoptosis. This obviously has far reaching implications for inflammation as the selective removal of cells (by apoptosis) without spillage of potentially harmful and pain-producing cellular components may be an important aspect of the anti-inflammatory effects of NSAIDs. Whether this effect can be substantiated in models of inflammation has yet to be determined.

D. Nitric Oxide and Nociception

An increasing body of evidence shows the modulatory effects of PGs on NO (see Sect. D.IV). NO is a free radical involved in the homeostasis of vascular function, neurotransmission, host defence mechanisms and numerous patho-physiological events (for review see Moncada et al. 1991). It is formed by the action of nitric oxide synthase (NOS) on l-arginine, with l-citrulline as a by product. Several cell type specific isoforms of NOS have been identified, which fall into three categories: calcium-dependent NOS as found constitutively in neurones (nNOS), calcium-independent NOS as found in hepatocytes and macrophages (iNOS) and calcium-dependent NOS as discovered in endothe-lial cells (eNOS).

In the CNS elevated levels of cyclic guanosine monophosphate (cGMP) are associated with neurotransmission by glutamate and other EAAs (Garthwaite 1990) via activation of the NMDA receptor (for review of second messengers and the NMDA-NO-cGMP system see Coderre 1994). Treatment with the NOS inhibitor, N^G-monomethyl-l-arginine, decreases cGMP in rat cerebral cells stimulated with NMDA, indicating that activation of NMDA receptors and the resultant increase in cGMP are mediated via NO (Bredt and Snyder 1989; Garthwaite et al. 1989). In the spinal cord noci-ceptive processing also involves NMDA receptors (Salt and Hill 1983; Watkins and Evans 1981; Meller and Gebhart 1993), again mediated via NO and elevation of cGMP.

The interaction between PGs and NO are complex and contradictory, as both stimulatory and inhibitory effects of PGs on NO and vice versa have been reported (see Sect. D.IV). In light of the fact that PGs can modulate NO, and NO can affect PGs, the role of NO in nociception must be addressed along with the possible effects, either direct or indirect, of NSAIDs on NO.

I. Analgesic Properties of NO

Analgesia induced by acetylcholine injection into rat paws is mediated by NO and the cGMP system (Durate et al. 1990). In carrageenan-induced hyperalgesia injection of l-arginine results in analgesia (Kawabata et al. 1992a) whilst inhibition of NOS decreases the action of peripheral morphine analgesia (Ferreira et al. 1991). Similar studies as to the central role of NO are also documented. For example, the parenteral administration of L-arginine in animals (Kawabata et al. 1992a,b) and humans (Harima et al. 1991) and topical application to the spinal cord of rats results in analgesia (Kawabata et al. 1992b).

II. Hyperalgesic Properties of NO

The evidence concerning the hyperalgesic effects of NO are based mainly on studies using NOS inhibitors. Topical administration to the spinal cord and intracerebroventricular administration of the NOS inhibitor Nw-nitro-L-arginine methyl ester (L-NAME) attenuates the behavioral response to pain, indicating a hyperalgesic role for NO (Kitto et al. 1992; Meller and Gebhart 1993; Moore et al. 1991). Injection of NO solutions into the forearms of humans evokes pain (Holthusen and Arndt 1994). Carrageenan injected into a rat hindpaw increases NADPH-diaphorase staining (indicative of NOS) in both ipsilateral and contralateral neurones of the lumbar spinal cord (Traub et al. 1994). Intraperitoneal injection of LPS induces hyperalgesia by activating the NMDA-NO system at the level of the spinal cord (Wiertelak et al. 1994). Acute thermal hyperalgesia by NMDA is mediated by NO (Kitto et al. 1993; Malmberg and Yaksh 1993) as is thermal hyperalgesia in neuropathic pain (Meller et al. 1992). Additional evidence as to the role of NO in neuropathic pain is provided by the finding of immunoreactivity to NOS in dorsal root neurones following ligation of L5 and L6 spinal nerves (Steel et al. 1994).

The discrepancies between hypoalgesic and hyperalgesic effects of NO may be attributed to the local tissue levels. This was demonstrated by Kawabata et al. (1994). It has been found that increasing the levels of NO with low doses of L-arginine result in an enhancement of the second phase of the formalin-induced behavioural nociception in mice. Conversely, inhibition of NOS with L-NAME results in antinociception. However, high doses of L-arginine also result in hypoalgesia, possibly due to inhibition of nociceptors. It is concluded that the nociceptive effects of NO, either hypo- or hyperalgesia, depend on the relative levels in the tissue. However, a note of caution as to the interpretation of these results must be made. This is based on the fact that NOS inhibitors as well as having effects on NOS also inhibit COX (Peterson et al. 1992). Thus as the second component of the formalin test has a large nociceptive component due to PGs, the use of L-NAME may also modulate PGs resulting in alteration of nociception.

1. Nitric Oxide in Thermal and Mechanical Hyperalgesia

It has been shown that activation of ionotropic α-amino-3-hydroxy-5-methyl-4-isoxazoleproprionate and metabotropic glutamate receptors does not involve the induction of NO (Meller and Gebhart 1994; Meller et al. 1993b). Additionally, mechanical hyperalgesia induced by intraplantar injection of zymosan or carrageenan in the rat is not mediated through NO, but the maintenance of thermal hyperalgesia in these models is (MELLER et al. 1993a, 1994a,b). Recent evidence between the dissociation of the mechanisms involved in thermal and hyperalgesia has implicated carbon monoxide. Carbon monoxide is formed by the action of hemeoxygenase (HO) on heme. MELLER et al. (1994a,b) have shown that whilst NOS inhibitors block thermal hyperalgesia they have no effect on mechanical hyperalgesia. In contrast, Sn protoporphyrin IX, an inhibitor of HO, have no effect on thermal hyperalgesia but attenuate mechanical hyperalgesia.

III. Effect of NSAIDs on NOS

Aspirin can inhibit iNOS expression in LPS-stimulated J774 macrophages whilst sodium salicylate, indomethacin and acetaminophen have no effect (AMIN et al. 1995). AEBERHARD et al. (1995) have reported similar findings. It is demonstrated that aspirin, sodium salicylate, indomethacin and ibuprofen inhibit iNOS gene induction in LPS and interferon-τ stimulated rat alveolar macrophages. In contrast, work in our Department using therapeutic doses of aspirin has demonstrated an increase in nitrite production in LPS stimulated J774 macrophages (Colville-Nash, personal communication). The effect of NSAIDs on the constitutive form of NOS as found in the brain have yet to be determined, as does the effect on NO-mediated nociception. However, a peripheral effect of NSAIDs on nitric oxide has been reported by TONUSSI and FERREIRA (1994). It was found that diclofenac-induced analgesia can be blocked by inhibition of NOS. This suggests that the mechanism of action of diclofenac-induced analgesia is not due to inhibition of the sensitising effects of peripherally formed PGs on nociceptors but rather a functional down-regulation of sensitised pain receptors.

IV. Interaction of PGs and NO

PGs can affect the activity of NOS and similarly NO can affect COX activity. These effects are contradictory as both stimulatory and inhibitory actions are reported in the literature. PGE2 can inhibit the IL-1 stimulated induction of NOS in rat mesangial cells (TETSUKA et al. 1994). PGE_2 and PGI_2 can inhibit LPS-induced iNOS in J774 macrophages (MAROTTA et al. 1992). In contrast endogenously formed PGE_2 increases NO synthesis in LPS-stimulated rat kupffer cells (GAILLARD et al. 1992). The effects of NO on COX activity are just as complex. NO can activate COX in rat islets of Langerhans (CORBETT et al. 1993). Inhibition of NOS results in a decrease in PGI_2 production in LPS-treated rat lungs (SAUTEBIN and DI ROSA 1994), suggesting that NO can stimulate COX. This has also been shown in vivo. In the rat hydronephrotic kidney NOS inhibition attenuates the BK-induced release of PGE_2 (SALVEMINI et al. 1994).

Nitric oxide can also inhibit COX, although the evidence as to which isoform of COX is affected is sparse. Habib et al. (1994) have shown that NO specifically downregulates COX-2 in LPS-stimulated rat peritoneal macrophages, whilst COX-2 derived PGs stimulates NO production. The actions of NO on COX may be explained by the relative concentrations of NO. Low levels of NO can stimulate PG production whereas high levels of NO derived from sodium nitroprusside, a nitric oxide donor, inhibit PG production (Swierkosz et al. 1995).

V. Interactions Between NOS and HO

The enzyme HO is constitutively expressed in the brain where it is believed to play a part in neurotransmission (Verma et al. 1993). Recent work in our Department has shown the modulatory effects of NOS on HO. In brain homogenates addition of L-arginine decreases HO activity whilst L-NAME increases HO activity (Willis et al. 1995). Given the fact that in the brain both NOS and HO exist constitutively, interactions between these two enzyme systems can therefore occur. Furthermore, as NSAIDs can modulate NOS activity (see Sect. D.III), these could have additional effects on HO. Whether NSAIDs have a direct effect on HO has yet to be determined.

E. Conclusion

The recent finding of a second mitogen-inducible isoform of COX, COX-2, has led to a resurgence of interest in the field of NSAIDs. It has been established that COX-2 is the predominant isoform of COX in a number of models of inflammation and in human pathologies. By sparing COX-1 these drugs would theoretically have anti-inflammatory and analgesic activity with fewer side effects than traditional NSAIDs. In models of inflammation and pain these drugs have proved to be equipotent with or of greater efficacy than conventional NSAIDs. However, the observation that COX-2 is present constitutively in the brain and female reproductive system may give rise to other side effects separate from effects on the stomach and kidney. In conclusion, the therapeutic potential of COX-2 inhibitors for the control of inflammation and pain relief has yet to be proven.

Acknowledgements. The author is indebted to Dr Annette Tomlinson and Dr Paul Colville-Nash for help in the preparation of this manuscript. Dr I. Appleton is a Royal Society, Smith and Nephew Foundation Research Fellow.

References

Abramson SB, Weissmann G (1989) The mechanism of action of nonsteroidal antiinflammatory drugs. Arthritis Rheum 32:1–9

Aeberhard EE, Henderson SA, Arabolos NS, Griscavage JM, Castro FE, Barrett CT, Ignarro L (1995) Nonsteroidal anti-inflammatory drugs inhibit expression of the inducible nitric oxide synthase gene. Biochem Biophys Res Commun 208(3):1053–1059

Amin AR, Vyas P, Attur M, Leszczynska-Piziak J, Patel IR, Weissmann G, Abramson SB (1995) The mode of action of aspirin-like drugs: effect on inducible nitric oxide synthase. Proc Natl Acad Sci USA 92(17):7926–7930

Appleton I, Tomlinson A, Mitchell JA, Willoughby DA (1995) Distribution of cyclooxygenase isoforms in murine chronic granulomatous inflammation. Implications for future anti-inflammatory therapy. J Pathol 176:413–420

Appleton I, Tomlinson A, Willoughby DA (1996) Induction of cyclooxygenase and nitric oxide synthase in inflammation. Adv Pharmacol 35:27–78

Barrachina MD, Calatayud S, Canet A, Bello R, Diaz de Rojas F, Guth PH, Espluges JV (1995) Transdermal nitroglycerin prevents nonsteroidal anti-inflammatory drug gastropathy. Eur J Pharmacol 282 (2):R3–R4

Bjorkman R (1995) Central antinociceptive effects of non-steroidal anti-inflammatory drugs and paracetamol. Experimental studies in the rat. Acta Anaesth Scand [Suppl] 103(39):1–44

Bredt DS, Snyder SH (1989) Nitric oxide mediated glutamate-linked enhancement of cGMP levels in the cerebellum. Proc Natl Acad Sci USA 86:9030–9033

Brune K, Alpermann H (1983) Non-acidic pyrazoles: inhibition of prostaglandin production, carrageenan oedema and yeast fever. Agents Actions 13:360–363

Brune K, Rainsford KD, Wagner K, Peskar BA (1981) Inhibition by anti-inflammatory drugs of prostaglandin production in cultured macrophages. Naunyn Schmiedebergs Arch Pharmacol 315:269–276

Brune K, Beck WS, Geisslinger G, Menzel-Soglowek S, Peskar BM, Peskar BA (1991) Aspirin-like drugs may block pain independently of prostaglandin synthesis inhibition. Experentia 47(3):257–161

Buritova J, Honore P, Chapman V, Besson J-M (1995) Carrageenan oedema and spinal Fos-LI neurones reduced by piroxicam in the rat. Neuroreport 6(10):1385–1388

Chan CC, Gordon R, Brideau C, Rodger IW, Li CS, Prasit P, Tagari P, Ethier D, Vickers P, Boyce S, Rupniak N, Webb J, Hill R, Ford-Hutchinson AW (1994) In vivo pharmacology of L-745,337: a novel non steroidal antiinflammatory agent (NSAID) with an ulcerogenic sparing effect in rat and monkey stomach. Proceedings of the XIIth Congress of Pharmacology (IUPHAR), Montreal, Canada

Coderre TJ (1994) The role of excitatory amino acid receptors and intracellular messengers in persistent nociception afer tissue injury in rats. Mol Neurobiol 7:229–246

Corbett JA, Kwon G, Turk J, McDaniel ML (1993) IL-1β induces the coexpression of both nitric oxide synthase and cyclooxygenase by islets of Langerhans: activation of cyclooxygenase by nitric oxide. Biochemistry 32:13767–13770

Crofford LJ, Wilder RL, Ristimaki AP, Sano H, Remmers EF, Epps HR, Hla T (1994) Cyclooxygenase-1 and -2 expression in rheumatoid synovial tissues. Effects of interleukin-1b, phorbol ester and corticosteroids. J Clin Invest 93:1095–1101

Cruwys SC, Garrett NE, Kidd BL (1995) Sensory denervation with capsaicin attenuates inflammation and nociception in arthritic rats. Neurosci Lett 193(3):205–207

Cunha FQ, Poole S, Lorenzetti BB, Ferreira SH (1992) The pivotal role of tumour necrosis factor alpha in the development of inflammatory hyperalgesia. Br J Pharmacol 107(3):660–664

Cuzzolin L, Covforti A, Donini M, Adami A, DelSoldato P, Benoni G (1994) Effects of intestinal microflora, gastrointestinal tolerability and antiinflammatory efficacy of diclofenac and nitrofenac in adjuvant arthritic rats. Pharmacol Res 29:89–97

DeWitt DL, Meade EA (1993) Serum and glucocorticoid regulation of gene transcription and expression of the prostaglandin H synthase-1 and prostaglandin H synthase-2 isozymes. Arch Biochem Biophys 306(1):94–102

DeWitt DL, Smith WL (1988) Primary structure of prostaglandin G/H synthase from sheep vesicular gland determined from complementary DNA sequence. Proc Natl Acad Sci USA 85:1412–1416

DeWitt DL, El-Harith EA, Kraemer SA, Andrews MJ, Yao EF, Armstrong RL, Smith
    WL (1990) The aspirin and heme-binding sites of ovine and murine prostaglandin
    endoperoxide synthases. J Biol Chem 265:5192–5198
Dubuisson D, Dennis SG (1977) The formalin test: a quantitative study of the analgesic
    effects of morphine, meperidine and brain stem stimulation in rats and cats. Pain
    4:161–174
Dubourdieu C, Dray F (1989) Central analgesic action of ketoprofen through
    prostaglandins and substance P inhibition in rats. Proceedings of the 3rd
    Interscience World Conference on Inflammation, Antirheumatics, Analgesics,
    Immunomodulators
Dumuis A, Pin J-P, Oomagari K, Sebben M, Bockaert J (1990) Arachidonic acid
    released from striatal neurons by joint stimulation of ionotropic and metabotropic
    quisaualate receptors. Nature 347:182–184
Durate ID, Lorenzetti BB, Ferreira SH (1990) Peripheral analgesia and activation of
    the nitric oxide-cyclic GMP pathway. Eur J Pharmacol 186(2–3):289–293
Evett GE, Xie W, Chapman JG, Robertson DL, Simmons DL (1993) Prostaglandin G/
    H synthase isoenzyme 2 expression in fibroblasts: regulation by dexamethasone,
    mitogens, and oncogenes. Arch Biochem Biophys 306(1):169–177
Ferguson WW, Edmonds AW, Starling JR, Wangensteen SL (1973) Protective effect of
    prostaglandin E1 (PGE1) on lysosomal enzyme release in serotonin-induced gas-
    tric ulceration. Ann Surg 177:648–654
Ferreira SH (1972) Prostaglandins, aspirin-like drugs and analgesia. Nature 240:200–
    203
Ferreira SH, Nakamura M, Abreu Castro MS (1978) The hyperalgesic effects of
    prostacyclin and PGE2. Prostaglandins 16:31–37
Ferreira SH, Duarte IDG, Lorenzetti M (1991) The molecular mechanism of action of
    peripheral morphine analgesia: stimulation of the cGMP system via nitric oxide
    release. Eur J Pharmacol 210:121–122
Flower RJ, Vane JR (1974) Inhibition of prostaglandin biosynthesis. Biochem
    Pharmacol 23:1439–1450
Fogh K, Hansen ES, Herlin T, Knudsen V, Henriksen TB, Ewald H, Bunger C,
    Kragballe K (1989) 15-Hydroxy-eicosatetraenoic acid (15-HETE) inhibits carrag-
    eenan-induced experimental arthritis and reduces synovial fluid leukotriene B4
    (LTB4). Prostaglandins 37:213–228
Funk CD, Funk LB, Kennedy AS, Pong AS, FitzGerald GA (1991) Human platelet/
    erythroleukemia cell prostaglandin G/H synthase: cDNA cloning, expression and
    gene chromosomal assignment. FASEB J 5:2304–2312
Futaki N, Arai I, Hamasaki Y, Takahashi S, Higuchi S, Otomo S (1993a) Selective
    inhibition of NS-398 on prostanoid production in inflamed tissue in rat carrag-
    eenan–air pouch inflammation. J Pharm Pharmacol 45:753–755
Futaki N, Yoshikawa K, Hamasaka Y, Arai I, Higuchi S, Iizuka H, Otomo S (1993b)
    NS-398, a novel non-steroidal anti-inflammatory drug with potent analgesic and
    anti-pyretic effects, which causes minimal stomach lesions. Gen Pharmacol
    24:105–110
Futaki N, Yoshikawa K, Hamasaka Y, Arai I, Higuchi S, Iizuka H, Otomo S (1993c)
    NS-398, a novel non-steroidal anti-inflammatory drug with potent analgesic and
    antipyretic effects, which causes minimal stomach lesions. Gen Pharmacol
    24(1):105–110
Futaki N, Takahashi S, Yokoyama M, Arai I, Higuchi S, Otomo S (1994) NS-398, a
    new anti-inflammatory agent, selectively inhibits prostaglandin G/H synthase/
    cyclooxygenase (COX-2) activity in vitro. Prostaglandins 47:55–59
Gaillard T, Mulsch A, Klein H, Decker K (1992) Regulation of prostaglandin E2 of
    cytokine-elicited nitric oxide synthesis in rat liver macrophages. Biol Chem
    373:897–902
Gammon CM, Allen ACC, Morell P (1989) Bradykinin stimulates phosphoinisotide
    hydrolysis and mobilization of arachidonic acid in dorsal root ganglion neurons.
    J Neurochem 53:95–101

Garthwaite J (1990) Nitric oxide synthesis linked to activation of excitatory neurotrans-
    mitter receptors in the brain. In: Moncada N, Higgs EA (eds) Nitric oxide from L-
    arginine: a bioregulatory system. Elsevier, Amsterdam, pp 115–137
Garthwaite J, Garthwaite G, Palmer RMJ, Moncada S (1989) NMDA receptor activa-
    tion induces nitric oxide synthesis in rat brain slices. Eur J Pharmacol 172:413–416
Grilli M, Chiu JJ-S, Lenardo MJ (1993) NF-kappa B and Rel: participants in a multi-
    form transcriptional regulatory system. Int Rev Cytol 143:1–62
Grossman CJ, Wiseman J, Lucas FS, Travethick MA, Birch PJ (1995) Inhibition of
    constitutive and inducible cyclooxygenase activity in human platelets and mono-
    nuclear cells by NSAIDs and COX 2 inhibitors. Inflamm Res 44:253–257
Habib A, Bernard C, Tedgui A, Maclouf J (1994) Evidence of cross-talks between
    inducible nitric oxide synthase and cyclooxygenase II in rat peritoneal macroph-
    ages. Proceedings of the 9th International Conference on Prostaglandins and
    Related Compounds, Florence
Harima A, Shimizu H, Takagi H (1991) Analgesic effect of L-arginine in patients with
    persistent pain. Eur Neuropsychopharmacol 1:529–533
Herschmann HR, Xie W, Andersen RD, Fletcher BS, Reddy S, Gilbert R (1994)
    Regulation and function of the inducible prostaglandin synthase TIS10/PGS2.
    Proceedings of the 9th International Conference on Prostaglandins and Related
    Compounds, Florence
Higgs GA, Salmon JA, Henderson B, Vane JR (1987) Pharmacokinetics of aspirin and
    salicylate in relation to inhibition of arachidonate cyclooxygenase and anti-
    inflammatory activity. Proc Natl Acad Sci USA 84:1417–1420
Holthusen H, Arndt JO (1994) Nitric oxide evokes pain in humans on intracutaneous
    injection. Neurosci Lett 165:71–74
Holtzman MJ, Turk J, Shornick LP (1991) Alteration of a novel prostaglandin endop-
    eroxide synthase by aspirin to 15-hydroxyeicosatetraenoic acid and not prostag-
    landin is the major product (abstract). Clin Res 39:182
Hunskaar S, Hole K (1987) The formalin test in mice: dissociation between inflamma-
    tory and non-inflammatory pain. Pain 30:103–114
Hunskaar S, Fasmer OB, Hole K (1985) Acetylsalicyclic acid, paracetamol and mor-
    phine inhibit behavioral responses to intrathecally administered substance P or
    capsaicin. Life Sci 37:1835–1841
Juhlin S, Michaelson G (1969) Cutaneous vascular reactions to prostaglandins in
    healthy subjects and in patients with urticaria and atopic dermatitis. Acta
    Dermatol Venereol 49:251–161
Katori M, Harada Y, Hatanaka K, Majima M, Kawamura M, Ohno T, Aizawa A,
    Yamamoto S (1995) Induction of prostaglandin H synthase-2 in rat carrageenin-
    induced pleurisy and effect of selective COX-2 inhibition. Adv Prost Thromb
    Leukoc Res 23:345–348
Kawabata A, Fukuzumi Y, Fukushima Y, Takagi H (1992a) Antinociceptive effect of
    l-arginine on the carrageenin-induced hyperalgesia of the rat: possible involve-
    ment of central opiod systems. Eur J Pharmacol 218:153–158
Kawabata A, Nishimura Y, Takagi T (1992b) L-Leucyl-L-arginine, naltrindole and D-
    arginine block antinociception elicited by L-arginine in mice with carrageenin-
    induced hyperalgesia. Br J Pharmacol 107:1096–1101
Kawabata A, Manabe S, Manabe Y, Takagi H (1994) Effect of topical administration
    of L-arginine on formalin-induced nociception in the mouse: a dual role of periph-
    erally formed NO in pain modulation. Br J Pharmacol 112:547–550
Kitto KF, Haley JE, Wilcox GL (1992) Involvement of nitric oxide in spinally mediated
    hyperalgesia in the mouse. Neurosci Lett 148:1–5
Kitto F, Haley JE, Wilcox GL (1993) Characterization of the role of spinal NMDA
    receptors on thermal nociception in the rat. Neurosci Lett 148:1–5
Kopp E, Ghosh S (1994) Inhibition of NF-KB by sodium salicylate and aspirin. Science
    265:956–959
Kubes P, Suzuki M, Granger DM (1991) Nitric oxide: an endogenous modulator of
    leucocyte adhesion. Proc Natl Acad Sci USA 88:4651–4655

Kujubu DA, Fletcher BS, Varnum BC, Lim RW, Herschman HR (1991) TIS10, a phorbol ester tumor promoter-inducible mRNA from Swiss 3T3 cells, encodes a novel prostaglandin synthase/cyclooxygenase homologue. J Biol Chem 266:12866–12872

Lee YH, Cheng WD, Bianchi RG, Mollison K, Hansen J (1973) Effects of oral administration of PGE2 on gastric secretion and experimental peptic ulcerations. Prostaglandins 3:29–45

Lu X, Xie W, Reed D, Bradshaw WS, Simmons DL (1995) Nonsteroidal antiinflammatory drugs cause apoptosis and induce cyclooxygenases in chicken embryo fibroblasts. Proc Natl Acad Sci USA 92(17):7961–7965

Malmberg AB, Yaksh TL (1992) Hyperalgesia mediated by spinal glutamate or substance P receptor blocked by spinal cyclooxygenase inhibition. Science 257:1276–1279

Malmberg AB, Yaksh TL (1993) Spinal nitric oxide synthesis inhibition blocks NMDA induced thermal hyperalgesia and produces antinociception in the formalin test in rats. Pain 54:291–300

Marotta P, Sautebin L, DiRosa M (1992) Modulation of the induction of nitric oxide synthase by eicosanoids in the murine macrophage cell line J774. Br J Pharmacol 107:640–641

Masferrer JL, Seibert K, Zweifel B, Needleman P (1992) Endogenous glucocorticoids regulate an inducible cyclooxygenase enzyme. Proc Natl Acad Sci USA 89:3917–3921

Masferrer JL, Zweifel BS, Manning PT, Hauser SD, Leahy KM, Smith WG, Isakson PC, Seibert K (1994) Selective inhibition of inducible cyclooxygenase 2 in vivo is antiinflammatory and nonulcerogenic. Proc Natl Acad Sci USA 91:3228–3232

Matsumura H, Honda K, Goh Y, Ueno R, Sakai T, Inoue S, Hayaishi O (1989) Awaking effect of prostaglandin E2 in freely moving rats. Brain Res 481:242–249

McCormack K (1994) Non-steroidal anti-inflammatory drugs and spinal nociceptive processing. Pain 59:9–43

McCormack K, Brune K (1991) Dissociation between the anti-nociceptive and anti-inflammatory effeects of the nonsteroidal anti-inflammatory drugs: a survey of their analgesic efficacy. Drugs 41:533–547

McEwan BS, DeKloet ER, Rostene W (1986) Adrenal steroid receptors and actions in the nervous system. Physiol Rev 66:1121–1188

Meller ST, Gebhart GF (1993) Nitric oxide (NO) and nociceptive processing in the spinal cord. Pain 52:127–136

Meller ST, Gebhart GF (1994) The role of nitric oxide in spinal hyperalgesia. In: Urban L (ed) The cellular mechanisms of sensory processing. Springer, Berlin Heidelberg New York, pp 401–419

Meller ST, Pechman PS, Gebhart GF, Maves TJ (1992) Nitric oxide mediates the thermal hyperalgesia produced in a model of neuropathic pain in the rat. Neuroscience 50:7–10

Meller ST, Dykstra C, Gebhart GF (1993a) Characterization of the spinal mechanisms of thermal and mechanical hyperalgesia following intraplantar zymosan. Soc Neurosci Abstr 19:967

Meller ST, Dykstra C, Gebhart GF (1993b) Mechanisms of mechanical hyperalgesia: receptor subtypes and cellular events. Proceedings of the 7th World Congress on Pain. ISAP, Seattle, pp 224–225

Meller ST, Cummings CP, Traub RJ, Gebhart GF (1994a) The role of nitric oxide in the development and maintenance of the hyperalgesia produced by intraplantar injection of carrageenan in the rat. Neuroscience 60:367–374

Meller ST, Dykstra CL, Gebhart GF (1994b) Investigations of the possible role of carbon monoxide (CO) in the thermal and mechanical hyperalgesia in the rat. Neuroreport 5:2337–2341

Moncada S, Ferreira SH, Vane JR (1975) Inhibition of prostaglandin biosynthesis as the mechanism of analgesia of aspirin-like drugs in the dog knee joint. Eur J Pharmacol 31:250–260

Moncada S, Palmer RMJ, Higgs EA (1991) Nitric oxide: physiology, pathophysiology and pharmacology. Pharmacol Rev 43:109–142

Moore AR, Willis D, Gilroy DW, Tomlinson A, Appleton I, Willoughby DA (1995) Cyclooxygenase in rat pleural hypersensitivity reactions. Adv Prost Thromb Leukoc Res 23:349–351

Moore PK, Oluyomi AO, Babbedge RC, Wallace P, Hart SL (1991) L-Ng-nitro arginine methyl estaer exhibits antinociceptive activity in the mouse. Br J Pharmacol 102:198–202

Ojeda SR, Campbell WB (1982) An increase in hypothalamic capacity to synthesize prostaglandin E_2 precedes the first preovulatory surge of gonadotropins. Endocrinology 110:409–412

O'Neill GP, Ford-Hutchinson AW (1993) Expression of mRNA for cyclooxygenase-1 and cyclooxygenase-2 in human tissues. FEBS Lett 330:156–160

Peterson DA, Peterson DC, Archer S, Weir EK (1992) The non specificity of specific nitric oxide synthase inhibitors. Biochem Biophys Res Commun 187(2):797–801

Picot D, Loll PJ, Garavito N (1994) The X-ray crystal structure of the membrane protein prostaglandin H2 synthase-1. Nature 367:243–249

Reuter BK, Cirino G, Wallace JL (1994) Markedly reduced intestinal toxicity of a diclofenac derivative. Life Sci 55:PL1–PL8

Safieh-Garabedian B, Poole S, Allchorne A, Winter J, Woolfe CJ (1995) Contribution of interleukin-1β to the inflammation-induced increase in nerve growth factor levels and inflammatory hyperalgesia. Br J Pharmacol 115(7):1265–1275

Salt TE, Hill RG (1983) Neurotransmitter candidates of somatosensory primary afferent fibers. Neuroscience 10:1083–1103

Salvemini D, Seibert K, Masferrer JL, Misko TP, Currie MG, Needleman P (1994) Endogenous nitric oxide enhances prostaglandin production in a model of renal inflammation. J Clin Invest 93:1940–1947

Sandrini G, Ruiz L, Capararo M, Garofoli F, Beretta A, Nappi G (1992) Central analgesic activity of ibuprofen. A neurophysiological study in humans. Int J Clin Parmacol Res 12(4):197–204

Sautebin L, Di Rosa M (1994) Nitric oxide regulates PGI2 production by lungs from LPS-treated rats. Proceedings of the 9th International Conference on Prostaglandins and Related Compounds, Florence

Seibert K, Zhang Y, Leahy K, Hauser S, Masferrer J, Perkins W, Lee LN, Isakson P (1994) Pharmacological and biochemical demonstration of the role of cyclooxygenase 2 in inflammation and pain. Proc Natl Acad Sci USA 91:12013–12017

Simmons DL, Xie W, Chipman JG, Evett GE (1991) Multiple cyclooxygenases: Cloning of a mitogen-inducible form. In: Bailey JM (ed) Prostaglndins, leukotrienes, lipoxins and PAF. Pleneum, New York, pp 67–78

Smith WL, Marnett LJ, DeWitt DL (1991) Prostaglandin and thromboxane biosynthesis. Pharmacol Ther 49:153–179

Smith WL, Regier MK, Morita I, Schindler M, DeWitt DL, Laneuville O, Lecomte M, Bhattacharyya D, Otto JC (1994) Structure, function and regulation of PGH synthase isozymes. Proceedings of the 9th International Conference on Prostaglandins and Related Compounds, Florence

Steel JH, Terenghi G, Chung JM, Na HS, Carlton SM, Pollack JM (1994) Increased nitric oxide synthase immunoreactivity in rat dorsal root ganglion in a neuropathic pain model. Neurosci Lett 169:81–84

Swierkosz TA, Mitchell JA, Warner TD, Botting RM, Vane JR (1995) Co-induction of nitric oxide synthase and cyclo-oxygenase: interactions between nitric oxide and prostanoids. Br J Pharmacol 114:1335–1342

Taiwo YO, Bjerknes LK, Goetzl EJ, Levine JD (1989) Mediation of primary afferent peripheral hypoeralgesia by the cAMP second messenger system. Neuroscience 32(3):577–580

Tetsuka T, Daphna-Iken D, Srivastava SK, Baier LD, DuMaine J, Morrison AR (1994) Cross-talk between cyclooxygenase and nitric oxide pathways: prostaglandin E2

negatively modulates induction of nitric oxide synthase by interleukin-1. Proc Natl
    Acad Sci USA 91:12168–12172
Tomlinson A, Appleton I, Moore AR, Gilroy DW, Willis D, Mitchell JA, Willoughby
    DA (1994) Cyclo-oxygenase and nitric oxide synthase isoforms in rat carrageenin-
    induced pleurisy. Br J Pharmacol 113:693–698
Tonussi CR, Ferreira SH (1994) Mechanism of diclofenac analgesia: direct blockade of
    inflammatory sensitization. Eur J Pharmacol 251:173–179
Traub RJ, Solodkin A, Gebhart GF (1994) NADPH diaphorase histochemistry pro-
    vides evidence for a bilateral somatotopically inappropriate response to unilateral
    hind paw inflammation in the rat. Brain Res 647:113–123
Ueno R, Honda K, Inoue S, Hayaishi O (1983) Prostaglandin D2, a cerebral sleep-
    inducing substance in rats. Proc Natl Acad Sci USA 80:1735–1737
Urquhart E (1993) Central analgesic activity of nonsteroidal anti-inflammatory drugs
    in animal and human pain models. Semin Arthritis Rheum 23:198–205
Vane JR (1971) Inhibition of prostaglandin synthesis as a mechanism of action for
    aspirin-like drugs. Nature 231:232–235
Vane JR, Botting RM (1994) Biological properties of cyclooxygenase products. Lipid
    Med: 61–97
Vane JR, Mitchell JA, Appleton I, Tomlinson A, Bishop-Bailey D, Croxtall J,
    Willoughby DA (1994) Inducible isoforms of cyclooxygenase and nitric oxide
    synthase in inflammation. Proc Natl Acad Sci USA 91:2046–2050
Verma A, Hirsch DJ, Glatt CE, Ronnett GV, Snyder SH (1993) Carbon monoxide: a
    putative neural messenger. Science 259:381–384
Wang L-H, Hajibeige A, Xu X-M, Loose-Mitchell D, Wu KK (1993) Characterization
    of the promoter of human prostaglandin H synthase-1 gene. Biochem Biophys Res
    Commun: 406–411
Watkins JC, Evans RH (1981) Pharmacology of excitatory amino acid transmitters.
    Annu Rev Pharmacol Toxicol 21:165–204
Weissman G (1991) The actions of NSAIDs. Hosp Pract 26:60–76
Weissman G (1992) Prostaglandins as modulators of inflammation. New Stand Arth
    Care 3:3–5
Whittle BJR (1976) Relationship between the prevention of rat gastric erosions and the
    inhibition of acid secretion by prostaglandins. Eur J Pharmacol 40:233–239
Wiertelak EP, Furness LE, Watkins LR, Maier SF (1994) Illness-induced hyperalgesia
    is mediated by a spinal NMDA-nitric oxide cascade. Brain Res 664:9–16
Wilborn J, De Witt DL, Peters-Golden (1995) Expression and role of cyclooxygenase
    isoforms in alveolar and peritoneal macrophages. Am J Physiol 268:L294–230
Willis AL (1969) Parrallel assay of prostaglandin-like activity in rat inflammatory
    exudate by means of cascade superfusion. J Pharm Pharmacol 21:216–218
Willis D, Tomlinson A, Frederick R, Paul-Clark M, Willoughby DA (1995) Modulation
    of hemeoxygenase activity in brain and spleen homogenates by nitric oxide and
    NO donors. Biochem Biophys Res Commun 214:1152–1156
Xie W, Chapman JG, Robertson DL et al (1991) Expression of a mitogen-responsive
    gene encoding prostaglandin synthase is regulated by mRNA splicing. Proc Natl
    Acad Sci USA 88:2692–2696
Xu X-M, Hajibeige A, Tazawa D, Loose-Mitchell D, Wang L-H, Wu KK (1995)
    Characterization of human prostaglandin H synthase genes. Adv Prost Thromb
    Leukoc Res 23:105–107
Yamagata K, Andreasson KI, Kaufmann WE, Barnes CA, Worley PF (1993) Expres-
    sion of a mitogen-inducible cyclooxygenase in brain neurones: regulation by syn-
    aptic activity and glucocorticoids. Neuron 11:371–386
Yashpal K, Coderre TJ (1993) Contribution of nitric oxide arachidonic acid and
    proteiin kinase C to persistent pain following tissue injury in rats. 7th World
    Congress on Pain. International Association for the Study of Pain, Seattle, p 24

CHAPTER 4

The Sympathetic Nervous System and Pain

M. Koltzenburg

A. Introduction

The sympathetic nervous system is involved in the control of virtually all bodily homeostatic regulations. Powerful changes in sympathetic function occur in both acute and chronic pain states. Early concepts portrayed the sympathetic nervous system as a rather primitive system that reacts in a uniform way to stressful conditions including pain with a generalised "fight and flight" reaction (LANGLEY 1903; CANNON 1929; HESS and BRUGGER 1943). More recently it has been recognised that the autonomic nervous system consists of networks of peripheral and central neurones that respond rather specifically to painful stimuli (JÄNIG 1985; LOEWY and SPYER 1990; JÄNIG and MCLACHLAN 1992). Furthermore, neurobiological investigations and clinical studies now demonstrate that the sympathetic nervous system not only reacts to noxious stimuli but also is in some conditions directly involved in the generation and maintenance of pain. It is the purpose of this review to focus on this enigmatic aspect of the sympathetic nervous system.

B. The Emergence of the Concept of an Interaction Between the Sympathetic and the Somatosensory System

We have arrived at the present concepts of a sympathetic influence on pain processing by a convoluted route of clinical conjectures. As some patients in chronic pain present with obvious malfunctions of sympathetic effector organs such as blood flow or sweating abnormalities, clinicians have, perhaps out of sheer desperation, tried sympatholytic procedures in patients with otherwise intractable pain. While the rationale for these therapeutic interventions may have been obscure and rooted in medical folklore, some procedures have nonetheless provided astonishing pain relief (LIVINGSTONE 1943; LOH and NATHAN 1978; BONICA 1990; STANTON-HICKS et al. 1996). These remarkable reports sparked off a more global interest in pain and the sympathetic nervous system, especially among those in clinical professions who earn a living out of sympatholytic procedures. However, judging the relative importance of the sympathetic nervous system in various pain states has been difficult as diagnostic criteria have been vague and inconsistent over time, and terminology the

Tower of Babel. In the absence of knowledge about pathophysiology, clinicians have resorted to the use of a wide range of ornate but often ill-defined diagnostic labels such as reflex sympathetic dystrophy, algodystrophy, causalgia, shoulder-hand syndrome or Sudeck's disease.

However, these labels have done little but camouflage our ignorance and have even been positively misleading by prejudicing the views on the pathobiology of the disease. It is therefore not surprising that the findings of many of the studies are often difficult, if not impossible, to interpret given that they are heavily tainted by patient selection drawn from a rag bag of conditions. Moreover, there is little agreement on the precipitating factors, which are thought to range from trivial injury to severe nerve damage or soft tissue trauma. Reports on the natural history of these conditions have often been heavily biased by unsystematic observations and preferences of the various clinical specialities treating these patients. Furthermore, the incidence of these disorders is touted by some to be exquisitely rare, whereas other authorities consider it to be frequent. This unsatisfactory situation has led some to an indiscriminate overuse, if not abuse, of sympatholytic procedures. Conversely, the inevitable failures to cure many patients has led other researchers in the field to flatly deny the existence of a sympathetic component in the generation of any pain (OCHOA 1993; OCHOA and VERDUGO 1993; SCHOTT 1994). However, on a balanced view most clinical investigators now agree that the sympathetic nervous system can – in a group of chronic pain patients – contribute significantly to the pain.

The prevailing chaos has now been acknowledged by the International Association for the Study of Pain and has led to several proposals that are aimed to clarify the issue. First, the neutral term "complex regional pain syndromes" (CRPS) has now been introduced to describe those painful conditions that usually follow injury, occur regionally, have a distal predominance of abnormal findings and exceed in both magnitude and duration the expected clinical course of the inciting clinical event (MERSKEY and BOGDUK 1994; STANTON-HICKS et al. 1995). Diagnostic criteria have now been formulated to facilitate and unify future studies on the epidemiology, pathophysiology and treatments (STANTON-HICKS et al. 1995; JÄNIG and STANTON-HICKS 1996). Second, the umbrella term "sympathetically maintained pain" (SMP) has been chosen for pains that are maintained by sympathetic efferent innervation or by circulating catecholamines (MERSKEY and BOGDUK 1994; STANTON-HICKS et al. 1995; JÄNIG and STANTON-HICKS 1996). A major conceptual advance over the past years has been the emerging consensus amongst most investigators that SMP is a feature of several types of pain disorder and does not constitute a disease in its own right (Fig. 1A). In other words, SMP does not equal reflex sympathetic dystrophy or complex regional pain syndrome but may be one of the many factors contributing to the generation of clinically relevant pain states.

Most investigators now concur that the sympathetically maintained pain component may vary within one etiologically defined disease, such as periph-

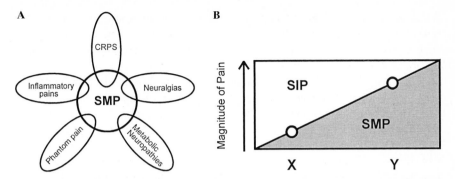

Fig. 1. A Sympathetically maintained pain (*SMP*) may be a symptom in many disease states. **B** Schematic illustration that the ratio of SMP or sympathetically independent pain (*SIP*) may vary between different disease states (*X, Y*) or at different time points (*X, Y*) during the natural history of a disease

eral nerve trauma, and that it may do so over time (Fig. 1B). Two diagnostic tests, each with its own weaknesses and strengths, are used in current clinical practice to determine whether SMP is present, namely local anaesthetic block of appropriate sympathetic ganglia or intravenous infusion with the non-selective α-adrenoceptor antagonist phentolamine. Although it is currently not carved into stone as to what constitutes a positive result, most investigators would diagnose SMP if a greater than 50% reduction in the magnitude of pain occurs during sympatholysis. However, this cut-off point is somewhat arbitrary, and there may be a continuum of responses (Fig. 1B).

The recognition of sympathetically maintained pain states has two major implications. First, it is attractive for the development of clinical treatment strategies that harness sympatholytical procedures for the relief of pain states that fail to respond to conventional analgesic therapies. Second, the development of a novel interaction between the sympathetic nervous system and sensory processing is of general neurobiological interest because it is an example of the plasticity and long-term changes in the peripheral and central nervous system that are involved in the processing of nociceptive information. The present review puts forward evidence that the acquisition of an abnormally increased sensitivity of nociceptors to catecholamines is in many cases the primary cause of SMP. This nociceptor excitation not only signals the ongoing pain but also precipitates subsequent changes in the CNS that are collectively known as central sensitisation, which is the basis of various forms of stimulus-induced pains.

I. The Key Clinical Findings in Patients with SMP

The most valuable body of clinical evidence comes from few careful studies of small groups of patients suffering from focal nerve injury. It is in this group of disorders that a case for a significant sympathetic component of the pain can most convincingly been made. Prevailing clinical wisdom does not support the notion of a significant contribution of the sympathetic nervous system in other chronic painful disorders, although only few systematic studies are available at the present time.

Patients suffering from focal peripheral nerve lesions often present with ongoing background pain and a combination of variable stimulus-induced pains (hyperalgesias) to mechanical or thermal stimuli (FRUHSTORFER et al. 1976; PRICE et al. 1989, 1992; CAMPBELL et al. 1992; TOREBJÖRK 1990; WAHREN et al. 1991; GRACELY et al. 1992; VERDUGO and OCHOA 1992; OCHOA and YARNITZKY 1993; KOLTZENBURG et al. 1994b). These findings are essentially the same in patients whose pain is either sympathetically maintained or sympathetically independent, and there is presently no independent diagnostic test that predicts the response to sympatholytical procedures (LINDBLOM and VERRILLO 1979; WAHREN and TOREBJÖRK 1992; KOLTZENBURG et al. 1994b; TOREBJÖRK et al. 1995).

Three lines of evidence now converge to indicate that the ongoing stimulus-independent pain is caused by the development of a persistent excitation of nociceptors that have normally no spontaneous activity. First, pain is abolished or at least significantly reduced by local anaesthetic block of the damaged peripheral nerve or its innervation territory (KIBLER and NATHAN 1960; ROWBOTHAM and FIELDS 1989; ROWBOTHAM et al. 1995; ARNÉR et al. 1990; BONICA 1990; NURMIKKO et al. 1991; CAMPBELL et al. 1992; CHABAL et al. 1992; GRACELY et al. 1992; TOREBJÖRK et al. 1995), indicating that activity arising distally in the nerve or at the receptive terminals causes pain. Second, the stimulus-independent pain persists during differential blockade of myelinated afferents suggesting that unmyelinated fibres can signal the ongoing pain (CAMPBELL et al. 1988, 1992; OCHOA and YARNITZKY 1993; KOLTZENBURG et al. 1994b; TOREBJÖRK et al. 1995). Third, psychophysical experiments suggest that different levels of nociceptor activity are correlated with the corresponding magnitudes of pain (GRACELY et al. 1992; KOLTZENBURG et al. 1994b). These clinical findings are supported by animal experiments that have directly demonstrated the development of ongoing nociceptor activity in damaged peripheral nerves (see below).

In some patients catecholamines are critically involved in the maintenance of this abnormal nociceptor excitation, although at this time it remains unclear why only a fraction of patients develop SMP while others with apparently identical peripheral nerve lesions do not. Sympatholytic interventions can significantly reduce pain and hyperalgesia in these individuals, either by local anaesthetic block of sympathetic ganglia (PRICE et al. 1989; BONICA 1990; STANTON-HICKS et al. 1996) or by regional depletion of catecholamines with local guanethedine treatment (HANNINGTON-KIFF 1974; LOH and NATHAN 1978; WAHREN et al. 1991; HORD et al. 1992; STANTON-HICKS et al. 1996). By contrast, electrical stimulation of the decentralised thoracic sympathetic chain in conscious patients undergoing surgery under local anaesthesia has been reported to cause pain (WALKER and NULSEN 1948; WHITE and SWEET 1969).

Moreover, blockade of α-adrenoceptors (ABRAM and LIGHTFOOT 1981; GHOSTINE et al. 1984; ARNÉR 1991; RAJA et al. 1991; TREEDE et al. 1992a; DELLIMIJN et al. 1994), but not of β-adrenoceptors (SCADDING et al. 1982; RAJA et al. 1991) can confer pain relief. Furthermore, pain can sometimes be aggravated by local injection of noradrenaline or the α_1-selective adrenoceptor agonist phenylephrine (WALLIN et al. 1976; DAVIS et al. 1991; CHABAL et al. 1992; TOREBJÖRK et al. 1995; ALI et al. 1996) but not by the α_2-adrenoceptor agonist clonidine (DAVIS et al. 1991).

This astonishing effect is probably best illustrated in those patients in whom intracutaneous injection of noradrenaline can rekindle the pain and hyperalgesias during a period of temporary pain relief afforded by sympatholysis (Fig. 2; WALLIN et al. 1976; DAVIS et al. 1991; TOREBJÖRK et al. 1995). As evidenced by a differential block of peripheral nerves, both the ongoing sympathetically maintained pain and the rekindled pain following injections of catecholamines are conducted by unmyelinated nociceptive primary afferent neurones (KOLTZENBURG et al. 1994b; TOREBJÖRK et al. 1995). Moreover, noradrenaline-evoked pain can be observed in patients after surgical sympathectomy, indicating that the excitation of nociceptors does not require the presence of postganglionic fibres (WALLIN et al. 1976). Although results from these careful clinical studies and a vast number of animal experiments (see below) together conclude that nociceptive primary afferent neurones can acquire an abnormal sensitivity to catecholamines, the hypoth-

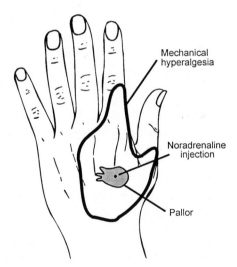

Fig. 2. Intracutaneous injection of noradrenaline rekindled ongoing pain and mechanical hyperalgesia in a patient with SMP who had suffered a partial nerve lesion of the superficial radial nerve, and who was temporarily relieved from pain by a sympathetic block. Whereas ongoing pain was conducted by unmyelinated nociceptors, brush-evoked pain was conducted by large myelinated fibres. (Modified from TOREBJÖRK et al. 1995)

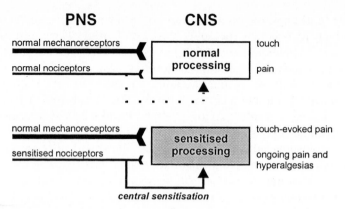

Fig. 3. Schematic representation that a nociceptor-mediated central sensitisation causes touch-evoked pain which is conducted by large myelinated (Aβ) fibres

esis still awaits its final proof by direct microneurographic recordings in patients.

If we accept that the ongoing activity of nociceptor is maintained in some patients by catecholamines, it becomes clear why sympatholytical procedures can result in the abolition of both ongoing pain and stimulus-induced hyperalgesias (Fig. 3). Studies on patients suffering from neuralgia have determined that the central sensitisation which is thought to be the basis of several kinds of hyperalgesia such as brush-evoked pain is dynamically maintained by a persistent nociceptor excitation (GRACELY et al. 1992; KOLTZENBURG et al. 1994b; TOREBJÖRK et al. 1995). Therefore these hyperalgesias and the stimulus-independent background pain usually resolve in parallel after abolition of nociceptor excitation (PRICE et al. 1989, 1992; GRACELY et al. 1992; TREEDE et al. 1992a; DELLIMIJN et al. 1994; KOLTZENBURG et al. 1994b). This indicates that abnormal nociceptor excitation is the primary cause of neuralgia, and that many forms of clinically apparent hyperalgesias are secondary consequences of the persistent nociceptor excitation.

C. Sympathetic Activation Has a Negligible Effect on Normal Sensory Processing

The effect of the sympathetic nervous system on somatosensory processes had already attracted the interest of the great physiologist and founder of experimental medicine, Claude Bernard. In a classical experiment he removed the superior cervical ganglion of a cat and studied the subsequent effects on autonomic effector organs and sensation (BERNARD 1851). As many others who later performed similar experiments, he found that there is normally no acute sympathetic effect on sensation.

Many neurophysiological studies have also directly investigated the influence of sympathetic stimulation on the receptive properties of primary afferents in normal mammals including humans. In animals single units were recorded from teased filaments of the desheathed nerve and tested with electrical stimulation of sympathetic neurones or administration of catecholamines. The findings of these extensive studies are summarised in Table 1, and the gist of these investigations is that sympathetic fibres have no demonstrable effects on the functional properties of normal nociceptors and little effect of questionable significance on non-nociceptive afferents. Most of the changes in non-nociceptive fibres were only observed with prolonged synchronous high-frequency stimulation of sympathetic fibres that are far beyond the biologically relevant discharge activity of sympathetic fibres. Furthermore, sympathetically evoked responses were quantitatively very small compared to the excitation that could be elicited by adequate natural mechanical or thermal stimulation.

Many studies could not completely rule out that the observed effects were simply the consequence of secondary tissue alterations following activation of autonomic effector organs. Indeed, several studies found that the responses of sympathetic stimulation were mimicked by occlusion of the vascular supply (ELDRED et al. 1960; BHOOLA et al. 1962; CALMA and KIDD 1962; EDWALL and SCOTT 1971; MATTHEWS 1976; FREEMAN and ROWE 1981; HUNT et al. 1982). It is also clear that some mechanosensitive afferents are indirectly excited by movements of hairs and adjacent skin during contraction of the piloarrector muscles. Finally, cooling that accompanies forceful vasoconstriction could influence the firing of thermoreceptors, and it is well known that even small temperature changes can modify the stimulus response functions of mechanoreceptors (KONIETZNY 1984; JÄNIG and KOLTZENBURG 1992). Where tested, the weak effects of sympathetic stimulation were usually blocked by α-selective adrenoceptor antagonists (NILSSON 1972; MATTHEWS 1976; CASH and LINDEN 1982; ROBERTS et al. 1985; ROBERTS and ELARDO 1985a).

At this time there is no information about possible long-term effects of postganglionic sympathetic fibres on the function of primary sensory neurones under normal conditions. However, it is known that nociceptive afferents and sympathetic efferents compete for limited amounts of growth factors such as nerve growth factor, and that its availability can strongly regulate the receptive properties of nociceptors over a period of days to weeks in adult animals in vivo (KOLTZENBURG et al. 1996).

D. Several Interactions Between the Sympathetic and the Nociceptive Systems Develop After Nerve Injury

While animal studies have convincingly shown that sympathetic modulation of receptive properties of afferent fibres is negligible under physiological conditions, they have also determined beyond reasonable doubt that an interaction between primary afferent neurones and postganglionic sympathetic fibres can

Table 1. Effects of sympathetic activation by electrical stimulation of sympathetic fibres or administration of catecholamines on the receptive properties of primary afferent neurones

Receptor type	Species	Effect of sympathetic stimulation	References
Cutaneous mechanoreceptors			
Rapidly adapting mechanoreceptor type I (Meisner corpuscles)	Human	0 ($n = 12$)	Dotson et al. 1990
Pacini corpuscle	Human	0 ($n = 5$), + (20%, $n = 20$)	Hallin and Wiesenfeld-Hallin 1983; Wiesenfeld-Hallin and Hallin 1984a,b; Dotson et al. 1990
	Cat	− (54%) + (31%, $n = 13$)	Freeman and Rowe 1981
Hair follicle afferents	Cat	− (90%, $n = 40$)	Nilsson 1972; Pierce and Roberts 1981; Roberts and Levitt 1982
	Rabbit	− (100%, $n = 15$)	Barasi and Lynn 1986
Slowly adapting mechanoreceptors type I (Merkel cell complexes)	Human	0 ($n = 5$), + (15%, $n = 13$)	Hallin and Wiesenfeld-Hallin 1983; Wiesenfeld-Hallin and Hallin 1984a,b; Dotson et al. 1990
	Cat	+ (37%, $n = 68$)	Roberts et al. 1985
Slowly adapting mechanoreceptors type II (Ruffini endings)	Human		Dotson et al. 1990
	Cat	+ (100%, $n = 17$)	Pierce and Roberts 1981
Low-threshold mechanoreceptors with unmyelinated axons	Cat		Roberts and Elardo 1985a
	Rabbit	+ (90%, $n = 10$)	Barasi and Lynn 1986

Cutaneous nociceptors			
Thin myelinated (Aδ) nociceptors	Cat	0 ($n = 44$)	ROBERTS and ELARDO 1985b
	Rabbit	0 ($n = 8$)	BARASI and LYNN 1986
	Rat	0 ($n = 4$)	LANG et al. 1990
	Human	0 ($n = 7$)	ELAM et al. 1996
	Monkey	0	SELIG et al. 1993
Unmyelinated (C) nociceptors	Rabbit	0 ($n = 28$), – ($n = 12$)	SHEA and PERL 1985; BARASI and LYNN 1986; SATO and PERL 1991; BOSSUT and PERL 1995
	Rat	0	SANJUE and JUN 1989; SATO et al. 1993
Muscle receptors			
Primary or secondary muscle spindles (group Ia, II)	Cat	+, –	ELDRED et al. 1960; HUNT 1960; BHOOLA et al. 1962; CALMA and KIDD 1962; PASSATORE and FILIPPI 1981; HUNT et al. 1982
	Rat	–	MATSUO et al. 1995
Golgi tendon organs (group Ib)	Cat	0	HUNT 1960
Nociceptors (group III, IV)	Rat	+	MENSE 1986; KIESCHKE et al. 1988
Dental receptors			
Tooth pulp receptors	Cat	+	EDWALL and SCOTT 1971; MATTHEWS 1976
Peridontal receptors	Cat	– (50%, $n = 64$)	CASH and LINDEN 1982
	Rabbit	+ (30%, $n = 132$)	PASSATORE and FILIPPI 1983

+, Excitation or facilitation of an evoked response; –, inhibition or depression of an evoked response; 0, no effect. Where available, the numbers in parenthesis give the percentage of affected units and the total number of afferents tested.

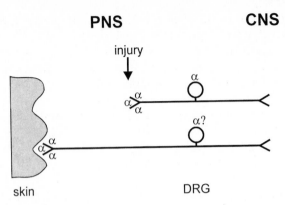

Fig. 4. Possible sites (α) where nociceptors become responsive to sympathetic stimulation following partial nerve lesion

develop after nerve lesions. Because of its anatomical structure it is obvious that any possible interaction between the sensory system and the sympathetic nervous system is confined to the peripheral nervous system. This interaction has been shown to occur at three points of a sensory neurone, namely at the soma in the dorsal root ganglion, at the tips of regenerating sprouts of severed afferent neurones or in undamaged fibres that run in a partially transected nerve (Fig. 4). These interactions appear to occur to a various extent in different animal models of neuralgia.

I. Animal Models of Neuropathic and Sympathetically Maintained Pain

The animal models that have been used to investigate nociceptive mechanisms after nerve injury can be divided into two major groups. One of the first models that was developed was the stump neuroma created by complete transection of a major peripheral nerve and the prevention of regeneration (WALL and GUTNICK 1974; CODERRE et al. 1986; JÄNIG 1988; DEVOR 1994). Rats and mice, but not higher mammals, start to mutilate the denervated limb during the weeks that follow. This behaviour has (not without dispute) been taken as behavioural evidence for the presence of pain. The neuroma model mimics the clinical condition of a phantom limb pain or anaesthesia dolorosa that can develop after amputations or denervation of a limb in humans. Since nerve fibres lose contact with their peripheral targets, the model is not suited to study stimulus-induced pains and therefore does not adequately model the situation that is the hallmark of many neuralgias in humans. To overcome these short-comings several investigators have developed various models of partial injury of the sciatic nerve using a chronic constriction (BENNETT and XIE 1988; SHERBOURNE et al. 1992; SOMMER et al. 1993), partial transection (SELTZER et al. 1990), ligation of its spinal roots (KIM and CHUNG 1992;

CARLTON et al. 1994), cryoneurolisis (DeLEO et al. 1994) or inflammation (MAVES et al. 1992, 1993; ELIAV and BENNETT 1996).

The common denominator of these models is the combination of a considerable degree of nerve damage and the retention of some innervation of the peripheral tissue that can carry the signals for stimulus-induced pains. In these models animals usually exhibit behavioural signs of ongoing pain and mechanical hyperalgesia, but hyperalgesia to thermal stimuli seems to be more variable (BENNETT 1993). There are several reports that sympatholytical procedures reduce the nociceptive behaviour (KIM and CHUNG 1991; NEIL et al. 1991; SHIR and SELTZER 1991; KIM et al. 1993; PERROT et al. 1993; DESMEULES et al. 1995; KINNMAN and LEVINE 1995; TRACEY et al. 1995a). However, it is presently not entirely clear why other studies have failed to provide evidence for an involvement of the sympathetic nervous system in these models (WAKISAKA et al. 1991; WILLENBRING et al. 1995a,b; FONTANA and HUNTER 1996; GRETHEL et al. 1996). Some discrepancies may be explained by strain differences, differences in the timing of the intervention, by variances in the pharmacological or surgical sympatholytical procedures or by different behavioural test paradigms.

II. Sprouts of Axotomised Afferents Projecting into a Neuroma

Neurophysiological studies have extensively studied the properties of primary afferent neurones projecting into a stump neuroma after complete nerve transection. A common finding in damaged peripheral nerves is electrical cross-talk between axons of all diameters (JÄNIG 1988; LISNEY 1989; DEVOR 1994). The basis of these short circuits are so-called ephapses that allow a tight one-to-one coupling between axons. Although rarely present in seemingly normal nerves (MEYER and CAMPBELL 1987), they are found in up to 20% of the fibres in the stump neuroma of the cat (BLUMBERG and JÄNIG 1982a, 1984). The presence of such ephapses between unmyelinated axons has invited speculations that sympathetic fibres could directly couple to primary afferent neurones. However, despite an intensive search such electrical interaction has never been demonstrated (JÄNIG and KOLTZENBURG 1991; BLUMBERG and JÄNIG 1984; MEYER and CAMPBELL 1987).

Sprouts that are issued by axotomised afferent fibres are exquisitely sensitive to many stimuli. Many develop ongoing activity and often respond to a variety of mechanical, thermal or chemical stimuli (JÄNIG 1988; LISNEY 1989; DEVOR 1994). The mechanical sensitivity of regenerating fibres is the basis for the Hofmann-Tinel sign that has been used since the beginning of the century by neurologists to detect axon tips in focal nerve damage. The development of adrenergic sensitivity among afferent neurones is the basis for a sympathetic-afferent coupling. Sprouts of regenerating sensory neurones that are trapped in a stump neuroma frequently respond to electrical stimulation of postganglionic sympathetic fibres or to systemic or local administration of catecholamines (DEVOR and JÄNIG 1981; KORENMAN and DEVOR 1981; SCADDING 1981;

BLUMBERG and JÄNIG 1982b, 1984; HÄBLER et al. 1987; JÄNIG 1990; WELK et al. 1990). Since the afferents have been disconnected from the periphery, it is not possible to unequivocally determine the receptive function that these neurones have had.

However, primary afferents of all conduction velocities can acquire such responsiveness including afferent fibres with thin myelinated or unmyelinated axons that are presumably the processes of erstwhile nociceptors (DEVOR and JÄNIG 1981; BLUMBERG and JÄNIG 1984; HÄBLER et al. 1987; JÄNIG 1990). The degree of responsiveness varies with species and the time interval after nerve damage. Where tested, the sympathetic effects on nociceptors were usually blocked by administration of α-selective adrenoceptor antagonists although a detailed breakdown into the relative contribution of different receptor sub-types has not yet been performed. There is also some evidence that sympathetic stimulation can excite primary afferent neurones through a non-adrenergic mechanism (JÄNIG 1990). A candidate substance is neuropeptide Y which is found in many noradrenergic sympathetic fibres and whose injection into the paw aggravates mechanical and thermal hyperalgesia, after partial sciatic nerve transection probably via the Y2 receptor (TRACEY et al. 1995b).

Although these excitatory effects have been studied mainly after transection of major nerve trunks, it is reasonable to assume that damage to the terminal branches of a nerve can cause similar consequences. Supposing that many forms of penetrating tissue injury produce such minor nerve damage, an interaction between sympathetic and primary afferents may develop under conditions where even meticulous clinical examination would probably fail to demonstrate nerve injury. Moreover, in models of partial nerve injury many axons form a neuroma-in-continuity (CARLTON et al. 1991; MUNGER et al. 1992; SOMMER et al. 1993), and these afferents have by and large similar electrophysiological properties as those in a nerve end neuroma (HÄBLER et al. 1987; KAJANDER and BENNETT 1992; KOLTZENBURG et al. 1994a; XIE et al. 1995).

III. Primary Afferents Projecting into a Partially Damaged Nerve

An interaction between nociceptors and sympathetic fibres has also been shown to develop in non-transected nerve fibres running in a partially lesioned nerve. Following chronic constriction or partial transection of the nerve or transections of some nerve roots (SATO and PERL 1991; SELIG et al. 1993; KOLTZENBURG et al. 1994a; BOSSUT and PERL 1995; RINGKAMP et al. 1996) unmyelinated and thin myelinated nociceptive afferents that had either low or no ongoing activity responded with a weak irregular discharge to local administrations of catecholamines to the receptive field (Fig. 5). There is also evidence that a subpopulation of rapidly adapting mechanoreceptors with large myelinated fibres have an unusually strong response to mechanical stimuli that can be abolished by sympathetic blockade (NA et al. 1993). In rodents the

A

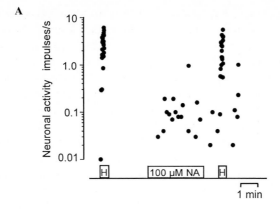

B

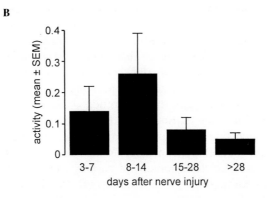

Fig. 5. A Excitation of a non-axotomised nociceptor recorded from a partially injured nerve during superfusion of the cutaneous receptive field with noradrenaline. *H*, Heat response. **B** Time dependence of the average discharge evoked in a population of nociceptors with no or low ongoing activity. These nociceptors (whose axons had not been transected) had receptive fields within the nerve territory of a partially damaged nerve. (Modified from KOLTZENBURG et al. 1994a)

interactions appear to involve an α_2-adrenoceptor whereas in primates the excitation is apparently mediated by α_1-adrenoceptors. Little information is presently available about the subtypes of the α_1- or α_2-adrenoceptor, the ionic mechanisms or the intracellular messengers that mediate the excitation. Furthermore, the mechanism by which functional adrenoceptors appear is unknown. However, the theoretical possibilities include the upregulation of receptors that are already expressed in sensory neurones or the synthesis of novel adrenoceptors. It is also conceivable that changes in the intracellular transduction pathways are necessary to permit an adrenoceptor-mediated excitation of sensory neurones. When tested, the adrenergic excitation of nociceptors were quantitatively most prominent two weeks after partial nerve damage and gradually disappeared thereafter (Fig. 5).

Catecholamines also produce a weak sensitisation of some nociceptors to heat. However, nociceptive afferents with moderate or high ongoing activity are either not affected or display a slight inhibition of the ongoing activity during administration of noradrenaline. This indicates that a high degree of excitability – as judged by their level of ongoing activity – is not the prerequisite for an excitatory sympathetic-afferent interaction, but that other mechanisms may be required. As a proportion of nociceptors develop an adrenergic sensitivity after sympathectomy (PERL 1994), it has been suggested that mechanisms which induce the typical denervation super-sensitivity of autonomic effector organs following sympathetic denervation might also be responsible for an upregulation of adrenoceptors on nociceptors. Indeed, there are now several reports using autoradiographic binding techniques (MCMAHON 1991) or in situ hybridisation (PERL 1994; DAVAR et al. 1996) that provide morphological evidence for an upregulation of adrenoceptors on dorsal root ganglion cells.

The results of these studies now provide experimental support for a number of enigmatic clinical findings. First, after nerve damage non-injured nociceptors that innervate partially denervated tissue can develop a sensitivity to catecholamines. Second, the adrenoceptor-mediated excitation can occur distal to a nerve lesion. Third, the magnitude of the effect develops within days, but often decreases as time goes by. Fourth, removal of a number of sympathetic neurones may provide the signal for an upregulation of adrenoceptor. This suggests that a critical density of the sympathetic innervation is required for the development of a sympathetic-afferent interaction: a necessary reduction to trigger the abnormal catecholamine-sensitivity of nociceptors, yet at the same time a sufficient density to provide enough noradrenaline for this excitation. Fifth, the catecholamine sensitivity of nociceptors appears to be present on afferents with no or very low ongoing activity. Thus the clinical effectiveness of a sympatholytical procedure may depend on the ratio of responsive and non-responsive fibres at a given moment of time, and therefore significant relief can be expected only if other factors do not cause a persistent discharge of nociceptors.

IV. Interactions Between Sympathetic Fibres and Primary Afferent Neurones in the Dorsal Root Ganglion

A further site where sympathetic efferent neurones can excite primary afferents is the dorsal root ganglion. Several days after axotomy many cells with large myelinated fibres start to discharge (LISNEY and DEVOR 1987; DEVOR and WALL 1990). This ectopic discharge can be modulated by two different mechanisms (Fig. 6). First, electrical or natural excitation of neighbouring cells within the ganglion can increase the discharge. This effect has been termed crossed afterdischarge and is probably mediated by an increase in extracellular concentration of potassium (UTZSCHNEIDER et al. 1992). The crossed afterdischarge is not tightly locked to the stimulus, indicating that it is not

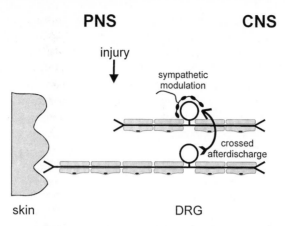

Fig. 6. A crossed afterdischarge and sympathetic activation can excite cells with large myelinated axons in the dorsal root ganglion

mediated through an ephaptic mechanism. The interaction is found primarily in axotomised cells with myelinated axons and only rarely in neurones with unmyelinated axons. Although not studied in detail, most of the neurones probably subserved non-nociceptive functions prior to their axotomy. Interestingly, the electrical or natural excitation of intact nerve cells that have their soma in the same ganglion can evoke the crossed afterdischarge in axotomised ectopically discharging neurones. The intact neurones that were capable to induce the crossed afterdischarge had usually large myelinated fibres. Thus, crossed afterdischarges are predominately an interaction between non-nociceptive sensory neurones with large myelinated neurones that could lead to a temporal and spatial distortion of sensory information, although its role in the generation of pain remains unclear.

The second modulatory influence of the ectopic discharge of neurones in the dorsal root ganglion is mediated by postganglionic sympathetic fibres (McLachlan et al. 1993; Devor et al. 1994). Several days after axotomy electrical stimulation of sympathetic fibres or systemic administration of adrenaline can modulate the ectopic discharge of cells that had presumably non-nociceptive function prior to their axotomy. Slightly more than half of the responses are excitatory, while the remaining cases display an inhibition of the ongoing ectopic activity. While the sympathetic effects are blocked by the α-selective adrenoceptor antagonist phentolamine, the crossed afterdischarges that are evoked in these cells are unaffected by phentolamine. Similar effects on dorsal root ganglion cells also appear to occur following partial injury of the sciatic nerve (Kajander and Bennett 1992; Kajander et al. 1992; Xie et al. 1995). There is also morphological evidence for a sympathetic-afferent interaction at the level of the dorsal root ganglion. Under normal instances there are only few postganglionic fibres that innervate blood vessels (Stevens et al. 1983; Risling et al. 1985; McLachlan et al. 1993).

However, after axotomy there is a profuse growth of sympathetic neurones into the dorsal root ganglion and postganglionic sympathetic fibres start to encircle dorsal root ganglion cells to form "baskets" (McLACHLAN et al. 1993; CHUNG et al. 1994). Nevertheless, the formation of sympathetic baskets around ganglion cells takes several weeks after axotomy of the rat sciatic nerve at middle-thigh level, in contrast to the development of a functional coupling that can be detected within days. It has been suggested that an increase of retrogradely transported nerve growth factor is the signal for the ingrowth of sympathetic fibres into the dorsal root ganglion because transgenic mice that overexpress the gene encoding for nerve growth factor in the skin show the same dramatic formation of sympathetic baskets around sensory neurones (DAVIS et al. 1994). Thus the dorsal root ganglion is an unexpected site for an interactions between the soma of sensory neurones and postganglionic sympathetic efferent fibres. However, as mainly neurones with large myelinated axons appear to be excited by sympathetic stimulation, and as sympathetic baskets are usually found around large sensory neurones, the possible clinical importance of this kind of interaction between sympathetic fibres and mainly non-nociceptive afferents for the generation of pain remains to be determined.

V. Are Changes in the Sympathetic Nervous System Necessary To Permit the Interaction with Primary Afferent Fibres?

While primary afferent neurones undergo a host of changes that permit an interaction with postganglionic sympathetic fibres, much less is known about the necessary changes in the sympathetic nervous system that allow the contact with the afferent fibres. Because of the obvious malfunction of autonomic effector organs in some patients presenting with SMP, many texts have maintained that an excessive sympathetic discharge is a decisive factor in the generation of pain. However, several lines of evidence from clinical studies and animal experiments now converge to indicate that this is probably not the case. In patients with SMP direct microneurographic recordings have demonstrated normal or decreased neural sympathetic discharge (WALLIN et al. 1976). This is also supported by the reduced levels of noradrenaline that have been measured in the venous outflow of a symptomatic extremity (DRUMMOND et al. 1991). It is therefore more likely that a denervation supersensitivity (ARNOLD et al. 1993; KURVERS et al. 1995) overcompensates for the reduced sympathetic activity, resulting in a seemingly exaggerated autonomic response.

Clinical investigations have also shown a complex deterioration of the sympathetic reflex patterns of an affected extremity (BLUMBERG et al. 1994; BARON et al. 1996; KURVERS et al. 1996a). While several sympathetic reflexes were normal, the sympathetic control of thermoregulation was often altered so that the limb was usually cooler than on the contralateral unaffected side. However, it seems unlikely that these reflex changes are the cause of the pains although they might indirectly contribute to the sensory abnormalities in the presence of cold hyperalgesia. Rather, the asymmetrical sympathetic vasoconstrictor responses could be the physiological response to a strong pain stimulus that also occurs in normal humans (MAGERL et al. 1996). The clinical findings are fully corroborated by animal experiments. After peripheral nerve lesion there is an atrophy of sympathetic cell bodies and their postganglionic fibres (JÄNIG 1988; LISNEY 1989). This involution extends to the ability of sympathetic neurones to synthesise and store catecholamines (KARLSTRÖM and DAHLSTRÖM 1973; GOLDSTEIN et al. 1988; WAKISAKA et al. 1991). It is clear that the depletion of catecholamines and a reduced release of the transmitter could greatly impair the ability of sympathetic fibres to interact with primary afferents even if the latter were responsive. As in patients, a denervation supersensitivity of blood vessels appears to be important to mediate an exaggerated vasoconstrictor response after nerve injury (JOBLING et al. 1992; KOLTZENBURG et al. 1995; KURVERS et al. 1996b) and there are also considerable changes of the sympathetic reflex patterns after nerve damage in animals (BLUMBERG and JÄNIG 1985; JÄNIG and KOLTZENBURG 1991).

In summary, a number of critical changes of primary afferent neurones and in the sympathetic nervous system appear to be necessary to permit an interaction that results in the generation of sympathetically maintained pain. The different temporal and spatial profiles of these changes may explain why the magnitude of SMP may vary over time, and why it develops to a variable extent in different individuals with seemingly identical lesions.

E. Can the Sympathetic Nervous System Modulate Pain and Hyperalgesia Under Inflammatory Conditions?

In recent years a large number of animal studies have provided evidence that the sympathetic nervous system can modulate the inflammatory response and the nociceptive behaviour in rodents (Fig. 7). Since there is a profound change of the receptive properties of nociceptors under inflammatory conditions (TREEDE et al. 1992b; MEYER et al. 1994; KOLTZENBURG 1995; REEH and KRESS 1995), it is conceivable that changes of the inflammatory response could indirectly affect the nociceptive system. Although many animal studies clearly point towards a contribution of the sympathetic nervous system in inflammatory pain states, prevailing clinical wisdom does not endorse a significant contribution of the sympathetic nervous system for the generation and maintenance of the pains in patients suffering from chronic inflammatory diseases. One study of patients with rheumatoid arthritis found a small reduction in some pain measurements after local intravenous treatment of an affected extremity with guanethedine (LEVINE et al. 1986b).

Studies in normal human volunteers using experimental models of inflammatory pain confirm that sympathetic responses on pain perception are small and possibly indirect. The thermal hyperalgesia evoked by intradermal injec-

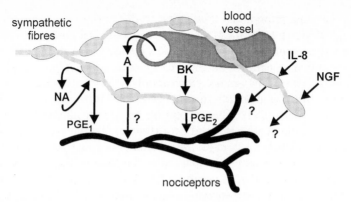

Fig. 7. Mechanisms that have been proposed how postganglionic sympathetic endings interact with inflammatory mediators or catecholamines

tion of capsaicin can be slightly aggravated by concomitant administration of noradrenaline (DRUMMOND 1995) while the administration of phentolamine can produce a mild decrease of the mechanical hyperalgesia (LIU et al. 1996). Some studies are confounded by the fact that changes in the local blood flow appear to be responsible for the sympathetic effect (DRUMMOND 1996), and that administration of high doses of noradrenaline on its own causes (by yet unknown mechanisms) a small but significant drop in the heat pain threshold (MEYER and RAJA 1996). By contrast, the sympathetic nervous system plays no appreciable role in modulating the pain and heat hyperalgesia after bradykinin injections (MEYER et al. 1992). Thus the few currently available investigations in humans indicate that the sympathetic nervous system is not invariably involved in the generation of inflammatory pain, and that the magnitude of the effects are, if present, small.

I. The Contribution of Sympathetic Fibres to Inflammation

The role of the sympathetic nervous system for inflammatory reactions has been extensively studied by Levine and colleagues in the knee joint of rats (CODERRE et al. 1989; GREEN et al. 1992, 1993a–d, 1995; LEVINE and TAIWO 1994; PIERCE et al. 1995). Using the Evans blue technique they measured the plasma extravasation of plasma proteins into the knee joint cavity after intra-articular injection of a variety of compounds. Intra-articular infusion of brady-kinin, serotonin or the mast cell degranulating compound 48/80 resulted in a profound plasma extravasation that was strongly reduced by a preceding denervation of the joint or by surgical or pharmacological sympathectomy. Since abolition of the discharge of sympathetic fibres by decentralisation of the lumbar sympathetic chain or local anaesthetic block of the sympathetic nerve endings in the joint did not modify this response, neural activity in postgangli-onic sympathetic fibres appears to be not important for the sympathetic-mediated plasma extravasation. Instead, the mere presence of postganglionic terminals appears to be crucial for the pro-inflammatory effect. This conclusion is also supported by the finding that intra-articular administration of 6-hydroxydopamine, a neurotoxin that acutely destroys adrenergic neurones, causes plasma extravasation probably by the release of mediators from sympathetic varicosities. It is unlikely that plasma extravasation is brought about by the release of noradrenalin or neuropeptide Y, as intra-articular infusion of these substances diminishes the plasma extravasation. Alternatively, ATP or prostaglandin E2 which can both be released from sympathetic terminals, have been suggested to play an important role for the sympathetically dependent plasma extravasation in the knee joint. Unfortunately, no studies have so far been carried out to determine the relative importance of the sympathetic nervous system in the neurogenic inflammation in other tissues.

The role of the sympathetic nervous system in modulating the severity of the joint lesions in Freund's adjuvant arthritis of the rat, has also been assessed by X-ray studies (LEVINE et al. 1986a). Joint lesions were reportedly attenuated in chemically sympathectomised rats, after adrenal medullectomy or by systemic treatment with β_2-selective adrenoceptor antagonists but were enhanced by treatment with β_2-selctive adrenoceptor agonists (LEVINE et al. 1988; CODERRE et al. 1990). Since the enhancement was prevented by a preceding sympathectomy, it was hypothesised that circulating adrenaline acts on the terminals of postganglionic sympathetic fibres to release a detrimental factor which has so far not been identified.

The dominant theme that runs through these and other behavioural studies (see below) is that postganglionic sympathetic fibres are – independently of their ongoing discharge – an important source of algesic and pro-inflammatory mediators. These compounds are thought to be non-adrenergic substances, possibly prostaglandins, that mediate plasma extravasation and aggravate inflammatory joint lesions. Presently it is unclear whether the mechanims that have been demonstrated for joints also operate in other tissues. Although these studies report that postganglionic sympathetic fibres mediate and aggravate some inflammatory responses in the knee joint, it has not been directly determined by neurophysiological recordings whether the receptive properties of nociceptors innervating the inflamed joint are altered by sympathectomy (SCHAIBLE and GRUBB 1993). On the contrary, neurogenic plasma extravasation has been shown not to alter the receptive properties of nociceptors (REEH et al. 1986; MEYER et al. 1988), and therefore the relationship between the sympathetically dependent extravasation and nociception remains unclear.

II. The Contribution of Sympathetic Fibres to Nociceptive Behaviour

In another series of experiments Levine and colleagues used the Randall-Sellito paw pressure test to study the effects of the sympathetic nervous system on the nociceptive behaviour of rats rendered hyperalgesic by intracutaneous of bradykinin or cutaneous administration of chloroform (LEVINE et al. 1986c; TAIWO et al. 1987, 1989, 1990; TAIWO and LEVINE 1988, 1989, 1990; KHASAR et al. 1995). After chloroforme treatment, but not in normal animals, the injection of noradrenaline aggravated the hyperalgesia. This ability of noradrenaline was prevented by the pre-treatment with the α_2-selective adrenoceptor antagonist yohimbine or a preceding sympathectomy, but not by the α_1-selective adrenoceptor antagonist prazosin. Likewise, the bradykinin-induced hyperalgesia appeared to depend on postganglionic sympathetic fibres as chemical sympathectomy prevented this response. It was therefore concluded that noradrenaline and bradykinin act presynaptically on the varicosities of postganglionic sympathetic fibres to release other compounds, notably prostaglandins, that then directly sensitise the receptive endings of nociceptors.

However, the general applicability of these conclusions has been questioned. In humans intracutaneous injection of bradykinin causes hyperalgesia to heat but not to mechanical stimuli (MANNING et al. 1991), and neither pain nor hyperalgesia is abolished by surgical sympathectomy (MEYER et al. 1992). A major weakness in the behavioural studies is that the postulated cellular changes have so far not been confirmed by direct neurophysiological recordings. By contrast, careful neurophysiological studies in rodents and primates have determined that bradykinin does neither sensitise nociceptors to mechanical stimuli (MEYER et al. 1994; REEH and KRESS 1995), nor is the excitation or the heat sensitisation of nociceptors prevented by a preceding surgical sympathectomy in the rat (KOLTZENBURG et al. 1992).

Other behavioural experiments in rats also suggest that the sympathetic nervous system contributes to the inflammatory hyperalgesia in cutaneous inflammation induced by intradermal injection of carrageenan. The behavioural signs of hyperalgesia are reduced by pre-treatment with guanethidine but aggravated by local treatment with catecholamine re-uptake inhibitors or high doses of noradrenaline or adrenaline (NAKAMURA and FERREIRA 1987). Hyperalgesia was also reduced by neutralisation of interleukin 8 (CUNHA et al. 1991) or nerve growth factor (LEWIN et al. 1994; WOOLF et al. 1994; MCMAHON et al. 1995; SIUCIAK et al. 1996). Conversely, injections of either interleukin 8 or nerve growth factor produces an hyperalgesia that can be reduced by sympathectomy (CUNHA et al. 1991; ANDREEV et al. 1995; WOOLF et al. 1996). Apart from kinins and arachidonic acid derivatives, other mediators such as tumor necrosis factor-α, interleukin 1β or interleukin 6 have been implicated to contribute to the hyperalgesia of inflamed skin through mechanisms that may require sympathetic fibres (CUNHA et al. 1991, 1992; SAFIEH GARABEDIAN et al. 1995; WOOLF et al. 1996). However, the interactions between these mediators and the role of the sympathetic nervous system are at present not completely understood.

Few electrophysiological studies have directly examined the possibility that the receptive properties of nociceptors are influenced by sympathetic activity in inflamed tissue. After creation of a mild burn injury or injection of inflammatory mediators some mechano-heat sensitive nociceptors are excited by high-frequency stimulation of sympathetic efferent fibres (ROBERTS and ELARDO 1985b; SANJUE and JUN 1989). However, the excitation has been quantitatively very small, not maintained throughout the sympathetic stimulation and achieved only by a non-physiologically synchronous high-frequency stimulation (Fig. 8). Where tested, the excitatory effects have been blocked by phentolamine, suggesting that they are mediated by an α-adrenoceptor. Sympathetic stimulation or close arterial injection of noradrenaline also excite about one-third of the unmyelinated nociceptive afferents innervating chronically inflamed skin of the rat (SATO et al. 1993). The effects are blocked by the α_2-selective adrenoceptor antagonist yohimbine. Since they were also observed in sympathectomised animals, it is likely that the nociceptors were excited by a direct action of catecholamines on α_2-adrenoceptors (SATO et al. 1994).

In conclusion, the sympathetic effects on nociceptive afferents innervating inflamed tissue contrast with the results in normal animals where sympathetic modulation of the properties of nociceptive afferents is negligible. However, the fast changes that can be observed in many behavioural experiments and in

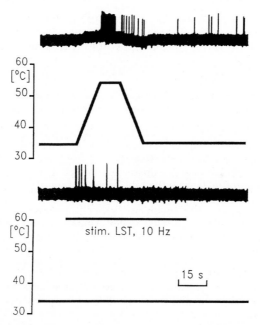

Fig. 8. Recording of a nociceptor innervating the hairy skin of the cat. The unit did initially not respond to electrical stimulation of sympathetic fibres (not shown); however it is excited by a mild burn injury evoked by heating of the receptive field above 50°C. After the heat injury synchronous high-frequency electrical stimulation of sympathetic fibres in the lumbar sympathetic trunk (*stim. LST*) evoked a weak response. (Modified from ROBERTS and ELARDO 1985b)

some electrophysiological studies suggest that the sympathetic nervous system can in principle rapidly affect nociceptive processes. This rapid sympathetic modulation of nociceptive activity in inflamed tissue contrasts with the time course of a sympathetic afferent coupling after nerve damage which takes days to develop. This could mean that different mechanisms are responsible. The effects in inflamed tissue appear partially to be mediated indirectly through the release of mediators from the varicosities of sympathetic terminals, or they may be the consequence of a rapid alteration of the cellular transduction properties within the receptive terminals of nociceptors. By contrast, the sympathetic effects on primary afferents after nerve damage are probably mediated directly. The slower development of this responsiveness suggests that changes in the synthesis of adrenoceptors or of molecules that are relevant for the subsequent intracellular transduction pathways are required.

References

Abram SE, Lightfoot RW (1981) Treatment of long-standing causalgia with prazosin. Reg Anesth 6:79–81

Ali Z, Wesselmann U, Meyer RA, Campbell JN, Raja SN (1996) Pain induced by intradermal norepinephrine and phenylephrine in patients with neuropathic pain. Abstracts of the 8th World Congress on Pain, p 398

Andreev NY, Dimitrieva N, Koltzenburg M, McMahon SB (1995) Peripheral administration of nerve growth factor in the adult rat produces a thermal hyperalgesia that requires the presence of sympathetic post-ganglionic neurones. Pain 63:109–115

Arnér S (1991) Intravenous phentolamine test: diagnostic and prognostic use in reflex sympathetic dystrophy. Pain 46:17–22

Arnér S, Lindblom U, Meyerson BA, Molander C (1990) Prolonged relief of neuralgia after regional anesthetic blocks. A call for further experimental and systematic clinical studies. Pain 43:287–297

Arnold JMO, Teasell RW, MacLeod AP, Brown JE, Carruthers SG (1993) Increased venous alpha-adrenoceptor responsiveness in patients with reflex sympathetic dystrophy. Ann Intern Med 118:619–621

Barasi S, Lynn B (1986) Effects of sympathetic stimulation on mechanoreceptive and nociceptive afferent units from the rabbit pinna. Brain Res 378:21–27

Baron R, Blumberg H, Jänig W (1996) Clinical characteristics of patients with complex regional pain syndrome in Germany with special emphasis on vasomotor function. In: Jänig W, Stanton-Hicks M (eds) Reflex sympathetic dystrophy: a reappraisal. International Association for the Study of Pain, Seattle, p 25

Bennett GJ (1993) Animal models of neuropathic pain. In: Gebhart GF, Hammond DL, Jensen TS (eds) Proceedings of the 7th World Congress on Pain. International Association for the Study of Pain, Seattle, p 495

Bennett GJ, Xie YK (1988) A peripheral mononeuropathy in rat that produces disorders of pain sensation like those seen in man. Pain 33:87–107

Bernard C (1851) Influence du grand sympathique sur la sensibilité et sur calorification. C R Soc Biol 3:163–164

Bhoola KD, Diete-Spiff K, Webster RA (1962) The effect of adrenaline on mammalian muscle spindles. J Physiol (Lond) 164:16P–17P

Blumberg H, Hoffmann U, Mohadjer M, Scheremet R (1994) Clinical phenomenology nd mechanisms of reflex sympathetic dystrophy: emphasis on edema. In: Gebhart GF, Hammond DL, Jensen TS (eds) Proceedings of the 7th World Congress on Pain. International Association for the Study of Pain, Seattle, p 455

Blumberg H, Jänig W (1982a) Activation of fibres via experimentally produced stump neuromas of skin nerves: ephaptic transmission or retrograde sprouting. Exp Neurol 76:468–482

Blumberg H, Jänig W (1982b) Changes in unmyelinated fibers including sympathetic postganglionic fibers of a skin nerve after peripheral neuroma formation. J Auton Nerv Syst 6:173–183

Blumberg H, Jänig W (1984) Discharge pattern of afferent fibers from a neuroma. Pain 20:335–353

Blumberg H, Jänig W (1985) Reflex patterns in postganglionic vasoconstrictor neurons following chronic nerve lesions. J Auton Nerv Syst 14:157–180

Bonica JJ (1990) The management of pain, 2nd edn. Lea and Febiger, Philadelphia

Bossut DF, Perl ER (1995) Effects of nerve injury on sympathetic excitation of $A\delta$ mechanical nociceptors. J Neurophysiol 73:1721–1723

Calma I, Kidd GL (1962) The effect of adrenaline on muscle spindle in cat. Arch Ital Biol 100:381–393

Campbell JN, Raja SN, Meyer RA, Mackinnon SE (1988) Myelinated afferents signal the hyperalgesia associated with nerve injury. Pain 32:89–94

Campbell JN, Meyer RA, Raja SN (1992) Is nociceptor activation by alpha-1 adrenoreceptors the culprit in sympathetically maintained pain. APS J 13:344–350

Cannon WB (1929) Bodily changes in pain, hunger fear and rage, 2nd edn. Appleton, New York

Carlton SM, Dougherty PM, Pover CM, Coggeshall RE (1991) Neuroma formation and numbers of axons in a rat model of experimental peripheral neuropathy. Neurosci Lett 131:88–92

Carlton SM, Lekan HA, Kim SH, Chung JM (1994) Behavioral manifestations of an experimental model for peripheral neuropathy produced by spinal nerve ligation in the primate. Pain 56:155–166

Cash RM, Linden RWA (1982) Effects of sympathetic nerve stimulation on intra-oral mechanoreceptor activity in the cat. J Physiol (Lond) 329:451–463

Chabal C, Jacobson L, Russell LC, Burchiel KJ (1992) Pain response to perineuromal injection of normal saline, epinephrine, and lidocaine in humans. Pain 49:9–12

Chung K, Kim HJ, Na HS, Yoon YW, Chung JM (1994) Changes in the sympathetic innervation to the sensory ganglia at variable times after a neuropathic nerve injury. Soc Neurosci Abstr 20:760

Coderre TJ, Grimes RW, Melzack R (1986) Deafferentation and chronic pain in animals: an evaluation of evidence suggesting autotomy is related to pain. Pain 26:61–84

Coderre TJ, Basbaum AI, Levine JD (1989) Neural control of vascular permeability: interactions between primary afferents, mast cells, and sympathetic efferents. J Neurophysiol 62:48–58

Coderre TJ, Basbaum AI, Dallman MF, Helms C, Levine JD (1990) Epinephrine exacerbates arthritis by an action at presynaptic β2-adrenoceptors. Neuroscience 34:521–523

Cunha FQ, Lorenzetti BB, Poole S, Ferreira SH (1991) Interleukin-8 as a mediator of sympathetic pain. Br J Pharmacol 104:765–767

Cunha FQ, Poole S, Lorenzetti BB, Ferreira SH (1992) The pivotal role of tumour necrosis factor alpha in the development of inflammatory hyperalgesia. Br J Pharmacol 107:660–664

Davar G, Fareed M, Lee DH, Noh HR, Chung JM (1996) Identification and increased expression of a novel alpha 2-adrenoreceptor mRNA in dorsal root ganglia in a rat model of experimental painful neuropathy. Abstracts of the 8th World Congress on Pain, p 29

Davis KD, Treede R-D, Raja SN, Meyer RA, Campbell JN (1991) Topical application of clonidine relieves hyperalgesia in patients with sympathetically maintained pain. Pain 47:309–317

Davis BM, Albers KM, Seroogy KB, Katz DM (1994) Overexpression of nerve growth factor in transgenic mice induces novel sympathetic projections to primary sensory neurons. J Comp Neurol 349:464–474

DeLeo JA, Coombs DW, Willenbring S, Colburn RW, Fromm C, Wagner R, Twitchell BB (1994) Characterisation of a neuropathic pain model: sciatic cryoneurolysis in the rat. Pain 56:9–16

Dellimijn PLI, Fields HL, Allen RR, McKay WR, Rowbotham MC (1994) The interpretation of pain relief and sensory changes follwoing sympathetic blockade. Brain 117:1475–1487

Desmeules JA, Kayser V, Weil Fuggaza J, Bertrand A, Guilbaud G (1995) Influence of the sympathetic nervous system in the development of abnormal pain-related behaviours in a rat model of neuropathic pain. Neuroscience 67:941–951

Devor M (1994) Pathophysiology of injured nerve. In: Wall PD, Melzack R (eds) Textbook of pain, 3rd edn. Churchill Livingstone, Edinburgh, p 79

Devor M, Jänig W (1981) Activation of myelinated afferents ending in a neuroma by stimulation of the sympathetic supply in the rat. Neurosci Lett 24:43–47

Devor M, Wall PD (1990) Cross-excitation in dorsal root ganglia of nerve-injured and intact rats. J Neurophysiol 64:1733–1746

Devor M, Jänig W, Michaelis M (1994) Modulation of activity in dorsal root ganglion neurons by sympathetic activation in nerve-injured rats. J Neurophysiol 71:38–47

Dotson R, Ochoa J, Cline M, Roberts W, Yarnitzky D, Simone D, Marchettini P (1990) Sympathetic effects on human low threshold mechanoreceptors. Soc Neurosci Abstr 16:1280

Drummond PD (1995) Noradrenaline increases hyperalgesia to heat in skin sensitized by capsaicin. Pain 60:311–315

Drummond PD (1996) Noradrenaline and ischaemia increase hyperalgesia to heat in capsaicin-treated skin. Abstracts of the 8th World Congress on Pain, p 35

Drummond PD, Finch PM, Smythe GA (1991) Reflex sympathetic dystrophy: the significance of differing plasma catecholamine concentrations in affected and unaffected limbs. Brain 114:2025–2036

Edwall L, Scott D (1971) Influence of changes in microcirculation on the excitabilty of the sensory unit in the tooth of the cat. Acta Physiol Scand 82:555–556

Elam M, Skarphedinsson JO, Olausson B, Wallin BG (1996) No apparent sympathetic modulation of single C-fiber afferent transmission in human volunteers. Abstracts of the 8th World Congress on Pain, pp 398–399

Eldred E, Schnitzlein HN, Buchwald J (1960) Responses of muscle spindles to stimulation of the sympathetic trunk. Exp Neurol 2:187–195

Eliav E, Bennett GJ (1996) An experimental neuritis of the rat sciatic nerve that produces unilateral allodynia and hyperalgesia in the hind paw. Abstracts of the 8th World Congress on Pain, p 26

Fontana DJ, Hunter JC (1996) Evidence against involvement of the sympathetic nervous system in the maintenance of mechanical allodynia following spinal nerve ligation (SNL). Abstracts of the 8th World Congress on Pain, p 31

Freeman B, Rowe M (1981) The effect of sympathetic nerve stimulation on responses of cutaneous Pacinian corpuscles in the cat. Neurosci Lett 22:145–150

Fruhstorfer H, Lindblom U, Schmidt WG (1976) Method for quantitative estimation of thermal thresholds in patients. J Neurol Neurosurg Psychiatry 39:1071–1075

Ghostine SY, Comair YG, Turner DM, Kassell N, Azar CG (1984) Phenoxybenzamine in the treatment of causalgia. J Neurosurg 60:1263–1268

Goldstein RS, Raber P, Govrin Lippmann R, Devor M (1988) Contrasting time course of catecholamine accumulation and of spontaneous discharge in experimental neuromas in the rat. Neurosci Lett 94:58–63

Gracely RH, Lynch SA, Bennett GJ (1992) Painful neuropathy: altered central processing, maintained dynamically by peripheral input. Pain 51:175–194

Green PG, Basbaum AI, Levine JD (1992) Sensory neuropeptide interactions in the production of plasma extravasation in the rat. Neuroscience 50:745–749

Green PG, Luo J, Hammond ER, Levine JD (1993a) Trypsin enhances sympathetic neuron-dependent plasma extravasation in the rat knee joint. Neurosci Lett 158:117–119

Green PG, Luo J, Heller P, Levine JD (1993b) Modulation of bradykinin-induced plasma extravasation in the rat knee joint by sympathetic co-transmitters. Neuroscience 52:451–458

Green PG, Luo J, Heller PH, Levine JD (1993c) Neurogenic and non-neurogenic mechanisms of plasma extravasation in the rat. Neuroscience 52:735–743

Green PG, Luo J, Heller PH, Levine JD (1993d) Further substantiation of a significant role for the sympathetic nervous system in inflammation. Neuroscience 55:1037–1043

Green PG, Miao FJ, Jänig W, Levine JD (1995) Negative feedback neuroendocrine control of the inflammatory response in rats. J Neurosci 15:4678–4686

Grethel EJ, Ringkamp M, Meyer RA, Raja SN (1996) Intraplantar administration of alpha-adrenergic antagonists does not alter responses of neuropathic rats to mechanical and cold stimuli. Abstracts of the 8th World Congress on Pain, pp 348–349

Häbler H-J, Jänig W, Koltzenburg M (1987) Activation of unmyelinated afferents in chronically lesioned nerves by adrenaline and excitation of sympathetic efferents in the cat. Neurosci Lett 82:35–40

Hallin RG, Wiesenfeld-Hallin Z (1983) Does sympathetic activity modify afferent inflow at the receptor level in man? J Auton Nerv Syst 7:391–397

Hannington-Kiff JG (1974) Intravenous regional sympathetic block with guanethedine. Lancet 1:1019–1020

Hess WR, Brugger M (1943) Das subkorticale Zentrum der affektiven Abwehrreaktion. Helv Physiol Acta 1:33–52

Hord AH, Rooks MD, Stephens BO, Rogers HG, Fleming LL (1992) Intravenous regional bretylium and lidocaine for treatment of reflex sympathetic dystrophy: a randomized, double-blind study. Anesth Analg 74:818–821

Hunt CC (1960) The effect of sympathetic nerve stimulation on mammalian muscle spindles. J Physiol (Lond) 151:332–341

Hunt CC, Jami L, Laporte Y (1982) Effects of stimulating the lumbar sympathetic trunk on cat hindlimb muscle spindles. Arch Ital Biol 120:371–384

Jänig W (1985) Organization of the lumbar sympathetic outflow to skeletal muscle and skin of the cat hindlimb and tail. Rev Physiol Biochem Pharmacol 102:119–213

Jänig W (1988) Pathophysiology of nerve following mechanical injury. In: Dubner R, Gebhart GF, Bond MR (eds) Proceedings of the 5th World Congress on Pain. Elsevier, Amsterdam, p 89

Jänig W (1990) Activation of afferent fibers ending in an old neuroma by sympathetic stimulation in the rat. Neurosci Lett 111:309–314

Jänig W, Koltzenburg M (1991) Plasticity of sympathetic reflex organization following cross-union of inappropiate nerves in the adult cat. J Physiol (Lond) 436:309–323

Jänig W, Koltzenburg M (1992) Possible ways of sympathetic-afferent interactions. In: Jänig W, Schmidt RF (eds) Pathophysiological mechanisms of reflex sympathetic dystrophy. VCH, Weinheim, p 213

Jänig W, McLachlan EM (1992) Characteristics of function-specific pathways in the sympathetic nervous system. Trends Neurosci 15:475–481

Jänig W, Stanton-Hicks M (1996) Reflex sympathetic dystrophy: a reappraisal. International Association for the Study of Pain, Seattle

Jobling P, McLachlan EM, Jänig W, Anderson CR (1992) Electrophysiological responses in the rat tail artery during reinnervation following lesions of the sympathetic supply. J Physiol (Lond) 454:107–128

Kajander KC, Bennett GJ (1992) Onset of a painful peripheral neuropathy in rat: a partial and differential deafferentation and spontaneous discharge in Aβ and Aδ primary afferent neurons. J Neurophysiol 68:734–744

Kajander KC, Wakisaka S, Bennett GJ (1992) Spontaneous discharge originates in the dorsal root ganglion at the onset of a painful peripheral neuropathy in the rat. Neurosci Lett 138:225–228

86   M. KOLTZENBURG

Karlström L, Dahlström A (1973) The effect of different typers of axonal trauma on the synthesis and transport of amine storage granules in rat sciatic nerve. J Neurobiol 4:191–200

Khasar SG, Miao FJ, Levine JD (1995) Inflammation modulates the contribution of receptor-subtypes to bradykinin-induced hyperalgesia in the rat. Neuroscience 69:685–690

Kibler RF, Nathan PW (1960) Relief of pain and paraesthesiae by nerve block distal to a lesion. J Neurol Neurosurg Psychiatry 23:91–98

Kieschke J, Mense S, Prabhakar NR (1988) Influence of adrenaline and hypoxia on rat muscle receptors in vitro. Prog Brain Res 74:91–97

Kim SH, Chung JM (1991) Sympathectomy alleviates mechanical allodynia in an experimental animal model for neuropathy in the rat. Neurosci Lett 134:131–134

Kim SH, Chung JM (1992) An experimental model for peripheral neuropathy produced by segmental spinal nerve ligation in the rat. Pain 50:355–363

Kim SH, Na HS, Sheen K, Chung JM (1993) Effects of sympathectomy on a rat model of peripheral neuropathy. Pain 55:85–92

Kinnman E, Levine JD (1995) Sensory and sympathetic contributions to nerve injury-induced sensory abnormalities in the rat. Neuroscience 64:751–767

Koltzenburg M (1995) The stability and plasticity of the encoding properties of peripheral nerve fibres and their relationship to provoked and ongoing pain. Semin Neurosci 7:199–210

Koltzenburg M, Kress M, Reeh PW (1992) The nociceptor sensitization by bradykinin does not depend on sympathetic neurones. Neuroscience 46:465–473

Koltzenburg M, Kees S, Budweiser S, Ochs G, Toyka KV (1994a) The properties of unmyelinated afferents change in a chronic constriction neuropathy. In: Gebhart GF, Hammond DL, Jensen TS (eds) Proceedings of the 7th World Congress on Pain. International Association for the Study of Pain, Seattle, p 511

Koltzenburg M, Torebjörk HE, Wahren LK (1994b) Nociceptor modulated central plasticity causes mechanical hyperalgesia in chronic neuropathic and acute chemogenic pain. Brain 117:579–591

Koltzenburg M, Häbler H-J, Jänig W (1995) Functional reinnervation of the vasculature of the adult cat paw pad by axons originally innervating vessels in hairy skin. Neuroscience 67:245–252

Koltzenburg M, Bennett DLH, McMahon SB, Shelton DL, Toyka KV (1996) Sequestration of endogenous nerve growth factor (NGF) reduces the sensitivity of nociceptors. Abstracts of the 8th World Congress on Pain, p 120

Konietzny F (1984) Peripheral neural correlates of temperature sensation in man. Human Neurobiol 3:21–32

Korenman EMD, Devor M (1981) Ectopic adrenergic sensitivity in damaged peripheral nerve axons in the rat. Exp Neurol 72:63–81

Kurvers HA, Jacobs MJ, Beuk RJ, Van den Wildenberg FA, Kitslaar PJ, Slaaf DW, Reneman RS (1995) Reflex sympathetic dystrophy: evolution of microcirculatory disturbances in time. Pain 60:333–340

Kurvers HA, Jacobs MJ, Beuk RJ, Van den Wildenberg FA, Kitslaar PJ, Slaaf DW, Reneman RS (1996a) The spinal component to skin blood flow abnormalities in reflex sympathetic dystrophy. Arch Neurol 53:58–65

Kurvers HAJM, Stassen F, Slaaf DW, Daemen MARC, van den Wildenberg FAJM, Kitslaar PJEHM, Jacobs MJHM, De Mey J (1996b) Loose ligation of the rat sciatic nerve induces autonomic denervation and hypersensitivity to catecholamines. Abstracts of the 8th World Congress on Pain, p 31

Lang E, Novak A, Reeh PW, Handwerker HO (1990) Chemosensitivity of fine afferents from rat skin in vitro. J Neurophysiol 63:887–901

Langley JN (1903) Das sympathische und verwandte nervöse System der Wirbeltiere (autonomes nervöses System). Ergeb Physiol 2:818–872

Levine J, Taiwo Y (1994) Inflammatory pain. In: Wall PD, Melzack R (eds) Textbook of pain, 3rd edn. Churchill Livingstone, Edinburgh, p 45

Levine JD, Dardick SJ, Roizen MF, Helms C, Basbaum AI (1986a) Contribution of sensory afferents and sympathetic efferents to joint injury in experimental arthritis. J Neurosci 6:3423–3429

Levine JD, Fye K, Heller P, Basbaum AI, Whiting OK (1986b) Clinical response to regional intravenous guanethidine in patients with rheumatoid arthritis. J Rheumatol 13:1040–1043

Levine JD, Taiwo YO, Collins SD, Tam JK (1986c) Noradrenaline hyperalgesia is mediated through interaction with sympathetic postganglionic neurone terminals rather than activation of primary afferent nociceptors. Nature 323:158–160

Levine JD, Coderre TJ, Helms C, Basbaum AI (1988) Beta 2-adrenergic mechanisms in experimental arthritis. Proc Natl Acad Sci USA 85:4553–4556

Lewin GR, Rueff A, Mendell LM (1994) Peripheral and central mechanisms of NGF-induced hyperalgesia. Eur J Neurosci 6:1903–1912

Lindblom U, Verrillo RT (1979) Sensory functions in chronic neuralgia. J Neurol Neurosurg Psychiatry 42:422–435

Lisney SJ (1989) Regeneration of unmyelinated axons after injury of mammalian peripheral nerve. Q J Exp Physiol 74:757–784

Lisney SJ, Devor M (1987) Afterdischarge and interactions among fibers in damaged peripheral nerve in the rat. Brain Res 415:122–136

Liu M, Max MB, Parada S, Robinovitz E, Bennett GJ (1996) Sympathetic blockade with intravenous phentolamine inhibits capsaicin-evoked mechanical allodynia in humans. Abstracts of the 8th World Congress on Pain, p 400

Livingstone WK (1943) Pain mechanisms: a physiological interpretation of Causalgia and its related states. Macmillan, New York

Loewy AD, Spyer KM (1990) Central regulation of autonomic functions. Oxford University Press, Oxford

Loh L, Nathan PW (1978) Painful peripheral states and sympathetic blocks. J Neurol Neurosurg Psychiatry 41:664–671

Magerl W, Koltzenburg M, Schmitz J, Handwerker HO (1996) Asymety and time course of cutaneous sympathetic reflex responses following sustained excitation of chemosensitive nociceptors in humans. J Auton Nerv Syst 57:63–72

Manning DC, Raja SN, Meyer RA, Campbell JN (1991) Pain and hyperalgesia after intradermal injection of bradykinin in humans. Clin Pharmacol Ther 50:721–729

Matsuo R, Ikehara A, Nokubi T, Morimoto T (1995) Inhibitory effect of sympathetic stimulation on activities of masseter muscle spindles and the jaw jerk reflex in rats. J Physiol (Lond) 483:239–250

Matthews B (1976) Efect of sympathetic stimulation on the response of intradermal nerves to chemical stimulation. In: Bonica JJ, Albe Fessard DG (eds) Proceeding of the 1st World Congress on Pain. Raven, New York, p 195

Maves TJ, Pechman PS, Gebhart GF, Meller ST (1992) Possible chemical contribution from chromic gut sutures produces disorders of pain sensation like those seen in man. Pain 54:57–69

Maves TJ, Pechman PS, Gebhart GF, Meller ST (1993) Continuous infusion of acidified saline around the rat sciatic nerve produces a reversible thermal hyperalgesia. Abstracts of the 7th World Congress on Pain. International Association for the Study of Pain, Seattle, p 31

McLachlan EM, Jänig W, Devor M, Michaelis M (1993) Peripheral nerve injury triggers noradrenergic sprouting within dorsal root ganglia. Nature 363:543–546

McMahon SB (1991) Mechanisms of sympathetic pain. Br Med Bull 47:584–600

McMahon SB, Bennett DL, Priestley JV, Shelton DL (1995) The biological effects of endogenous nerve growth factor on adult sensory neurons revealed by a trkA-IgG fusion molecule. Nat Med 1:774–780

Mense S (1986) Slowly conducting afferent fibres from deep tissues: neurobiological properties and central nervous actions. Prog Sens Physiol 6:139–219

Merskey H, Bogduk M (1994) Classification of chronic pain, 2nd edn. International Association for the Study of Pain, Seattle

Meyer RA, Campbell JN (1987) Coupling between unmyelinated peripheral nerve fibers does not involve sympathetic efferent fibers. Brain Res 437:181–182

Meyer RA, Raja SN (1996) Intradermal norepinephrine produces a dose-dependent hyperalgesia to heat in humans. Abstracts of the 8th World Congress on Pain, p 398

Meyer RA, Campbell JN, Raja SN (1988) Antidromic nerve stimulation in monkey does not sensitize unmyelinated nociceptors to heat. Brain Res 441:168–172

Meyer RA, Davis KD, Raja SN, Campbell JN (1992) Sympathectomy does not abolish bradykinin-induced cutaneous hyperalgesia in man. Pain 51:323–327

Meyer RA, Campbell JN, Raja SN (1994) Peripheral neural mechanisms of nociception. In: Wall PD, Melzack R (eds) Textbook of pain, 3rd edn. Churchill Livingstone, Edinburgh, p 13

Munger BL, Bennett GJ, Kajander KC (1992) An experimental painful peripheral neuropathy due to nerve constriction. I. Axonal pathology in the sciatic nerve. Exp Neurol 118:204–214

Na HS, Leem JW, Chung JM (1993) Abnormalities of mechanoreceptors in a rat model of neuropathic pain: possible involvement in mediating mechanical allodynia. J Neurophysiol 70:522–528

Nakamura M, Ferreira SH (1987) A peripheral sympathetic component in the inflammatory hyperalgesia. Eur J Pharmacol 135:145–153

Neil A, Attal N, Guilbaud G (1991) Effects of guanethidine on sensitization to natural stimuli and self-mutilating behaviour in rats with a peripheral neuropathy. Brain Res 565:237–246

Nilsson BY (1972) Effects of sympathetic stimulation on mechanoreceptors of cat vibrissae. Acta Physiol Scand 85:390–397

Nurmikko T, Wells C, Bowsher D (1991) Pain and allodynia in postherpetic neuralgia: role of somatic and sympathetic nervous systems. Acta Neurol Scand 84:146–152

Ochoa JL (1993) Guest editorial: essence, investigation, and management of "neuropathic" pains: hopes from acknowledgment of chaos. Muscle Nerv 16:997–1008

Ochoa JL, Verdugo RJ (1993) Reflex sympathetic dystrophy: definitions and history of the ideas with a critical review of human studies. In: Low P (ed) Clinical autonomic disorders. Little Brown, Boston, p 473

Ochoa JL, Yarnitzky D (1993) Mechanical hyperalgesias in neuropathic pain patients: dynamic and static subtypes. Ann Neurol 33:465–472

Passatore M, Filippi CM (1981) On whether there is a direct sympathetic influence on jaw muscle spindles. Brain Res 219:162–165

Passatore M, Filippi CM (1983) Sympathetic modulation of peridontal mechanoreceptors. Arch Ital Biol 121:55–65

Perl ER (1994) Causalgia and reflex sympathetic dystrophy revisited. In: Boivie J, Hansson P, Lindblom U (eds) Touch, temperature, and pain in health and disease: mechanisms and assessments. International Association for the Study of Pain, Seattle, p 231

Perrot S, Attal N, Ardid D, Guilbaud G (1993) Are mechanical and cold allodynia in mononeuropathic and arthritic rats relieved by systemic treatment with calcitonin or guanethidine? Pain 52:41–47

Pierce JP, Roberts WJ (1981) Sympathetic induced changes in the response of guard hair and type II receptors in the cat. J Physiol (Lond) 314:411–428

Pierce PA, Xie GX, Peroutka SJ, Green PG, Levine JD (1995) 5-Hydroxytryptamine-induced synovial plasma extravasation is mediated via 5-hydroxytryptamine 2a receptors on sympathetic efferent terminals. J Pharmacol Exp Ther 275:502–508

Price DD, Bennett GJ, Rafii A (1989) Psychophysical observations on patients with neuropathic pain relieved by a sympathetic block. Pain 36:273–288

Price DD, Long S, Huitt C (1992) Sensory testing of pathophysiological mechanisms of pain in patients with reflex sympathetic dystrophy. Pain 49:163–173

Raja SN, Treede R-D, Davis KD, Campbell JN (1991) Systemic alpha-adrenergic blockade with phentolamine: a diagnostic test for sympathetically maintained pain. Masui 74:691–698

Reeh PW, Kress M (1995) Effect of classic algogens. Semin Neurosci 7:221–226

Reeh PW, Kocher L, Jung S (1986) Does neurogenic inflammation alter the sensitivty of unmyelinated nociceptors in the rat? Brain Res 384:42–50

Ringkamp M, Ali Z, Chien HF, Campbell JN, Flavahan NA, Meyer RA (1996) Alpha-one adrenergic sensitivity in cutaneous C-fiber nociceptors following an L6 nerve ligation in monkey. Abstracts of the 8th World Congress on Pain, p 349

Risling M, Dalsgaard CJ, Terenius L (1985) Neuropeptide Y-like immunoreactivity in the lumbosacral pia mater in normal cats and after sciatic neuroma formation. Brain Res 358:372–375

Roberts WJ, Elardo SM (1985a) Sympathetic activation of unmyelinated mechanore-ceptors in cat skin. Brain Res 339:123–125

Roberts WJ, Elardo SM (1985b) Sympathetic activation of A-delta nociceptors. Somatosens Res 3:33–44

Roberts WJ, Levitt GR (1982) Histochemical evidence for sympathetic innervation of hair receptor afferents in cat skin. J Comp Neurol 210:204–209

Roberts WJ, Elardo SM, King KA (1985) Sympathetically induced changes in the responses of slowly adapting type I receptors in cat skin. Somatosens Res 2:223–236

Rowbotham MC, Fields HL (1989) Topical lidocaine reduces pain in post-herpetic neuralgia. Pain 38:297–301

Rowbotham MC, Davies PS, Fields HL (1995) Topical lidocaine gel relieves postherpetic neuralgia. Ann Neurol 37:246–253

Safieh Garabedian B, Poole S, Allchorne A, Winter J, Woolf CJ (1995) Contribution of interleukin-1 beta to the inflammation-induced increase in nerve growth factor levels and inflammatory hyperalgesia. Br J Pharmacol 115:1265–1275

Sanjue H, Jun Z (1989) Sympathetic fascilitation of sustained discharges of polymodal nociceptors. Pain 38:85–90

Sato J, Perl ER (1991) Adrenergic excitation of cutaneous pain receptors induced by peripheral nerve injury. Science 251:1608–1610

Sato J, Suzuki S, Iseki T, Kumazawa T (1993) Adrenergic excitation of cutaneous nociceptors in chronically inflamed rats. Neurosci Lett 164:225–228

Sato J, Suzuki S, Tamura R, Kumazawa T (1994) Norepinephrine excitation of cutane-ous nociceptors in adjuvant-induced inflamed rats does not depend on symathetic neurons. Neurosci Lett 177:135–138

Scadding JW (1981) Development of ongoing activity, mechanosensitivity, and adrena-line sensitivity in severed peripheral nerve axons. Exp Neurol 73:345–364

Scadding JW, Wall PD, Parry CB, Brooks DM (1982) Clinical trial of propranolol in post-traumatic neuralgia. Pain 14:283–292

Schaible H-G, Grubb BD (1993) Afferent and spinal mechanisms of joint pain. Pain 55:5–54

Schott GD (1994) Visceral afferents: their contribution to 'sympathetic dependent' pain. Brain 117:397–413

Selig DK, Meyer RA, Campbell JN (1993) Noradrenaline excitation of cutaneous nociceptors two weeks after ligation of spinal nerve L7 in monkey. Soc Neurosci Abstr 19:326

Seltzer Z, Dubner R, Shir Y (1990) A novel behavioral model of neuropathic pain disorders produced in rats by partial sciatic nerve injury. Pain 43:205–218

Shea VK, Perl ER (1985) Failure of sympathetic stimulation to affect responsiveness of rabbit polymodal nociceptors. J Neurophysiol 54:513–519

Sherbourne CD, Gonzales R, Goldyne ME, Levine JD (1992) Norepinephrine-induced increase in sympathetic neuron-derived prostaglandins is independent of neuronal release mechanisms. Neurosci Lett 139:188–190

Shir Y, Seltzer Z (1991) Effects of sympathectomy in a model of causalgiform pain produced by partial sciatic nerve injury in rats. Pain 45:309–320

Siuciak JA, Lewis D, Lindsay RM (1996) Blockade of NGF hyperalgesia with TrkA-IgG receptor body. Abstracts of the 8th World Congress on Pain, p 120

Sommer C, Galbraith JA, Heckman HM, Myers RR (1993) Pathology of experimental compression neuropathy producing hyperesthesia. J Neuropathol Exp Neurol 52:223–233

Stanton-Hicks M, JΣnig W, Hassenbusch S, Haddox JD, Boas R, Wilson P (1995) Reflex sympathetic dystrophy: changing concepts and taxonomy. Pain 63:127–133

Stanton-Hicks M, Raj PP, Racs GB (1996) Use of regional anesthetics for diagnosis of reflex sympathetic dystrophy and sympathetically maintained pain: a critical evaluation. In: Jänig W, Stanton-Hicks M (eds) Reflex sympathetic dystrophy: a repraisal. International Association for the Study of Pain, Seattle, p 217

Stevens RT, Hodge CJ, Apkarian V (1983) Catecholamine varicosities in cat dorsal root ganglion and spinal ventral roots. Brain Res 261:151–154

Taiwo YO, Levine JD (1988) Characterization of the arachidonic acid metabolites mediating bradykinin and noradrenaline hyperalgesia. Brain Res 458:402–406

Taiwo YO, Levine JD (1989) Prostaglandin effects after elimination of indirect hyperalgesic mechanisms in the skin of the rat. Brain Res 492:397–399

Taiwo YO, Levine JD (1990) Direct cutaneous hyperalgesia induced by adenosine. Neuroscience 38:757–762

Taiwo YO, Goetzl EJ, Levine JD (1987) Hyperalgesia onset latency suggests a hierarchy of action. Brain Res 423:333–337

Taiwo YO, Bjerknes LK, Goetzl EJ, Levine JD (1989) Mediation of primary afferent peripheral hyperalgesia by the cAMP second messenger system. Neuroscience 32:577–580

Taiwo YO, Heller PH, Levine JD (1990) Characterization of distinct phospholipases mediating bradykinin and noradrenaline hyperalgesia. Neuroscience 39:523–531

Torebjörk E (1990) Clinical and neurophysiological observations relating to pathophysiological mechanisms in reflex sympathetic dystrophy. In: Stanton-Hicks M, Jänig W, Boas RA (eds) Reflex sympathetic dystrophy. Kluwer Academic, Boston, p 71

Torebjörk E, Wahren LK, Wallin G, Hallin R, Koltzenburg M (1995) Noradrenaline-evoked pain in neuralgia. Pain 63:11–20

Tracey DJ, Cunningham JE, Romm MA (1995a) Peripheral hyperalgesia in experimental neuropathy: mediation by alpha 2-adrenoreceptors on post-ganglionic sympathetic terminals. Pain 60:317–327

Tracey DJ, Romm MA, Yao NN (1995b) Peripheral hyperalgesia in experimental neuropathy: exacerbation by neuropeptide Y. Brain Res 669:245–254

Treede R-D, Davis KD, Campbell JN, Raja SN (1992a) The plasticity of cutaneous hyperalgesia during sympathetic ganglion blockade in patients with neuropathic pain. Brain 115:607–621

Treede R-D, Meyer RA, Raja SN, Campbell JN (1992b) Peripheral and central mechanisms of cutaneous hyperalgesia. Prog Neurobiol 38:397–421

Utzschneider D, Kocsis J, Devor M (1992) Mutual excitation among dorsal root ganglion neurons in the rat. Neurosci Lett 146:53–56

Verdugo R, Ochoa JL (1992) Quantitative somatosensory thermotest. A key method for functional evaluation of small calibre afferent channels. Brain 115:893–913

Wahren LK, Torebjörk E (1992) Quantitative sensory tests in patients with neuralgia 11 to 25 years after injury. Pain 48:237–244

Wahren LK, Torebjörk E, Nyström B (1991) Quantitative sensory testing before and after regional guanethidine block in patients with neuralgia in the hand. Pain 46:23–30

Wakisaka S, Kajander KC, Bennett GJ (1991) Abnormal skin temperature and abnormal sympathetic vasomotor innervation in an experimental painful peripheral neuropathy. Pain 46:299–313

Walker AE, Nulsen F (1948) Electrical stimulation of the upper thoracic portion of the sympathetic chain in man. Arch Neurol Psychiatry 59:559–560

Wall PD, Gutnick M (1974) Properties of afferent nerve impulses originating from a neuroma. Nature 248:740–743

Wallin BG, Torebjörk HE, Hallin RG (1976) Preliminary observations on the patho-physiology of hyperalgesia in the causaligic pain syndrome. In: Zotterman Y (ed) Sensory functions of the skin in primates. Pergamon, Oxford, p 489

Welk E, Leah JD, Zimmermann M (1990) Characteristics of A-fibers and C-fibers ending in a sensory nerve neuroma in the rat. J Neurophysiol 63:759–766

White JC, Sweet WH (1969) Pain and the neurosurgeon: a forty year experience. Thomas, Springfield

Wiesenfeld-Hallin Z, Hallin RG (1984a) Can sympathetic outflow influence afferent activity in man? In: von Euler C, Franzén O, Lindblom U, Ottoson D (eds) Somatosensory mechanisms. Macmillan, London, p 197

Wiesenfeld-Hallin Z, Hallin RG (1984b) The influence of the sympathetic system on mechanoreception and nociception. A review. Human Neurobiol 3:41–46

Willenbring S, Beauprie IG, DeLeo JA (1995a) Sciatic cryoneurolysis in rats: a model of sympathetically independent pain. I. Effects of sympathectomy. Anesth Analg 81:544–548

Willenbring S, DeLeo JA, Coombs DW (1995b) Sciatic cryoneurolysis in rats: a model of sympathetically independent pain. II. Adrenergic pharmacology. Anesth Analg 81:549–554

Woolf CJ, Safieh Garabedian B, Ma QP, Crilly P, Winters J (1994) Nerve growth factor contributes to the generation of inflammotory sensory hypersensitivity. Neuro-science 62:327–331

Woolf CJ, Ma QP, Allchorne A, Poole S (1996) Peripheral cell types contributing to the hyperalgesic action of nerve growth factor in inflammation. J Neurosci 15:2716–2723

Xie Y, Zhang J, Petersen M, LaMotte RH (1995) Functional changes in dorsal root ganglion cells after chronic nerve constriction in the rat. J Neurophysiol 73:1811–1820

White JC, Sweet WH (1969) Pain and the neurosurgeon: a forty year experience. Thomas, Springfield

CHAPTER 5

Excitability Blockers: Anticonvulsants and Low Concentration Local Anesthetics in the Treatment of Chronic Pain

H.L. FIELDS, M.C. ROWBOTHAM, and M. DEVOR

A. Introduction

The major use of anticonvulsants is in the treatment of epileptic seizures. Local anesthetics are used primarily to block peripheral nerves for temporary anesthesia or diagnostic purposes to temporarily relieve pain or to enable minor surgery. In recent years a new use for systemic administration of local anesthetics and anticonvulsants has emerged: the treatment of specific chronically painful conditions. This use permits anticonvulsants and local anesthetics to be rationally grouped together as specialized analgesics. While neither class of drug has a clearly established analgesic efficacy for most common pains, both can dramatically relieve patients with severe neuropathic pain. The weight of evidence suggests that their effectiveness is greatest for those painful conditions associated with abnormal neuronal discharge. The basis for this action appears to be correction of the pathophysiological disturbance initiated by the neural injury. Specifically, they stabilize abnormally excitable nerve membranes.

Recent research on animal models of neuropathic pain and on human pain patients, and the completion of clinical trials of anticonvulsants and subanesthetic concentrations of local anesthetics, has brought us a new appreciation of a clinically important mechanism for the production of neuropathic pain: ectopic impulse generation by damaged, dysfunctional primary sensory neurons and their axons. This abnormal, ectopic discharge can be suppressed by drugs that have been used as membrane stabilizers in other contexts: anticonvulsants and local anesthetics used at concentrations far too low to block the propagation of action potentials in normal nerves (GLAZER and PORTENOY 1991; TANELIAN and VICTORY 1995). Because the process of ectopic impulse generation is far more sensitive to these drugs than is normal impulse conduction, it is possible to give them systemically or topically without massive failure of other systems that depend on normal nerve conduction.

This chapter discusses anticonvulsants and systemic local anesthetics in the context of current concepts of the pathophysiology of neuropathic pain. First, we review the clinical literature relating to their use and efficacy in the treatment of neuropathic pain. We then summarize the basic animal and human research that has given rise to these concepts.

B. Anticonvulsants in the Treatment of Neuropathic Pain

I. Trigeminal Neuralgia (Tic Douloureux)

Long before there was any certain knowledge of the mechanisms of neuropathic pain BERGOUIGNAN (1942) reported that the anticonvulsant diphenylhydantoin (phenytoin, Dilantin) can abort the severe, lancinating pain of trigeminal neuralgia. Carbamazepine (Tegretol) was later found to be even more effective (IANNONE et al. 1958; ROCKLIFF and DAVIS 1966) and is currently the treatment of choice for this condition. Trigeminal neuralgia is a very distinctive and easily diagnosed condition. It occurs mainly in the distribution of the mandibular and/or maxillary branches of the trigeminal nerve, primarily in elderly patients with no other neurological abnormalities. Pain consists of one or a cluster of spontaneous brief (<1s) "lightning" stabs of sharp pain, separated by pain free intervals. The pain may remit spontaneously for months or even years (RAPPAPORT and DEVOR 1994). A similar condition occurs in the sensory distribution of the 9th cranial nerve (glossopharyngeal neuralgia).

In over 70% of patients with trigeminal neuralgia pain is initially controlled rapidly and completely on standard anticonvulsant doses of carbamazepine. This is all the more impressive since the pain is cripplingly severe and is thought resistant to even high doses of opioid analgesics. Although many drugs with anticonvulsant activity are effective in patients with trigeminal neuralgia, others, such as pentobarbital, are not (SWERDLOW 1984). The mechanism of anticonvulsant action apparently makes a difference (see below).

There is currently no satisfactory animal model for trigeminal neuralgia, and underlying neural mechanisms remain uncertain (FROMM et al. 1984; DUBNER et al. 1987; RAPPAPORT and DEVOR 1994). Damage to primary afferent neurons is thought to play a major role in the generation of pain (KERR 1979). Typical tic-like pain is seen in some patients with demyelinating disease (multiple sclerosis) and is occasionally caused by tumors that compress the trigeminal nerve or root. At surgery most patients with idiopathic trigeminal neuralgia are found to have blood vessels that impinge intradurally on the trigeminal root, resulting in local demyelination (JANNETTA 1967). Removing the vessel from direct contact with the root provides prolonged relief (JANNETTA 1976). This suggests that compression and/or local demyelination of trigeminal axons causes abnormal afferent discharge that results in pain. Sites at which afferent axons are experimentally compressed and demyelinated are known to become sources of abnormal ectopic discharge (BURCHIEL 1980; CALVIN et al. 1982, 1977). This discharge is highly sensitive to anticonvulsant concentrations of carbamazepine and phenytoin (BURCHIEL 1988; YAARI and DEVOR 1985).

Suppression of ectopic impulses by excitability blockers is discussed in detail below as a way of explaining their analgesic effectiveness in neuropathic pain. However, patients with trigeminal neuralgia have characteristic clinical features that are not explained by spontaneous ectopic impulses. First is the brief, electric-like quality of the pain, and, second, tic patients have highly sensitive localized trigger points on their face or gums. This hypersensitivity is often disabling as it may preclude normal eating or speaking. An intriguing proposal to explain these characteristic clinical features of trigeminal neuralgia is "cross-excitation" among adjacent primary afferents. A strategically located excitation may activate neighboring afferents, which, in turn, would activate their neighbors, and so forth, resulting in a positive-feedback "chain reaction" (RAPPAPORT and DEVOR 1994). Such spread of ectopic firing can occur among axons at the trigeminal root compression site and/or within the trigeminal ganglion proper. There are several ways that this cross-excitation could occur. These include electric fields ("ephaptic cross-talk"), and ion- or neurotransmitter-mediated interaction (LISNEY and DEVOR 1987; RAPPAPORT and DEVOR 1994; RASMINSKY 1980; SELTZER and DEVOR 1979).

In addition to accounting for trigger points, cross-excitation might also explain the paroxysmal nature of sensation in tic douloureux. Specifically, bursts would be expected if the chain reaction proceeds rapidly and if it includes a spread of activity from touch sensitive afferents to adjacent nociceptors (RAPPAPORT and DEVOR 1994). Finally, cross-excitation can account for the peculiar "electric shock-like" quality of the sensation in tic, and other neuropathic pain states. Both cross-excitation in an injured nerve and electric shocks differ from natural stimuli in that both can simultaneously activate all types of afferents at high frequency.

II. Other Painful Conditions Responding to Anticonvulsants

Because of its dramatic success in the treatment of trigeminal neuralgia carbamazepine has been used by neurologists to treat a variety of other painful conditions. Table 1 lists painful conditions that have been reported to respond to anticonvulsants (DUNSKER and MAYFIELD 1976; ESPIR and MILLAC 1970; FIELDS and RASKIN 1976; LEIJON and BOIVIE 1989; McQUAY et al. 1995; SHIBASAKI and KUROIWA 1975; SWERDLOW 1984). In several of these conditions a lancinating or shooting component is present. In one of the most common, diabetic neuropathy, the pain is often steady and burning, but some patients have a "shooting" component (RULL et al. 1969). SWERDLOW and CUNDILL (1981) reported their experience with 170 patients treated for "lancinating" pain. In their uncontrolled study the pains were due to a variety of causes. These authors reported that each of four anticonvulsants: phenytoin, carbamazepine, clonazepam, and valproic acid were helpful for some patients. A clear exception to this generalization is that some anticonvulsants are effective in the prophylaxis of migraine headaches, a painful condition which has no paroxysmal component (McQUAY et al. 1995).

III. Clinical Use of Anticonvulsants

The range of plasma levels required for therapy of trigeminal neuralgia and epilepsy are the same for carbamazepine, and although it has not been system-

Table 1. Painful conditions responsive to anticonvulsants and local anesthetics

Condition	Drugs	Evidence for efficacy
Trigeminal neuralgia	Carbamazepine	A
	Tocainide	B
	Phenytoin, clonazepam, valproate, lidocaine i.v., gabapentin	C
Other cranial neuralgias	Phenytoin, carbamazepine, valproate, clonazepam	C
Diabetic neuropathy	Phenytoin, carbamazepine, mexiletine, i.v. lidocaine	A
	Topical lidocaine	C
Mono- and polyneuropathies	Carbamazepine, lidocaine i.v., mexiletine, gabapentin, topical lidocaine	C
Fabry's disease	Phenytoin	B
Radiculopathy	Lidocaine i.v.	C
Postherpetic neuralgia	Topical lidocaine	A
	Lidocaine i.v.	B
	Clonazepam, valproate[a], phenytoin, carbamazepine[b]	C
Central poststroke pain	Phenytoin, mexiletine	C
	Carbamazepine[b]	C
Multiple sclerosis	Carbamazepine	B
	Mexiletine	C
Stump pain	Carbamazepine	C
Complex regional pain syndrome	Lidocaine i.v., gabapentin	C

A, Multiple randomized controlled trials show efficacy; B, single randomized controlled trial shows efficacy; C, uncontrolled studies or anecdotal reports of multiple patients.
[a] Valproate combined with amitriptyline.
[b] Controlled study showed no benefit compared to placebo.

atically studied, there is no reason to think that this is not the case for the other anticonvulsants. This does not mean, however, that neuropathic pain necessarily results from seizure activity in the CNS. The processes whereby carbamazepine and phenytoin suppress abnormal CNS activity may also be relevant to abnormal ectopic firing in the peripheral nervous system (PNS; BURCHIEL 1988; CATTERALL 1987; YAARI and DEVOR 1985). Readers are referred to RALL and SCHLEIFER (1985) and LEVY et al. (1995) for a detailed account of the pharmacology of anticonvulsants.

1. Carbamazepine

Carbamazepine is the first-line drug for the treatment of trigeminal neuralgia and is worth trying for other neuropathic pain conditions. Because of individual variation in the pharmacokinetics of carbamazepine and the fact that signs of toxicity appear near the upper end of the therapeutic range of plasma concentrations, it is important to carefully adjust the dose when initiating long-term therapy. Therapy is initiated with a dose of 100 mg twice daily. The dose should be increased in 100 mg increments every few days until either complete relief is obtained or signs of toxicity appear (LEVY et al. 1995). For most patients therapeutic plasma concentrations are between 5 and 10 μg/ml, and side effects usually appear at levels above 8 μg/ml (TOMSON et al. 1980). In a given patient there may be a very sharp threshold for the plasma level required to obtain relief. For example, in one patient of ours a plasma level of 5.6 μg/ml gave no relief, whereas a level of 6.4 μg/ml gave complete relief. A possible explanation for such threshold behavior is provided below.

Dose-related side effects include sedation, ataxia, vertigo, and blurred vision. Nausea and vomiting are also common. A mild leukopenia occurs in about 10% of patients and persists in one-quarter of these. Because of rare cases of irreversible aplastic anemia, regular monitoring of hematological function is recommended. Since trigeminal neuralgia typically undergoes spontaneous remissions, it is worthwhile trying to taper the drug after 3–6 months and reinstituting therapy if the pain returns.

Carbamazepine is the first-line anticonvulsant for long-term treatment of trigeminal neuralgia. Other drugs are available as a second line or add-on drug if side effects or a drug reaction limits the use of carbamazepine. No comparative studies are available to rank-order these alternatives: phenytoin, baclofen, valproic acid, and clonazepam.

2. Phenytoin

Phenytoin was the first anticonvulsant to be utilized in pain management. Uncontrolled studies on a total of 49 patients reported phenytoin to be effective in the treatment of trigeminal neuralgia (IANNONE et al. 1958). Double-blind placebo controlled studies have demonstrated analgesia with diphenylhydantoin in both diabetic neuropathy and Fabry's disease (a small fiber neuropathy). Phenytoin is available for parenteral administration and can be used in patients who are having severe (CHADDA and MATHUR 1978; LOCKMAN et al. 1973) and frequent attacks. In such patients intravenous administration of phenytoin may provide immediate relief. For intravenous administration the commercially prepared phenytoin should be diluted by one-half in normal saline immediately before use and injected in boluses of 50 μg or less each minute, to a total dose of 600–1000 mg.

3. Clonazepam

Clonazepam should be considered as a third-line drug for lancinating neuropathic pain, especially in patients who require plasma levels of carbamazepine or phenytoin approaching the toxic range in order to obtain pain relief. Unlike the other anticonvulsants reviewed here, clonazepam is structurally and pharmacologically related to the benzodiazepine family. Its antiepileptic mechanism is uncertain but is presumed to involve potentiation of inhibitory GABA neurotransmission. The reduction in pain intensity with clonazepam may be due to its antianxiety and antispasticity effects rather that to its anticonvulsant effect. There is limited evidence for pain relief with other benzodiazepines (DELLEMIJN and FIELDS 1994).

Successful treatment of a variety of cranial neuralgias with clonazepam has been reported in uncontrolled studies that include a total of 46 trigeminal neuralgia patients, and a small number suffering from sphenopalatine ganglion neuralgia, malignant skull base neuralgia, glossopharyngeal neuralgia, and cluster headache (CACCIA 1975; COURT and KASE 1976; SMIRNE and SCARLATO 1977). Effective daily doses ranged from 3 to 8 mg. Conversely, MAX and coworkers (1988) studied lorazepam, another benzodiazepine with anticonvulsant properties, in a double-blind cross-over comparison with amitriptyline and placebo in patients with postherpetic neuralgia. Lorazepam was ineffective compared to amitriptyline.

To lessen sedation the initial dose of clonazepam should be as low as 0.5 mg taken at bedtime. The dose is then titrated to effect by adding 0.5 mg every 3–5 days and dividing the total daily dose so that it is given two to four times per day. The maximum dose recommended for the treatment of epilepsy is 20 mg per day, but significant analgesia or intolerable side effects, usually sedation, should be apparent at doses below 8 mg per day. Clonazepam's elimination half-life is 18–39 h. Catabolism is by first-order kinetics. Being a CNS depressant, acute toxicity of clonazepam produces confusion, somnolence, hypotension, and even coma. Patients should be warned that their ability to perform hazardous activities such as driving may be impaired. Transiently elevated serum aminotransferase and alkaline phosphatase, anemia, leukopenia, thrombocytopenia, and eosinophilia have all been reported. Periodic complete blood counts, platelet count, and liver function tests should be performed. Clonazepam should be discontinued with a gradual taper, as abrupt stoppage may result in severe withdrawal symptoms, including seizures. Because clonazepam is a benzodiazepine, patients with a history of substance abuse or alcoholism should be warned and monitored closely for signs of psychological dependence.

4. Valproic Acid

Valproic acid may be useful for chronic headache but has been little studied for neuropathic pain. In an open label study PEIRIS et al. (1980) reported partial or complete control of trigeminal neuralgia in 9/20 patients with valproic acid in doses of up to 1200 mg/day.

Valproic acid and divalproex sodium are structurally unrelated to any of the other anticonvulsants. Valproic acid is most often prescribed as divalproex sodium (Depakote), an equal combination of valproic acid an sodium valproate. Its anticonvulsant mechanism of action is unknown, but valproic acid is known to increase brain γ-aminobutyric acid (GABA). No plasma level therapeutic range has been established for pain control with valproic acid.

Similar to the treatment of seizures, the starting dose for the treatment of pain is 250 mg twice per day, and the dose is gradually titrated to effect. Side effects and potentially serious toxicity have greatly limited the use of valproic acid for chronic pain. The combination of sedation, gastrointestinal side effects, hair loss (usually reversible), abnormal liver function tests, potentially fatal hepatotoxicity, inhibition of platelet aggregation, and numerous other potential hematological and nonhematological effects make pre-treatment screening and close follow-up mandatory.

5. Gabapentin

Gabapentin was approved for marketing in the United States in 1995 as adjunctive therapy in the treatment of seizures. The drug is structurally related to the neurotransmitter GABA but does not interact with GABA receptors and is not converted into GABA or another GABA agonist. Although it does not appear to block GABA reuptake, it does enhance the release of GABA from nerve terminals (HONMOU et al. 1995).

Because of its apparently benign side effect profile and relative lack of drug interactions, gabapentin is currently entering widespread use for pain management as an alternative to the best established anticonvulsant, carbamazepine. A recent report suggests that gabapentin is useful in treating reflex sympathetic dystrophy (MELLICK et al. 1995), and a small series of patients with neuropathic pain has recently been reported (ROSNER et al. 1996). However, as of this writing, there are no published controlled clinical studies on gabapentin as an analgesic agent.

Unlike carbamazepine, clinical trials do not indicate that routine monitoring of clinical laboratory parameters is necessary for safe use of gabapentin. Furthermore, the drug may be used in combination with other anticonvulsant drugs; it is not appreciably metabolized, bioavailability is high, and kinetics are straightforward, with an elimination half-life of 5–7 h. The dose must be adjusted in patients with renal failure, but no adjustment is necessary in patients with hepatic disorders because the drug is not appreciably metabolized. The most common side effects are related to CNS depression, such as dizziness or somnolence. Dosage recommendations for adults are a starting dose of 300 mg per day, increasing in 300 mg/day increments as tolerated to 300–600 mg three times a day. Doses of 2400–3600 mg/day have been used for short periods or in clinical trials. Acute oral overdoses of up to 49 g have been reported without fatality. Because of the short half-life, doses should not be given more than 12 h apart and discontinuation of the drug should be spread over a 1 week (or longer) period.

6. Lamotrigine

As with gabapentin, lamotrigine is approved for use in addition to other anticonvulsant drugs in the treatment of partial seizures. Lamotrigine is similar to phenytoin and carbamazepine in blocking voltage-dependent sodium channels (CHEUNG et al. 1992), and it reduces the release of the excitatory transmitters glutamate and aspartate (TEOH et al. 1995). Lamotrigine is well absorbed from the gastrointestinal tract, with peak plasma levels in 1.5–5h. It is metabolized by glucuronidation and has a single-dose half-life of 24h. Unlike gabapentin, there are significant interactions of lamotrigine with other anticonvulsants. Concurrent use of carbamazepine and lamotrigine increases carbamazepine levels and can produce clinical toxicity. Valproate concentrations are decreased and lamotrigine half-life more than doubles when lamotrigine is used concurrently with valproic acid. Concurrent use of lamotrigine with phenobarbital, phenytoin, or primidone leads to shortening of the lamotrigine half-life because of induction of hepatic glucuronidation enzymes.

Although it reportedly has an analgesic action in rodents with nerve damage (NAKAMURA-CRAIG and FOLLENFANT 1995), there are no published clinical trials of lamotrigine for pain. Dizziness, diplopia, ataxia, blurred vision, nausea, vomiting, and rash are the most common adverse effects when the drug is added to other anticonvulsants, with rash occurring in 10% of patients. Starting doses depend on other drugs being used concurrently but range from 25 mg every other day to 50 mg/day. The usual maintenance dose is 300–500 mg/day, divided twice daily.

In summary, anticonvulsant drugs are dramatically effective for trigeminal neuralgia and are useful for other, usually neuropathic pain states. Clinical experience suggests that they are most effective in conditions in which the pain has a lancinating component. This point has not been examined quantitatively, however, and the apparent usefulness of these drugs in migraine prophylaxis may be an important exception.

C. Systemically Administered Local Anesthetics in the Treatment of Neuropathic Pain

I. Conditions Responding to Systemic Local Anesthetics

Systemic administration of local anesthetics for analgesia has a long history (BONICA 1953). In recent years analgesic efficacy for systemic local anesthetics has been demonstrated in prospective controlled studies for diabetic neuropathy (DEJGARD et al. 1988; KASTRUP et al. 1987; STRACKE et al. 1992), Dercum's disease (ATKINSON et al. 1985; PETERSEN et al. 1986) and postherpetic neuralgia (ROWBOTHAM et al. 1991). In each of these neuropathic pain conditions patients often, but not always, report a lancinating component to their pain. In two large uncontrolled series, systemic local anesthetics were most often effective for patients with pain due to peripheral nerve injury (EDWARDS et al. 1985; GALER et al. 1993). Other groups of patients have been reported to show excellent responses to systemic local anesthetic administration include cranial neuralgias, multiple sclerosis, cancer pain, thalamic pain, and arachnoiditis (for reviews see BONICA 1953; CHABAL 1994; GLAZER and PORTENOY 1991; TANELIAN and VICTORY 1995).

Despite this evidence for broad spectrum analgesia there is conflicting evidence as to the efficacy of systemic local anesthetics in conditions without obvious nerve damage. For example, CASSUTO et al. (1985) reported significant analgesic efficacy for intravenous lidocaine in postoperative pain, and JONSSON et al. (1991) reported its efficacy for burn pain. On the other hand, others have reported systemic local anesthetics to have minimal or no analgesic effectiveness for postoperative (TANELIAN and VICTORY 1995) and experimental pain (MARCHETTINI et al. 1992). It may well be that the selectivity of systemic local anesthetics for neuropathic versus "physiological" pain is relative and depends upon the plasma concentrations achieved. In fact, a lower plasma concentration of local anesthetic is apparently required to relieve neuropathic versus nonneuropathic pain (BOAS et al. 1982; ROWLINGSON et al. 1980). This relative selectivity may be due to the fact that the ability of local anesthetics to block action potentials depends on the axon's firing frequency and on the relative "safety factor" of impulse generation at normal sensory endings versus ectopic firing sites (RAYMOND and THALHAMMER 1987, and see below).

II. Which Local Anesthetic To Choose?

1. Intravenous Lidocaine

The protocol used at the University of California San Francisco Pain Management Center is to administer lidocaine intravenously at a dose of 5 mg/kg over 1 h, without a bolus. The infusion may be continued at the same rate for an additional 15–30 min if pain relief is incomplete. Side effects are mild, and cardiovascular changes are minimal. End-infusion blood levels are typically in the range of 1–3 μg/ml range. Most commonly, if significant analgesia is reported, the pain returns to baseline within several hours, although patients occasionally report pain relief lasting several days to weeks.

Alternative methods of delivering lidocaine intravenously may be utilized. For instance, MARCHETTINNI et al. (1992) utilized only a 60 s injection of 1.5 mg/kg as a successful test procedure. Others have used computer-controlled infusion pump systems to target and maintain stable plasma lidocaine concentrations (FERRANTE et al. 1955; TANELIAN and BROSE 1991; WALLACE et al. 1995). Although serious adverse effects are uncommon with the administration of parenteral lidocaine, continuous ECG, heart rate and blood pressure monitoring is required, and resuscitative equipment must be immediately available. Patients with preexisting cardiac conduction defects should be screened by a cardiologist before intravenous administration of lidocaine.

After an intravenous bolus of 50–100 mg lidocaine antiarrhythmic effects begin in 45–90 s and last 10–20 min. The terminal phase half-life of lidocaine is 1.5–2 h. Approximately 90% of an intravenous lidocaine dose is rapidly metabolized by the liver. The procedure should be used with caution in patients with sinus bradycardia and incomplete heart block. An increase in ventricular rate may occur in patients with atrial fibrillation. If an arrhythmia develops or prolongation of the PR interval or the QRS complex occurs, the infusion should be discontinued. Intravenous lidocaine is contraindicated in patients with a known hypersensitivity to amide-type local anesthetics, Adams-Stokes syndrome and severe heart block. Severe liver disease impairs lidocaine metabolism and clearance, resulting in higher plasma levels at any given dose. The most common side effects, albeit transient and dose dependent, are associated with intravenous lidocaine's CNS effects. These adverse effects include drowsiness, dizziness, tremulousness, euphoria, blurring of vision, parasthesias, and dysarthria. In the doses normally used lidocaine is an anticonvulsant. At high blood levels, usually exceeding 10 mg/ml, lidocaine may cause seizures. If a patient is concurrently taking another local anesthetic antiarrhythmic, adverse effects could appear earlier in the infusion. Cimetidine and propranolol each may diminish the systemic clearance of lidocaine, resulting in higher plasma lidocaine levels.

Although there is good evidence that intravenous lidocaine reduces pain in a variety of disorders, its usefulness in chronic pain management, remains unclear (EDWARDS et al. 1985; GALER et al. 1993). Animal models suggest that a brief pulse of systemic lidocaine can produce prolonged analgesia (CHAPLAN et al. 1995). In a few patients relief from each administration is sufficiently long lasting that they prefer periodic intravenous lidocaine to daily oral medications. More commonly, a lidocaine infusion is used to either further explore the nature of the pain (MARCHETTINI et al. 1992) or to predict response to an oral antiarrhythmic or anticonvulsant agent that also blocks sodium channels (EDMONDSON et al. 1993; GALER et al. 1996). The response to intravenous lidocaine partially predicts response to oral local anesthetics for arrhythmia control (MURRAY et al. 1989); however, the evidence that the lidocaine infusion test is useful in predicting response to analogous oral medications is limited to one small prospective study (GALER et al. 1996).

2. Oral Local Anesthetic Antiarrhythmics

At present mexiletine and flecainide are available for oral use as local anesthetic type antiarrhythmics. Of the two the use of mexiletine is much more extensive for pain management. A third oral local-anesthetic type antiarrythmic, tocainide, had accumulated evidence for efficacy in animal studies and in a double-blind clinical trial in trigeminal neuralgia (LINDSTROM and LINDBLOM 1987). However, its use has been severely restricted because of a higher than expected incidence of aplastic anemia.

A randomized double-blind placebo, controlled cross-over study by DEJGARD et al. (1988) showed that mexiletine significantly reduces pain, dysesthesias, and paresthesias in patients with chronic painful diabetic neuropathy. A second blinded study showed mexiletine to be especially beneficial in those diabetic neuropathy patients with pain descriptors of stabbing, burning, heat, and formication (STRACKE et al. 1992). An intermediate dose of

450 mg /day was felt best overall. In open-label trials mexiletine has been reported effective for a variety of painful neuropathies, poststroke pain, multiple sclerosis pain, and phantom pain (AWERBUCH and SANDY 1990; CHABAL et al. 1992a).

Mexiletine, structurally similar to lidocaine, is a local anesthetic and a class IB antiarrhythmic. The initial dose is 150 or 200 mg once per day with food. The dose is then increased as tolerated by one capsule every 3–7 days up to a ceiling of 1200 mg total per day, divided into three or four doses. ECG and plasma levels should be monitored closely at the higher doses. Mexiletine plasma levels peak in 2–3 h. The elimination half-life is 10–12 h, but in patients with abnormal liver function it may be delayed up to 25 h. Therapeutic plasma levels for antiarrhythmic effects range from 0.5 to 2 mg/ml. Plasma levels of mexiletine may be reduced with concomitant therapy with phenytoin, rifampin, and phenobarbital; cimetidine therapy may result in elevated mexiletine levels. Mexiletine is contraindicated in patients with preexisting second- or third-degree AV blockade, but patients with first degree AV block may be treated safely. Hypotension and bradycardia may occur with overdosage. Mexiletine may worsen arrhythmias but uncommonly affects less serious arrhythmias, such as frequent premature beats and nonsustained ventricular tachycardia. In fewer than 10% of patients mexiletine causes palpitations and chest pain. In controlled studies upper gastrointestinal distress occurs in 40%, and tremor, lightheadedness, and incoordination each occur in about 10%. Gastrointestinal effects can be reduced by taking the medication with meals, an antacid, or carafate. Ataxia and seizures are reported to occur in 2 of 1000 patients. Dose-limiting sedation and dysequilibrium appear to be less of a problem than with carbamazepine. Flecainide may be worth considering as an alternative therapy for neuropathic pain (DUNLOP et al. 1991; SINNOTT et al. 1991) if the use of mexiletine is limited by side effects.

III. Topical Local Anesthetics for Chronic Pain

Subcutaneous local anesthetic infiltration into the area of greatest pain is effective for postherpetic neuralgia pain (PHN; ROWBOTHAM and FIELDS 1989; SECUNDA et al. 1941). Two double-blind, vehicle-controlled studies have demonstrated the efficacy of topical lidocaine in PHN (ROWBOTHAM et al. 1995, 1996). Importantly, by using active drug at a site remote from the affected area in PHN patients ROWBOTHAM and coworkers (1995) demonstrated that part of the analgesic effect of topically applied lidocaine is at the cutaneous terminals of the affected sensory nerves. Anecdotally, topical local anesthetics have also been reported effective for burn pain, diabetic neuropathy, and miscellaneous chronic pain complaints (GALER et al. 1996).

Skin thickness and vascularity influence the time of onset and duration of analgesia with topical agents (ARENDT-NEILSEN et al. 1990). Areas with thick stratum corneum, such as the hand and antecubital fossa, have a slower onset of analgesia than the back, which has a thinner epidermis but similar blood flow. Areas of high vascularity, such as the forehead, have a rapid onset of analgesia but reduced efficacy and short duration. Cutaneous free nerve endings are located primarily at the dermal-epidermal junction, close to the papillary capillaries. If the vascular uptake of local anesthetic is high, the concentration around the nerve endings remains low and produces inadequate analgesia. In areas of relatively low blood flow analgesia may continue for a time after the drug is removed from the skin surface because the skin acts as as a drug reservoir. In areas of high vascularity the rate of vascular uptake may be equal to influx of drug through the skin and the analgesic effect begins to decline as soon as the drug is removed from the skin.

The mechanism of action of topically applied local anesthetics for relieving the pain of PHN is uncertain. It is possible that they act by blocking normal impulse conduction.

The base form of lidocaine in relatively high concentration blocks experimentally induced sunburn and painful electrical stimulation (DALILI and ADRIANI 1971). Furthermore, lidocaine base 3% in cream form produces sufficient anesthesia to allow minor skin operations (NIAMTU et al. 1984). After a 1-h application under occlusion, Eutectic Mixture of Local Anesthetics or (EMLA), a 2.5% lidocaine base and 2.5% xylocaine base combination in emulsion cream form, produces sufficient sensory blunting to significantly reduce the pain of venipuncture, lumbar puncture, minor skin operations, and harvesting skin for split-thickness skin grafts (EHRENSTROM REIZ and REIZ 1982).

On the other hand, topical local anesthetics relieve PHN pain by a cutaneous action (ROWBOTHAM et al. 1995) but with minimal sensory loss (ROWBOTHAM and FIELDS 1996). For example, sensory testing 6h after lidocaine patch application has indicated that cutaneous C nociceptors are still able to function (ROWBOTHAM et al. 1993). Because this treatment does not produce dense local analgesia or thermanesthesia, it is unlikely that the intracutaneous drug concentration achieved by topical application climbs high enough to produce complete axon conduction block. Rather, it is likely that the pain relief results from suppression of firing in damaged, sensitized primary afferents.

D. Mechanisms of Action: Anticonvulsants and Local Anesthetics Suppress Abnormal Primary Afferent Firing

I. Evidence that Abnormal Afferent Firing Contributes to Neuropathic Pain, and that Membrane-Stabilizing Drugs Suppress This Activity

1. Sources of Ectopic Firing

In teased axon recordings from dorsal roots in rats and rabbits with chronic nerve injury, WALL and GUTNICK (1974) and KIRK (1974) demonstrated a higher increased level of ongoing discharge in afferent A and C fibers than in intact dorsal root or after acute nerve section. Subsequent studies identified two principle sources of this activity: the nerve injury site (e.g., neuroma or nerve compression zone; GOVRIN-LIPPMANN and DEVOR 1978; HABLER et al. 1987; reviewed in DEVOR 1994) and the associated dorsal root ganglia (DRGs; KAJANDER et al. 1992; WALL and DEVOR 1983; XIE et al. 1995). In addition to spontaneous firing, ectopic discharge at both of these locations is produced by normally ineffective gentle mechanical displacement (Tinel sign) and by a range of chemical stimuli. Perhaps the most interesting of the latter is the response to circulating adrenaline and sympathetic efferent stimulation

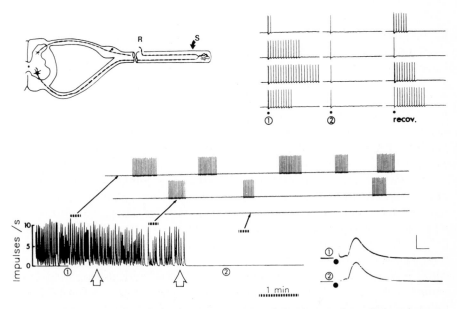

Fig. 1. Lidocaine suppresses ongoing discharge originating at sites of chronic nerve injury. *Upper left,* experimental setup. Recordings (*R*) were made from a single axon from a rat's sciatic nerve that had been cut across 8 days previously. The axon, which had a conduction velocity of 37.5 m/s as measured by its response latency to stimulation at (*S*), fired spontaneously in a bursty (on-off) pattern as shown (period indicated by *encircled 1*). *First arrow,* 100 μl 1% lidocaine (1 mg) was injected into the bloodstream. This caused the bursts to become shorter, and less frequent. After a second such injection (*second arrow*) firing ceased altogether (*encircled 2*). During the time that ectopic firing was abolished the axon continued to conduct impulses normally. *Lower right,* spike responses to single electrical pulses delivered at (*S*) before the lidocaine injections (*encircled 1*) and after (*encircled 2*). Before lidocaine injection the axon frequently responded to electrical stimulus pulses with a brief burst of up to ca. 20 spikes (afterdischarge). *Upper right,* four such responses are shown (*encircled 1*). Following lidocaine injection such afterdischarge bursts ceased, although the axon continued to respond with a single spike (*encircled 2*). By 40 min after the 2nd lidocaine injection spontaneous bursting and afterdischarge had recovered (*recov.*). Calibrations: 1.5 mV, 0.5 ms (*lower right*), 200 ms (*upper right*). Ratemeter time constant, 0.5 s. (Data from DEVOR et al. 1992)

(Devor 1994; Devor and Janig 1981). The resulting "sympathetic-sensory coupling" may explain the fact that some chronic pain syndromes, for example, causalgia, are relieved by adrenoreceptor antagonists or sympathetic ganglion block.

A variety of "membrane-stabilizing" drugs have been shown to suppress abnormal discharge originating at nerve injury sites and associated DRGs (Fig. 1). These include anticonvulsants (carbamazepine, phenytoin Burchiel 1988; Yaari and Devor 1985), the antiarrhythmic mexiletine (Chabal et al. 1989a), local anesthetics (lidocaine, Devor et al. 1992), and corticosteroids (dexamethasone, triamcinolone, Devor et al. 1985). Each of these prevented the generation of spontaneous ectopic impulses at much lower concentrations than are required to block normal impulse propagation. Although this review does not consider the actions of corticosteroids, we point out that in addition to their being anti-inflammatory, they have long been known to possess "membrane-stabilizing" properties and, unlike the membrane-stabilizing local anesthetics and anticonvulsants, are available in depot formulations.

2. Ectopic Firing and Pain

Ectopic firing contributes to pain in two ways. First, abnormal afferent barrages that propagate into the CNS directly elicit abnormal sensations, including paresthesias and, when nociceptors are involved, dysesthesias and pain. These may be spontaneous, or evoked by movement, or by endogenous chemical events (e.g., changes in sympathetic outflow). Second, ectopic nociceptor activity can trigger and maintain "central sensitization." Central sensitization is a CNS hyperexcitability state in the presence of which afferent input, normal or ectopic, entering along low-threshold $A\beta$ fibers, is interpreted by the brain as pain (Campbell et al. 1988; Torebjork et al. 1992; Woolf 1992). This dual role of ectopic firing in neuropathic pain is best illustrated under conditions in which a well localized focus of abnormal firing can be identified. Sheen and Chung (1993), for example, severed the spinal nerve of DRGs L5 and L6 in rats, creating a focus of ectopic discharge in the L5 and L6 neuromas and DRGs. The result was behavioral signs of ongoing pain, presumably due to the ectopic firing, and allodynia in the hindlimb skin served by the neighboring L4 root, presumably due to central sensitization triggered by the ectopic firing. Blocking central propagation of the abnormal, ectopic discharge by secondarily cutting the L5 and L6 dorsal roots both eliminated the ongoing pain and normalized sensation in the l4 territory. Other means of reducing the abnormal neuroma and DRG discharge are also effective at relieving cutaneous allodynia in these animals. These include sympathectomy (Kim et al. 1993) and systemic administration of local anesthetics (Chaplan et al. 1995). Interestingly, just as in clinical experience, systemic lidocaine sometimes relieves cutaneous hypersensitivity in animal models of neuropathic pain for a longer time than would be expected from the serum half-life of the drug (Chaplan et al. 1995).

There is some clinical evidence that ectopic impulse generation contributes to central sensitization. Thus GRACELY et al. (1992) reported a patient with a focally painful scar near the knee and allodynia extending up the thigh and down the calf. Local anesthetic block of the scar eliminated the extended allodynia as well as the scar pain for the duration of the block. The interpretation offered was that noxious input originating in the scar triggered a spinal central sensitization state which amplified, and rendered painful, Aβ touch input from the thigh and calf. Similar observations have been reported in patients with postherpetic neuralgia (ROWBOTHAM and FIELDS 1989).

II. Clinical Evidence that Abnormal Afferent Firing Contributes to Neuropathic Pain

The method of percutaneous microneurographic recording from single nerve fibers in conscious man (VALLBO et al. 1979) permits a direct comparison of neural discharge and sensation. A small number of such studies in patients with neuropathic pain has appeared (CLINE et al. 1989; NORDIN et al. 1984; NYSTROM and HAGBARTH 1981; OCHOA et al. 1982; OCHOA and TOREBJORK 1980). In each a striking correlation was found between spontaneous and evoked discharges, on the one hand, and neuropathic paresthesias and pain, on the other.

Evidence that spontaneous activity in damaged unmyelinated afferents contributes to pain was provided by CLINE and colleagues (1989). They reported patients who complained of burning pain and hyperalgesia and had warm skin. These patients had spontaneous activity in unmyelinated primary afferents which presumably contributed to their pain. Even more dramatically, NYSTROM and HAGBARTH (1981) documented ongoing discharge in the peroneal nerve in a lower extremity amputee. The patient had ongoing phantom foot pain which was augmented by percussion of the neuroma. The same percussion elicited an intense burst of spike activity, mostly in slowly conducting axons. This was eliminated, along with the evoked pain, by local anesthetic block of the neuroma. In a related study dysesthesias referred to the foot were triggered by straight-leg lifting (Lasegue's sign) in a patient with radicular pain related to surgery for disk herniation. This maneuver evoked ectopic impulse bursts in the sural nerve, the intensity of which waxed and waned in close correlation with the abnormal sensation (NORDIN et al. 1984).

There are also studies demonstrating sensory changes evoked by the injection of test substances at foci of neuropathic pain. In rodents, adrenaline injected into a neuroma augments ectopic firing while lidocaine suppresses it. Correspondingly, adrenaline injected into a nerve injury site in humans evokes pain, while lidocaine blocks it (CHABAL et al. 1989b, 1992b). Likewise, α-adrenoreceptor agonists evoke pain when injected into skin in patients whose hyperalgesia was previously relieved by sympatholytic treatments (DAVIS et al. 1991; TOREBJORK et al. 1995). This implies that in some patients with sympathetically dependent pain primary afferents are abnormally adrenosensitive.

The same conclusion is supported by the observation that direct electrical stimulation of sympathetic efferent fibers in man evokes pain, but only in patients with sympathetically dependent pain (WALKER and NULSEN 1948; WHITE and SWEET 1969). These clinical observations are in keeping with the electrophysiological observations of sympathetic-sensory coupling noted in experimental nerve injury (DEVOR 1994; DEVOR and JANIG 1981).

In contrast to the nerve injury site, the DRG has not yet been investigated as a potential source of ectopic firing in humans despite the strong experimental evidence in animals. There are, however, positive hints in man. For example, in the microneurographic study of NYSTROM and HAGBARTH (1981), although anesthetic block of the neuroma eliminated the Tinel response, it failed to eliminate much of the ongoing nerve activity. This persistent activity may well have originated in the DRG and propagated centrifugally to the recording electrode. Another indication comes from studies by FEINSTEIN et al. (1954). They injected hypertonic (6%) saline into the interspinous tissue in amputees. Within seconds this evoked a natural painful phantom limb sensation, and "filled out" phantoms that had faded with time following amputation and become incomplete. In animal preparations, axons do not fire on topical application of 6% saline, but DRG neurons do (DEVOR 1996). FEINSTEIN et al. (1954) may have been activating the DRG nearest to their injection needle.

III. Mechanisms by Which Membrane-Stabilizing Drugs Suppress Ectopic Neural Activity

1. Na⁺ Channels

The development of ectopic hyperexcitability is thought to be due to remodeling of the axon membrane's local electrical properties (DEVOR 1994; DEVOR et al. 1994; RIZZO et al. 1995). A major contributing mechanism appears to be the accumulation of excess voltage sensitive Na^+ channels in terminal swellings (neuroma endbulbs) and sprouts in the region of injury, and in patches of demyelination. In addition, axonal injury appears to trigger the upregulation of Na^+ channel synthesis in sensory cell bodies in the DRG, and the expression of previously silent Na^+ channel types (WAXMAN et al. 1994). Computer simulation predicts that an increase in the density of Na^+ channels increases the electrical excitability of nerve cells (DEVOR et al. 1994).

The common denominator among the membrane-stabilizing drugs that we have been discussing, carbamazepine, phenytoin, mexiletine, and local anesthetics, is that they block the functioning of Na^+ channels (CATTERALL 1987). This appears to be the reason that they suppress abnormal neural discharge. Another class of highly effective anticonvulsants, the barbiturates, do not have this effect and are not known to be effective for neuropathic pain. They are thought to suppress seizure activity by enhancing inhibitory GABAergic neurotransmission. That is, they act synaptically rather than directly on membrane excitability. Likewise, antiarrhythmic drugs that act by mechanisms other than

Na$^+$ channel blockade do not have any known analgesic efficacy. Even baclofen, a drug known to act synaptically at the GABAB receptor and which is effective for trigeminal neuralgia (FROMM et al. 1984), has recently been shown to have a membrane-stabilizing action (DOLPHIN and SCOTT 1987).

2. Basis for Selectivity

Impulse propagation along axons is known to depend on the functioning of Na$^+$ channels. How, then, can systemic and regional use of the membrane-stabilizing drugs under examination suppress abnormal neural firing without also globally blocking nerve conduction? The apparent answer is that the sensitivity of these two processes to Na$^+$ channel block, their respective "safety factor," is very different (DEVOR 1995; DEVOR et al. 1994). That is, the impulse-generating process is far more sensitive to membrane-stabilizing drugs than is the process of conduction of already formed impulses. For example, in experimental animals, abnormal impulse generation in DRG cells was 100% arrested by a systemic dose of 1 mg/kg lidocaine, and ectopic afferent firing originating at sites of nerve injury required 5 mg/kg for blockade. Neither dose, however, had a detectable effect on normal nerve impulse conduction, which persisted even in the presence of plasma concentrations which were lethal to the animal (DEVOR et al. 1992).

3. Does Analgesia Result from Suppression of PNS or CNS Activity or Both?

As with ectopic impulse generation in injured peripheral axons and DRG cells, the firing of many spinal cord neurons is suppressed by concentrations of Na$^+$ channel blockers significantly below those required to block impulse propagation in axons. Some dorsal horn neurons operate at low "safety factor," near their "threshold for repetitive firing." This means that slight suppression may be enough to tilt their activation balance toward silence. Data from experimental animals show that under some circumstances plasma levels of lidocaine sufficient to suppress ectopic firing in the PNS also suppresses CNS activity (SOTGIU et al. 1991; WOOLF and WIESENFELD-HALLIN 1985). The possibility must therefore be considered that at clinically relevant doses membrane-stabilizing drugs may act in the CNS as well as in the PNS.

ABRAM and YAKSH (1994) examined this issue by comparing the effect of systemic lidocaine in three rat pain models: the formalin test (which uses a chemical stimulus to produce a two phase nociceptive response), partial ligation of the sciatic nerve (which produces neuropathic hyperalgesia), and normal paw withdrawal to noxious heat. At doses of lidocaine which markedly reduced the neuropathic hyperalgesia lidocaine had no significant effect on withdrawal latency in the normally innervated paw or on either phase of the formalin-induced response. At higher doses lidocaine reduced only the second phase of the formalin test, which is thought to be due in part to the development of a state of central sensitization. These results indicate that depending on dose systemic lidocaine can suppress impulses generated by damaged PNS and also affect CNS pain transmission processes, either directly or indirectly.

4. Strategies for Reducing Dose-Limiting Side Effects of Systemic Membrane-Stabilizing Drugs

The dose-limiting side effects involved in the systemic use of Na+ channel blockers include sedation, ataxia, vertigo, blurred vision, nausea and vomiting. All are CNS effects. It is very often dizziness and loss of alertness that limit titrating to higher, and presumably more effective, analgesic doses. This limitation might be overcome by regional infusion of a dilute solution of carbamazepine, lidocaine, etc. into a suspected source of ectopic firing, an injured brachial plexus, for example, or a few adjacent DRGs. The use of concentrations well below those that block nerve conduction would ensure intact motor and residual sensory function.

Another potential approach to avoiding dose-limiting CNS toxicity would be to produce a carbamazepine or lidocaine-like agent in a form that preserves membrane-stabilizing properties of the parent drug but does not cross the blood-brain barrier. No such drug exists at present.

Pharmacological agents that block Na^+ channels by binding to the extracellular mouth of the channel are known and used widely as reagents in basic neuroscience research (e.g., tetrodotoxin and saxitoxin). They differ from the local anesthetics and anticonvulsants, however, in that their potency does not depend on the firing rate of the neuron (i.e., they are not use-dependent blockers). To our knowledge, neither tetrodotoxin nor saxitoxin has been tested in the context of neuropathic pain. They are highly toxic substances, but in sufficiently low concentration they might be both safe and effective. In a first attempt, perhaps Helsinki approval could be obtained for use of these agents in a Bier block.

Finally, mention should be made of the likelihood that nociceptive afferents use a complement of Na^+ channel molecules subtly different from those present in low-threshold afferents and those present in the heart and the brain. This difference might permit the creation of novel Na^+ channel blockers that selectively target and silence nociceptors.

E. Summary

The weight of clinical evidence is consistent with a role of abnormal spontaneous activity in primary afferents in neuropathic pain. Since such activity is relatively selectively sensitive to certain anticonvulsants and to low concentrations of local anesthetics, it is likely that the efficacy of such drugs in neuropathic pain depends at least partly on their blocking of ectopic activity.

Acknowledgements. The work of M.D. on this subject is supported primarily by the U.S.-Israel Binational Science Foundation, German-Israel Foundation for Research and Development, and Israel Ministry of Science and Arts. The contributions of H.L.F. and M.C.R. were supported primarily by NIH grant NS 21445 and a gift from Harry Hind.

References

Abram SE, Yaksh TL (1994) Systemic lidocaine blocks nerve injury-induced hyperalgesia and nociceptor-driven spinal sensitization in the rat. Anesthesiology 80:383–391 (discussion 325A)

Arendt-Neilsen L, Bjerring P, Nielsen J (1990) Regional variations in analgesic efficacy of EMLA cream. Quantitatively evaluated by argon laser stimulation. Acta Derm Venereol 70:314–318

Atkinson JH Jr, Kremer EF, Garfin SR (1985) Psychopharmacological agents in the treatment of pain. J Bone Joint Surg [Am] 67:337–342

Awerbuch GI, Sandy KR (1990) Mexiletine for thalamic pain syndrome. Int J Neurosci 55:129–133

Bergouignan M (1942) Successful cure of essential facial neuralgias by sodium iphenylhydantoinate. Rev Laryngol Otol Rhinol 63:34–41

Boas RA, Covino BG, Shahnarian A (1982) Analgesic responses to i.v. lignocaine. Br J Anaesth 54:501–505

Bonica JJ (1953) The management of pain, with special emphasis on the use of analgesic block in diagnosis, prognosis, and therapy. Lea and Febiger, Philadelphia

Burchiel KJ (1980) Abnormal impulse generation in focally demyelinated trigeminal roots. J Neurosurg 53:674–683

Burchiel KJ (1988) Carbamazepine inhibits spontaneous activity in experimental neuromas. Exp Neurol 102:249–253

Caccia MR (1975) Clonazepam in facial neuralgia and cluster headache. Clinical and electrophysiological study. Eur Neurol 13:560–563

Calvin WH, Howe JF, Loeser JD (1977) Ectopic repetitive firing in focally demyelinated axons and some implications for trigeminal neuralgia. In: Anderson DJ, Matthews B (eds) Pain in the trigeminal region: proceedings of a symposium held in the Department of Physiology, University of Bristol, England on 25–27 July 1977. Elsevier/North-Holland, Amsterdam

Calvin WH, Devor M, Howe JF (1982) Can neuralgias arise from minor demyelination? Spontaneous firing, mechanosensitivity, and afterdischarge from conducting axons. Exp Neurol 75:755–763

Campbell JN, Raja SN, Meyer RA, Mackinnon SE (1988) Myelinated afferents signal the hyperalgesia associated with nerve injury. Pain 32:89–94

Cassuto J, Wallin G, Hogstrom S, Faxen A, Rimback G (1985) Inhibition of postoperative pain by continuous low-dose intravenous infusion of lidocaine. Anesth Analg 64:971–974

Catterall WA (1987) Common modes of drug action on Na+ channels: local anaesthetics, antiarrhythmics and anti-convulsants. Trends Pharmacol Sci 8:57–65

Chabal C (1994) Membrane stabilizing agents and experimental neuromas. In: Fields HL, Liebeskind JC (eds) Pharmacological approaches to the treatment of chronic pain: new concepts and critical issues. International Association for the Study of Pain, Seattle, pp 205–210

Chabal C, Jacobson L, Russell LC, Burchiel KJ (1989a) Pain responses to perineuromal injection of normal saline, gallamine, and lidocaine in humans. Pain 36:321–325

Chabal C, Russell LC, Burchiel KJ (1989b) The effect of intravenous lidocaine, tocainide, and mexiletine on spontaneously active fibers originating in rat sciatic neuromas. Pain 38:333–338

Chabal C, Jacobson L, Mariano A, Chaney E, Britell CW (1992a) The use of oral mexiletine for the treatment of pain after peripheral nerve injury. Anesthesiology 76:513–517

Chabal C, Jacobson L, Russell LC, Burchiel KJ (1992b) Pain response to perineuromal injection of normal saline, epinephrine, and lidocaine in humans. Pain 49:9–12

Chadda VS, Mathur MS (1978) Double blind study of the effects of diphenylhydantoin sodium on diabetic neuropathy. J Assoc Physicians India 26:403–406

Chaplan SR, Bach FW, Shafer SL, Yaksh TL (1995) Prolonged alleviation of tactile allodynia by intravenous lidocaine in neuropathic rats. Anesthesiology 83:775–785

Cheung H, Kamp D, Harris E (1992) An in vitro investigation of the action of lamotrigine on neuronal voltage-activated sodium channels. Epilepsy Res 13:107–112

Cline MA, Ochoa J, Torebjork HE (1989) Chronic hyperalgesia and skin warming caused by sensitized C nociceptors. Brain 112:621–647

Court JE, Kase CS (1976) Treatment of tic douloureux with a new anticonvulsant (clonazepam). J Neurol Neurosurg Psychiatry 39:297–299

Dalili H, Adriani J (1971) The efficacy of local anesthetics in blocking the sensations of itch, burning, and pain in normal and "sunburned" skin. Clin Pharmacol Ther 12:913–919

Davis KD, Treede RD, Raja SN, Meyer RA, Campbell JN (1991) Topical application of clonidine relieves hyperalgesia in patients with sympathetically maintained pain (see comments). Pain 47:309–317

Dejgard A, Petersen P, Kastrup J (1988) Mexiletine for treatment of chronic painful diabetic neuropathy. Lancet 1:9–11

Dellemijn PL, Fields HL (1994) Do benzodiazepines have a role in chronic pain management? Pain 57:137–152

Devor M (1994) Pathophysiology of injured nerve. In: Wall PD, Melzack R (eds) Textbook of pain, 3rd edn. Churchill Livingstone, London, pp 79–100

Devor M (1995) Neurobiological basis for selectivity of Na+ channel blockers in neuropathic pain. Pain Forum 4:83–86

Devor M (1996) Phantom limb phenomena and their neural mechanism. In: Myslobodsky MS (ed) Mythomanias. Erlbaum, London

Devor M, Janig W (1981) Activation of myelinated afferents ending in a neuroma by stimulation of the sympathetic supply in the rat. Neurosci Lett 24:43–47

Devor M, Govrin-Lippmann R, Raber P (1985) Corticosteroids suppress ectopic neural discharge originating in experimental neuromas. Pain 22:127–137

Devor M, Wall PD, Catalan N (1992) Systemic lidocaine silences ectopic neuroma and DRG discharge without blocking nerve conduction. Pain 48:261–268

Devor M, Lomazov P, Matzner O (1994) Na+ channel accumulation in injured axons as a substrate for neuropathic pain. In: Boivie J, Hansson P, Lindblom U (eds) Touch, temperature, and pain in health and disease: mechanisms and assessments: a Wenner-Gren center international symposium. International Association for the Study of Pain, Seattle, pp 207–230

Dolphin AC, Scott RH (1987) Calcium channel currents and their inhibition by (−)-baclofen in rat sensory neurones: modulation by guanine nucleotides. J Physiol (Lond) 386:1–17

Dubner R, Sharav Y, Gracely RH, Price DD (1987) Idiopathic trigeminal neuralgia: sensory features and pain mechanisms. Pain 31:23–33

Dunlop RJ, Hockley JM, Tate T, Turner P (1991) Flecainide in cancer nerve pain (letter; comment). Lancet 337:1347

Dunsker SB, Mayfield FH (1976) Carbamazepine in the treatment of the flashing pain syndrome. J Neurosurg 45:49–51

Edmondson EA, Simpson RK Jr, Stubler DK, Beric A (1993) Systemic lidocaine therapy for poststroke pain. South Med J 86:1093–1096

Edwards WT, Habib F, Burney RG, Begin G (1985) Intravenous lidocaine in the management of various chronic pain states – a review of 211 cases. Regional Anesth 10:1–6

Ehrenstrom Reiz GM, Reiz SL (1982) EMLA – a eutectic mixture of local anaesthetics for topical anaesthesia. Acta Anaesthesiol Scand 26:596–598

Espir ML, Millac P (1970) Treatment of paroxysmal disorders in multiple sclerosis with carbamazepine (Tegretol). J Neurol Neurosurg Psychiatry 33:528–531

Feinstein B, Luce JC, Langton JNK (1954) The influence of phantom limbs. In: Klopsteg PE, Wilson PD (eds) Human limbs and their substitutes; presenting results of engineering and medical studies of the human extremities and application of the data to the design and fitting of artifical limbs and to the care and training of amputees. In: Summary and correlation of a research program for the Department of Medicine and Surgery, US Veterans Administration, and for the Office of the Surgeon General, Department of the Army. McGraw-Hill, New York, p 844

Ferrante FM, Paggioli J, Cherukuri S, Arthur GR (1955) The analgesic response to intravenous lidocaine in the treatment of neuropathic pain. Anesth Analg 82:91–97

Fields HL, Raskin NH (1976) Anticonvulsants and pain. In: Klawans HL (ed) Clinical neuropharmacology. Raven, New York, pp 173–184

Fromm GH, Terrence CF, Chattha AS (1984) Baclofen in the treatment of trigeminal neuralgia: double-blind study and long-term follow-up. Ann Neurol 15:240–244

Galer BS, Miller KV, Rowbotham MC (1993) Response to intravenous lidocaine infusion differs based on clinical diagnosis and site of nervous system injury. Neurology 43:1233–1235

Galer BS, Harle J, Rowbotham MC (1996) Response to intravenous lidocaine infusion predicts subsequent response to oral mexiletine: a prospective study. J Pain Symptom Manage 12:1–7

Glazer S, Portenoy RK (1991) Systemic local anesthetics in pain control. J Pain Symptom Manage 6:30–39

Govrin-Lippmann R, Devor M (1978) Ongoing activity in severed nerves: source and variation with time. Brain Res 159:406–410

Gracely RH, Lynch SA, Bennett GJ (1992) Painful neuropathy: altered central processing maintained dynamically by peripheral input (published erratum appears in Pain 1993 Feb;52(2):251–253; see comments). Pain 51:175–194

Habler HJ, Janig W, Koltzenburg M (1987) Activation of unmyelinated afferents in chronically lesioned nerves by adrenaline and excitation of sympathetic efferents in the cat. Neurosci Lett 82:35–40

Honmou O, Kocsis JD, Richerson GB (1995) Gabapentin potentiates the conductance increase induced by nipecotic acid in CA1 pyramidal neurons in vitro. Epilepsy Res 20:193–202

Iannone A, Baker AB, Morrell F (1958) Dilantin in the treatment of trigeminal neuralgia. Neurology 8:126–128

Jannetta PJ (1967) Arterial compression of the trigeminal nerve at the pons in patients with trigeminal neuralgia. J Neurosurg 26 [Suppl]:159–162

Jannetta PJ (1976) Microsurgical approach to the trigeminal nerve at the pons in patients with trigeminal neuralgia. Prog Neurol Surg 7:180–200

Jonsson A, Cassuto J, Hanson B (1991) Inhibition of burn pain by intravenous lignocaine infusion. Lancet 338:151–152

Kajander KC, Wakisaka S, Bennett GJ (1992) Spontaneous discharge originates in the dorsal root ganglion at the onset of a painful peripheral neuropathy in the rat. Neurosci Lett 138:225–228

Kastrup J, Petersen P, Dejgard A, Angelo HR, Hilsted J (1987) Intravenous lidocaine infusion – a new treatment of chronic painful diabetic neuropathy? Pain 28:69–75

Kerr FWL (1979) Craniofacial neuralgias. Adv Pain Res Ther 4:283–295

Kim SH, Na HS, Sheen K, Chung JM (1993) Effects of sympathectomy on a rat model of peripheral neuropathy. Pain 55:85–92

Kirk EJ (1974) Impulses in dorsal spinal nerve rootlets in cats and rabbits arising from dorsal root ganglia isolated from the periphery. J Comp Neurol 155:165–175

Leijon G, Boivie J (1989) Central post-stroke pain – a controlled trial of amitriptyline and carbamazepine. Pain 36:27–36

Levy RH, Mattson RH, Meldrum BS (1995) Antiepileptic drugs, 4th edn. Raven, New York

Lindstrom P, Lindblom U (1987) The analgesic effect of tocainide in trigeminal neuralgia. Pain 28:45–50

Lisney SJ, Devor M (1987) Afterdischarge and interactions among fibers in damaged peripheral nerve in the rat. Brain Res 415:122–136

Lockman LA, Hunninghake DB, Krivit W, Desnick RJ (1973) Relief of pain of Fabry's disease by diphenylhydantoin. Neurology 23:871–875

Marchettini P, Lacerenza M, Marangoni C, Pellegata G, Sotgiu ML, Smirne S (1992) Lidocaine test in neuralgia. Pain 48:377–382

Max MB, Schafer SC, Culnane M, Smoller B, Dubner R, Gracely RH (1988) Amitriptyline, but not lorazepam, relieves postherpetic neuralgia. Neurology 38:1427–1432

McQuay H, Carroll D, Jadad AR, Wiffen P, Moore A (1995) Anticonvulsant drugs for management of pain: a systemic review. BMJ 311:1047–1052

Mellick GA, Mellicy LB, Mellick LB (1995) Gabapentin in the management of reflex sympathetic dystrophy (letter). J Pain Symptom Manage 10:265–266

Murray KT, Barbey JT, Kopelman HA, Siddoway LA, Echt DS, Woosley RL, Roden DM (1989) Mexiletine and tocainide: a comparison of antiarrhythmic efficacy, adverse effects, and predictive value of lidocaine testing. Clin Pharmacol Ther 45:553–561

Nakamura-Craig M, Follenfant RL (1995) Effect of lamotrigine in the acute and chrnoic hyperalgesia induced by PGE2 and in the chronic hyperalgesia in rats with streptozotocin-induced diabetes. Pain 63:33–37

Niamtu JD, Campbell RL, Garrett MS (1984) The anesthetic skin patch for topical anesthesia. J Oral Maxillofac Surg 42:839–840

Nordin M, Nystrom B, Wallin U, Hagbarth KE (1984) Ectopic sensory discharges and paresthesiae in patients with disorders of peripheral nerves, dorsal roots and dorsal columns. Pain 20:231–245

Nystrom B, Hagbarth KE (1981) Microelectrode recordings from transected nerves in amputees with phantom limb pain. Neurosci Lett 27:211–216

Ochoa JL, Torebjork HE (1980) Paraesthesiae from ectopic impulse generation in human sensory nerves. Brain 103:835–853

Ochoa J, Torebjork HE, Culp WJ, Schady W (1982) Abnormal spontaneous activity in single sensory nerve fibers in humans. Muscle Nerve 5:S74–77

Peiris JB, Perera GL, Devendra SV, Lionel ND (1980) Sodium valproate in trigeminal neuralgia. Med J Aust 2:278

Petersen P, Kastrup J, Zeeberg I, Boysen G (1986) Chronic pain treatment with intravenous lidocaine. Neurol Res 8:189–190

Rall TW, Schleifer LS (1985) Drugs effective in the therapy of neuropathic pain. In: Gilman AG (ed) The pharmacological basis of therapeutics. Macmillan, New York, pp 446–472

Rappaport ZH, Devor M (1994) Trigeminal neuralgia: the role of self-sustaining discharge in the trigeminal ganglion. Pain 56:127–138

Rasminsky M (1980) Ephaptic transmission between single nerve fibres in the spinal nerve roots of dystrophic mice. J Physiol (Lond) 305:151–169

Raymond SA, Thalhammer JG (1987) Endogenous activity dependent mechanisms for reducing hyperexcitability of axons: effects of anesthetics and CO_2. In: Chalazonitis N, Gola M (eds) Inactivation of hypersensitive neurons: proceedings of a satellite symposium of the 30th Congress of the International Union of Physiological Sciences, Vancouver, 11–13 July 1986. Liss, New York, pp 331–343

Rizzo MA, Kocsis JD, Waxman SG (1995) Selective loss of slow and enhancement of fast Na+ currents in cutaneous afferent dorsal root ganglion neurones following axotomy. Neurobiol Dis 2:87–96

Rockliff BW, Davis EH (1966) Controlled sequential trials of carbamazepine in trigeminal neuralgia. Arch Neurol 15:129–136

Rosner H, Rubin L, Kestenbaum A (1996) Gabapentin adjunctive therapy in neuropathic pain states. Clin J Pain 12(1):56–58

Rowbotham MC, Fields HL (1989) Post-herpetic neuralgia: the relation of pain complaint, sensory disturbance, and skin temperature. Pain 39:129–144

Rowbotham MC, Fields HL (1996) The relationship of pain, allodynia, and thermal sensation in post-herpetic neuralgia. Brain 119:347–354

Rowbotham MC, Reisner-Keller LA, Fields HL (1991) Both intravenous lidocaine and morphine reduce the pain of postherpetic neuralgia. Neurology 41:1024–1028

Rowbotham MC, Galer BS, Allen RR, Davies PJ, Verkempinck CM, Keller LR (1993) Lidocaine patch for post-herpetic neuralgia: results of a double-blind, placebo controlled trial. Congress abstracts, 7th World Congress on Pain, International Association for the Study of Pain, Seattle

Rowbotham MC, Davies PS, Fields HL (1995) Topical lidocaine gel relieves postherpetic neuralgia. Ann Neurol 37:246–253

Rowbotham MC, Davies PS, Verkempinck CV, Galer BS (1996) Lidocaine patch: double-blind controlled study of a new treatment method for post-herpetic neuralgia. Pain 65:39–4

Rowlingson JC, DiFazio CA, Foster J, Carron H (1980) Lidocaine as an analgesic for experimental pain. Anesthesiology 52:20–22

Rull JA, Quibrera R, Gonzalez-Millan H, Lozano Castaneda O (1969) Symptomatic treatment of peripheral diabetic neuropathy with carbamazepine (Tegretol): double blind crossover trial. Diabetologia 5:215–218

Secunda L, Wolf W, Price J (1941) Herpes zoster: local anesthesia in the treatment of pain. N Engl J Med 224:501–503

Seltzer Z, Devor M (1979) Ephaptic transmission in chronically damaged peripheral nerves. Neurology 29:1061–1064

Sheen K, Chung JM (1993) Signs of neuropathic pain depend on signals from injured nerve fibers in a rat model. Brain Res 610:62–68

Shibasaki H, Kuroiwa Y (1975) Painful tonic seizure in multiple sclerosis. Arch Neurol 30:47–51

Sinnott C, Edmonds P, Cropley I, Hanks G (1991) Flecainide in cancer nerve pain (letter; comment). Lancet 337:1347

Smirne S, Scarlato G (1977) Clonazepam in cranial neuralgias. Med J Aust 1:93–94

Sotgiu ML, Lacerenza M, Marchettini P (1991) Selective inhibition by systemic lidocaine of noxious evoked activity in rat dorsal horn neurons. Neuroreport 2:425–428

Stracke H, Meyer UE, Schumacher HE, Federlin K (1992) Mexiletine in the treatment of diabetic neuropathy. Diabetes Care 15:1550–1555

Swerdlow M (1984) Anticonvulsant drugs and chronic pain. Clin Neuropharmacol 7:51–82

Swerdlow M, Cundill JG (1981) Anticonvulsant drugs used in the treatment of lancinating pain. A comparison. Anaesthesia 36:1129–1132

Tanelian DL, Brose WG (1991) Neuropathic pain can be relieved by drugs that are use-dependent sodium channel blockers: lidocaine, carbamazepine, and mexiletine. Anesthesiology 74:949–951

Tanelian DL, Victory RA (1995) Sodium channel-blocking agents. Pain Forum 4:75–80

Teoh H, Fowler LJ, Bower NG (1995) Effect of lamotrigine on the electrically-evoked release of endogenous amino acids from slices of dorsal horn of the rat spinal cord. Neuropharmacology 34:1273–1278

Tomson T, Tybring G, Bertilsson L, Ekbom K, Rane A (1980) Carbamazepine therapy in trigeminal neuralgia: clinical effects in relation to plasma concentration. Arch Neurol 37:699–703

Torbejork E, Wahr LK, Wallin G, Hallin R, Koltzenberg M (1995) Noradrenaline-evoked pain in neuralgia. Pain 63:11–20

Torebjork HE, Lundberg LE, LaMotte RH (1992) Central changes in processing of mechanoreceptive input in capsaicin-induced secondary hyperalgesia in humans. J Physiol (Lond) 448:765–780

Vallbo AB, Hagbarth KE, Torebjork HE, Wallin BG (1979) Somatosensory, proprioceptive, and sympathetic activity in human peripheral nerves. Physiol Rev 59:919–957

Walker AE, Nulsen F (1948) Electrical stimulation of the upper thoracic portion of the
    sympathetic chain in man. Arch Neurol Psychiatry 59:559–560
Wall PD, Devor M (1983) Sensory afferent impulses originate from dorsal root ganglia
    as well as from the periphery in normal and nerve injured rats. Pain 17:321–339
Wall PD, Gutnick M (1974) Properties of afferent nerve impulses originating from a
    neuroma. Nature 248:740–743
Wallace MS, Dyck JB, Rossi SS, Yaksh TL (1995) Computer controlled lidocaine
    infusion for the evaluation of neuropathic pain after peripheral nerve injury. Pain
    (in press)
Waxman SG, Kocsis JD, Black JA (1994) Type III sodium channel mRNA is expressed
    in embryonic but not adult spinal sensory neurons, and is reexpressed following
    axotomy. J Neurophysiol 72:466–470
White JC, Sweet WH (1969) Pain and the neurosurgeon; a forty-year experience.
    Thomas, Springfield
Woolf CJ (1992) Excitability changes in central neurons following peripheral damage.
    In: Willis WDJ (ed) Hyperalgesia and allodynia: the Bristol-Myers Squibb sym-
    posiumon pain research. Raven, New York, pp 221–243
Woolf CJ, Wiesenfeld-Hallin Z (1985) The systemic administration of local anaes-
    thetics produces a selective depression of C-afferent fibre evoked activity in the
    spinal cord. Pain 23:361–374
Xie Y, Zhang J, Petersen M, LaMotte RH (1995) Functional changes in dorsal root
    ganglion cells after chronic nerve constriction in the rat. J Neurophysiol 73:1811–
    1820
Yaari Y, Devor M (1985) Phenytoin suppresses spontaneous ectopic discharge in rat
    sciatic nerve neuromas. Neurosci Lett 58:117–122

Tachykinins: Central and Peripheral Effects

P.J. BIRCH

A. Introduction

The neurobiology of tachykinins and tachykinin receptors has been studied for several decades (GUARD and WATSON 1991; NAKANISHI 1991). The tachykinins are a family of peptides that are broadly distributed in the mammalian central nervous system. This neuropeptide family includes substance P (SP), neurokinin A and neurokinin B, and these act preferentially on three major neurokinin receptors, NK-1, NK-2 and NK-3, respectively (PATACCHINI and MAGGI 1995). Substance P and NK-1 receptors represent the most extensively studied sensory neuropeptide system, and this chapter reviews the central and peripheral effects of this tachykinin and discusses the therapeutic potential of drugs designed to interact specifically with this system.

B. Substance P and NK-1 Receptors

I. Association with Sensory Systems

A large body of evidence strongly implicates a role for SP and NK-1 receptors in the processing of sensory information. This evidence has been obtained from studies investigating the biochemistry, pharmacology and pathology of this neuropeptide system in both the peripheral and central nervous systems. At peripheral sites SP is believed to play a pro-inflammatory role, and at central (spinal) sites it is involved in modulation of the transfer of nociceptive information.

Biochemical approaches have shown that SP is present in both the peripheral and central terminals of primary afferent C fibres (HOKFELT et al. 1975; JU et al. 1987), and ultrastructural analysis has identified afferent SP-positive terminals apposed to nociceptive-specific neurones in the spinal cord dorsal horn (DE KONINCK et al. 1992). SP is also present in interneurones and descending pathways which terminate within the spinal cord dorsal horn. Release of SP from each of these pathways could influence sensory transmission. NK-1 receptors have been localised in the peripheral receptive field of sensory nerves and within specific laminae of the spinal cord dorsal horn. This has been demonstrated using a variety of techniques including receptor auotradiography (MANTYH and HUNT 1985; YASHPAL et al. 1990), in situ hydbridisation (MAENO et al. 1993) and receptor immuno-mapping (LIU et al. 1994).

Antibody microprobe technology has enabled the release of SP to be measured in sensory systems. For example, SP is released into the rat and cat spinal cord following electrical stimulation of C fibres (DUGGAN and HENDRY 1986) and by the peripheral administration of noxious thermal, mechanical and chemical (inflammatory) stimuli (DUGGAN et al. 1987, 1988; SCHAIBLE et al. 1990; GARRY and HARGREAVES 1992).

The functional properties of SP in sensory systems have also been studied. Electrophysiological experiments have revealed that spinal administration of SP produces a slow depolarisation of nociceptive dorsal horn neurones (HENRY 1976; DE KONINCK and HENRY 1991) and enhancement of noxious reflexes (WOOLF and WIESENFELD-HALLIN 1986). In behavioural studies in rodents the intrathecal injection of SP and of SP analogues reduce nociceptive thresholds (PICARD et al. 1993; YASHPAL et al. 1982; YASHPAL and HENRY 1983) and produce aversive behaviours indicative of nociception (HYLDEN and WILCOX 1983).

II. Pathophysiology

Changes in the expression of SP and its receptor have been measured following inflammation and nerve injury. For instance, synthesis and peripheral transport of SP in dorsal root ganglion cells and spinal cord is increased following induction of inflammatory hyperalgesia in rat (MINAMI et al. 1989; DONNERER et al. 1992; SMITH et al. 1992; HANESCH et al. 1993; SLUKA and WESTLUND 1993). A role for nerve growth factor in the upregulation of SP following peripheral inflammation has also been described (LESLIE et al. 1995). Dorsal horn NK-1 receptor expression is altered during inflammatory pain. A two-fold increase in NK-1 receptor number is observed following formalin-induced nociception (MCCARSON and KRAUSE 1994) whereas both increases and decreases in receptor number have been observed in persistent inflammatory models (SCHAFER et al. 1993; STUCKY et al. 1993; MCCARSON and KRAUSE 1994). During the development of neuropathic hyperalgesia dorsal root ganglia and dorsal horn SP levels are decreased, most probably reflecting damage to afferent fibres (CAMERON et al. 1991; MUNGLANI et al. 1995) and increases in NK-1 receptor number have been observed (AANONSEN et al. 1992; PALMER et al. 1995).

III. Substance P and NK-1 Receptors in Man

Importantly, SP and NK-1 receptors have been detected in dorsal root ganglion cells and in the superficial laminae of the human spinal cord (DIETL et al. 1989; TOMOKANE et al. 1991) and show a very similar distribution to that observed in rat. It is also well-known that peripheral injection of SP into human forearm causes wheal, flare and cutaneous pain which can last for up to 2 h (FOREMAN 1988; FULLER et al. 1987; PEDERSEN-BJERGAARD et al. 1989).

Several tissue biopsy and pathology investigations have been reported. SP-positive nerve fibres are detectable in patella, peri-patella soft tissue and lumbar facet joints surgically removed form patients with painful joint pathologies but are not easily detectable in cortical of trabecular bone, cartilage, or subchondral bone of normal patellas or facets (BEAMAN et al. 1993; GILES and HARVE 1987; WOJTYS et al. 1990). Patients with rheumatoid arthritis, osteoarthritis, Reiter's syndrome and post-traumatic arthritis have increased plasma and synovial fluid levels of SP compared to controls (MARSHALL et al. 1990). Interestingly, SP levels are much higher in the synovial fluid of rheumatoid patients than in that of patients with osteoarthritis (ARNALICH et al. 1994; MENKES et al. 1993), suggesting that SP may be more associated with inflammatory arthritis. Also of interest is a recent report which shows that a 9-year-old child with congenital insensitivity to pain had no detectable SP in articular nerve fibres and extremely low levels of SP in synovial fluid, suggesting the the pain insensitivity was due to the SP deficit (DERWIN et al. 1994).

C. NK-1 Receptor Antagonists

Animal and human data suggest that SP plays an important role in the modulation of sensory function. However, definitive evidence has awaited the development of specific and selective NK-1 receptor antagonists which can block the actions of SP.

Peptide antagonists selective for the NK-1 receptor have been available for over a decade. These agents have been used mainly for pharmacological characterisation of NK-1 receptor mechanisms in vitro, although certain studies in vivo have also been of value (BIRCH et al. 1992a; FLEETWOOD-WALKER et al. 1990). More recently, several non-peptide antagonists have been described: CP-96345 (SNIDER et al. 1991), CP-99994 (MCLEAN et al. 1993), RP-67580 (GARRET et al. 1991), RPR-100893 (LEE et al. 1994), SR-140333 (EMONDS-ALT et al. 1993; OURY-DONAT et al. 1994), GR-203040 (BEATTIE et al. 1995), LY-303870 (GITTER et al. 1995), and L-737488 (MACLOED et al. 1995). Although these non-peptide antagonists have high affinity for NK-1 receptors, marked species differences exist (BERESFORD et al. 1991), and the choice of pre-clinical animal species is important for therapeutic modelling. In addition, some compounds have ion channel blocking activity which must be taken into consideration when interpreting data (GUARD et al. 1993). For this reason many investigators have evaluated enantiomeric pairs of these compounds (stereoselectivity) as these have differing affinities for the NK-1 receptor but are equipotent at blocking ion channels. The discovery of these antagonists has facilitated greatly the study of the neurobiology of SP and such compounds appear to have therapeutic potential in several areas.

D. Therapeutic Potential of Drugs Acting at NK-1 Receptors

I. Acute and Chronic Pain

The models which have been used to investigate the potential antinociceptive activity of non-peptide NK-1 receptor antagonists can be broadly categorised into three types: extravasation/inflammation models, electrophysiological models, and behavioural pain models.

1. Extravasation/Inflammation Models

A range of non-peptide compounds and a variety of species have been investigated in models in which extravasation/inflammation has been induced by exogenous agents or by electrical stimulation of peripheral C fibre afferents (Table 1). In models in which a specific C fibre activation occurs (mustard oil, capsaicin, electrical stimulation) a stereoselective action of the NK-1 antagonist is observed, indicating that substance P is important for neurogenic inflammation. However, in other models which involve the release of a range of mediators from afferent and non-afferent sites (e.g. the carrageenan model) stereoselectivity was not observed. This may indicate that the channel-blocking action of these drugs also contributes to the anti-oedema activity under certain conditions.

Table 1. NK-1 receptor antagonists: extravasation/inflammation models

Stimulus/model	Species	Tissue	Antagonist	Reference
Capsaicin or mustard oil induced plasma protein extravasation	Rat, guinea-pig, mouse	Skin, viscera, lung, dura	CP-96345, CP-99994, RP-67580, RPR-100893, SR-140333	McLean et al. 1993a; Nagahisa et al. 1992b; Lembeck et al. 1992; Shepheard et al. 1993; Lee et al. 1994; Amann et al. 1995
Electrically induced (neurogenic) plasma protein extravasation	Rat, guinea-pig	Skin; dura	CP-96345, CP-99994, RP-67580, RPR-100893, SR-140333, GR-203040	Lembeck et al. 1992; Wiesenfeld-Hallin and Xu 1993; Xu et al. 1992; Emonds-Alt et al. 1993; Garret et al. 1991; Lee et al. 1994; Beattie et al. 1995
Mustard oil induced oedema	Mouse	Paw	CP-96345, CP-99994	Lembeck et al. 1992
Carrageenan-induced oedema	Rat	Paw	CP-96345	Nagahisa et al. 1992a, 1993; Yamamoto et al. 1993

In summary, the experiments performed with neurogenic inflammation support the hypothesis that blockade of peripheral NK-1 receptors produces anti-inflammatory effects. However, the ability of these compounds to produce such effects in humans depends entirely on the degree to which neurogenic inflammation contributes to the pathology of human inflammatory disease, and this is currently unknown.

2. Electrophysiological Models

A wide variety of electrophysiological preparations have been used to investigate the role of NK-1 receptors in nociception (Table 2). The electrophysiological correlates used in these studies are different manifestations of spinal hyperexcitability. Stereospecific effects have been observed in the majority of studies, indicating that blockade of spinal NK-1 receptors has the potential to produce antinociception. In addition, one study indicated the potential for a supraspinal NK-1 mechanism (EMONDS-ALT et al. 1993).

Table 2. NK-1 receptor antagonists: electrophysiological models

Electrophysiological correlate	Species	Antagonist	Stereoselectivity	Reference
Noxious mechanical and thermal excitation of dorsal horn neurones	Cat	CP-96345, CP-99994	Yes	RADHAKRISHNAN and HENRY 1991; DE KONINCK and HENRY 1991
Formalin-induced excitation of dorsal horn neurones	Rat	RP-67580	Yes	CHAPMAN and DICKENSON 1993
C fibre dependent facilitation of the flexor reflex	Rat, rabbit	CP-96345 CP-99994 RP-67580	Yes	WIESENFELD-HALLIN and XU 1993; XU et al. 1992; LAIRD et al. 1993
Electrically and mustard oil induced cutaneous mechanical allodynia of spinal flexor motoneurones	Rat	RP-67580	Yes	MA and WOOLF 1995
NGF- or UV irradiation-induced prolongation of C fibre evoked ventral root potential; NGF or UV irradiation-induced A and C fibre evoked wind-up of ventral root potential	Rat	CP-96345 RP-67580	Not reported	THOMSON et al. 1994, 1995
Noxious mechanical excitation of thalamic neurones	Rat	SR-140333	Yes	EMONDS-ALT et al. 1993

Of particular significance is the report of Ma and Woolf (1995), which investigated hyperexcitability in posterior biceps femoris-semitendinosus spinal flexor motoneurones. In this study only pre-treatment, and not post-treatment, with RP-67580 was effective at reducing the electrophysiological correlate of cutaneous mechanical allodynia. This suggests that NK-1 receptors plays a role in the initiation but not in the maintenance of spinal hyperexcitability. In the same series of experiments muscle C fibre conditioning inputs were not blocked by RP-67580, indicating that an involvement of NK-1 receptors is further restricted to cutaneous hypersensitivity. This may have important clinical implications for the therapeutic use of NK-1 antagonists. The above information is derived from studies measuring the development of acute hyperexcitability, and these studies do not provide information about a possible role for NK-1 receptors in persistent pain, which is manifest over a longer time period. It is conceivable that regenerative hyperexcitability processes occur during persistent pain, and hence NK-1 receptor mechanisms may be operational even during the apparent maintenance phase.

3. Behavioural Models

Several behavioural models have been used to investigate the potential antinociceptive activity of non-peptide NK-1 antagonists. These can be grouped into threshold tests, acute-tonic pain and acute hyperalgesia models, and persistent hyperalgesia models.

a) Threshold Tests

In rodent threshold nociceptive tests employing either mechanical (paw-pressure) or thermal (paw-flick, hot-plate, tail-flick) stumuli, non-peptide NK-1 antagonists are ineffective, at least at doses that are free of profound motor side effects (Garces et al. 1992; Yamamoto et al. 1993; Rupniak et al. 1993; Amann et al. 1995; Seguin et al. 1995). This is in agreement with the observation that SP is not released following the application of such brief stimuli.

b) Acute-Tonic Pain and Acute Hyperalgesia Models

Tables 3 and 4 summarise data from formalin-induced nociception and abdominal constriction assays. Acute-tonic tests revealed robust antinociceptive effects although consistent stereospecific effects were not observed. Thus the ion channel blocking activity may account for some of these actions, as discussed above.

The actions of the NK-1 antagonist CP-96345 in an acute thermal hyperalgesia paradigm has been evaluated. In this paradigm the prior administration of a noxious thermal stimulus reduces subsequent thermal nociceptive thresholds. The antagonist is reported to reverse thermal hyperalgesia in a stereospecific manner (Yashpal et al. 1993). Similarly, Yamamoto et al. (1993) have reported that subcutaneous pretreatment with CP-96345 produces

Table 3. NK-1 receptor antagonists: acute tonic tests

Compound	Species	Efficacy	Stereoselectivity	Reference
Formalin-induced nociception				
RP-67580	Mouse, rat, guinea-pig	Where evaluated, active against both phases	Stereoselectivity claimed in majority of studies	SEGUIN and MILLAN 1994; GARRET et al. 1991; SEGUIN et al. 1995
CP-96345	Mouse, rat	Poorly active against first phase, more effective against second phase	Stereoselectivity claimed in some studies, but not observed in others	SAKARUDA et al. 1993; NAGAHISA et al. 1993; YASHPAL et al. 1993; YAMAMOTO and YAKSH 1991
CP-99994	Mouse, rat, gerbil	More effective against second phase compared to first phase	Where evaluated, little stereoselectivity observed	SEGUIN and MILLAN 1994; SMITH et al. 1995; SEGUIN et al. 1995
SR-140333	Mouse	Equi-effective against both phases	Not evaluated	SEGUIN et al. 1995
Abdominal constriction				
RP-67580	Mouse, rat	Phenylbenzoquinone, acetic acid	Where evaluated, stereoselectivity observed	GARRET et al. 1991; SEGUIN et al. 1995
CP-96345	Mouse	Acetic acid	Not evaluated	NAGAHISA et al. 1992b
CP-99994	Mouse	Acetylcholine, acetic acid	Where evaluated, no stereoselectivity observed	SMITH et al. 1995; SEGUIN et al. 1995
SR-140333	Mouse	Acetic acid	Not evaluated	SEGUIN et al. 1995

Table 4. NK-1 receptor antagonists: anti-emetic profile in animal models

Compound	Species	Emetogen	Activity	Reference
CP-99994	Ferret	Loperamide, apomorphine, morphine, Ipecacuanha, copper sulphate, cisplatin, radiation	Potent blockade of retching and vomiting; enantiomeric specificity observed	Bountra et al. 1993; Tattersall et al. 1993, 1994; Watson et al. 1995
CP-99994	Dog	Apomorphine, copper sulphate	Reduction of retching and vomiting	Watson et al. 1995
GR-203040	Ferret	Morphine, ipecacuanha, copper sulphate, cyclophosphamide, cisplatin, radiation	Potent blockade of retching and vomiting	Gardner et al. 1995
GR-203040	Dog	Ipecacuanha	Potent blockade of emesis	Gardner et al. 1995
GR-203040	*Suncus murinus*	Motion	Blockade of emesis and increase in latency to first emetic episode	Gardner et al. 1995

a stereoselective block of carrageenan-induced thermal hyperalgesia in rat, whereas intrathecal pretreatment or post-treatment by either route was ineffective. These authors concluded that blockade of peripheral NK-1 receptors is responsible for the anti-hyperalgesic effect, and that this mechanism is operational only during the initiation of the hyperalgesic response. Similar effects have been reported for ±CP-96345 against carrageenan-induced mechanical hyperalgesia (Birch et al. 1992b), although Nagahisa et al. (1992a) subsequently reported a lack of stereospecificity in this model when the individual enantiomers were evaluated. A subsequent study showed SR140333 to be ineffective against prostaglandin E2 induced thermal hyperalgesia at doses that block neurogenic plasma extravasation (Amann et al. 1995).

The results from evaluation of non-peptide NK-1 antagonists in behavioural models of acute-tonic pain and acute hyperalgesia appear inconclusive.

c) Persistent Hyperalgesia Models

Only two reports have appeared assessing the effects of NK-1 receptor antagonists in persistent hyperalgesia models. The first study evaluated the activity of intrathecal CP-96345 against thermal hyperalgesia induced by loose ligation of the sciatic nerve (mononeuropathy). The antagonist was given 7 days after ligation, and no reversal of hyperalgesia was observed (YAMAMOTO and YAKSH 1992). The second study evaluated the activity of RP-67580 against mechanical hyperalgesia in a rat diabetic neuropathy model. In the latter study the compound was given 4 weeks after the injection of streptozocin, and a full reversal of hyperalgesia was reported (COURTIEX et al. 1993). Importantly, a stereospecific effect was observed.

4. Visceral Pain

The preceding sections describe the role of SP and NK-1 receptors predominantly in models of somatic pain. However, another very important but perhaps overlooked area of clinical need is in the effective treatment of pain of visceral origin. The clinical features of somatic and visceral pain differ from one another. Somatic pain is often associated with the presence and evolution of an injury, whereas visceral pain is dull, poorly localised, referred to other areas, and not always associated with an obvious internal lesion. Although differences in the neural organisation and integration of somatic and visceral pain mechanisms may exist, the key to understanding visceral pain, and hence the design of therapeutic agents, must rely on progress in understanding the underlying pathophysiology of functional and inflammatory bowel disorders.

Neurotransmitters which play a role in somatic pain or in the control of intestinal motility could be involved in the alterations of sensory perception associated with visceral pain. SP fibres are found in myenteric and submucous plexus and also in circular and longitudinal muscle layers, and NK-1 receptors have been identified in gastrointestinal smooth muscle cells (BURCHER et al. 1986).

Current hypotheses on the pathogenesis of visceral hyperalgesia and visceral allodynia incorporate a role for gastrointestinal infection. Interestingly, certain gastrointestinal infections have been shown to produce an upregulation of intestinal mast cells, particularly those in close association with SP-containing sensory nerves, and it has been suggested that this plays a role in the initiation of visceral sensory abnormalities (BIENENSTOCK et al. 1991). In addition, rectal mucosal levels of SP and NK-1 receptors located on intestinal blood vessels and lymphoid follicles are upregulated in patients with inflammatory bowel disease (BERNSTEIN et al. 1993; MANTYH et al. 1988), again suggesting that enhanced transmission at this receptor system contributes to the inflammatory pathology.

Although several animal models of visceral pain have been developed, there have been few studies with NK-1 antagonists. CP-96345 and RP67580 are reported to inhibit the rectocolonic inhibitory reflex in rats but are unable to influence the distension-induced enhancement of abdominal contractions (JULIA et al. 1994). Additional studies are required to ascertain the role of substance P and NK-1 receptors in visceral nociception.

II. Migraine

Migraine is characterised by a severe, pulsatile-type headache often accompanied by several sensory disturbances such as photophobia, phonophobia, nausea and vomiting. The pain of migraine headache appears to be associated with inflammation of the pain-sensitive trigeminal nerve fibres in cerebral and dural vasculature (Moskowitz 1992). These sensory fibres pass via trigeminal ganglia to the trigeminal nucleus caudalis, and this brainstem area projects to the thalamus and cerebral cortex, where the pain of migraine is experienced. Trigeminal afferents also project to the nucleus tractus solitarius which is involved in control of nausea and vomiting.

Current evidence supports a role for SP in the pathogenesis of migraine. Cerebral and dural blood vessels from several species, including humans, receive a dense innervation of SP-like immunoreactive nerve fibres from trigeminal ganglia, and SP has been detected at the central terminals of these fibres within the trigeminal nuclues caudalis (Edvinsson et al. 1983, 1989). Release of SP from the peripheral and central terminals of the trigeminal system has been reported (Goadsby et al. 1988; Yonehara et al. 1991). Functional studies have shown SP to dilate cerebral blood vessels via an NK-1 receptor mechanism (Beattie et al. 1993) and to induce plasma protein leakage in dura mater (Buzzi and Moskowitz 1990). The latter effect is also induced by the electrical or capsaicin stimulation of trigeminal ganglia, and antagonist studies have shown that this is mediated by activation of NK-1 receptors (O'Shaughnessy and Connor 1993; Shepheard et al. 1993; Lee et al. 1994). Similar studies have indicated a functional NK-1 receptor mechanism at central trigeminal terminals. For instance, RPR 100893 blocks stimulation-induced c-*fos* mRNA and Fos protein expression in trigeminal nucleus caudalis (Cutrer et al. 1995).

In summary, NK-1 receptors, activated by SP, appear to play an important role in dural vasodilatation, in dural plasma protein extravasation, and in sensory transmission within the trigeminal nucleus caudalis. Thus non-peptide NK-1 antagonists have the potential to provide a novel treatment for migraine. As 10% of the adult population suffer from migraine headache, clinical evaluation is fully warranted.

III. Emesis

Nausea and vomiting can occur in a number of clinical and non-clinical settings. The most significant of these include chemotherapy- and radiotherapy-induced nausea and vomiting, emesis in anticipation of cytotoxic treatment, post-operative nausea and vomiting, and motion sickness. Although serotonin type 3 receptor antagonists have provided some clinical benefit in relieving nausea and vomiting, more effective, broad-spectrum anti-emetic treatments are required.

SP-immunoreactive fibres and NK-1 receptors have been detected in hindbrain areas (e.g. nucleus tractus solitarius, dorsal motor nucleus of the vagus) that are involved in the emetic reflex in several animal species and in man (McRITCHIE and TORK 1994; WATSON et al. 1995). SP is also co-localised with serotonin in the enterochromaffin cells in the gastrointestinal tract (SJOLUND et al. 1983), a known site for cytotoxic agents to initiate the emetic reflex. As a consequence of this, non-peptide NK-1 receptor antagonists have been evaluated in animal models of emesis (Table 4), and profound anti-emetic activity has been observed against a range of emetogens. Preliminary studies have also indicated a central site of action is involved in anti-emetic effects of NK-1 antagonists (GARDNER et al. 1994; WATSON et al. 1995).

In summary, there is considerable evidence that SP plays a critical role in the emetic response induced by a range of clinically-relevant stimuli. Thus NK-1 receptor antagonists may offer a novel, efficacious and broad-spectrum anti-emetic treatment in man. Clinical studies sponsored by several pharmaceutical companies are currently underway.

E. Summary

The tachykinin substance P plays a major role in sensory transmission at both central and peripheral sites. Current evidence suggests that blockade of the action of SP at the NK-1 receptor may provide novel therapeutic treatments for acute pain, chronic pain, migraine headache and emesis. Currently a number of potent, selective non-peptide NK-1 receptor antagonists are undergoing clinical evaluation and clinical data is eagerly awaited.

References

Aanonsen LM, Kajander KC, Bennett GJ, Seybold V (1992) Autoradiographic analysis of 125I-substance P binding in rat spinal cord following chronic constriction injury of the sciatic nerve. Brain Res 596:259–268

Amann R, Schuligoi R, Holzer P, Donnerer J (1995) The nonpeptide NK-1 receptor antagonist SR140333 produces long-lasting inhibition of neurogenic inflammation but does not influence acute chemo- or thermonociception in rats. Naunyn Schmiedebergs Arch Pharmacol 352:201–205

Arnalich F, de Miguel E, Perez-Ayala C, Martinez M, Vazquez JJ, Gijon-Banos J, Hernanz A (1994) Neuropeptides and interleukin-6 in human joint inflammation relationship between intraarticular substance P and interleukin-6 concentrations. Neurosci Lett 170:251–254

Beaman DN, Graziano GP, Glover RA, Wojtys EM, Chang V (1993) Substance P innervation of lumbar spine facet joints. Spine 18:1044–1049

Beattie DT, Stubbs CM, Connor HE, Feniuk W (1993) Neurokinin-induced changes in pial artery diameter in the anaesthetized guinea-pig. Br J Pharmacol 108:146–149

Beattie DT, Beresford IJM, Connor HE, Marshall FH, Hawcock AB, Hagan RM, Bowers JS, Birch PJ, Ward P (1995) The pharmacology of GR203040, a novel, potent and selective non-peptide NK1 receptor antagonist. Br J Pharmacol 116:3158–3163

Beresford IJ, Birch PJ, Hagan RM, Ireland SJ (1991) Investigation into species variants in tachykinin NK1 receptors by use of the non-peptide antagonist, CP-96,345. Br J Pharmacol 104:292–293

Bernstein CN, Robert ME, Eysselein VE (1993) Rectal substance P concentrations are increased in ulcerative colitis but not in Crohn's disease. Am J Gastroenterol 88:908–913

Bienenstock J, MacQueen G, Sestini P, Marshall JS, Stead RH, Perdue MH (1991) Mast cell/nerve interactions in vitro and in vivo. Am Rev Respir Dis 143:S55–S58

Birch PJ, Beresford IJM, Rogers H, Hagan RM, Bailey F, Hayes AG, Harrison SM, Ireland SJ (1992a) Profile of activity of the peptide NK1 receptor antagonist GR82334 in acute nociceptive tests. Br J Pharmacol 105:134P

Birch PJ, Harrison SM, Hayes AG, Rogers H, Tyers MB (1992b) The nonpeptide NK-1 receptor antagonist ±-CP-96345 produces antinociceptive and anti-oedema effects in rat. Br J Pharmacol 105:508–510

Bountra C, Bunce K, Dale T, Gardner C, Jordan C, Twissell D, Ward P (1993) Antiemetic profile of a non-peptide neurokinin NK1 receptor antagonist, CP-99,994, in ferrets. Eur J Pharmacol 249:R3–R4

Burcher E, Buck SH, Lovenberg W, O'Donohue TL (1986) Characterization and autoradiographic localization of multiple tachykinin binding sites in gastrointestinal tract and bladder. J Pharmacol Exp Ther 236:819–831

Buzzi MG, Moskowitz MA (1990) The antimigraine drug, sumatriptan (GR43175), selectively blocks neurogenic plasma extravasation from blood vessels in dura mater. Br J Pharmacol 99:202–206

Cameron AA, Cliffer KD, Dougherty PM, Willis WD, Carlton SM (1991) Changes in lectin, GAP-43 and neuropeptide staining in the rat superficial dorsal horn following experimental peripheral neuropathy. Neurosci Lett 131:249–252

Chapman V, Dickenson AH (1993) The effect of intrathecal administration of RP67580, a potent NK-1 antagonist on nociceptive transmission in the rat spinal cord. Neurosci Lett 157:149–152

Courteix C, Lavarenne J, Eschalier A (1993) RP-67580 a specific tachykinin NK1 receptor antagonist, relieves chronic hyperalgesia in diabetic rats. Eur J Pharmacol 241:267–270

Cutrer FM, Moussaoui S, Garret C, Moskowitz MA (1995) The non-peptide neurokinin-1 antagonist, RPR 100893, decreases c-fos expression in trigeminal nucleus caudalis following noxious chemical meningeal stimulation. Neuroscience 64:741–750

De Koninck Y, Henry JL (1991) Substance P-mediated slow excitatory postsynaptic potential elicited in dorsal horn neurons in vivo by noxious stimulation. Proc Natl Acad Sci USA 88:11344–11348

De Koninck Y, Ribeiro-da-Silva A, Henry JL, Cuello AC (1992) Spinal neurons exhibiting a specific nociceptive response receive abundant substance P-containing synaptic contacts. Proc Natl Acad Sci USA 89:5073–5077

Derwin KA, Glover RA, Wojtys EM (1994) Nociceptive role of substance-P in the knee joint of a patient with congenital insensitivity to pain. J Paediatr Orthop 14:258–262

Dietl MM, Sanchez M, Probst A, Palacios JM (1989) Substance P receptors in the human spinal cord: decrease in amyotrophic lateral sclerosis. Brain Res 483:39–49

Donnerer J, Schuligoi R, Stein C (1992) Increased content and transport of substance P and calcitonin gene-related peptide in sensory nerves innervating inflamed tissue: evidence for a regulatory function of nerve growth factor in vivo. Neuroscience 49:693–698

Duggan AW, Hendry IA (1986) Laminar localization of the sites of relese of immunoreactive substance P in the dorsal horn with antibody-coated microelectrodes. Neurosci Lett 68:134–140

Duggan AW, Morton CR, Zhao ZQ, Hendry IA (1987) Noxious heating of the skin releases immunoreactive substance P in the substantia gelatinosa of the cat: a study with antibody microprobes. Brain Res 403:345–349

Duggan AW, Hendry IA, Morton CR, Hutchison WD, Zhao ZQ (1988) Cutaneous stimuli releasing immunoreactive substance P in the dorsal horn of the cat. Brain Res 451:261–273

Emonds-Alt X, Doutremepuich JD, Heaulme M, Neliat G, Santucci V, Steinberg R, Vilain P, Bichon D, Ducoux J-P, Proietto V, Van Broeck D, Soubrie P, Le Fur G, Breliere J-C (1993) In vitro and in vivo biological activities of SR140333, a novel potent non-peptide tachykinin NK-1 receptor antagonist. Eur J Pharmacol 250:403–413

Edvinsson L, Rosendal-Helgesen S, Uddman R (1983) Substance P: localisation, concentration and release in cerebral arteries, choroid plexus and dura mater. Cell Tissue Res 234:1–7

Edvinsson L, Hara H, Uddman R (1989) Retograde tracing of nerve fibres to the rat middle cerebral artery with True Blue: colocalisation with different peptides. J Cereb Blood Flow Metab 9:212–218

Fleetwood-Walker SM, Mitchell R, Hope PJ, El-Yassir N, Molony V, Bladon CM (1990) The involvement of neurokinin receptor subtypes in somatosensory processing in the superficial dorsal horn of the cat. Brain Res 519:169–182

Foreman JC (1988) The skin as an organ for the study of the pharmacology of neuropeptides. Skin Pharmacol 1:77–83

Fuller RW, Conradson TB, Dixon CM, Crossman DC, Barnes PJ (1987) Sensory neuropeptide effects in human skin. Br J Pharmacol 92:781–788

Garces YI, Rabito SF, Minshall RD, Sagen J (1992) Lack of potent antinociceptive activity by substance P antagonist CP-96,345 in the rat spinal cord. Life Sci 52:353–360

Gardner CJ, Bountra C, Bunce KT, Dale TJ, Jordan CC, Twissell DJ, Ward P (1994) Anti-emetic activity of neurokinin NK-1 receptor antagonists is mediated centrally in the ferret. Br J Pharmacol 112:516P

Gardner CJ, Twissell DJ, Dale TJ, Jordan CC, Kilpatrick GJ, Bountra C, Ward P (1995) The broad-spectrum anti-emetic activity of the novel non-pepitde tachykinin NK-1 receptor antagonist GR203040. Br J Pharmacol 116:3158–3163

Garret C, Carruette A, Fardin V, Moussaoui S, Peyronel JF, Blanchard JC, Laduron PM (1991) Pharmacological properties of a potent and selective nonpeptide substance P antagonist. Proc Natl Acad Sci USA 88:10208–10212

Garry MG, Hargreaves KM (1992) Enhanced release of immunoreactive CGRP and substance P spinal dorsal horn slices occurs during carrageenan inflammation. Brain Res 582:139–142

Giles LG, Harvey AR (1987) Immunohistochemical demonstration of nociceptors in the capsule and synovial folds of human zygapophyseal joints. Br J Rheumatol 26:362–364

Gitter BD, Bruns RF, Howbert J, Waters DC, Threlkeld PG, Cox LM, Nixon JA, Lobb KL, Mason NR, Stengel PW, Cockerham SL, Silbaugh SA, Gehlert DR, Schober DA, Iyengar S, Calligaro DO, Regoli D, Hipskind PA (1995) Pharmacological characterisation of LY303870: a novel potent and selective non-peptide substance P (NK-1) receptor antagonist. J Pharmacol Exp Ther 275: 737–744

Goadsby PJ, Edvinsson L, Ekman R (1988) Release of vasoactive peptides in the extracerebral circulation of man and cat during activation of the trigeminovascular system. Ann Neurol 23:193–196

Guard S, Watson SP (1991) Tachykinin receptor types: classification and membrane signalling mechanisms. Neurochem Int 18:149–165

Guard S, Boyle SJ, Tang KW, Watling KJ, McKnight AT, Woodruff GN (1993) The interaction of the NK-1 receptor antagonist CP-96345 with L-type calcium channels and its functional consequences. Br J Pharmacol 110:385–391

Hanesch U, Pfrommer U, Grubb BD, Heppelmann B, Schaible H-G. (1993) The proportion of CGRP-immunoreactive and SP-mRNA containing dorsal root ganglion cells is increased by a unilateral inflammation of the ankle joint of the rat. Regul Pept 46:202–203

Henry JL (1976) Effects of substance P on functionally identified units in cat spinal cord. Brain Res 114:439–451

Hokfelt T, Kellerth JO, Nilsson G, Pernow B (1975) Experimental immunohistochemical studies on the localization and distribution of substance P in cat primary
sensory neurons. Brain Res 100:235–252

Hylden JLK, Wilcox GL (1983) Pharmacological characterization of substance P-
induced nociception in mice: modulation by opioid and noradrenergic agonists at
the spinal level. J Pharmacol Exp Ther 226:398–404

Ju G, Hokfelt T, Brodin E, Fahrenkrug J, Fischer JA, Frey P, Elde RP, Brown JC
(1987) Primary sensory neurons of the rat showing calcitonin gene-related peptide
immunoreactivity and their relation to substance P-, somatostatin-, galanin-, vasoactive intestinal polypeptide- and cholecystokinin-immunoreactive ganglion cells.
Cell Tissue Res 247:417–431

Julia V, Morteau O, Bueno L (1994) Involvement of neurokinin 1 and 2 receptors in
viscerosensitive response to rectal distension in rats. Gastroenterology 107:94–102

Laird JMA, Hargreaves RJ, Hill RG (1993) Effect of RP67580, a non-peptide
neurokinin1 receptor antagonist, on facilitation of a nociceptive spinal flexion
reflex in the rat. Br J Pharmacol 109:713–718

Lee WS, Moussaoui SM, Moskowitz MA (1994) Blockade by oral or parenteral
RPR100893 (a nonpeptide NK-1 receptor antagonist) of neurogenic plasma protein extravasation within the guinea-pig dura mater and conjunctiva. Br J Pharmacol 112:920–924

Lembeck FJ, Donnerer M, Tsuchiya M, Nagahisa A (1992) The nonpeptide antagonist
CP-96345 is a potent inhibitor of neurogenic inflammation. Br J Pharmacol 105:
527–530

Leslie TA, Emson PC, Dowd PM, Woolf CJ (1995) Nerve growth factor contributes to
the up-regulation of GAP43 and preprotachykinin A messenger RNAs in primary
sensory neurones following peripheral inflammation. Neuroscience 67:753–761

Liu H, Brown JL, Jasmin L, Maggio JE, Vigna SR Mantyh PW, Basbaum A (1994)
Synaptic relationship between substance P and the substance P receptor: light and
electron microscopic characterization of the mismatch between neuropeptides and
their receptors. Proc Natl Acad Sci USA 91:1009–1013

Ma QP, Woolf CJ (1995) Involvement of neurokinin receptors in the induction but not
the maintenance of mechanical allodynia in rat flexor motoneurones. J Physiol
(Lond) 486:769–777

MacLeod AM, Cascieri MA, Merchant KJ, Sadowski S, Hardwicke S, Lewis RT,
MacIntyre DE, Metzger JM, Fong TM, Shepheard S, Tattershall FD, Hargreaves
R, Baker R (1995) Synthesis and biological evaluation of NK1 antagonists derived
from l-tryptophan. J Med Chem 38:934–941

Maeno H, Kiyama H, Tohyama M (1993) Distribution of the substance P receptor
(NK-1 receptor) in the central nervous system. Mol Brain Res 18:43–58

Mantyh PW, Hunt SP (1985) The autoradiographic localization of substance P receptors in the rat and bovine spinal cord and the rat and cat spinal trigeminal nucleus
pars caudalis and the effects of neonatal capsaicin. Brain Res 332:315–324

Mantyh CR, Gates TS, Zimmerman RP, Welton ML, Passaro EP, Vigna SR, Maggio
JE, Kruger L, Mantyh PW (1988) Receptor binding sites for substance P, but not
substance K or neuromedin K, are expressed in high concentrations by arterioles,
venules, and lymph nodules in surgical specimens obtained from patients with
ulcerative colitis and Crohn disease. Proc Natl Acad Sci USA 85:3235–3239

Marshall KW, Chiu B, Inman RD (1990) Substance P and arthritis: analysis of plasma
and synovial fluid levels. Arthritis Rheum 33:87–90

McCarson KE, Krause JE (1994) NK-1 and NK-3 type tachykinin receptor mRNA
expression in the rat spinal cord dorsal horn is increased during adjuvant or
formalin-induced nociception. J Neurosci 14:712–720

McLean S, Ganong A, Seymour PA, Snider RM, Desai MC, Rosen, T, Bryce DK,
Longo KP, Reynolds LS, Robinson G, Scmidt AW, Siok C, Heym J (1993a)
Pharmacology of CP-99,994; a nonpeptide antagonist of the tachykinin
neurokinin-1 receptor. J Pharmacol Exp Ther 267:472–479

McRitchie DA, Tork I (1994) Distribution of substance P-like immunoreactive neurons and terminals throughout the nucleus of the solitary tract in the human brainstem. J Comp Neurol 343:83–101

Menkes CJ, Renoux M, Laoussadi S, Mauborgne A, Bruxelle J, Cesselin FJ (1993) Substance P levels in the synovium and synovial fluid from patients with rheumatoid arthritis and osteoarthritis. Rheumatology 20:714–717

Minami M, Kuraishi Y, Kawamura M, Yamaguchi T, Masu Y, Nakanishi S, Satoh M (1989) Enhancement of preprotachykinin A gene expression by adjuvant-induced inflammation in the rat spinal cord: possible involvement of substance P-containing spinal neurons in nociception. Neurosci Lett 98:105–110

Moskowitz MA (1992) Neurogenic versus vascular mechanisms of sumatriptan and ergot extravasation in dura mater: proposed action in vascular headaches. Trends Pharmacol Sci 13:307–311

Munglani R, Bond A, Smith GD, Harrison SM, Elliott P, Birch PJ, Hunt SP (1995) Changes in neuronal markers in a mononeuropathic rat model: relationship between neuropeptide Y, pre-emptive drug treatment and long term mechanical hyperalgesia. Pain 63:21–31

Nagahisa A, Asai R, Kanai Y, Murase A, Tsuchiya-Nakagaki M, Nakagaki T, Shieh TC, Taniguchi K (1992a) Non-specific activity of ±CP-96,345 in models of pain and inflammation. Br J Pharmacol 107:273–275

Nagahisa A, Kanai Y, Suga O, Taniguchi K, Tsuchiya M, Lowe JA, Hess HJ (1992b) Anti-inflammatory and analgesic activity of a non-peptide substance P receptor antagonist. Eur J Pharmacol 217:191–195

Nagahisa A, Kanai Y, Suga O, Taniguchi K, Tsuchiya M, Lowe JA, Hess HJ (1993) Antiinflammatory and analgesic activity of CP-96,345: an orally active non-peptide substance P receptor antagonist. Regul Pept 46:433–436

Nakanishi S (1991) Mammalian tachykinin receptors. Annu Rev Neurosci 14:123–126

O'Shaughnessy CT, Connor HE (1993) Neurokinin NK-1 receptors mediate plasma protein extravasation in guinea-pig dura. Eur J Pharmacol 236:319–321

Oury-Donat F, Lefevre IA, Thurneyssen O et al (1994) SR140333, a novel, selective and potent nonpeptide antagonist of the NK1 tachykinin receptor: characterization on the U373MG cell line. J Neurochem 62:1399–1407

Palmer JA, Munglani R, Smith GD, Birch PJ, Hunt SP (1995) NK-1 receptor on lamina 1 neurones of the spinal cord: distribution, relation to substance P and response to peripheral stimulation. Soc Neurosci Abstr 21:1413

Patacchini R, Maggi CA (1995) Tachykinin receptors and receptor subtypes. Arch Int Pharmacodyn Ther 329:161–184

Pedersen-Bjergaard U, Nielsen LB, Jensen K, Edvinsson L, Jansen I, Olesen J (1989) Algesia and local responses induced by neurokinin A and substance P in human skin and temporal muscle. Peptides 10:1147–1152

Picard P, Boucher S, Regoli D, Gitter BD, Howbert JJ, Couture R (1993) Use of non-peptide tachykinin receptor antagonists to substantiate the involvement of NK-1 and NK-2 receptors in a spinal nociceptive reflex in the rat. Eur J Pharmacol 232:255–261

Radhakrishnan V, Henry JL (1991) Novel substance P antagonist, CP-96,345, blocks responses of cat spinal dorsal horn neurons to noxious cutaneous stimulation and to substance P. Neurosci Lett 132:39–43

Rupniak NMJ, Boyce S, Williams AR, Cook G, Longmore J, Seabrook GR, Caeser M, Iversen SD, Hill RG (1993) Antinociceptive activity of NK-1 receptor antagonists: non-specific effects of racemic RP-67580. Br J Pharmacol 110:1607–1613

Sakaruda T, Katsuma K, Yogo H, Tan-No K, Sakaruda S, Kisara K (1993) Antinociception induced by CP-96345 a non-peptide NK-1 receptor antgonist in the mouse formalin and capsaicin tests. Neurosci Lett 151:142–145

Schafer MK, Nohr D, Krause JE, Weihe E (1993) Inflammation-induced upregulation of NK-1 receptor mRNA in dorsal horn neurones. Neuroreport 4:1007–1010

Schaible H-G, Jarrott B, Hope PJ, Duggan AW (1990) Release of immunoreactive substance P in the spinal cord during development of acute arthritis in the knee joint of the cat: a study with antibody microprobes. Brain Res 529:214–223

Seguin L, Millan MJ (1994) The glycine B receptor partial agonist (+) HA966, enhances induction of antinociception by RP67480 and CP-99-994. Eur J Pharmacol 253:R1–R3

Seguin L, Le Marouille-Girardon S, Millan MJ (1995) Antinociceptive profile of non-peptidergic NK-1 and NK-2 receptor antagonists: a comparison to other classes of antinociceptive agent. Pain 61:325–343

Shepheard SL, Williamson DJ, Hill RG, Hargreaves RJ (1993) The nonpeptide NK-1 receptor antagonist RP-67580 blocks neurogenic plasma extravasation in the dura mater of rats. Br J Pharmacol 238:421–424

Sjolund K, Sanden G, Hakanson R, Sundler F (1983) Endocrine cells in human intestine: an immunocytochemical study. Gastroenterology 85:1120–1130

Smith GD, Harmar AJ, McQueen DS, Seckl JR (1992) Increase in substance P and CGRP but not somatostatin content of innervating dorsal root ganglia in adjuvant monoarthritis in the rat. Neurosci Lett 137:257–260

Smith GD, Harrison SM, Bowers J, Wiseman J, Birch PJ (1995) Non-specific effects of the tackykinin NK-1 receptor antagonist CP-99994 in antinociceptive tests in rat, mouse and gerbil. Eur J Pharmacol 271:481–487

Sluka KA, Westlund KN (1993) Behavioural and immunohistochemical changes in an experimental arthritis model in rats. Pain 55:367–377

Snider RM, Constantine JW, Lowe JA, Longo KP, Lebel WS, Woody HA, Drozda SE, Desai MC, Vinick FJ, Spencer RW, Hess HJ (1991) A potent nonpeptide antagonist of the substance P (NK-1) receptor. Science 251:435–437

Stucky CL, Galeazza MT, Seybold VS (1993) Time-dependent changes in Bolton-Hunter-labeled 125I-substance P binding in rat spinal cord following unilateral adjuvant-induced peripheral inflammation. Neuroscience 57:397–409

Tattersall FD, Rycroft W, Hargreaves RJ, Hill RG (1993) The tachykinin NK1 receptor antagonist CP-99,994 attenuates cisplatin induced emesis in the ferret. Eur J Pharmacol 250:R5–R6

Tattersall FD, Rycroft W, Hill RG, Hargreaves RJ (1994) Enantioselective inhibition of apomorphine-induced emesis in the ferret by the neurokinin1 receptor antagonist CP-99,994. Neuropharmacology 33:259–260

Thomson SWN, Dray A, Urban L (1994) Injury-induced plasticity of spinal reflex activity: NK-1 neurokinin receptor activation and enhanced A- and C-fibre mediated responses in the rat spinal cord in vitro. J Neurosci 14:3672–3687

Thomson SWN, Dray A, McCarson KE, Krause JE, Urban L (1995) Nerve growth factor induces mechanical allodynia associated with novel A fibre-evoked spinal reflex activity and enhanced NK-1 receptor activation in the rat. Pain 62:219–231

Tomokane N, Kitamoto T, Tateishi J, Sato Y (1991) Immunohistochemical quantification of substance P in spinal dorsal horns of patients with multiple system atrophy. J Neurol Neurosurg Psychiatry 54:535–541

Watson JW, Gonsalves SF, Fossa AA, McLean S (1995) The anti-emetic effects of CP-99,994 in the ferret and the dog: role of the NK1 receptor. Br J Pharmacol 115:84–94

Wiesenfeld-Hallin Z, Xu X-J (1993) The differential roles of substance P and neurokinin A in spinal cord hyperexcitability and neurogenic inflammation. Regul Pept 46:165–173

Wojtys EM, Beaman DN, Glover RA, Janda D (1990) Innervation of the human knee joint by substance-P fibers. Arthroscopy 6:254–263

Woolf C, Wiesenfeld-Hallin Z (1986) Substance P and calcitonin gene-related peptide synergistically modulate the gain of the nociceptve flexor withdrawal in the rat. Neurosci Lett 66:226–230

Xu X-J, Dalsgaard CJ, Maggi CA, Wiesenfeld-Hallin Z (1992) NK-1, but not NK-2 tachykinin receptors mediate plasma extravasation induced by antidromic C-fiber stimulation in rat hindpaw: demonstrated with the NK-1 antagonist CP-96,345 and the NK-2 antagonist Men10207. Neurosci Lett 139:249–252

Yamamoto T, Yaksh TL (1991) Stereospecific effects of a nonpeptidic NK-1 selective antagonist, CP-96,345: antinociception in the absence of motor dysfunction. Life Sci 49:1955–1963

Yamamoto T, Yaksh TL (1992) Effects of intrathecal capsaicin and an NK-1 antagonist, CP,96-345, on the thermal hyperalgesia observed following unilateral constriction of the sciatic nerve in the rat. Pain 51:329–334

Yamamoto T, Shimoyama N, Mizuguchi (1993) Effects of FK224, a novel cyclopeptide NK1 and NK2 antagonist, and CP-96,345, a nonpeptide NK1 antagonist, on development and maintenance of thermal hyperesthesia evoked by carrageenan injection in the rat paw. Anaesthesiology 79:1042–1050

Yashpal K, Henry JL (1983) Endorphins mediate overshoot of substance P-induced facilitation of a spinal nociceptive reflex. Can J Physiol Pharmacol 61:303–307

Yasphal K, Wright DM, Henry JL (1982) Substance P reduces tail-click latency: implications for chronic pain syndromes. Pain 14:155–167

Yashpal K, Dam TV, Quirion R (1990) Quantitative autoradiographic distributions of multiple neurokinin binding sites in rat spinal cord. Brain Res 506:259–266

Yashpal K, Radhakrishnan V, Coderre TJ, Henry JL (1993) CP-96345, but not its stereoisomer CP-96344, blocks the nociceptive responses to intrathecally administered substance P and to noxious thermal and chemical stimuli in the rat. Neuroscience 52:1039–1047

Yonehara N, Shibutani T, Imai Y, Ooi Y, Sawada I, Inoki R (1991) Serotonin inhibits the release of substance P evoked by tooth pulp stimulation in trigeminal nucleus caudalis in rabbits. Neuropharmacology 30:5–13

CHAPTER 7

Growth Factors and Pain

S.B. McMahon and D.L.H. Bennett

A. Introduction

The past decade has seen increasing interest in the mechanisms of persistent pain and the growing awareness that these mechanisms differ significantly from those of acute and transient phenomena so often utilised in earlier laboratory studies. In two particular areas, inflammatory pain and neuropathic pain, laboratory efforts have been intensive. In the case of the former considerable efforts have been made to identify the peripheral mediators for responsible abnormal sensibility of inflamed tissues. The first half of this chapter reviews evidence that one particular molecule, nerve growth factor (NGF), is ubiquitously expressed in inflamed tissues and may play a central and critical role in the generation of sensory abnormalities. In the case of the latter, neuropathic pain states, studies of animal models have revealed multiple pathophysiological mechanisms. The second half of this review considers the possibility that many of these abnormalities arise from decreased availability of peripherally produced growth factors as a consequence of damage to primary sensory neurones. Although potentially confusing, it is not paradoxical that an excess of a factor (in this case NGF) is pain-producing in one context while its lack leads to pain in another.

B. NGF and Its Receptors

NGF belongs to a family of proteins termed the neurotrophins which also includes brain-derived neurotrophic factor (BDNF), neurotrophin 3, neurotrophin 4/5 (Lindsay et al. 1994) and neurotrophin 6 (Gotz et al. 1994; Fig. 1). Most of the information available about the structure of NGF comes from the study of NGF extracted from adult mouse submandibular gland (for review see Bradshaw et al. 1993). The active form of NGF exists as a dimer of two identical polypeptide chains of 118 amino acids. Each subunit contains three intrachain disulphide bonds, and X-ray diffraction studies of crystals of NGF (McDonald et al. 1991) show that each protomer consists of three antiparallel β-sheets. There are three hairpin loops at the top of each protomer, and it is in these regions that many of the residues that are variable between different members of the neurotrophin family are found. It is thought that these residues that may be important in determining the different biologi-

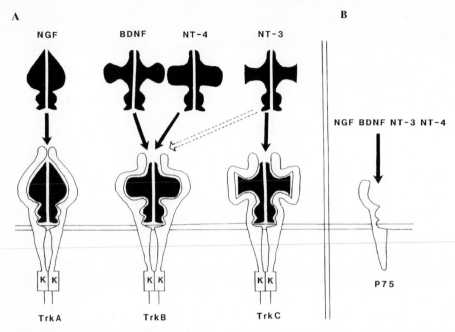

Fig. 1A,B. Schematic illustration of the neurotrophin family and its receptors. See text for details

cal properties of the members of the neurotrophin family, such as specificity of receptor interaction.

Two different types of receptor for the neurotrophins have been described (for reviews see Meakin and Shooter 1992; Barbacid 1994; Chao and Hempstead 1995). There is a low-affinity receptor termed p75 which binds equally well to all the neurotrophins. Additionally, there is a family of high-affinity receptors, trks (Kaplan et al. 1991), which are tyrosine kinase receptors. The p75 receptor is widely expressed in the CNS, sympathetic neurones, sensory neurones and Schwann cells. The p75 receptor contains a single trans-membrane segment flanked by extracellular and intracellular domains. It is still unclear as to how important the p75 receptor is in mediating the response of cells to NGF. A number of in vitro assays indicate that the importance of this receptor is limited, although animals that lack p75 do show deficits in the development of the nervous system (Lee et al. 1992). The p75 receptor may interact with trk receptors and modulate their sensitivity and specificity for the different neurotrophins.

There are three known members of the trk family of receptors, termed trkA, trkB and trkC, which show different specificities for the neurotrophins. The trk family is characterised by IgG-C2 domains, repeats that are rich in leucine and cysteine residues and a consensus tyrosine-kinase domain. NGF interacts specifically with the trkA receptor. It is the trkA receptor that is thought to mediate the biological actions of NGF such as neurite outgrowth and cell survival. This has been demonstrated by both in vitro assay systems and the marked deficits that occur in neuronal development in animals that lack the trkA receptor (SMEYNE et al. 1994). The two populations of peripheral neurones that express the trkA receptor (and hence are NGF responsive) are sympathetic neurones and many neural crest derived sensory neurones.

Increasing information is now available about the events that occur after binding of NGF to the trkA receptor. Following NGF binding the tyrosine-kinase domain of the receptor is activated, and a number of substrates are phosphorylated, and autophosphorylation of the receptor also occurs. Proteins which contain an SH2 domain are recruited to the phosphorylated residues on the receptor (SCHLESSLINGER 1994). After this interaction has occurred, a wide number of intracellular pathways become activated (see MARSHALL 1995), including the protein kinase C pathway, the *ras* pathway and the phosphinositide 3-kinase pathway (GREENE and KAPLAN 1995). Recently a further pathway has been described involving the juxtamembrane sequence of the receptor and the tyrosine phosphorylation of a protein termed SNT (PENG et al. 1995). It is now apparent that differential activation of these signalling pathways is possible, thus producing different cellular responses under different circumstances of receptor activation (for instance, sustained versus transient activation; GREENE and KAPLAN 1995).

No antagonists are available at present which show specificity between different members of the trk family. However, a group of alkaloids including K252a and b show non-specific antagonism at trk receptors. These agents prevent trk-dependent tyrosine phosphorylation and thus block cellular responses to NGF (BERG et al. 1992). This will be an area of important development in the future.

Early studies on the role of NGF in the sympathetic and sensory nervous system gave rise to the neurotrophic concept. This is that a target produces a limiting amount of neurotrophin which binds to receptors on the neurones innervating that target and is internalised and retrogradely transported by these neurones. The retrograde transport of neurotrophin is important in regulating the survival and differentiated function of responsive neurones (CROWLEY et al. 1994). Indeed, it is these findings which have given rise to the hope that the neurotrophins will prove beneficial in treating peripheral neuropathies (as reviewed in McMAHON and PRIESTLEY 1995).

C. NGF as A Mediator of Persistent Pain

There is now a large body of experimental work suggesting that NGF interacts with pain-signalling systems. Some of the evidence is correlative, relating to levels of endogenously produced NGF or the distribution of its high-affinity receptor trkA, and some is related to the effects of exogenously administered NGF. Some of the evidence is circumstantial, or simply consistent with the proposed role for NGF as a mediator of inflammatory pain, while some is direct. The major lines of evidence are summarised in the sections below.

I. NGF Maintains Nociceptor Sensitivity In Vivo

NGF is constitutively expressed in the adult animal in many peripheral tissues of the body, usually at very low levels (Shelton and Reichardt 1984). A variety of cell types produce NGF. The major supply in normal skin appears to originate from keratinocytes (Albers et al. 1994), but it is clear that fibroblasts, immune cells and smooth muscle cells can also manufacture the protein (Steers et al. 1991). The low levels produced in normal adult tissues are sufficient to exert strong biological effects on the peripheral innervation of the body. One piece of evidence is that peripherally produced NGF protein is retrogradely transported by peripheral nerves (Otten 1991; Donnerer et al. 1992; DiStefano et al. 1992). More compellingly, autoimmunisation experiments (Otten et al. 1979; Gorin and Johnson 1980; Rich et al. 1984; Johnson et al. 1982) have shown that the levels of neurotransmitters in sympathetic neurones depend upon constitutively produced NGF. These experiments also suggest that in the adult, unlike the developing animal, NGF is not necessary for the survival of sensory neurones.

We have recently examined the normal biological role of NGF using a synthetic fusion protein, a trkA-IgG, capable of acting as a 'ligand trap' and sequestering NGF (McMahon et al. 1995a). The molecule, consisting of two extracellular domains of trkA dimerised via the association of their respective Fc regions, was constructed recombinantly (Shelton et al. 1995). The molecule blocked the survival-promoting effects of NGF (but not neurotrophin 3 or BDNF) in an in vitro survival assay of embryonic sensory neurones (McMahon et al. 1995a). We infused this anti-NGF 'receptorbody' subcutaneously into the hindpaw of adult rats using mini-osmotic pumps. After continuous treatment for 4–5 days the treated animals started to show prolonged latencies of response to noxious thermal stimuli. That is, they became hypoalgesic. After 2 weeks of treatment they also showed greatly reduced responsiveness to a chemical irritant, capsaicin. Together these results suggest that normal levels of NGF are important regulators of the sensitivity of pain-signalling systems. The mechanism is not clear. One possibility is that NGF deprivation leads to death of primary sensory neurones. However, this would not explain the fact that the behavioural hypoalgesia produced by trkA-IgG treatment shows a complete recovery some days after treatment finishes. Auto-immunisation data, quoted above, also speak against it. Another possibility is that the production of the appropriate transducers/receptors by the sensory neurones depends upon the supply of NGF. In support, it is known that the capsaicin sensitivity of cultured sensory neurones is regulated by the levels of NGF in the medium (Winter et al. 1988; Bevan and Winter 1995). A third possibility is that NGF regulates the morphology of terminal arbors of sensory neurones in skin, and that these retract after sequestering NGF. The work of DIAMOND and colleagues (1987, 1992a,b) suggests just this action in other contexts. We now have preliminary evidence to support this claim (BENNETT et al. 1995). A final possibility is that NGF regulates the expresion of neuropeptides in sensory neurones, which would have implications for the central connectivity of these neurones. Whatever the mechanism of the effect, the implication is that the availability of NGF has the capacity to regulate strongly the responsiveness of nociceptive systems

II. Expression of NGF in Inflammatory States

An essential feature of the hypothesis that NGF is a mediator of inflammatory pain is that the levels of the protein are increased in appropriate tissues at appropriate times in inflammatory conditions. There is now considerable and compelling evidence that this occurs. In a variety of animal models of inflammation, including those produced by Freund's adjuvant (DONNERER et al. 1992; SAFIEH-GARABEDIAN et al. 1995), subcutaneous carrageenan (WESTKAMP and OTTEN 1987; OTTEN 1991; ALOE et al. 1992), and in a rat model of cystitis (ANDREEV et al. 1993; ODDIAH et al. 1995), NGF expression is increased. NGF also appears to be upregulated in the synovium of human arthritic patients (ALOE et al. 1992). The increased NGF expression has been documented in various ways, including increased NGF protein in inflamed tissue, increased NGF protein retrogradely transported in nerves supplying the affected tissues, increased mRNA levels for NGF measured by in situ hybridisation and by reverse-transcriptase polymerase chain reaction. The increased levels of NGF seen in inflamed tissue may derive from a variety of sources. Immune cells (lymphocytes, macrophages, mast cells) appear a rich potential source (BROWN et al. 1991; ALOE et al. 1992; LEON et al. 1994; SANTAMBROGIO et al. 1994), although fibroblasts or Schwann cells in nerve in the inflamed tissue are other possibilities (HEUMANN et al. 1987b; MATSUOKO et al. 1991).

We have looked in some detail at NGF expression in one animal model, a rat model of cystitis. An acute sterile inflammation is precipitated by the brief intravesical administration of turpentine oil in anaesthetised female rats (McMAHON and ABEL 1987; McMAHON et al. 1995b). Within 1 h plasma extravasation and oedema are seen, and leucocytes then migrate into the tissue. The inflamed animals show features typical of cystitis is humans: increased bladder motility and frequency of micturition, and signs of abdominal hyperalgesia and ongoing discomfort. These behavioural and reflex changes also begin within about 1 h, and persist for up to 24 h. Electrophysiological experiments have shown sensitisation of primary afferent and spinal cord neurones innervating the inflamed bladder, with a similarly rapid onset (HÄBLER et al. 1988, 1993; McMAHON 1988; see also McMAHON et al. 1995b). In the same model in situ hybridisation showed a very marked increase in NGF mRNA, apparent within 2 h, peaking shortly thereafter and returning to baseline levels within 24 h (Andreev et al. 1993). More recently we have also seen equivalent increases with reverse-transcriptase polymerase chain reaction and a sensitive enzyme-linked immunosorbent assay for NGF protein (Oddiah et al. 1995). Thus NGF upregulation closely parallels the sensory and reflex abnormalities in this model.

III. Expression of NGF Receptors on Nociceptors

Since the biological effects of NGF are believed to be mediated largely or exclusively through the high-affinity trkA receptor, the expression of this receptor is likely to indicate those neuronal populations which might be directly affected by the neurotrophin. Evidence from a number of laboratories suggests that the trkA receptors are expressed in adult animals selectively by small-calibre, predominantly nociceptive afferents.

A number of techniques have been employed to study trkA expression, including in situ hybridisation for trkA mRNA (Carroll et al. 1992; Verge et al. 1992; Mu et al. 1993; McMahon et al. 1994; Wright and Snider 1995), high-affinity binding of labelled NGF (Richardson et al. 1986; Verge et al. 1989a,b, 1990a,b, 1992), retrograde transport from peripheral nerve to dorsal root ganglia (DRG) of iodinated NGF (Richardson and Riopelle 1984; DiStefano et al. 1992) and immunohistochemistry (Averill et al. 1995). These studies all agree that in the L4 and L5 DRG about 45% of adult neurones express trkA. These cells are mostly of small diameter.

In a recent study we examined the possible relationship between the expression of trkA and various other neurochemical markers (Averill et al. 1995). DRG cells can be divided into three minimally overlapping subgroups. Firstly, the population traditionally described as "large light" can be identified by the anti-neurofilament antibody RT97 (Lawson et al. 1984). These cells, about 30% of the total, have mostly myelinated axons and in the periphery are likely to be connected to mechanosensitive endings such as Pacinian corpuscles, hair follicle afferents and muscle spindles (for reviews see Lawson 1992; Willis and Coggeshall 1991). A second population of DRG cells contain cell surface glycoconjugates with terminal D-galactose residues and can be identified with markers such as the monoclonal antibody LA4 (Alvarez et al. 1989) and the lectin *Griffonia simplicifolia* IB4 (Silverman and Kruger 1990). These neurones, about 30% of the total (Alvarez et al. 1991), have unmyelinated axons, do not show RT97 immunoreactivity, and are likely to innervate predominantly nociceptors and thermoreceptors (Willis and Coggeshall 1991). The third population of DRG cells consists of those that constitutively synthesise neuropeptides. The best marker for this group is the neuropeptide that is expressed by the largest number of DRG cells, namely calcitonin gene related peptide (CGRP). About 45% of lumbar DRG cells contain CGRP immunoreactivity (Lawson 1992). Peptides such as substance P, somatostatin and galanin coexist with CGRP. CGRP immunoreactive cells are predominantly small with unmyelinated axons and hence form the other half of the "small dark" population, again, likely to innervate predominantly nociceptors and thermoreceptors.

A striking feature is that trkA expression corresponds almost perfectly with the CGRP population (AVERILL et al. 1995). The non-peptide LA4/IB4 population, in contrast, is largely not trkA expressing (with only 6% overlap). In fact, the overlap observed between trkA and the markers RT97, IB4 and LA4 corresponds closely to the known overlap between CGRP and these markers.

The expression of trkA receptors is also related to the functional properties of sensory neurones. Using in situ hybridisation for trk mRNAs, we recently observed that relatively few afferent neurones innervating skeletal muscle expressed trkA, whereas those innervating a visceral target, the urinary bladder, were nearly all trkA expressing (MCMAHON et al. 1994). Interestingly, the latter population also appeared to co-express trkB, the high-affinity receptor for two other members of the neurotrophin family, BDNF and neurotrophin 4/5. In all cases, however, trkA was found predominantly in small neurones which are known to be responsive to nociceptive stimuli.

Together these results strongly suggest that altered levels of NGF have the capacity to directly interact with specifically pain-signalling peripheral sensory systems.

IV. Hyperalgesic Effects of Exogenous NGF

LEWIN et al. (1993, 1994) studied the effects of a single systemic dose of 1 mg/ kg NGF on the sensitivity of the animals to noxious thermal and mechanical stimuli. They found that this dose elicited two phases of hyperalgesia. The first appeared within 30 min, while the second took several hours to emerge and persisted for several days. Thermal hyperalgesia was present in both phases, but mechanical hyperalgesia was found only during the delayed, second, phase. LEWIN et al. suggested that the first phase arose because of a peripheral action of NGF while the second required changes in the central processing of nociceptive information. These conclusions were based partly on arguments relating to the timing of the effects and partly on the effects of pharmacological manipulations (see LEWIN 1995).

We have recently undertaken related studies in which small doses of NGF are injected subcutaneously into the hindpaws of adult rats (ANDREEV et al. 1995). Injections of 50–500 ng NGF produced a dose-dependent thermal hyperalgesia which appeared within 30 min of treatment and lasted for a number of hours. The effect was large in magnitude and observed in experiments in which the experimenter was blinded to the treatment. NGF was probably acting at the site of injection and not systemically in these experiments since the hyperalgesia was seen only ipsilaterally.

Injections of NGF to human volunteers is also reported to produce a rapid onset and marked increased sensitivity to painful stimuli (PETTY et al. 1994).

Intravenous injections of very small amounts (1 μg/kg) produced a widespread aching pain in deep tissues. Subcutaneous injections produced hyperalgesia at the site of injection. These effects developed quickly (within 60 min in some cases) and persisted for hours or a few days.

The hyperlagesia produced by NGF can be sustained. Transgenic animals which continuously over-express NGF in skin from mid-developmental stages are hyperalgesic when tested as adults (Davis et al. 1993). We have examined the effects of chronic (2-week) subcutaneous infusions of NGF into adult animals (Al-Sahili et al. 1995) or repeated daily subcutaneous injections. In both cases the thermal hyperalgesia associated with these low-dose treatments was maintained throughout the treatment period.

V. Sensitisation of Nociceptors by Exogenous NGF

One would expect that the ability of NGF to induce behavioural hyperalgesia, described above, would be reflected in physiological changes in nociceptive systems. We now have supporting evidence from several sources. One observation is that local administration of NGF leads to a restricted neurogenic extravasation of plasma proteins into the tissue. We have monitored this following NGF treatment of skin and bladder using the Evan's blue technique (Andreev et al. 1995; Dmitrieva and McMahon 1995). In both tissues NGF produces a modest extravasation at short latency. Since this extravasation is absent in animals treated neonatally with capsaicin (and therefore lacking most unmyelinated afferent fibres), it is likely to be neurogenic in origin. That is, NGF is capable of inducing a response analogous to a component of the triple response of Lewis. It is known that neurogenic extravasation depends upon neuropeptides released from the peripheral terminals of nociceptors following their activation. Thus NGF appears capable of acutely activating some primary sensory nociceptors.

There is also direct electrophysiological evidence of peripheral activation and sensitisation of thin-calibre afferent fibres by NGF. In anaesthetised rats we characterised the response properties of thin (Aδ and C) fibres innervating the urinary bladder (Dmitrieva and McMahon 1995). We then exposed the peripheral terminals of these afferents to NGF by injecting it intravesically. We found that within 30 min sensory neurones were sensitised to bladder distension. This was true for both Aδ and C fibres, and included some fibres that initially had no mechanosensitivity (i.e. were of the type known as 'silent' nociceptors; McMahon and Koltzenburg 1994). The sensitisation persisted for the duration of recordings (up to 3 h). Many fibres also developed low levels of ongoing activity. These changes were very similar to those reported following chemical inflammation of the urinary bladder. That is, the time course and nature of changes in bladder primary afferent neurones in a model of cystitis are consistent with their mediation by NGF.

Other data suggest that NGF can activate and sensitise peripheral nociceptive fibres. Firstly, the administration of NGF into the urinary bladder, as described above, leads to induction of the proto-oncogene c-fos in dorsal horn neurones (Dmitrieva et al., unpublished observations). The number of cells in which c-*fos* was induced, and their lamina distribution, was very similar to that seen after chemical inflammation of the urinary bladder. We have also examined electrophysiological changes after NGF treatment of somatic tissues (ANDREEV et al. 1994). We recorded from dorsal horn neurones with receptive fields on the hindpaw and activated by noxious heating. Small doses of NGF (500 ng) were then injected subcutaneously into the centre of the receptive fields. Within 20 min most neurones showed a progressive increase in ongoing activity and responsiveness to noxious heating. The most parsimonious explanation for these findings is that the NGF caused a peripheral sensitisation of nociceptors which was then reflected in enhanced responses of dorsal horn neurones.

Recently RUEFF and MENDELL (1995) have studied the responsiveness of cutaneous nociceptors using an in vitro preparation and have found that topical administration of NGF produces a heat sensitisation in a about 20% of afferent nociceptors.

Thus experiments using very different techniques all suggest that increased levels of NGF are capable of rapidly sensitising peripheral terminals of nociceptors.

VI. Anti-hyperalgesic Effects of NGF "Antagonism"

The evidence presented above is consistent with the hypothesis that NGF is a mediator of inflammatory pain states. However, in order to demonstrate the biological role of endogenous NGF, one requires pharmacological 'antagonism'. We currently have no selective antagonists of the trkA receptor. However, we have utilised, in vivo experiments, a synthetic trkA-IgG fusion molecule capable of sequestering and neutralising NGF but not other neurotrophins (McMAHON et al. 1995a).

We asked whether this molecule can block the sensory abnormalities that develop in two models of inflammation – that produced by subcutaneous carrageenan and the rat model of cystitis described previously. In the model of cystitis we measured the progressive increase in bladder reflex excitability that occurs with inflammation. Normally, slow filling of the bladder results initially in gradual increases in intravesical pressure. At some level of distension a series of large CNS-generated micturition contractions begin. These micturition contractions are initiated by activity in afferent neurones innervating the urinary bladder, and thus indirectly reflect the sensitivity of sensory systems (McMAHON 1986). At the onset of experimental inflammation the excitability of bladder reflexes rises, and micturition contractions are initiated at lower distending volumes. When animals are pre-treated systemically with the NGF sequestering molecule (1 mg/kg) the hyper-reflexia associated with inflammation fails to develop (DMITRIEVA et al. 1995). Pretreatment with trkB-IgG (a similar molecule without NGF-sequestering capacity) does not have this effect. Since the trk-IgGs do not appear to cross the blood-brain barrier, these data suggest that the sensory changes occurring with inflammation are critically dependent on peripheral upregulation of NGF.

We have also studied another model of inflammation, that produced by subcutaneous injections of carrageenan into a rat hindpaw. This treatment produces a marked and persistent thermal hyperalgesia of the treated paw. When we mixed the inflammatory agent with trkA-IgG, most of the expected hyperalgesia did not develop (McMahon et al. 1995a). The block of carrageenan hyperlagesia by trkA-IgG was dose dependent and not seen with control IgG molecules. The conclusion from these experiments is, again, that these sensory abnormalities developing with inflammation is critically dependent upon the production of NGF in the inflamed tissue.

Similar conclusions have been reached in two other recent studies that have used neutralising antibodies to NGF (Lewin et al. 1994; Woolf et al. 1994). Both report that hyperalgesia associated with experimental inflammation is blocked when NGF is sequestered. These experiments provide the most compelling reasons for believing that upregulation of NGF in inflammatory states is of key functional importance for the abnormal pain sensations that arise. The way(s) in which this might come about are discussed in the following section.

D. Mechanisms of NGF-Induced Hyperalgesia

The evidence presented above strongly implicates NGF in the genesis of pain and hyperalgesia in inflammatory states. However, it only incidentally addresses the issue of the mechanism of this effect. There are two broad ways in which the data fits into our framework of understanding of mechanisms of persistent pain. These are described below and illustrated schematically in Fig. 2.

I. Peripheral Sensitisation

There is now a large body of evidence (reviewed in Koltzenburg 1995; Reeh and Kress 1995) that the encoding properties of primary sensory nociceptors are modifiable. Most notably, a number of pathophysiological states, particularly those caused by tissue injury or inflammation, are associated with the tonic activation and sensitisation of these sensory neurones. Under these conditions nociceptors have lowered thresholds for activation and respond more vigorously to suprathreshold stimuli. It is not difficult to see how this increased sensitivity of nociceptors can contribute to the ongoing pain and hyperlagesia seen in these pathophysiological states. It is also now clear that a wide variety of chemicals, including prostaglandins, bradykinin, serotonin, histamine and even hydrogen ions can induce this sensitisation of nociceptors. Many of these agents are released into damaged tissue.

Much of the data presented above is consistent with the suggestion that NGF itself produces peripheral sensitisation of nociceptors. The rapid onset of hyperalgesia after subcutaneous injections of NGF strongly suggests a peripheral action, as does the ability of NGF to induce neurogenic extravasation (ANDREEV et al. 1995; DMITRIEVA and McMAHON 1995). Finally, of course, the direct electrophysiological observations of sensitisation of primary sensory neurones demonstrates this effect (DMITRIEVA and McMAHON 1995; RUEFF and MENDELL 1995). Given that many nociceptors express the trkA receptor, it is possible that sensitisation occurs following the direct binding and activation of this receptor by NGF.

However there are other cellular elements in peripheral tissues which express the trkA receptor, and it is possible that sensitisation of nociceptors arises indirectly. TrkA receptors are known to be expressed by both sympathetic postganglionic neurones and by some mast cells (HORIGOME et al. 1993; THOENEN 1991), and indeed NGF is known to be a potent degranulator of mast cells (HORIGOME et al. 1993). There is good evidence that mast cell products (such as histamine and serotonin) are capable of sensitising nociceptors (see REEH and KRESS 1995). There is also a body of evidence that, in other contexts, the chemical activation of sympathetic postganglionic fibres can lead to the release of a number of products of arachidonic acid metabolism that are capable of producing hyperalgesia (reviewed in HELLER et al. 1994; KOLTZENBURG and McMAHON 1991). There is now experimental evidence suggesting that at a large component of the peripheral sensitising effect of NGF is indirect. Thus, the rapid onset hyperlagesia produced by NGF is largely blocked in sypathectomised animals (ANDREEV et al. 1995) or in animals pre-treated with the mast cell degranulator 48/80 (LEWIN et al. 1994). The cascade of events leading to peripheral sensitisation by NGF is illustrated schematically in Fig. 2.

Figure 2 also illustrates potential antecedent events leading to NGF production in inflammation. There is now some experimental evidence that two cytokines, tumour necrosis factor (TNF) α and interleukin (IL) 1β, are necessary intermediates. It is well recognised that both these cytokines are themselves released into inflamed tissues. We have now found (unpublished observations) that small doses of TNFα injected subcutaneously produce marked thermal and mechanical hyperlagesia that is blocked by sequestering NGF, and that antibodies to TNFα block the hyperlagesia seen in carrageenan inflammation. A similar repertoire of effects has been reported for IL-1β (SAFIEH-GARABEDIAN et al. 1995). Whether these two cytokines act serially or in parallel is not known.

II. Central Sensitisation

Notwithstanding the evidence presented in the preceding section, there are reasons to believe that NGF has an important impact on pain signalling systems other than by inducing peripheral sensitisation. One reason is that

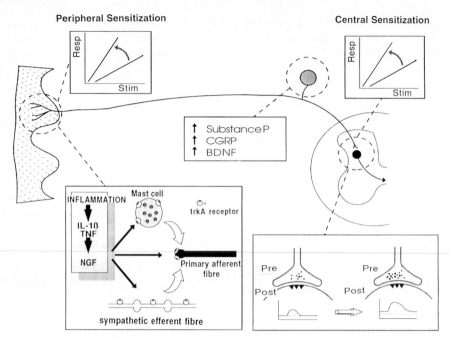

Fig. 2. Schematic illustration of the mechanisms by which NGF may affect pain-signalling systems. See text for details

NGF is retrogradely transported by trkA expressing sensory neurones and is known to exert major effects on gene expression in these cells (see below). A second is that the later components of hyperalgesia induced by systemic injections of NGF not readily explained by peripheral mechanisms and appear to have a central component (Lewin et al. 1994; Lewin 1995). A major development in pain research over the past decade or so is the recognition that the central relay of nociceptive information in the spinal cord is itself rather plastic. In particular, there are now many examples of increases in excitability of these central neurones triggered by peripheral injury. In these many different examples the central changes – dubbed central sensitisation – exhibit common physiological and pharmacological features (see McMahon et al. 1993). There is now some circumstantial and some direct evidence to suggest that peripheral increases in NGF levels can also activate this process.

This evidence, also illustrated in Fig. 2, comes in several parts. Firstly, NGF modulates levels of number of neurotransmitters/neuromodulators in sensory neurones. In vivo (Kuraishi et al. 1989; Donnerer et al. 1992; Leslie et al. 1995) and in vitro (see Lindsay 1992), substance P and CGRP levels are increased by NGF. Sequestration of NGF conversely leads to lowered expression of CGRP (McMahon et al. 1995a). Increased production of peptides is also reflected as increased levels in the central terminals of nociceptors. It is known that many forms of central sensitisation depend upon the sensory neuropeptides substance P and CGRP released from the central terminals of primary afferent nociceptors with activity (see McMahon et al. 1993). One can therefore hypothesise that the increased levels of these peptides by NGF is a key intermediate step in the generation of central sensitisation.

Increased retrograde transport of NGF also has other important effects on small-diameter sensory neurones. These include the apparent increased expression of receptors expressed by the neurones (e.g. capsaicin and γ-aminobutyric acid; Bevan and Winter 1995). Altered receptor expression on both peripheral and central terminations of nociceptors is likely to have important functional consequences for information processing. The expression of another neurotrophin, BDNF, is also known to be regulated by NGF (Apfel et al. 1996b; and unpublished observations). The consequences of this are only speculative at present, but there is the possibility of autocrine or paracrine actions (Acheson et al. 1995) and even of central release followed by post-synaptic actions (i.e. acting as a neurotransmitter)

We also have direct electrophysiological evidence of central sensitisation triggered by NGF. In one study (Lewin et al. 1992) we delivered NGF to a peripheral target for 2 weeks by mini-osmotic pumps and then evaluated the excitability of spinal cord neurones to activation of the treated afferents. We found a major increase in central excitability to inputs from both unmyelinated afferents (which are likely to retrogradely transport NGF) and also to activation of myelinated afferents, themselves likely not to be sensitive to NGF. A recent report by Thompson et al. (1995) utilised an in vitro preparation to assess the consequences of prior systemic NGF exposure. They too observed a generalised increase in spinal neurone excitability. They also found that the pharmacology of the NGF-induced central sensitisation was the same as other forms of central sensitisation in that it was blocked by antagonists of both the NMDA receptor and the substance P receptor.

The dual mechanisms of peripheral and central sensitisation are, of course, not mutually exclusive, but they may co-operate in the genesis of abnormal pain sensibility in cases of increased production of NGF. One would expect the time course of effect to differ, however, given the additional transport time required for effects mediated by altered gene expression.

E. Growth Factors and Neuropathic Pain

Neuropathic pain occurs as a consequence of nerve injury and is discussed more fully elsewhere in this volume (for a review see Bennett 1994). The causes of neuropathic pain are many and varied, ranging from physical trauma to metabolic conditions such as diabetes mellitus, but it is usually assumed that this type of pain is secondary to some injury to peripheral nerves. NGF may well have a role in the evolution of neuropathic pain, particularly as two populations of peripheral neurones implicated (primary sensory nociceptors and sympathetic neurones) are both NGF responsive. Nerve injury is known to reduce the retrograde transport of NGF in these neuronal populations, and therefore this is a very different concept from the role of NGF in the generation of inflammatory pain in which there is an acute overexpression of NGF in peripheral tissues. There is evidence, discussed in this chapter, that a balance in the retrograde supply of NGF is critical, and that an increase or a reduction in this supply result in the evolution of two different types of persistent pain state.

The first compelling reason that suggests NGF availability may be important in the evolution of neuropathic pain comes from recent studies on the effect of exogenous NGF administration on the behavioural consequences of two rat models of neuropathic pain. One of these employs the Chung model, involving transection of the L5 spinal nerve (Kinnman and Levine 1995). Administration of NGF via a mini-osmotic pump to the cut end of the spinal nerve delayed the onset of mechanical hyperalgesia which is normally associated with this lesion. This action of NGF was thought to be mediated by postganglionic sympathetic neurones as it was also present in capsaicin treated animals. The second study also used local administration of NGF, but to a sciatic nerve subjected to a chronic constriction injury (Ren et al. 1995). Chronic constriction injury is a well-characterised model resulting in both a mechanical and thermal hyperalgesia (Bennett and Xie 1988). Local infusion of NGF onto the ligated nerve abolished the thermal hyperalgesia following 5 days of administration, and the reduction in mechanical threshold that normally occurs was also prevented. This was a local effect as there was no change in nociceptive threshold on the contralateral side. Interestingly, once this persistent pain state was established, NGF could not influence the hyperalgesia. These results are the most convincing evidence to date that NGF may have therapeutic value in humans for the treatment of neuropathic pain. There is an ongoing clinical trial of the use of NGF in the treatment of small fibre neuropathy (e.g. diabetic neuropathy) in humans (Apfel et al. 1996a). A preliminary report claims some improvement in patients with neuropathic pain in terms of the incidence of painful symptoms. These interesting results raise the questions of the extent to which reduced NGF availability contributes to neuropathic pain and of the mechanisms by which exogenous NGF reverse this pathological state. We attempt to answer these questions in the following sections.

I. NGF Interacts with Adult Sensory and Sympathetic Neurones

NGF interacts with both primary sensory neurones and sympathetic neurones during development and in the adult. In the adult, as discussed above, both these populations continue to express the high-affinity receptor for NGF, trkA (McMahon et al. 1994; Wetmore and Olson 1995). It has also been demonstrated that both sympathetic and primary sensory neurones retrogradely transport NGF from the targets that they innervate (DiStefano et al. 1992; Hendry et al. 1974). It is now becoming increasingly obvious that in the adult

NGF can regulate many anatomical and functional characteristics of primary afferents and sympathetic neurones. NGF is important for regulation of the survival, morphology and neurotransmitter expression in adult sympathetic neurones in vitro (MAX et al. 1978) and in vivo (HENDRY 1977; PARAVICINI et al. 1975; RUIT et al. 1990). The interaction of NGF with adult primary sensory neurones and, in particular, nociceptive afferents is discussed above.

For this discussion we consider as examples two animal models of nerve injury to illustrate the possible role of NGF in the generation of neuropathic pain. These are axotomy and diabetic neuropathy. Axotomy and consequent neuroma formation produces widespread anatomical and functional abnormalities in the nervous system and in humans may be associated with persistent pain. Another neuropathic condition that may be associated with the development of chronic pain and dysaesthesias is diabetic neuropathy (HARATI 1987). Among patients with insulin-dependent diabetes mellitus 30% report hyperalgesia (ARCHER et al. 1983), and hyperalgesia has also been demonstrated in experimental diabetic neuropathy in animals (AHLGREN and LEVINE 1993). The most common type of neuropathy encountered in diabetes is a symmetric distal polyneuropathy, which is principally sensory-motor and often includes the autonomic system. There is now increasing interest in the role of NGF in diabetic neuropathy (for reviews see SCHMIDT 1993; BREWSTER et al. 1994).

Table 1 illustrates some of the anatomical and functional changes in sensory systems that occur in both of these conditions. It is apparent that after nerve injury abnormalities are not restricted to the peripheral nerve terminal but move centrally to involve the DRG and the dorsal horn (Fig. 3). Altered retrograde transport of NGF provides a powerful mechanism whereby changes in the environment of a peripheral nerve terminal could alter the function of the cell body and even central connectivity. There is now increasing evidence that many pathophysiological changes associated with these conditions either arise because of reduced NGF availability or at least may be ameliorated by exogenous NGF.

II. Altered Availability of NGF in Neuropathy

Nerve injury results in a reduced retrograde transport of NGF by primary afferent neurones. The level of NGF protein was reduced to 40% of control in the proximal portion of the nerve after sciatic nerve transection (HEUMANN et al. 1987a). After axotomy, perhaps as a compensatory response, there is an increase in the expression of NGF mRNA in non-neuronal cells of the proximal and particularly the distal nerve stumps. There are two peaks of increased expression, and these occur 1 day and then at 1 week following axotomy, after which NGF levels remain somewhat higher than control. The second phase of increased NGF expression is thought to be mediated by the invasion of macrophages and the release of Il-1 (HEUMANN et al. 1987b; LINDHOLM et al. 1987).

Table 1. Effects of axotomy and diabetic neuropathy on primary sensory neurones, sympathetic neurones and the dorsal horn

		Axotomy	Diabetic neuropathy	NGF deprivation
DRG cells	Cell death	⇑ [22]	↑ [12]	⇒ [11, 23]
	c-jun	⇑ [10]	?	⇐ [10]
	Neuropeptides: SP, CGRP	⇓ [8, 17, 30, 32]	⇓ [6, 7, 31]	⇓ [17, 23]
	Neuropeptides: galanin, VIP	⇑[a] [30]	↑	?
	GAP-43	⇑ [33]	→ [18]	?
	Neurofilament expression	⇓[a] [9, 28]	→ [18]	?
	trkA, p75 expression	⇓[a] [29]	?	⇓ [9]
	Axon calibre/cond. velocity	⇓[a] [9]	⇓ [16]	?
	Ongoing activity	↑ [5]	← [5]	
Post-ganglionic sympathetic neurones	Cell death	↑ [19]	→ [24, 25]	
	Noradrenaline synthesis	⇓ [13]	↑ [26]	⇓ [11]
	Dendritic arborisation	→ [9]	?	⇓ [27]
	Synaptic strength	⇓ [20]	?	?
Dorsal horn	Transganglionic degeneration	⇑ [4, 8]	?	?
	Afferent sprouting	↑ [34]	?	?
	Receptive field size	⇑ [8]	?	?
Behaviour		(Hyperalgesia, in CCI) [21]	(Hyperalgesia) [2]	(Hypoalgesia) [17]

Double-arrows, NGF-reversible effect. References: [1] Apfel et al. 1994; [2] Apfel et al. 1995; [3] Calcutt et al. 1993; [4] Apfel et al. 1995; [5] Devor 1994; [6] Diemel et al. 1992; [7] Diemel et al. 1994; [8] Fitzgerald et al. 1985; [9] Gold et al. 1991; [10] Gold et al. 1993; [11] Gorin and Johnson; 1980 [12] Harati 1987; [13] Hendry 1975; [14] Hokfelt et al. 1994; [15] Kinnman and Levine 1995; [16] Koltzenberg and McMahon 1991; [17] McMahon et al. 1995a; [18] Mohiuddin et al. 1995; [19] Purves 1975; [20] Purves and Nja 1976; [21] Ren et al. 1995; [22] Rich et al. 1987; [23] Schwartz et al. 1982; [24] Schmidt et al. 1981; [25] Schmidt et al. 1983; [26] Schmidt and Cogswell 1989; [27] Rutt et al. 1990; [28] Verge et al. 1990; [29] Verge et al. 1992; [30] Verge et al. 1995; [31] Willars et al. 1989; [32] Wong and Oblinger 1991; [33] Woolf et al. 1990; [34] Woolf et al. 1992.
[a] NGF-reversible effects only in small-diameter DRG cells, not in large-diameter DRG cells.

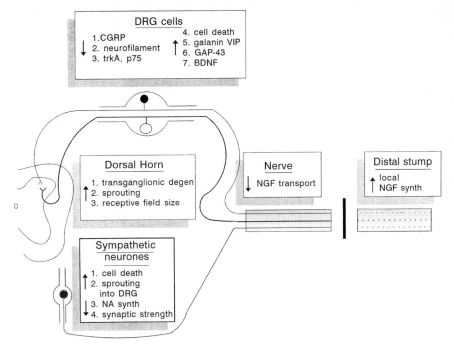

Fig. 3. Illustration of the effects of axotomy on DRG cells, sympathetic neurones and the dorsal horn. See Table 1 for further details

There is also an upregulation in the expression in the p75 receptor in non-neuronal cells of the distal segment which may modulate the availability of NGF for retrograde transport.

There is now a growing body of evidence that NGF levels are reduced in diabetes. In diabetic patients there is a decreased serum content of NGF which is related to an electrophysiological measurement of nerve function (FARADJI and SOTELO 1990). In experimental diabetes there is reduced NGF mRNA in the leg muscles, foot skin and sciatic nerve (FERNYHOUGH et al. 1994, 1995). There are also reduced levels of NGF protein in the submandibular gland, superior cervical ganglion and sciatic nerve in diabetic rats, and these reductions can be reversed by insulin treatment (HELLWEG and HARTUNG 1990; HELLWEG et al. 1991). Not only are NGF levels reduced in peripheral targets during experimental diabetes, but also the transport of endogenous or exogenous NGF is reduced in the sciatic nerve (JAKOBSEN et al. 1981; HELLWEG et al. 1994).

Thus there is much evidence suggesting a reduced production of NGF and/or reduced retrograde transport of this molecule during diabetes and following axotomy. The following sections ask to what extent this reduced availability of NGF contributes to changes believed to be important in the genesis of neuropathic pain.

III. Death of Injured Sensory Neurones

After axotomy cell death occurs in up to 30% of primary sensory neurones (Arvidsson et al. 1986), and this deafferentation may contribute to abnormal pain. Local administration of exogenous NGF to the site of axotomy can prevent the cell death of primary sensory neurones which occurs after axotomy (Rich et al. 1987). The rescue effect of NGF is not restricted to small-diameter DRG cells but also apparently includes large-diameter DRG cells, which is surprising as few large-diameter DRG cells express the trkA receptor. This may be a pharmacological effect of NGF as no cell death occurs in adult sensory neurones after auto-immunisation to NGF or following administration of anti-NGF antibodies (Schwartz et al. 1982).

Diabetic neuropathy is probably ultimately associated with a degree of cell death in DRG cells since in humans there is axon loss in nerve biopsies (Harati 1987). The ability of NGF to prevent such loss in animals has not been investigated.

IV. Altered Gene Expression in Damaged Sensory Neurones

The immediate early gene c-JUN is expressed in sensory neurones in response to nerve injury. This is a transcription factor and so may be upstream to other changes in gene expression that occur after axotomy. c-jun expression can be reduced in injured sensory neurones exposed to exogenous NGF and its expression is induced with anti-NGF treatment, indicating that the retrograde supply of NGF may regulate its expression (Gold et al. 1993). There is a marked alteration in the expression of neuropeptides by primary sensory neurones following axotomy (Hokfelt et al. 1994), which may have an important impact on spinal processing of sensory information (see McMahon et al. 1993). There is a reduction in the levels of substance P and CGRP whilst there is an increased expression of vasoactive intestinal polypeptide (VIP) and galanin in predominantly small-diameter primary sensory neurones. The administration of exogenous NGF can prevent the reduced substance P and CGRP expression that occurs in primary afferents following axotomy (Fitzgerald et al. 1985; Wong and Oblinger 1991; Verge et al. 1995). It has recently been shown that NGF administered intrathecally can partially prevent the upregulation of galanin and VIP in primary afferents that occurs after axotomy (Verge et al. 1995). Deprivation of NGF using anti-NGF treatments or NGF sequestration in adult animals has been shown to replicate some of the changes encountered after axotomy such as reduced substance P and CGRP expression (Schwartz et al. 1982; McMahon et al. 1995a) in primary afferents.

After axotomy there is also an increase in growth-associated protein (GAP) 43 expression in DRG cells (Woolf et al. 1990). GAP-43 is a phosphoprotein thought to be important in the development and plasticity of the nervous system. This effect may, however, be independent of NGF, which has been shown to positively regulate GAP-43 expression in culture (Mohiuddin et al. 1995a,b). This is at odds with the increased GAP-43 expression occurring after axotomy when the supply of NGF falls. It has been shown in vivo that administration of NGF does not alter GAP-43 expression in DRG cells. However, it may have a role in regulating GAP-43 expression in certain abnormal conditions such as inflammation (LESLIE et al. 1995). Another important consequence of axotomy is a reduced expression of both the p75 and trkA receptors in DRG cells (VERGE et al. 1992). After axotomy not only is there a reduction in the retrograde transport of NGF but also the ability of primary afferent neurones to respond to NGF also appears to be reduced. NGF infusion following axotomy can restore p75 expression (to supranormal levels) and partially restore trkA expression in primary sensory neurones.

There is also a reduced expression of neurofilament genes after axotomy which can be partially reversed after NGF administration in the population of DRG cells that have high-affinity binding sites for NGF (VERGE et al. 1990a,b). This change is not reversed in large-diameter afferents which do not express the trk receptor. This is further discussed below in relation to axonal calibre.

During diabetic neuropathy there is also reduced expression of the neuropeptides substance P and CGRP both in the sciatic nerve and the DRG (WILLARS et al. 1989; DIEMEL et al. 1994). The reduction in substance P, preprotachykinin mRNA and CGRP mRNA in the DRG and the decrease in substance P and CGRP in the sciatic nerve of diabetic rats can be corrected by treatment with NGF (APFEL et al. 1994, 1996b; DIEMEL et al. 1994). One functional outcome measure of neuropeptide expression in primary afferent neurones is Evan's blue extravasation. Evan's blue extravasation in response to cutaneous mustard oil administration is markedly reduced in diabetic rats. NGF administration can partially prevent this reduction (M. Koltzenberg, personal communication). Experimental diabetes also produces a reduction in the expression of neurofilament genes and GAP-43 mRNA (MOHIUDDIN et al. 1995a,b). Within the DRG the expression of VIP does not appear to be dramatically altered by experimental diabetes although interestingly the induction of VIP in response nerve injury is impaired (CALCUTT et al. 1993).

V. Axon Calibre/Conduction Velocity Changes with Damage

Axonal calibre is related to neurofilament expression (HOFFMAN et al. 1987). The reduced neurofilament expression and hence axon calibre that occurs after axotomy results in a reduction in conduction velocity in primary sensory neurones. NGF has been shown not only to partially reverse the reduced neurofilament expression occurring after axotomy (VERGE et al. 1990a,b; GOLD et al. 1991) but also to partially prevent the reduction in axonal calibre that occurs in primary sensory neurones (GOLD et al. 1991). Further evidence is that administration of NGF antiserum could produce a reduction in mean axonal calibre. There is some disagreement on this point in the literature as WONG and OBLINGER (1991) reported that NGF cannot rescue neurofilament expression after axotomy.

In diabetic neuropathy there is also a reduced axonal calibre and hence a conduction velocity slowing in primary afferent neurones. One study (Apfel et al. 1994, 1996b) has not shown any effect of NGF administration on this slowing as measured by compound action potentials. However, since this gives information only about conduction velocity in the most rapidly conducting primary afferent neurones, one might not expect NGF to be effective as only few of these fibres express trkA. A more recent study looking at conduction velocity in single units indicates that NGF may be able to prevent the slowing of unmyelinated primary afferents produced by experimental diabetes (Koltzenberg et al., unpublished observations).

VI. Changes in the Sympathetic Nervous System After Nerve Injury

NGF can prevent some of the biochemical and functional changes that occur in sympathetic neurones following injury (Hendry 1975; Purves and Nja 1976). Deprivation of NGF can also produce altered neurotransmitter expression, survival and morphology of sympathetic neurones (Gorin and Johnson 1980; Ruit et al. 1990) in a manner that is similar to that following axotomy. An important effect of axotomy and many other neuropathic conditions is the development of an abnormal connectivity between the sympathetic and sensory nervous systems whereby sympathetic activity can actually maintain the abnormal pain state (see Koltzenburg, this volume). One manifestation of this is the formation of abnormal basket-like terminations of sympathetic axons around sensory neurones within the DRG (McLachlan et al. 1993). It has recently been demonstrated that animals which actually overexpress NGF in the periphery also possess these abnormal sympathetic terminations within the DRG (Davis et al. 1994), and these animals are also hyperalgesic. This is a different situation to that of axotomy, where the retrograde supply of NGF is reduced, but demonstrates that an imbalance in NGF distribution can result in the development of this abnormal connectivity between the sympathetic and sensory nervous systems.

Diabetic neuropathy is associated with an axonopathy of sympathetic neurones although there appears to be little cell death in sympathetic ganglia (Schmidt et al. 1981, 1983). There is actually an increase in the activity in the enzyme tyrosine hydroxylase (the rate-limiting step in noradrenalin synthesis) within the superior cervical ganglion (Schmidt and Cogswell 1989). This is in the opposite direction to that expected but is suggested to be due to alterations in the target size of sympathetic neurones. Autonomic symptoms may be marked in diabetes, and given the importance of NGF in regulating sympathetic function this would be an important area of future research.

VII. Dorsal Horn Changes After Nerve Injury

Changes occur within the dorsal horn as a consequence of axotomy which reflect alterations at the level of the DRG. There is a reduced expression of substance P and CGRP and increased expression of galanin and VIP in nerve terminals within superficial laminae. The functional implications of this are thought to be a downregulation of excitatory peptides and an upregulation of inhibitory peptides potentially contributing to abnormal sensory processing (HOKFELT et al. 1994). A trans-ganglionic degeneration of nerve terminals within the dorsal horn is also associated with axotomy (JANCSO 1992). The increase in expression of GAP-43 in nerve terminals and the vacation of synaptic space due to the degeneration of other nerve terminals may be important in the generation of plasticity at the level of the dorsal horn. Indeed, sprouting of large myelinated afferents from laminae 3–4 into more superficial laminae has been demonstrated (WOOLF et al. 1992). This would result in dorsal horn neurones previously receiving an input from small-diameter nociceptive afferents now receiving an input from large-diameter, low-threshold mechanoreceptors. These anatomical abnormalities are accompanied by alterations in CNS function, such as altered somatotopy, reduced primary afferent depolarisation and increased spontaneous activity in dorsal horn neurones.

There is evidence that exogenous NGF can prevent many of the central changes associated with axotomy. The reduction in an enzyme, fluoride-resistant acid phosphatase, expressed by some small sensory neurones, which might represent transganglionic degeneration, can be partially prevented by administration of NGF (CSILLIK et al. 1985; FITZGERALD et al. 1985). The reduction in primary afferent depolarisation (which may represent a central disinhibition) and the appearance of abnormal receptive fields in dorsal horn cells that normally occur after axotomy are prevented by administration of exogenous NGF (FITZGERALD et al. 1985). We have recently demonstrated that administration of intrathecal NGF but not BDNF or neurotrophin 3 can completely prevent the sprouting of A fibres into lamina II of the dorsal horn following sciatic axotomy (BENNETT et al. 1996). This indicates that the sprouting phenomenon probably occurs secondarily to C fibre damage. By restoring C fibre function we prevented the A fibre sprouting. These findings also provide a strong rationale for the therapeutic use of NGF in the treatment of neuropathic pain.

In summary, we have described two different types of nerve injury, that produced by axotomy and that produced by diabetic neuropathy and have shown that in both of theses conditions there is a deficit in the peripheral synthesis and/or retrograde transport of NGF. The administration of exogenous NGF can prevent many of the anatomical, neurochemical and electrophysiological consequences of these insults. In general this "rescue" effect of NGF is limited to small-diameter primary afferents that express the trkA receptor and hence are NGF responsive. Some of the consequences of axotomy are not NGF reversible even in the population of small-diameter primary sensory neurones, for instance the increased GAP-43 expression. Another well-documented effect of nerve injury on primary afferent neurones is the development of ongoing activity in both unmyelinated and large myelinated afferents (DEVOR 1994), the role of NGF in the development of such ongoing activity has not been investigated. Deprivation of endogenous NGF can mimic some of the changes associated with nerve injury. NGF is therefore an important but certainly not the only factor involved in sensory and sympathetic neurones response to nerve injury. More recent studies both in animals and humans that have looked directly at the behavioural consequences of nerve injury indicate that the administration of NGF can prevent or ameliorate the persistent pain associated with these conditions.

VIII. Other Growth Factors and Neuropathic Pain

This discussion above concentrates on NGF since it is the best characterised member of the neurotrophin family. However, the interaction of other neurotrophic factors with sensory systems is now being more intensively studied. BDNF may be particularly interesting. It has been shown that this protein is actually synthesised by primary sensory neurones (WETMORE and OLSON 1995), and that it may have an autocrine or paracrine role in the survival of primary sensory neurones within the DRG (ACHESON et al. 1995). Such a survival role may be very important in relation to nerve injury. The effects of BDNF may not be restricted to the DRG as it is transported to the central terminals of primary sensory neurones. Indeed, it has recently been demonstrated that BDNF expression in primary sensory neurones can modulated by a number of factors. One of these is the administration of NGF, which increases BDNF expression within the DRG (APFEL et al. 1994, 1996b). In relation to this discussion it is interesting that both crush and axotomy can also increase BDNF expression particularly in small-diameter sensory neurones (ERNFORS et al. 1993; PRIESTLEY et al., unpublished observations). This increase in expression is reflected in an increase in BDNF immunostaining in the dorsal horn. The possible roles of this increased BDNF expression are still unclear but provide an exciting area of future research.

F. Conclusions

This chapter presents some lines of experimental evidence suggesting a role for NGF as a mediator of persistent pain states. We have discussed the role of growth factors, particularly NGF, in two distinct types of persistent pain, that associated with inflammation and that associated with neuropathy. In the former case there is now rather strong evidence from several laboratories converging on a common conclusion that upregulation of NGF is a critical event in the pathogenesis of pain. There is uncertainty about the events "downstream" to NGF production. The peripheral effects of NGF may be largely indirect. There is clear evidence that a variety of mediators, including prostaglandins and other products of arachidonic acid metabolism, bradykinin, histamine, and serotonin may contribute to inflammatory pain. Given the evidence for the involvement of both mast cells and post-ganglionic sympathetic terminals in NGF actions, it is feasible that NGF upregulation is simply "upstream" to the production of these classical mediators. The failure of existing analgesics to control adequately many forms of inflammatory pain may well stem from their targeting individual 'downstream' mediators. Therefore strategies aimed at controlling the means of production or action of NGF may represent an important new strategy in the treatment of inflammatory pain states.

There are still several unresolved issues. Firstly, most of the experimental studies have, often of necessity, utilised models of relatively short-lasting inflammation, typically measured only in days. In contrast, many forms of clinically relevant persistent pain have very much longer durations. We do not know whether the effects of NGF described in this chapter persist over such long time courses, or whether other actions of NGF arise only with time, for instance the anatomical remodelling of peripheral or even central terminals of nociceptive sensory neurones.

The second area discussed in this review, the role of growth factors in the genesis of neuropathic pain, is much less well established. However, there are now several strands of evidence implicating reduced NGF availability as the cause of some of the pathophysiological changes associated with nerve injury. The specific contribution of these changes to neuropathic pain remains largely unresolved. One might predict, however, that the use of NGF for the clinical treatment of neuropathic states (and trials to this end are underway), may be confounded by the systemic action of this protein on undamaged sensory systems.

Acknowledgements. Some of the work described in this chapter was supported by a Programme grant from the Medical Research Council of Great Britain. DLHB is supported by the special trustees of Guy's and St Thomas' hospitals.

References

Acheson A, Conover JC, Fandl JP, DeChlara TM, Russell M, Thadani A, Squinto SP, Yancopoulos GD, Lindsay RM (1995) A BDNF autocrine loop in adult sensory neurons prevents cell death. Nature 374:450–453

Ahlgren SC, Levine JD (1993) Mechanical hyperalgesia in streptozotocin-diabetic rats is not sympathetically maintained. Brain Res 616:171–175

Al-SalihiO, Averill S, Priestley JV, McMahon SB (1995) Subcutaneous infusions of NGF promote local heat and chemical hyperalgesia and increases in sensory neuron neuropeptides. J Physiol (Lond) 483:154P

Albers KM, Wright DE, Davis BM (1994) Overexpression of nerve growth factor in epidermis of transgenic mice causes hypertrophy of the peripheral nervous system. J Neurosci. 14:1422–1432

Aloe L, Tuveri MA, Levi Montalcini R (1992) Studies on carrageenan-induced arthritis in adult rats: presence of nerve growth factor and role of sympathetic innervation. Rheumatol Int 12:213–216

Alvarez FJ, Rodrigo J, Jessell TM, Dodd J, Priestley JV (1989) Ultrastructure of primary afferent fibres and terminals expressing alpha-galactose extended oligosaccharides in the spinal cord and brainstem of the rat. J Neurocytol 18:631–645

Alvarez FJ, Morris HR, Priestley JV (1991) Sub-populations of smaller diameter trigeminal primary afferent neurons defined by expression of calcitonin gene-related peptide and the cell surface oligosaccharide recognized by monoclonal antibody LA4. J Neurocytol 20:716–731

Andreev N, Inuishin M, McMahon SB (1994) Nerve growth factor acutely enhances the responsiveness of dorsal horn neurones to noxious heat. Soc Neurosci Abstr 20:1105

Andreev NY, Bennett D, Priestley JV, Rattray M, McMahon SB (1993) Synthesis of neurotrophins is upregulated by inflammation of urinary bladder in adult rats. Soc Neurosci Abstr 19:248

Andreev NY, Dmitrieva N, Koltzenburg M, McMahon SB (1995) Peripheral administration of nerve growth factor in the adult rat produces a thermal hyperalgesia that requires the presence of sympathetic post-ganglionic neurones. Pain 63:109–115

Apfel SC, Arezzo JC, Brownlee M, Federoff H, Kessler JA (1994) Nerve growth factor administration protects against experimental diabetic sensory neuropathy. Brain Res 634:7–12

Apfel SC, Adornato BT, Dyck PJ, Kessler JA, Vinik A, Rendell M, Griggs R, Barbano R, Rask C (1996a) Results of a double blind, placebo controlled trial of recombinant human nerve growth in diabetic polyneuropathy. Ann Neurol 40(3):194

Apfel SC, Wright DE, Wiideman AM, Dormiac, Snider WD, Kessler JA (1996b) Nerve growth factor regulates the expression of brain derived neurotrophic factor mRNA in the peripheral nervous system. MCN 7(2):134–142

Archer AG, Watkins PJ, Thomas PK, Sharma AK, Payan J (1983) The natural history of acute painful neuropathy in diabetes mellitus. J Neurol Neurosurg Psychiatry 46:491–499

Arvidsson J, Ygge J, Grant G (1986) Cell loss in lumbar dorsal root ganglia and transganglionic degeneration after sciatic nerve resection in the rat. Brain Res 373:15–21

Averill S, McMahon SB, Clary DO, Reichardt LF, Priestley JVP (1995) Immunocytochemical localization of trkA receptors in chemically identified subgroups of adult rat sensory neurons. Eur J Neurosci 7:1484–1494

Barbacid M (1994) The Trk family of neurotrophin receptors. J Neurobiol 25:1386–1403

Bennett D, Shelton D, Michael G, Priestley JV, McMahon SB (1995) The effect of chronic nerve growth factor (NGF) deprivation on pain-signalling systems in adult rats. Soc Neurosci Abst 21:227.11

Bennett DLH, French J, Priestley JV, McMahon SB (1996) NGF but NT-3 or BDNF prevents the A fiber sprouting into lamina II of the spinal cord that occurs following axotomy. MCN 8 (4):211–220

Bennett GJ (1994) Neuropathic pain. In: Wall PD, Melzack R (eds) Textbook of pain. Churchill Livingstone, Edinburgh, pp 201–224

Bennett GJ, Xie YK (1988) A peripheral mononeuropathy in rat that produces disorders of pain sensation like those seen in man. Pain 33:87–107

Berg MM, Sternberg DW, Parada LF, Chao MV (1992) K-252a inhibits nerve growth factor-induced trk proto-oncogene tyrosine phosphorylation and kinase activity. J Biol Chem 267:13–16

Bevan S, Winter J (1995) Nerve growth factor (NGF) differentially regulates the chemosensitivity of adult rat cultured sensory neurons. J Neurosci 15:4918–4926

Bradshaw RA, Blundell TL, Lapatto R, McDonald NQ, Murray-Rust J (1993) Nerve growth factor revisited. Trends Biochem Sci 18:48–52

Brewster WJ, Fernyhough P, Diemel LT, Mohiuddin L, Tomlinson DR (1994) Diabetic neuropathy, nerve growth factor and other neurotrophic factor. Trends Neurosci 17:321–325

Brown MC, Perry VH, Lunn ER, Gordon S, Heumann R (1991) Macrophage dependence of peripheral sensory nerve regeneration: possible involvement of nerve growth factor. Neuron 6:359–370

Calcutt NA, Mizisin AP, Yaksh TL (1993) Impaired induction of vasoactive intestinal polypeptide after sciatic nerve injury in the streptozotocin-diabetic rat. J Neurol Sci 119:154–161

Carroll SL, SilosSantiago I, Frese SE, Ruit KG, Milbrandt J, Snider WD (1992) Dorsal root ganglion neurons expressing trk are selectively sensitive to NGF deprivation in utero. Neuron 9:779–788

Chao MV, Hempstead BL (1995) p75 and trk: a two-receptor system. Trends Neurosci 18(7):321–326

Crowley C, Spencer SD, Nishimura MC, Chen KS, Pitts-Meek S, Armanini MP, Ling LH, McMahon SB, Shelton DL, Levinson AD, Phillips HS (1994) Mice lacking nerve growth factor display perinatal loss of sensory and sympathetic neurons yet develop basal forebrain cholinergic neurons. Cell 76:1001–1011

Csillik B, Schwab ME, Thoenen H (1985) Transganglionic regulation of central terminals of dorsal root ganglion cells by nerve growth factor (NGF). Brain Res 331:11–15

Davis BM, Lewin GR, Mendell LM, Jones ME, Albers KM (1993) Altered expression of nerve growth factor in the skin of transgenic mice leads to changes in response to mechanical stimuli. Neuroscience 56:789–792

Davis BM, Albers KM, Seroogy KB, Katz DM (1994) Overexpression of nerve growth factor in transgenic mice induces novel sympathetic projections to primary sensory neurones. J Comp Neurol 349:464–474

Devor M (1994) The pathophysiology of the damaged peripheral nerve. In: Wall PD, Melzack R (eds) Textbook of pain. Churchill Livingstone, Edinburgh, pp 79–100

Diamond J, Coughlin M, Macintyre L, Holmes M, Visheau B (1987) Evidence that endogenous NGF is responsible for the collateral sprouting, but not the regeneration, of nociceptive axons in adult rats. Proc Natl Acad Sci USA 84:6596

Diamond J, Foerster A, Holmes M, Coughlin M (1992a) Sensory nerves in adult rats regenerate and restore sensory function to the skin independently of endogenous NGF. J Neurosci 12:1467–1476

Diamond J, Holmes M, Coughlin M (1992b) Endogenous NGF and nerve impulses regulate the collateral sprouting of sensory axons in the skin of the adult rat. J Neurosci 12:1454–1466

DiStefano PS, Friedman B, Radziejewski C, Alexander C, Boland P, Schick CM, Lindsay RM, Wiegand SJ (1992) The neurotrophins BDNF, NT-3, and NGF display distinct patterns of retrograde axonal transport in peripheral and central neurons. Neuron 8:983–993

Diemel LT, Brewster WJ, Fernyhough P, Tomlinson DR (1994) Expression of neuropeptides in experimental diabetes; effects of treatment with nerve growth factor or brain-derived neurotrophic factor. Mol Brain Res 21:171–175

Dmitrieva N, McMahon SB (1995) Sensitisation of visceral afferents by nerve growth factor in the adult rat. Pain 66:87–97

Dmitrieva N, Rice ASC, Shelton DI, McMahon SB (1995) The role of NGF in a model of persistent visceral pain. Soc Neurosci Abstr 21:227.12

Donnerer J, Schuligoi R, Stein C (1992) Increased content and transport of substance P and calcitonin gene-related peptide in sensory nerves innervating inflamed tissue: evidence for a regulatory function of nerve growth factor in vivo. Neuroscience 49:693–698

Ernfors P, Rosario CM, Merlio JP, Grant G, Aldskogius H and Persson H (1993) Expression of mRNAs for neurotrophin receptors in the dorsal root ganglion and spinal cord during development and following peripheral or central axotomy. Mol Brain Res 17:217–226

Faradji V, Sotelo J (1990) Low serum levels of nerve growth factor in diabetic neuropathy. Acta Neurol Scand 81:402–406

Fernyhough P, Diemel LT, Brewster WJ, Tomlinson DR (1994) Deficits in sciatic nerve neuropeptide content coincide with a reduction in target tissue nerve growth factor messenger RNA in streptozotocin-diabetic rats: effects of insulin treatment. Neuroscience 62:337–344

Fernyhough P, Diemel LT, Brewster WJ, Tomlinson DR (1995) Altered neurotrophin mRNA levels in peripheral nerve and skeletal muscle of experimentally diabetic rats. J Neurochem 64:1231–1237

Fitzgerald M, Wall PD, Goedert M, Emson PC (1985) Nerve growth factor counteracts the neurophysiological and neurochemical effects of chronic sciatic nerve section. Brain Res 332:131–141

Gold BG, Mobley WC, Matheson SF (1991) Regulation of axonal caliber, neurofilament content, and nuclear localization in mature sensory neurons by nerve growth factor. J Neurosci 11:943–955

Gold BG, Storm-Dickerson T, Austin DR (1993) Regulation of the transcription factor c-JUN by nerve growth factor in adult sensory neurons. Neurosci Lett 124:144–147

Gorin PD, Johnson EM Jr (1980) Effects of long-term nerve growth factor deprivationon the nervous system of the adult rat: an experimental autoimmune approach. Brain Res 198:27–42

Gotz R, Koster R, Winkler C, Raulf F, Lottspeich F, Schartl M (1994) Neurotrophin-6 is a new member of the nerve growth factor family. Nature 372:266–269

Greene LA, Kaplan DR (1995) Early events in neurotrophin signalling via Trk and p75 receptors. Curr Opin Neurobiol 5:579–587

Häbler H-J, Jänig W, Koltzenburg M (1988) A novel type of unmyelinated chemosensitive nociceptor in the acutely inflamed urinary bladder. Agents Actions 25:219–221

Häbler H-J, Jänig W, Koltzenburg M (1993) Receptive properties of myelinated primary afferents innervating the inflamed urinary bladder of the cat. J Neurophysiol 69:395–405

Harati Y (1987) Diabetic peripheral neuropathies (review). Ann Intern Med 107:546–559

Heller PH, Green PG, Tanner KD, Miao FJ-P, Levine JD (1994) Peripheral neural contributions to inflammation. In: Fields HL, Liebeskind JC (eds) Pharmacological approaches to the treatment of chronic pain: new concepts and critical issues. International Association for the Study of Pain, Seattle, pp 31–42

Hellweg R, Hartung HD (1990) Endogenous levels of nerve growth factor (NGF) are altered in experimental diabetes mellitus: a possible role for NGF in the pathogenesis ofdiabetic neuropathy. J Neurosci Res 26:258–267

Hellweg R, Wohrle M, Hartung HD, Stracke H, Hock C, Federlin K (1991) Diabetes mellitus-associated decrease in nerve growth factor levels is reversed by allogeneic pancreatic islet transplantation. Neurosci Lett 125:1–4

Hellweg R, Raivich G, Hartung HD, Hock C, Kreutzberg GW (1994) Axonal transport of endogenous nerve growth factor (NGF) and NGF receptor in experimental diabetic neuropathy. Exp Neurol 130:24–30

Hendry IA (1975) The response of adrenergic neurones to axotomy and nerve growth factor. Brain Res 94:87–97

Hendry IA (1977) The effect of the retrograde axonal transport of nerve growth factor on the morphology of adrenergic neurones. Brain Res 134:213–223

Hendry IA, Stach R, Herrup K (1974) Characteristics of the retrograde axonal transport system for nerve growth factor in the sympathetic nervous system. Brain Res 82:117–128

Heumann R, Korsching S, Bandtlow C, Thoenen H (1987a) Changes of nerve growth factor synthesis in nonneuronal cells in response to sciatic nerve transection. J Cell Biol 104:1623–1631

Heumann R, Lindholm D, Bandtlow C et al (1987b) Differential regulation of mRNA encoding nerve growth factor and its receptor in rat sciatic nerve during development, degeneration, and regeneration: role of macrophages. Proc Natl Acad Sci USA 84:8735–8739

Hoffman PN, Cleveland DW, Griffin JW, Landes PW, Cowan NJ, Price DL (1987) Neurofilament gene expression: a major determinant of axonal caliber. Proc Natl Acad Sci USA 84:3472–3476

Hokfelt T, Zhang X, Wiesenfeld-Hallin Z (1994) Messenger plasticity in primary sensory neurons following axotomy and its functional implications. Trends Neurosci 17:22–30

Horigome K, Pryor JC, Bullock ED, Johnson EM (1993) Mediator release from mast cells by nerve growth factor. Neurotrophin specificity and receptor mediation. J Biol Chem 268:14881–14887

Jakobsen J, Brimijoin S, Skau K, Sidenius P, Wells D (1981) Retrograde axonal transport of transmitter enzymes, fucose-labeled protein, and nerve growth factor in streptozotocin-diabetic rats. Diabetes 30:797–803

Jancso G (1992) Pathobiological reactions of C-fibre primary sensory neurones to peripheral nerve injury. Exp Physiol 77:405–431

Johnson EM, Gorin PD, Osborne PD, Rydel RE, Pearson J (1982) Effects of autoimmune NGF deprivation in the adult rabbit and offspring. Brain Res 240:131–140

Kaplan DR, Hempstead BL, Martin-Zanca D, Chao MV, Parada LF (1991) The trk proto-oncogene product: a signal transducing receptor for nerve growth factor. Science 252:554–558

Kinnman E, Levine JD (1995) Sensory and sympathetic contributions to nerve injury-induced sensory abnormalities in the rat. Neuroscience 64:751–767

Kolzenburg M (1995) Stability and plasticity of nociceptor function and their relationship to provoked and ongoing pain. In: McMahon SB, Wall PD (eds) Seminars in the neurosciences, vol 7. Academic, Cambridge, pp 199–210

Koltzenburg M, McMahon SB (1991) The enigmatic role of the sympathetic nervous system in chronic pain. Trends Pharmacol Sci 12:399–402

Kuraishi Y, Nanayama T, Ohno H, Fujii N, Otaka A, Yajima H, Satoh M (1989) CGRP increases in the dorsal root ganglia of the adjuvant arthritic rat. Peptides 10:447–452

Lawson S, Harper AA, Harper E I, Garson JA, Anderton RH (1984) A monoclonal antibody against neurofilament protein specifically labels a subpopulation of rat sensory neurones. J Comp Neurol 228:263–272

Lawson SN (1992) Morphological and biochemical cell types of sensory neurons. In: Scott SA (ed) Sensory neurons. Diversity, development, and plasticity. Oxford University Press, New York, pp 27–59

Lee KF, Li E, Huber LJ et al (1992) Targeted mutation of the gene encoding the low affinity NGF receptor p75 leads to deficits in the peripheral sensory nervous system. Cell 69:737–749

Leon A, Buriani A, Dal Toso R, Fabris M, Romanello S, Aloe L (1994) Mast cells synthesize, store, and release nerve growth factor. Proc Natl Acad Sci USA 91:3739–3743

Leslie TA, Emson PC, Dowd PM, Woolf CJ (1995) Nerve growth factor contributes to the up-regulation of growth-associated protein 43 and preprotachykinin A messenger RNAs in primary sensory neurons following peripheral inflammation. Neuroscience 67:753–762

Lewin GR (1995) Neurotrophic factors and pain. In: McMahon SB, Wall PD (eds) Seminars in the neurosciences, vol 7. Academic, Cambridge, pp 227–232

Lewin GR, Winter J, McMahon SB (1992) Regulation of afferent connectivity in the adult spinal cord by nerve growth factor. Eur J Neurosci 4:700–707

Lewin GR, Ritter AM, Mendel LM (1993) Nerve growth factor induced hyperalgesia in the neonatal and adult rat. J Neurosci 13:2136–2148

Lewin GR, Rueff A, Mendell LM (1994) Peripheral and central mechanisms of NGF-induced hyperalgesia. Eur J Neurosci 6:1903–1912

Lindholm D, Heumann R, Meyer M, Thoenen H (1987) Interleukin-1 regulates synthesis of nerve growth factor in non-neuronal cells of rat sciatic nerve. Nature 330:658–659

Lindsay RM (1992) The role of neurotrophic factors in functional maintenance of mature sensory neurons. In: Scott SA (ed) Sensory neurons: diversity, development, and plasticity. Oxford University Press, New York, pp 404–420

Lindsay RM, Wiegand SJ, Altar CA, DiStefano PS (1994) Neurotrophic factors: from molecule to man. Trends Neurosci 17:182–190

Marshall CJ (1995) Specificity of receptor tyrosine kinase signaling: transient versus sustained extracellular signal-regulated kinase activation. Cell 80:179–185

Matsuoka I, Meyer M, Thoenen H (1991) Cell-type-specific regulation of nerve growth factor (NGF) synthesis in non-neuronal cells: comparison of Schwann cells with other cell types. J Neurosci 11:3165–3177

Max SR, Rohrer H, Otten U, Thoenen H (1978) Nerve growth factor-mediated induction of tyrosine hydroxylase in rat superior cervical ganglia in vitro. J Biol Chem 253:8013–8015

McDonald NQ, Lapatto R, Murray-Rust J, Gunning J, Wlodawer A (1991) New protein fold revealed by a 2.3-A resolution crystal structure of nerve growth factor. Nature 354:411–414

McLachlan EM, Janig W, Devor M, Michaelis M (1993) Peripheral nerve injury triggers noradrenergic sprouting within dorsal root ganglia. Nature 363:543–546

McMahon SB (1986) Sensory-motor integration in urinary bladder function. In: Cervero F, Morrison JFB (eds) Visceral sensation. Elsevier, Amsterdam, pp 245–253 (Progress in brain research, vol 67)

McMahon SB (1988) Neuronal and behavioural consequences of chemical inflammation of rat urinary bladder. Agents Actions 25:231–233

McMahon SB, Abel C (1987) A model for the study of visceral pain states: chronic inflammation of the chronic decerebrate rat urinary bladder by irritant chemicals. Pain 28:109–127

McMahon SB, Koltzenburg M (1994) Silent afferents and visceral pain. In: Fields HL, Liebeskind JC (eds) Pharmacological approaches to the treatment of chronic pain: new concepts and critical issues. International Association for the Study of Pain, Seattle, pp 11–30

McMahon SB, Priestley JV (1995) Peripheral neuropathies and neurotrophic factors: animal models and clinical perspectives. Curr Opin Neurobiol 5:616–624

McMahon SB, Lewin GR, Wall PD (1993) Central hyperexcitability triggered by noxious inputs. Curr Opin Neurobiol 3:602–610

McMahon SB, Armanini MP, Ling LH, Phillips HS (1994) Expression and coexpression of Trk receptors in subpopulations of adult primary sensory neurons projecting to identified peripheral targets. Neuron 12:1161–1171

McMahon SB, Bennett DLH, Priestley JV, Shelton D (1995a) The biological effects of endogenous NGF in adult sensory neurons revealed by a trkA-IgG fusion molecule. Nat Med 1(8):774–780

McMahon SB, Dmitrieva N, Koltzenburg M (1995b) Visceral pain. Br J Anaesth 75:132–144

Meakin SO, Shooter EM (1992) The nerve growth factor family of receptors. Trends Neurosci 15:323–331

Mohiuddin L, Fernandez K, Tomlinson DR, Fernyhough P (1995a) Nerve growth factorand neurotrophin-3 enhance neurite outgrowth and up-regulate the levels of messenger RNA for growth-associated protein GAP-43 and T alpha 1 alpha-tubulin in cultured adult rat sensory neurones. Neurosci Lett 185:20–23

Mohiuddin L, Fernyhough P, Tomlinson DR (1995b) Reduced levels of mRNA encoding endoskeletal and growth-associated proteins in sensory ganglia in experimental diabetes. Diabetes 44:25–30

Mu X, Silos-Santiago I, Carroll SL, Snider WD (1993) Neurotrophin receptor genes are expressed in distinct patterns in developing dorsal root ganglia. J Neurosci 13:4029–4041

Oddiah D, McMahon SB, Rattary M (1995) Inflammation produces an up-regulation of neurotrophin mRNAs in bladder. Soc Neurosci Abstr 21:604.15

Otten U (1991) Nerve growth factor: a signaling protein between the nervous and immune system. In: Basbaum AI, Besson J-M (eds) Towards a new pharmacotherapy of pain. Wiley, Chicester, pp 353–363

Otten U, Goedert M, Schwab M, Thibault J (1979) Immunisation of adult rats against 2.5S NGF: effects on the peripheral sympathetic nervous system. Brain Res 176:79–90

Paravicini U, Stoeckel K, Thoenen H (1975) Biological importance of retrograde axonal transport of nerve growth factor in adrenergic neurons. Brain Res 84:279–291

Peng X, Greene LA, Kaplan DR, Stephens RM (1995) Deletion of a conserved juxtamembrane sequence in Trk abolishes NGF-promoted neuritogenesis. Neuron 15:395–406

Petty BG, Cornblath DR, Adornato BT, Chaudhry V, Flexner C, Wachsman M, Sinicropi D, Burton LE, Peroutka SJ (1994) The effect of systemically administered recombinant human nerve growth factor in healthy human subjects. Ann Neurol 36(2):244–246

Purves D (1975) Functional and structural changes in mammalian sympathetic neurones following interruption of their axons. J Physiol (Lond) 252:429–463

Purves D, Nja A (1976) Effect of nerve growth factor on synaptic depression after axotomy. Nature 260:535–536

Reeh PW, Kress M (1995) Effects of classical algogens. In: McMahon SB, Wall PD (eds) Seminars in the neurosciences, vol 7. Academic, Cambridge, pp 221–226

Ren K, Thomas DA, Dubner R (1995) Nerve growth factor alleviates a painful peripheral neuropathy in rats. Brain Res 699(2):286–292

Rich KM, Yip KK, Osborne PA, Schmidt RE, Johnson EM (1984) Role of nerve growth factor in the adult dorsal root ganglia neuron and its response to injury. J Comp Neurol 230:110–118

Rich KM, Luszczynski JR, Osborne PA, Johnson EM Jr (1987) Nerve growth factor protects adult sensory neurons from cell death and atrophy caused by nerve injury. J Neurocytol 16:261–268

Richardson PM, Riopelle RJ (1984) Uptake of nerve growth factor along peripheral and spinal axons of primary sensory neurons. J Neurosci 4:1683–1689

Richardson PM, Issa VM, Riopelle RJ (1986) Distribution of neuronal receptors for nerve growth factor in the rat. J Neurosci 6:2312–2321

Rueff A, Mendell LM (1995) NGF-induced increas in thrmal sensitivity of nociceptive fibres in vitro. Soc Neurosci Abstr 21:605.16

Ruit KG, Osborne PA, Schmidt RE, Johnson EM Jr, Snider WD (1990) Nerve growth factor regulates sympathetic ganglion cell morphology and survival in the adult mouse. J Neurosci 10:2412–2419

Safieh-Garabedian B, Poole S, Allchorne A, Winter J, Woolf CJ (1995) Contribution of interleukin-1-beta to the inflammation induced increase in nerve growth factor levels and inflammatory hyperalgesia. Br J Pharmacol 115(7):1265–1275

Santambrogio L, Benedetti M, Chao MV, Muzaffar R, Kulig K, Gabellini N, Hochwald G (1994) Nerve growth factor production by lymphocytes. J Immunol 153:4888–4898

Schlessinger J (1994) SH2/SH3 signaling proteins. Curr Opin Gen Dev 4:25–30

Schmidt RE (1993) The role of nerve growth factor in the pathogenesis and therapy of diabetic neuropathy. Diabetic Med 10 [Suppl 2]:10S–13S

Schmidt RE, Cogswell BE (1989) Tyrosine hydroxylase activity in sympathetic nervoussystem of rats with streptozocin-induced diabetes. Diabetes 38:959–968

Schmidt RE, Nelson JS, Johnson EM Jr (1981) Experimental diabetic autonomic neuropathy. Am J Pathol 103:210–225

Schmidt RE, Modert CW, Yip HK, Johnson EM Jr (1983) Retrograde axonal transport of intravenously administered 125I-nerve growth factor in rats with streptozotocin-induced diabetes. Diabetes 32:654–663

Schwartz JP, Pearson J, Johnson EM (1982) Effect of exposure to anti-NGF on sensory neurons of adult rats and guinea pigs. Brain Res 244:378–381

Shelton DL, Reichardt LF (1984) Expression of the beta-nerve growth factor gene correlates with the density of sympathetic innervation of effector organs. Proc Natl Acad Sci USA 81:7951–7955

Shelton DL, Sutherland J, Gripp J, Camerato MP, Armanini MP, Phillips, Carroll K, Spencer SD, Levinson AD (1995) Human trks: molecular cloning, tissue distribution, and expression of extracellular domain immunoadhesins. J Neurosci 15:477–491

Silverman JD, Kruger L (1990) Selective neuronal glycoconjugate expression in sensory and autonomic ganglia: relation of lectin reactivity to peptide and enzyme markers. J Neurocytol 19:789–801

Smeyne RJ, Klein R, Schnapp A, Long LK, Bryant S, Lewin A, Lira SA, Barbacid M (1994) Severe sensory and sympathetic neuropathies in mice carrying a disrupted Trk/NGF receptor gene. Nature 368:246–249

Steers WD, Kolbeck S, Creedon D, Tuttle JB (1991) Nerve growth factor in the urinary bladder of the adult regulates neuronal form and function. J Clin Invest 88:1709–1715

Thoenen H (1991) The changing scene of neurotrophic factors. Trends Neurosci 14:165–170

Thompson SWN, Dray A, McCarson KE, Krause JE, Urban L (1995) NGF induces mechanical allodynia associated with novel A-fibre evoked spinal reflex activity and enhanced NK-1 receptor activation in the rat. Pain 62:219–332

Verge VM, Richardson PM, Benoit R, Riopelle RJ (1989a) Histochemical characterization of sensory neurons with high-affinity receptors for nerve growth factor. J Neurocytol 18:583–591

Verge VM, Riopelle RJ, Richardson PM (1989b) Nerve growth factor receptors on normal and injured sensory neurons. J Neurosci 9:914–922

Verge V M, Tetzlaff W, Richardson PM, Bisby MA (1990a) Correlation between GAP43 and nerve growth factor receptors in rat sensory neurons. J Neurosci 10:926–934

Verge VM, Tetzlaff W, Bisby MA, Richardson PM (1990b) Influence of nerve growth factor on neurofilament gene expression in mature primary sensory neurons. J Neurosci 10:2018–2025

Verge VM, Merlio JP, Grondin J et al (1992) Colocalization of NGF binding sites, trk mRNA, and low-affinity NGF receptor mRNA in primary sensory neurons: responses to injury and infusion of NGF. J Neurosci 12:4011–4022

Verge VM, Richardson PM, Wiesenfeld-Hallin Z, Hokfelt T (1995) Differential influence of nerve growth factor on neuropeptide expression in vitro: a novel role in peptide suppression in adult sensory neurons. J Neurosci 15(3):2081–2096

Westkamp G, Otten U (1987) An enzyme-linked immunoassay for nerve growth factor (NGF): a tool for studying regulatory mechanisms involved in NGF production in brain and in peripheral tissues. J Neurochem 12:4011–4022

Wetmore C, Olson L (1995) Neuronal and nonneuronal expression of neurotrophins and their receptors in sensory and sympathetic ganglia suggest new intercellular trophic interactions. J Comp Neurol 353:143–159

Willars GB, Calcutt NA, Compton AM, Tomlinson DR, Keen P (1989) Substance Plevels in peripheral nerve, skin, atrial myocardium and gastrointestinal tract of rats with long-term diabetes mellitus. Effects of aldose reductase inhibition. J Neurol Sci 91:153–164

Willis WD, Coggeshall RE (1991) Sensory mechanisms of the spinal cord. Plenum, New York

Winter J, Forbes A, Sternberg J, Lindsay R (1988) Nerve Growth Factor (NGF) regulates adult rat cultured dorsal root ganglion neuron responses to the excitotoxin capsaicin. Neuron 1:973–981

Wong J, Oblinger MM (1991) NGF rescues substance P expression but not neurofilament or tubulin gene expression in axotomized sensory neurons. J Neurosci 11:543–552

Woolf CJ, Reynolds ML, Molander C, O'Brien C, Lindsay RM, Benowitz LI (1990) The growth-associated protein GAP-43 appears in dorsal root ganglion cells and in thedorsal horn of the rat spinal cord following peripheral nerve injury. Neuroscience 34:465–478

Woolf CJ, Shortland P, Coggeshall RE (1992) Peripheral nerve injury triggers central sprouting of myelinated afferents. Nature 355:75–78

Woolf CJ, Safieh-Garabedian B, Ma Q-P, Crilly P, Winter J (1994) Nerve growth factor contributes to the generation of inflammatory sensory hypersensitivity. Neuroscience 62:327–331

Wright DE, Snider WD (1995) Neurotrophin receptor mRNA expression defines distinct populations of neurons in rat dorsal root ganglia. J Comp Neurol 351:329–338

Mechanisms of Central Hypersensitivity: Excitatory Amino Acid Mechanisms and Their Control

A. DICKENSON

There has been much evidence from clinical studies to support the idea that there are mechanisms for enhancing the transmission of pain. These events, underlying hyperalgesia – where the sensation of pain is greater than expected for a given stimulus, where the relationship between the stimulus and the response no longer holds – could be due to either peripheral or central mechanisms or indeed both. It is now clear that peripheral mechanisms are of great importance in this respect, and the primary hyperalgesia seen in damaged tissue is therefore explicable in terms of local mechanisms (see DRAY 1995). However, the secondary hyperalgesia around the damaged area is likely to involve central events, so-called central hypersensitivity. Arising from this is the idea that the ascending pain messages from the dorsal horn of the spinal cord are not the same under all circumstances but can be altered over short and long time courses. In addition, it is becoming clear that this plasticity, the ability of pain transmission and modulation systems to change, varies in different pain states (McQUAY and DICKENSON 1990). Thus there may be both common and unique alterations in different pain states.

A. Central Hypersensitivity

Understanding the spinal events that can enhance responses of neurones to low levels of afferent inputs starts to offer explanations for the extreme aberrations of pain transmission such as phantom limb pains, hyperalgesias and allodynias (touch-evoked pain) where the relationships between stimulus and response are markedly perturbed. The basis for this lack of strict concordance between stimulus and response appears to be the generation of central hypersensitivity (DICKENSON 1990, 1994a, 1995b; DRAY et al. 1994; DUBNER and RUDA 1992; McMAHON et al. 1993, 1995; PRICE et al. 1994a; WOOLF 1995; WOOLF and DOUBELL 1994; WOOLF and THOMPSON 1991). The mechanisms underlying this central hypersensitivity are discussed in this chapter, with emphasis on excitatory amino acid mechanisms.

I. Wind-Up and Central Hypersensitivity

There are two key observations on this subject. Firstly, high-frequency C fibre stimuli results in a marked and prolonged increase in the flexion withdrawal reflex in rats recorded from motoneurones in spinal animals (WOOLF 1983). Thus, noxious stimuli, applied at sufficient intensities can enhance spinal excitatory events by mechanisms that are restricted to the spinal cord. Secondly, the repetition of a constant-intensity C fibre stimulus induces the phenomenon of wind-up whereby the responses of certain dorsal horn nociceptive neurones suddenly increase markedly (in terms of both magnitude and duration) despite the constant input into the spinal cord (DAVIES and LODGE 1987; DICKENSON 1990, 1994a; DICKENSON and SULLIVAN 1987a, 1990; KING et al. 1988; MENDELL 1966; THOMPSON et al. 1990). Wind-up in normal animals is produced only by stimulation at C fibre strengths and possibly also Aδ stimulation but not by low-intensity stimuli. If a train of stimuli are given at frequencies of about 0.5 Hz or above, the responses of the neurone to the first few stimuli remain constant. However, as the stimulus continues, there is a rapid incremental increase in firing of the neurone from extracellular recordings or a cumulative long slow depolarization with intracellular records associated with increased action potentials (KING et al. 1988; THOMPSON et al. 1990). With extracellular recordings the neurone increases firing by up to 20-fold the initial rate.

Although wind-up is induced only by C fibre stimulation, once the process has occurred, all responses of the neurones are enhanced and a post-discharge following the C fibre latency band is evoked. This increase in response to a repeated constant stimulus is therefore thought to be one of the pivotal events in central hypersensitivity. Obviously there are likely to be many other causal factors, including changes in phenotype (HOKFELT et al. 1994), anatomical changes (WOOLF and DOUBELL 1994), which decrease neuronal thresholds and allow access of different afferent inputs to central nociceptive transmission. However, as a mechanism which enhances transmission without requring changes in afferent barrages, wind-up is clearly of prime importance (Fig. 1).

Not only can neuronal wind-up be observed under many forms of general anaesthesia (DICKENSON 1994a), but behavioural counterparts of this hypersensitivity are not blocked by volatile general anaesthesia such as with halothane (ABRAM and YAKSH 1993). That these spinal events are seen to be present during full anaesthesia suggests that the treatment of post-operative pain states needs to take into potential priming events occurring during the operations. This chapter discusses the possible pharmacological substrates underlying these changes and, as is shown, excitatory amino acids play a key role in these events.

B. Substrates for Central Hypersensitivity

I. Peptides

Historically substance P (SP) was the first transmitter to be related to the transmission of pain. SP release can be detected in the spinal cord following high- but not low-intensity peripheral stimulation, and the development of selective agonists and antagonists confirms a physiological role in the transmission of noxious messages (BIRCH et al. 1993; BRUGGER et al. 1990; CHAPMAN and DICKENSON 1993; CUMBERBATCH et al. 1995; SEGUIN et al. 1995; THOMPSON et al. 1993, 1994). The use of antibody microprobes to detect the spatial release of SP has shown that it is restricted essentially to the zones where the C fibres terminate (DUGGAN et al. 1988). In addition to SP, the release of neurokinin A and calcitonin gene related peptide (CGRP) has been demonstrated following C fibre activation. However, when CGRP is present, the subsequent release of SP is now extended to cover much of the dorsal horn. The interpretation of this finding is that the degradation of SP is reduced by CGRP binding to the peptidase that also cleaves SP. SP can therefore diffuse in an intact form over considerable distances (SCHAIBLE et al. 1992). The concept of actions at a distance from the release site, so-called volume transmission, has attracted interest as a basis for non-synaptic transmitter actions. Events such as these may have relevance to pain in that the peptides may diffuse to distant receptors, avoiding both peptidases and spatially restricted inhibitory influences. The induction of inflammation is accompanied by enhanced release of these peptides centrally (DRAY et al. 1994), due partly to the increases in production caused by agents such as nerve growth factor (MCMAHON et al. 1995; WOOLF 1995) which may then contribute to the central hypersensitivity by sole actions or interactions with other systems.

There is a consensus is that the conditions for release of SP from the fine afferents include a sufficiently long stimulus at an intensity sufficient to activate C fibres (URBAN et al. 1994). The acute responses of the neurones must therefore include some other transmitter, and the evidence implicates glutamate and aspartate. However, there is much evidence to suggest that peptides, especially SP, can allow or facilitate excitatory amino acid function in the spinal cord.

II. Excitatory Amino Acids

A large proportion of peripheral sensory fibres including both small and large fibres contain glutamate and aspartate (BATTAGLIA and RUSTIONI 1988; CLEMENTS et al. 1991; DEBIASI and RUSTIONI 1983; MAXWELL et al. 1990), and the localization of glutamate in the superficial spinal cord can be distinguished from that of γ-amino butyric acid (GABA) and aspartate (MERIGHI et al. 1991). There is good evidence that the glutamate seen in primary afferent terminals in laminae I, III and IV of the dorsal horn functions as a releasable transmitter (BROMAN et al. 1993; BROMAN and ADAHL 1994; MILLER et al. 1988). In the case of C fibres the coexistence of glutamate with peptides such as SP (BATTAGLIA and RUSTIONI 1988; DEBIASI and RUSTIONI 1983) and CGRP and/or SP (MERIGHI et al. 1991; MILLER et al. 1993) makes it highly likely that a noxious stimulus releases both peptides and excitatory amino acids from the afferent nociceptive fibres (JEFTINIJA et al. 1991; KANGRA and RANDIC 1991; SLUKA and WESTLUND 1993; SLUKA et al. 1994a). However, the subcellular organelles containing the amino acids differ from those with peptides, and therefore differential release from a single afferent can occur (MERIGHI et al. 1991). These anatomical studies suggest that glutamate is involved in the transmission of both high- and low-threshold information from afferents into the spinal cord although in pain states post-synaptic activation of both peptide receptors and receptors for the excitatory amino acids on nociceptive neurones occurs. In addition, there is further evidence from anatomical studies that transmission, at least from trigemino- and spinothalamic tract cells to certain thalamic areas, involves glutamate (ERICSON et al. 1995). There is an extensive literature from the 1950s to support the idea of important roles of excitatory amino acids in spinal sensory processing (CURTIS et al. 1959), which despite lack of any knowledge of the receptors or the availability of selective antagonists suggested important roles for these transmitters in spinal function (see HEADLEY and GRILLNER 1990).

1. Excitatory Amino Acid Receptors

The development of selective agonists and antagonists for the the excitatory amino acid receptors, the N-methyl-D-aspartate (NMDA), the metabotropic and the α-amino-3-hydroxy-5-methyl-isoxazole (AMPA) receptors (BARNARD and HENLEY 1990; FOSTER and FAGG 1987; LODGE and JOHNSON 1990; SEEBURG 1993; WATKINS and COLLINGRIDGE 1994; WILLETTS et al. 1990) now enables the roles of excitatory amino acids in the spinal processing of sensory information to be studied.

There is accumulating evidence that non-NMDA and NMDA receptors are expressed in the ganglia of primary afferents and therefore have functional roles at both the peripheral and central ends of the afferents. Two subunits of non-NMDA receptors (GluR4 and Glu5) have been found in dorsal root ganglia, as has NMDAR1 (SHIGEMOTO et al. 1992). High-affinity kainate receptors (containing GluR4) appear to have functional roles since nociceptive reflexes can be evoked by kainate administered peripherally (AULT and HILDEBRAND 1993) as well as uncharacterized receptors (CARLTON et al. 1995). In addition, there are data showing that the AMPA receptor (GluR1 and GluR2/3) and the metabotropic receptor (mGluR1) are also expressed on afferents (TOHYAMA et al. 1994). Furthermore, the NR1 subunit of the NMDA receptor is also found in afferents. There is a similarity between small- and large-diameter neurones in terms of this distribution except that the kainate receptor and the GluR1 subunit are not seen on small-diameter afferents. However, it needs to be borne in mind that many of these studies have been made in neonatal animals where developmental aspects may mean that the situation is not the same in the adult. For example, the developmental expression of AMPA and NMDA receptor subunits within the spinal cord shows remarkable change with the maturity of the animal (JAKOWEC et al. 1995; WATANABE et al. 1994) so that the subunit composition of the NMDA receptor is subject to rearrangement. However, in the adult rat not only are the NMDA,

AMPA and kainate receptors present, but as in young animals peripheral excitatory amino acids produce activation of nociceptors and behavioural responses. Thus there is evidence of functional receptors on the peripheral terminals of nociceptors (AULT and HILDEBRAND 1993), but it is not known whether they have a physiological role or whether the peripheral sensory nerve receptors function at the central terminals as well. A positive indication for a physiological role would require that antagonists administered peripherally have antinociceptive effects. Although this is not yet known, it is interesting to note that inflammation increases peripheral nerve levels of glutamate (WESTLUND et al. 1992).

The spinal receptors for the excitatory amino acids have been mapped using a number of techniques which include receptor binding autoradiography, in situ hybridization and receptor antisera in a number of species (CHINNERY et al. 1993; HENLEY et al. 1993; JAKOWEC et al. 1995; JANSEN et al. 1990; SHAW et al. 1991; TALLAKSEN-GREENE et al. 1992; TOHYAMA et al. 1994; TOLLE et al. 1993, WATANABE et al. 1994). There is relatively little information on the location of the receptors on neuronal processes except that in general they are found at higher levels on the dendrites than the soma of spinal neurones (ARANCIO et al. 1993).

The dorsal and ventral horns both contain all four receptors, but the distribution varies between areas, and the subunit composition of the receptors can differ, especially so for the AMPA receptor (TOHYAMA et al. 1994; TOLLE et al. 1993). There have been two extensive mapping studies in the rat using combinations of in situ and immunohistochemistry techniques, and the distribution of the receptor subunits agrees well between the two reports (TOHYAMA et al. 1994; TOLLE et al. 1993). The dorsal horn distribution of the AMPA receptor units is such that GluR4 expression is low in the superficial dorsal horn whereas GluR2 is strong and GluR1 and 3 is moderate. In the deeper dorsal horn the expression of all four units is moderate. By contrast to the dorsal horn distribution of the AMPA receptor, motoneurones express GluR3 and 4U at high levels whereas GluR2 is at moderate levels and GluR1 expression is weak. Interestingly, the expression pattern of GluR2 and GluR3 in the adult rat spinal cord is only about half that in the neonate, and the GluR1 unit declines by about 80% with development (JAKOWEC et al. 1995).

It is interesting to note the neuronal distribution of the receptors within areas of the spinal cord where interneurones predominate, namely the substantia gelatinosa. Here AMPA receptors are not found on spinothalamic neurones. In addition, a number of neurones that express GluR2 and GluR3 also contain enkephalin (TOHYAMA et al. 1994). Thus in addition to excitatory drives mediated by AMPA receptors, inhibitory neurones can also be potentially activated by afferent inputs using glutamate.

GluR5, the kainate receptor, is evenly distributed in a weak manner, and the NMDA NR1 receptor is strong throughout the spinal cord. The other members of the NMDA receptor family are only very low (NR2C and NR2D). However, there is a paradox in that the receptor binding studies, mainly autoradiography, for the two receptors show a similar situation for the AMPA receptor but quite a different distribution for the NMDA receptor which, from binding studies (CHINNERY et al. 1993; HENLEY et al. 1993; JANSEN et al. 1990; SHAW et al. 1991), is highly localized in the superficial dorsal horn in a number of species. Why is there a mismatch between the two studies? The receptor must make a complex, and the consensus is that NMDA receptors in vivo consist of an NR1/NR2 heterodimer. The wide distribution of the NR1 may mean that many of the NR1 receptors are not functional in mammalian neurones although dimeric receptors function in oocytes (LAMBOLEZ et al. 1991). However, there could be other yet unknown NMDA subunits, or low levels of expression of NR2 subunits may suggest that the NR1 predominates in the complex. For further discussion of this point see TOLLE et al. (1993).

The marked developmental changes in the receptors for the excitatory amino acids (JAKOWEC et al. 1995; WATANABE et al. 1994) means that great care must be taken in extrapolating from studies in young animals to the situation in the adult.

C. Mechanisms of Central Hypersensitivity

I. Wind-Up

Before discussing the roles of these different receptors in pain models it is important to reconsider briefly the two key events that really lead to the investigation of the roles of excitatory amino acids in spinal transmission of noxious events related to hypersensitivity. High-frequency stimulation of C fibres causes a marked and prolonged increase in the flexion withdrawal reflex in rats, the first evidence for the existence of central hypersensitivity (Woolf 1983). Here a brief series of C fibre stimuli cause enhanced reflex responses for about 40min. Even earlier, MENDELL (1966) had shown that the repetition of a constant-intensity C fibre stimulus induces the phenomenon of wind-up in spinal neurones where huge increases in the duration and the magnitude of the cell responses suddenly occur despite the input into the spinal cord remaining constant. Here the enhanced responses outlast the stimulus period (0.5min) by minutes rather than tens of minutes (DICKENSON 1990, 1994a). The differences in duration of the two events may be partly related to the intensity and frequency of the stimulation but also the presence of descending controls. The reflex studies were in spinalized animals whereas much of the work on wind-up has been in intact animals where supraspinal controls are operative and can act to curtail the responses in intact animals. Wind-up can be clearly demonstrated in human psychophysical studies with transcutaneous nerve stimulation leading to increases in pain ratings as the stimulus continues (PRICE et al. 1994b).

A clue to the underlying events behind these phenomena is that the response is both amplified and prolonged above the baseline response, and that wind-up is frequency dependent. Thus there must be mechanism(s) which increase excitability when summation occurs, and when the intensity and duration of the stimuli suffice to produce this. It turns out that the NMDA receptor is a major participant since the hypersensitive reflexes and wind-up both in animals and man are all are sensitive to NMDA receptor antagonists. However, some of the differences between various models and preparations may be due to differences in concurrent inhibitory controls. The roles of the main excitatory amino acid receptors are now considered and then the roles of inhibitory systems in controlling these events.

II. Evidence for a Role of the AMPA Receptor

The role played by the AMPA receptor for glutamate in the spinal transmission of noxious information can be investigated using the selective AMPA receptor antagonists 6-nitro-7-sulphamoylbenzo(f)quinoxaline-2,3-dione (NBQX) which has superseded the earlier antagonist 6-cyano-7-nitroquinoxaline-2,3-dione CNQX.

The phenomenon of wind-up in spinal neurones, whereby the neuronal response increases with repeated stimulation despite a constant stimulus intensity, was first described by MENDELL in 1966. In recent years there has been much interest in the mechanisms underlying wind-up in the spinal cord as a possible basis for much of the aberrant spinal processing of nociceptive messages in protracted pain states (see Sect. BI). A great deal of attention has focussed on the role played by the NMDA receptor for glutamate, activation of which has been shown to be critical to the manifestation of wind-up (BUDAI et al. 1992; DAVIES and LODGE 1987; DICKENSON and AYDAR 1991; DICKENSON and SULLIVAN 1987a). By contrast, the role played by the AMPA receptor in this phenomenon has not been specifically investigated. Although many attempts have been made to determine the role played by AMPA receptors in spinal nociceptive transmission, these have been hampered by a lack of selective antagonists for this receptor. CNQX, which was the drug of choice in many early studies, in addition to blocking the AMPA receptor, has been shown to antagonize NMDA receptor mediated responses in the cord via an action at the strychnine-insensitive glycine site (BIRCH et al. 1988; LONG et al. 1990). This makes it difficult to attribute the actions of CNQX on spinal nociceptive transmission solely to a blockade of AMPA receptors.

The ability of the much more selective AMPA receptor antagonist NBQX (PARSONS et al. 1994; SHEARDOWN et al. 1990) to reduce the C fibre evoked response of dorsal horn neurones is dependent upon the degree of wind-up evoked in the neurone by the stimulus. In neurones not displaying wind-up NBQX is able to produce at appropriate doses an almost complete inhibition of the electrically evoked nociceptive response of convergent dorsal horn neurones, showing the AMPA receptor plays a major role in sensory transmission in the dorsal horn of the spinal cord. However, in situations where wind-up occurs, the role played by AMPA receptors in overall nociceptive transmission in the spinal cord is diminished. In neurones which display wind-up following repetitive noxious stimulation the initial response of the neurone prior to the initiation of wind-up appears to be mediated predominantly if not entirely via the action of glutamate on AMPA receptors, evidenced by the complete block of this response by NBQX. However, the occurrence of wind-up is little influenced by the blockade of this initial response by NBQX. Indeed, the response of the neurone to the first few stimuli delivered at C fibre intensities can be abolished by NBQX, yet the cells wind up as normal. This suggests that neither the mechanisms underlying wind-up itself nor the mechanisms needed to initiate wind-up depend critically on the activation of AMPA receptors (STANFA and DICKENSON 1997). Importantly, by varying the frequency of stimulation wind-up of the neurones can be shown to be unaltered in neurones where complete NBQX blockade of the low-frequency C fibre responses has occurred. Thus wind-up is independent of AMPA-mediated baseline neuronal responses. This is consistent with findings that AMPA receptor antagonists are ineffective against behavioural manifestations of wind-up such as inflammatory hyperalgesia (HUNTER and SINGH 1994; REN et al. 1992a,b) and with studies showing nociceptive and other modalities of brief acute monosynaptic sensory transmission in the spinal cord are mediated via non-NMDA glutamate receptors (DAVIES and WATKINS 1983; MORRIS 1989; YOSHIMURA and JESSELL 1990).

In fact, early in vivo studies with the non-selective excitatory amino acid antagonists D-glutamyl-glycine and kynurenate showed that non-selective antagonists are more effective at blocking noxious evoked responses of dorsal horn neurones than more selective NMDA receptor antagonists (DAVIES and LODGE 1987; DICKENSON and SULLIVAN 1990). This fits with the idea that high-intensity stimuli activate both AMPA and NMDA receptors. The involvement of both non-NMDA and NMDA excitatory amino acid receptors in the nociceptive response of spinal dorsal horn neurones has also been shown in an in vitro spinal cord slice preparation. Here CNQX was shown to block the excitatory synaptic response in deep dorsal horn neurones following low-frequency stimulation of the dorsal roots. However, when the activation of NMDA receptors was facilitated, the evoked response was much less sensitive to CNQX (GERBER and RANDIC 1989a,b).

Where the role of AMPA receptors in spinal nociceptive transmission has been investigated using natural stimuli, NBQX and other antagonists have been shown to produce the expected reductions rather than an abolition of the responses to noxious stimuli but also innocuous stimuli (CUMBERBATCH et al. 1994). This was also seen in a study using CNQX, although here only one dose of CNQX was tested (NEUGEBAUER et al. 1993b). However, another study using CNQX (with the previously discussed problems of selectivity) has shown an almost complete blockade of the response to noxious pinch (DOUGHERTY et al. 1992). In an in vitro study using the hemisected spinal cord–hindlimb preparation CNQX abolished the modest neuronal response evoked by noxious pinch; here it could simply have been that the stimulus was insufficient to evoke NMDA receptor-mediated responses (KING and LOPEZ-GARCIA 1993).

In conclusion, the role of the AMPA receptor is to participate in the spinal transmission of both innocuous and noxious events where in the latter case it sets the baseline level of C fibre evoked responses. Subsequent NMDA receptor activation is independent of this baseline and is superimposed onto this activity, leading to enhancement of nociception, as has been described in many studies. Consequently the overall sensitivity of a nociceptive response to AMPA receptor blockade therefore depends on the extent to which spinal circuitry and the nature of the stimulus allow participation of the NMDA receptor in the nociceptive response.

III. Evidence for a Role of the Metabotropic Receptor

The metabotropic receptor has as yet an ill-defined role in pain states but may well contribute by acting to enhance NMDA and AMPA receptor function via intracellular actions (BLEAKMAN et al. 1992; BOND and LODGE 1995; CERNE and RANDIC 1992; WATKINS and COLLINGRIDGE 1994). There have been a limited number of studies on the role of this receptor. In general agonists at this site have been shown to produce hyperalgesia when combined with AMPA. Agonist and antagonist studies have illustrated physiological roles of the metabotropic receptor in acute behavioural (AANONSEN and WILCOX 1987; KOLHEKAR and GEBHART 1994) and more sustained nociception, in the latter case the responses of neurones to joint inflammation and to mustard oil (YOUNG et al. 1994, 1995). Using joint inflammation as a means of eliciting enhanced neuronal responses indicative of hyperalgesia, antagonists produce marked reductions in the neuronal responses (NEUGEBAUER et al. 1994). However, in contrast to studies showing excitatory effects mediated by the receptor, a metabotropic receptor agonist has been reported to depress monosynaptic transmission in the neonatal spinal cord (ISHIDA et al. 1993). Future studies on the metabotropic receptor(s) will be facilitated by full definition of the receptor subtypes and the development of selective antagonists (WATKINS and COLLINGRIDGE 1994)

IV. Evidence for a Role of the NMDA Receptor

The NMDA receptor has become an increasingly important target site as evidence accumulates for a role of the receptor in the enhancement of spinal processing of painful messages (see DICKENSON 1990, 1994b; DUBNER and RUDA 1992; McMAHON et al. 1993; PRICE et al. 1994a) and in many long term events in the brain (BASHIR and COLLINGRIDGE 1992; BLISS and COLLINGRIDGE 1993; COLLINGRIDGE and SINGER 1990; DAW et al. 1993; HEADLEY and GRILLNER 1990).

The reasons for the altered pain states produced when the NMDA receptor is activated stem from the high level of depolarizations produced by calcium influx through the channel and also the fact that the receptor-channel complex is not necessarily involved in synaptic transmission at all times and under all circumstances. This particular role is due to the complexity of the conditions needed for operation of the NMDA receptor-channel is consider-able. The release and binding of the excitatory amino acids is obviously needed, but in addition the co-agonist for the receptor, glycine, is required, in common with other NMDA-mediated plasticity. The latter condition appears to be ever present, due to the levels of glycine available in the spinal cord, and is borne out by the ability of antagonists at this site to produce inhibitions of NMDA-mediated nociception (BUDAI et al. 1992; DICKENSON and AYDAR 1990; KOLHEKAR et al. 1994; MILLAN and SEGUIN 1993, 1994; but see CODERRE 1993). Finally, a non-NMDA induced depolarization to remove the resting magnesium block of the channel is a prerequisite (LODGE and JOHNSON 1990; MAYER and WESTBROOK 1987; MACDONALD and NOWAK 1990; SEEBURG 1993). For these reasons the NMDA receptor-channel complex is not a partici-pant in "normal" synaptic transmission, but when the correct conditions are achieved, the complex suddenly becomes activated and adds a powerful depo-larizing or excitatory drive to transmission of pain in the spinal cord which then appears to lead to enhanced synaptic transmission or hypersensitivity (DICKENSON 1990, 1994a, 1995b; DUBNER and RUDA 1992; MCMAHON et al. 1993; NEUGEBAUER et al. 1993a,b; PRICE et al. 1994a; WOOLF and THOMPSON 1991).

A number of studies have demonstrated that glutamate is released from both low- and high-threshold afferents (see section) but electrophysiological studies indicate that in general only noxious events, at least under normal conditions, activate the NMDA receptor (BRUGGER et al. 1990; DOUGHERTY et al. 1992; RADAKRISHNAN and HENRY 1993b; SHER and MITCHELL 1990a; YASHPAL et al. 1991). As has been discussed, AMPA receptors are activated by both A and C fibre stimuli, and it has been suggested that peptides may differentiate between these fibre types since only C fibre stimulation elicits peptide release. Consequently C fibre induced release of excitatory peptides may provide the required depolarization to remove the block and allow NMDA receptor activation. Studies have shown (KING et al. 1988; THOMPSON et al. 1990, 1992) that the initiation of wind-up depends on the summation of prolonged depolarizations, such as those mediated by peptides including SP (BARANAUSKAS et al. 1995), which at appropriate frequencies of stimulation are capable of producing a cumulative depolarization sufficient to overcome and maintain the removal of the voltage-dependent Mg^{2+} block of the NMDA receptor channel. Given the transient nature of the current activated by AMPA receptors, the depolarizations produced by activation of this receptor would not be capable of summation over the 2s inter-stimulus interval (0.5 Hz stimulation) and hence would not be expected to contribute much to the initiation of wind-up.

That the summation of long, slow depolarizations is important for the initiation of wind-up is also demonstrated by the fact that reducing the fre-quency of stimulation, and hence reducing the possibility of a cumulative depolarization occurring, reduces the occurrence of wind-up. THOMPSON et al.

(1990) showed that prolonged post-synaptic depolarizations of 4–8 s can be evoked in ventral horn neurones following primary afferent stimulation at intensities sufficient to activate C fibres. The duration of this post-synaptic depolarization is such that, if this is also seen in the dorsal horn, it would allow summation of the potentials to occur following stimulation at 0.5 Hz but not following stimulation at 0.1 Hz, where the 10 s inter-stimulus interval exceeds the duration of the prolonged depolarization. Interestingly, when the frequency of stimulation is reduced to 0.1 Hz, the remaining response of the neurones is highly sensitive to AMPA receptor blockade (STANFA and DICKENSON 1997), suggesting that the contribution of peptides such as SP to the nociceptive response is made predominantly through the summation of their responses and subsequent permissive role for NMDA receptor activation. When this cumulative summation is prevented by reducing the frequency of stimulation, the underlying nociceptive response appears to be mediated almost entirely through activation of AMPA receptors.

Supporting the idea that the role of peptides can be minor in their own right, but that their actions are important for subsequent NMDA receptor activation, neurokinin receptor antagonists can reduce NMDA-mediated responses in the spinal cord. Furthermore, the administration of agonists, with most work having been done on SP, enhances the effects of NMDA or increases nociceptive responses (BRUGGER et al. 1990; CHAPMAN et al. 1994; MJELLEM-JOLY et al. 1992; NAGY et al. 1993; RANDIC et al. 1990; RUSIN et al. 1992, 1993; XU et al. 1992; YASHPAL et al. 1991; and see URBAN et al. 1994 for review). Furthermore, any increased release of afferent peptides or increased release of the excitatory amino acids themselves in, for example, inflammation (DRAY 1995; DRAY et al. 1994; MCMAHON et al. 1995; SORKIN et al. 1992; SLUKA and WESTLUND 1993; SLUKA et al. 1994a,b; WOOLF 1995) could facilitate NMDA transmission either directly via increased depolarizations removing the Mg^{2+} block of the channel or by alterations in intracellular messengers such as protein kinases (CHEN and HUANG 1992).

However, it has been shown that spinal neurones can be activated by NMDA administered iontophoretically or by pressure directly onto the cells (e.g. BIRCH et al. 1988; DOUGHERTY and WILLIS 1991a,b; NEUGEBAUER et al. 1993a,b; PARSONS et al. 1995), and that behavioural manifestations indicative of pain can be elicited in normal animals after spinal NMDA (AANONSEN and WILCOX 1987; AANONSEN et al. 1990; KOLHEKAR et al. 1993; MALMBERG and YAKSH 1992a,b, 1993b). Why this is the case when the Mg^{2+} block of the channel should be in place is unclear. The reasons may be related to the particular experimental situation causing levels of membrane potentials producing a submaximal Mg^{2+} block of the channel. It is not disputed that NMDA transmission is likely to be enhanced by prior excitatory drives onto neurones. Interestingly, the subunit composition of the NMDA receptor in the spinal cord is NR1/NR2D which in recombinant studies has lower sensitivity to Mg^{2+} block than other receptor units. This is borne out by studies on the native receptor, since at least in recordings from young rat spinal cords, the channel has reduced Mg^{2+} sensitivity (Momiyama et al. 1996). Possibly the situation with the spinal NMDA receptor in adults is similar.

In addition to the numerous spinal studies on the non-NMDA and NMDA receptors which are the focus of this chapter, it should be noted that supraspinal roles of the receptors are likely to be important in pain. For example, it has been shown that thalamic responses to sensory stimuli involve non-NMDA and NMDA receptors (Salt 1987; Salt and Eaton 1991), as do corticothalamic excitatory projections (Eaton and Salt 1996). Further evidence from behavioural approaches reveals excitatory amino acid evoked nociception from actions in the brainstem (Jensen and Yaksh 1992).

D. NMDA Antagonists and Spinal Hypersensitivity in Persistent Pain States

It is therefore now well established that wind-up and the reflex hypersensitivity are NMDA receptor mediated. Studies have shown that NMDA receptor antagonists (AP5), channel blockers (ketamine, MK-801, dextromethorphan) and glycine site antagonists (7CK) are indistinguishable in their ability to block wind-up at appropriate doses. Importantly, the baseline non-facilitated responses are unaltered by the antagonists (Davies and Lodge 1987; Dickenson and Aydar 1990; Dickenson and Sullivan 1987a; Dickenson et al. 1991; Fig. 1). The same NMDA mediation is seen with the hypersensitive

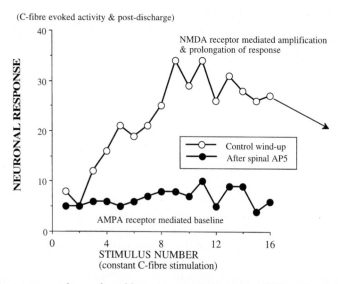

Fig. 1. The response of a rat dorsal horn to repeated constant C fibre simulation. Wind-up is exhibited in the control response and is blocked by the NMDA receptor antagonist AP5 leaving the AMPA receptor mediated constant baseline response to the stimuli

reflexes (WOOLF and THOMPSON 1991; XU et al. 1992) although here the NMDA antagonists do produce a partial reduction in the unconditioned reflex. Thus in both cases the enhanced responses are highly sensitive to NMDA antagonism, but there is a difference in the baseline sensitivity between dorsal horn neurones and motoneurones. The degree of reduction in the responses of the latter is likely to be due to NMDA receptors in the ventral horn (HEADLEY and GRILLNER 1990).

Wind-up, as indicated earlier, has attracted much interest as a central basis for longer term pathological and physiological or nociceptive pain states where hyperalgesia is present. However, the reason for this is simply that here is pharmacological system that when activated enhances the level of pain whilst the afferent input remains constant. It is therefore proposed that ongoing activity in afferents continually drives the receptor complex. Parallels have been sought with events in the brain, especially the hippocampus, related to memory, in particular to long-term potentiation (LTP; BLISS and COLLINGRIDGE 1993; COLLINGRIDGE and SINGER 1990; KOMBIAN and MALENKA 1994). Here some confusion may have arisen since LTP is but one of several forms of plasticity seen in the forebrain. LTP is a long-lasting enhancement of synaptic transmission which once induced by a tetanic stimulus endures for much longer periods of time than the spinal events and can even last for days. Once induced LTP does not need further inputs for maintenance. NMDA receptors are important in the induction of LTP. However, although there may be similarities, there is no reason to expect that the processes are identical, and in fact it would make little sense for sensory transmission to operate under the same conditions as memory. Furthermore, LTP is not the only process induced by high-frequency stimulation and inhibitory events can be triggered by similar mechanisms (BENARDO 1993; DUDEK and BEAR 1992; KOMBIAN and MALENKA 1994). These inhibitory events, activated by peripheral inputs are discussed below in the context of spinal controlling influences on NMDA-mediated events (Sect. FII).

I. Gene Induction

One of the intracellular changes associated with NMDA receptor activation is the influx of calcium into neurones, and thus an increase in intracellular levels of calcium (MAYER and WESTBROOK 1987). Furthermore, noxious stimuli which in turn could cause increased levels of intracellular calcium are known to stimulate the expression of the immediate-early gene, c-*fos* (FITZGERALD 1990; WISDEN et al. 1990), and many of the circumstances under which c-*fos* is induced in the nervous system involves NMDA receptor activation (see MORGAN 1991). However, from the view point of spinal nociceptive transmission the effect of NMDA receptor antagonism on c-Fos expression is not clear. Intrathecal administration of MK-801 (KEHL et al. 1991) and subcutaneous administration of dextromethorphan (ELLIOT et al. 1994), both NMDA receptor antagonists, have been shown to reduce spinal c-Fos expression evoked by peripheral injection of formalin. In addition, subcutaneous administration of HA966 an antagonist at the glycine site of the NMDA receptor has been shown to reduce carrageenan inflammation evoked spinal c-Fos expression (CHAPMAN et al. 1995). In contrast, systemic ketamine, also an NMDA receptor antagonist, has been shown not to reduce noxious heat evoked c-Fos expression (TÖLLE et al. 1991), but this may be due to the short-lasting effects of this drug.

Regardless of whether the induction of c-*fos* is entirely NMDA-dependent, the half-life of c-*fos* is short, and there is a rapid onset/offset of c-*fos* induction following noxious stimulation. Consequently the level of induction of c-*fos*, and therefore of the expression of the gene protein product c-Fos, closely mirrors the intensity and duration of the noxious stimulation. Numerous studies have demonstrated that the basal expression of c-Fos at the level of the spinal cord is extremely low. Following noxious stimulation there is a clear spatial and temporal expression of c-Fos in areas of the dorsal horn, the superficial and deep laminae, which contain neurones driven by nociceptive stimulation. Whether gene induction has consequences for pain transmission and modulation is still an unanswered question.

II. Inflammatory Hyperalgesia and NMDA Receptors

As the discussion above demonstrates, there is much evidence from behavioural, anatomical and electrophysiological approaches to support the importance of the NMDA receptor in nociception. However, it must be asked whether these NMDA-mediated events have physiological roles. The answer to this question is best provided by studies which show physiological states of nociception to be reduced by antagonists at the receptor. Does nociception require NMDA receptor activation? The answer is yes, but only when the intensity/duration or type of stimulus is such as to induce central hypersensitivity or hyperalgesia.

The first evidence for such a role used subcutaneous formalin as an inflammatory stimulus (HALEY et al. 1990). The peripheral injection of formalin has been widely used as a means of producing a more persistent but subchronic behavioural response to inflammation (DUBUISSON and DENNIS 1977; HUNSKAAR and HOLE 1987; PORRO and CAVAZZUTI 1993; TJOLSEN et al. 1988). Two phases of activity are produced, an initial response and then a more slowly developing second phase which results from peripheral inflammation. There is a remarkable concordance between behavioural and electrophysiological studies in that dorsal horn neurones exhibit the same two phases with very similar magnitudes and time courses (DICKENSON and SULLIVAN 1987b, 1989). The spinal neuronal responses to formalin are dose-dependently and markedly reduced (but not abolished) by blocking NMDA receptor function, here with systemic MK-801 and ketamine, the channel blockers, and also by the receptor antagonist AP-5, given spinally. With all agents there is a ceiling effect, and the maximal effects of the antagonists therefore did not exceed

80% inhibition. This fits with the idea that NMDA-dependent amplifications predominate in the second phase but are independent of baseline and first-phase AMPA-mediated responses (HUNTER and SINGH 1994). This is similar to the wind-up studies in which NMDA antagonists remove the amplification/ hyperalgesia without influencing the baseline responses. Studies with pre-treatments show that only the second phase of the neuronal responses, when tissue damage and inflammation occurs, of formalin-induced activity is sensitive to NMDA block (DICKENSON and AYDAR 1990; HALEY et al. 1990). This second phase of activity in electrophysiological studies is also sensitive to antagonists at the glycine modulatory site on the NMDA receptor channel complex (DICKENSON and AYDAR 1991). Importantly, the neuronal activity to this stimulus, which matches the behavioural responses perfectly in terms of magnitude and time course, is equally inhibited whether the NMDA antagonists are given as a pre-treatment or post-treatment, for example, once the activity is established. Thus the induction of the second-phase response must require NMDA receptor activation, but so too does the maintenance of the response.

Unlike the selective effect of NMDA antagonists on the second phase, D-glutamyl-glycine, the non-selective antagonist of all excitatory amino acid receptors reduces both phases of the responses, in line with the idea that the first phase is predominantly non-NMDA-mediated (HALEY et al. 1990).

Behavioural studies with formalin have reported similar findings. Thus the pre-administration of MK-801, other channel blockers and also glycine site antagonism are able selectively to reduce the second phase of the response (EISENBERG et al. 1993; VACCARINO et al. 1993). The ability of glycine site antagonists to reduce the late phase has also been by others, but importantly not only have they produced this action in the absence of motor deficits, but the channel blockers reduced both phases and could also lead to ataxia (MILLAN and SEGUIN 1993, 1994; SEGUIN et al. 1995). These studies underline the importance of monitoring motor actions of antagonists of the excitatory amino acids in behavioural studies. In addition, in the latter study no effect was seen in acute tests such as the tail-flick, supporting the idea that prolonged and high-intensity stimuli are needed to activate the NMDA receptor (MILLAN and SEGUIN 1993, 1994). At variance with a number of studies with glycine site antagonists is the report that they are ineffective in the formalin response, although MK-801 was able to reduce the second phase (CODERRE 1993; CODERRE and MELZACK 1992a,b). Furthermore, this study found that glycine site agonists enhance the effects of channel blockers. A potential reason for the differences is that the latter study used low concentrations of formalin, and the degree of inflammation may therefore have been insufficient for full NMDA receptor activation.

Carrageenan has been widely used as a model of peripheral inflammation where the hyperalgesia lasts for longer periods of time than the formalin response. In general, the hyperalgesia that can be observed in behavioural tests, peaks at about 3 h and then lasts for several days. In a behavioural study with carrageenan the thermal hyperalgesia seen at 3–4h was reduced dose-dependently by a number of NMDA receptor complex blockers with similar potencies. Thus receptor, glycine site and channel blockers were all effective after spinal administration whereas CNQX, the AMPA receptor antagonist was barely effective (EISENBERG et al. 1994; REN and DUBNER 1993; REN et al. 1992a,b; YAMAMOTO et al. 1993). Electrophysiological studies have found similar effects when increases in receptive field size were used as an index of hyperalgesia; MK-801 blocked these increases. Little or no effect of NMDA antagonists are seen in the absence of inflammation, suggesting again an involvement of the receptor only in enhanced responses (REN et al. 1992a).

Another approach to the study of excitatory amino acid mechanisms in hyperalgesia produced by inflammation has used arthritis as a model of inflammation. Arthritis produces inflammation that persists for weeks. A number of electrophysiological studies by Schaible and colleagues have used this model and by varying the timing between the induction of inflammation and the neuronal recordings have been able to study both early and late phases of the inflammation. There is evidence from these approaches, with local iontophoretic application and on occasions systemic administration, that NMDA receptor and channel blockers AP5 and ketamine reduce the enhanced responses to noxious and innocuous pressure to the inflamed joint. These authors also show that the doses of antagonists used are selective for the NMDA receptor. The same agents are effective only against noxious pressure in the normal joint. CNQX reduced the responses to both types of pressure in normal joints and also in the presence of inflammation. Both the NMDA and non-NMDA antagonists were able to reduce the established hypersensitivity and its induction as well as acute and more persistent stages of the inflammation (NEUGEBAUER et al. 1993a,b, 1994; SCHAIBLE et al. 1991). This ability of NMDA antagonists to be effective at all stages is similar to the results seen with the original description of NMDA involvement in formalin-induced inflammation. However, this group find that CNQX and also both metabotropic and the NMDA antagonists alone are able to almost completely abolish the responses after inflammation (NEUGEBAUER et al. 1993a, 1994; SCHAIBLE et al. 1991). It is difficult to explain how three independent receptors each appear to contribute almost fully to the observed responses.

Hypersensitivity in models of peripheral ischaemia is also reduced by NMDA antagonism (SHER and MITCHELL 1990a,b). In the first model the application of a tourniquet to the tail of a rat followed by reperfusion produces an enhanced neuronal response to pinch and an increase in spontaneous activity. Both receptor blockade and channel block by APV and ketamine, respectively, produce reductions in these responses without influencing the unconditioned responses to pinch or brush so that only the hyperalgesia is reduced only by NMDA block. Subsequent behavioural studies have shown that this central hyperalgesia, NMDA receptor mediated, was reduced by benzodiazepines (CARTMELL and MITCHELL 1993).

Although visceral nociception has been less extensively studied, there are reports of enhanced colo-rectal nociception after spinal NMDA administration (KOLHEKAR and GEBHART 1994). Furthermore, whereas AP5 has no effect on the behavioural responses to bladder inflation, after inflammation of the organ there is NMDA receptor mediated hypersensitivity of the reflex (RICE and McMAHON 1994).

In practically all these studies the emphasis has been on hyperalgesia and nociception, but after ultraviolet irradiation of the rat paw not only is there a hyperalgesia but allodynia also occurs. Here there are enhanced A fibre evoked and spontaneous neuronal activities which are partly peptide mediated (THOMPSON et al. 1994) and are sensitive to NMDA receptor antagonists (CHAPMAN and DICKENSON 1994). The roles of large fibres in pathological pain, especially allodynias, are important (WOOLF and DOUBELL 1994) and since these A fibre mediated pains can be difficult to control with classical analgesics, the ability of NMDA antagonists to control these pain states may be of clinical use.

III. Neuropathic Pain States and NMDA Receptors

Studies in animals with peripheral nerve damage provide evidence for a role of NMDA receptors in neuropathic pain states. Neuropathy can be accompanied by a constellation of symptoms and pain states which include spontaneous pain, hyperalgesia to thermal and/or mechanical stimuli, and finally allodynia, where normally innocuous stimuli induce pain. The models that have been used range from complete to partial nerve sections, partial ligation of certain nerve roots to loose ligation of the entire nerve (BENNETT 1994). One of the original studies on this topic used nerve section as a model of deafferentation neuropathic pain. The initial injury discharges after nerve damage were suggested to involve wind-up and NMDA activation and then to contribute to the subsequent pain states following nerve injuries (SELTZER et al. 1991a,b). The evidence showed that NMDA block during the nerve section delays subsequent pain-related behaviour. In addition to this pharmacological evidence for a role of the NMDA receptor, stimulation of the nerve at parameters able to induce wind-up were shown to worsen the nociception after section of the nerve (SELTZER et al. 1991a).

Behavioural studies in the BENNETT and XIE (1998) model of loose sciatic nerve ligation have shown that spinal administration of NMDA antagonists have beneficial effects weeks after occurrence of the injury against both the hyperalgesia and spontaneous pain (BANOS et al. 1994; DAVAR et al. 1991; MAO et al. 1992a,b, 1993; SMITH et al. 1994; TAL and BENNETT 1993; YAMAMOTO and YAKSH 1992a,b). In general these studies illustrate that early treatments delay hyperalgesia development, or when given after the ligation, that NMDA antagonists are still highly effective. Thus NMDA receptor activation is required for both the induction and then the maintenance of the pain-related behaviours. A range of drugs have been used and there appears to be little difference between receptor blockers such as AP-5 (YAMAMOTO and YAKSH 1992b) and channel blockers such as ketamine, dextrophan and MK-801 (DAVAR et al. 1991; MAO et al. 1993; TAL and BENNETT 1993; YAMAMOTO and YAKSH 1992a). Furthermore the ensemble of these results shows that NMDA receptors are critical for the spontaneous pain and heat hyperalgesia. However, MK-801 has been shown to be less effective against wind-up and C fibre induced reflex facilitation when given 2 weeks after axotomy in another model where the lesion is more extreme (XU et al. 1993, 1995).

Using the more recently developed model of tight ligation of two spinal nerves (CHOI et al. 1994; KIM and CHUNG 1992), it has been clearly shown that systemic ketamine can relieve all symptoms, including mechanical allodynia and hyperalgesia, cold allodynia and spontaneous pain (QIAN et al. 1996). Finally, in animal models of allodynia produced by block of spinal inhibitory amino acid controls, NMDA antagonists are effective against the tactile-evoked nociception (YAKSH 1989). In all these studies the agents were without obvious effects on the control responses.

Spinal ischaemia produced by photochemical lesions causes a prolonged allodynia-like syndrome (HAO et al. 1991a) which can be considered as a form of central neuropathic pain. NMDA receptor antagonists are able to reduce the allodynia only at very early stages in the process (HAO et al. 1991b).

Clearly then, as with inflammatory pain models, NMDA receptors are critical for the induction and the setting up of the hyperalgesia/allodynia and its subsequent maintenance in almost but not all of the experimental models. Antagonists acting to block the receptor, channel or other sites are highly effective in reducing or even abolishing the abnormal behaviours. Thus there is evidence for an involvement of the NMDA receptor in inflammatory pain, neuropathic pain, allodynia and ischaemic pain.

E. Controlling NMDA Receptor Activation

I. Clinical Use of NMDA Antagonists

The NMDA receptor therefore appears to be of great importance in the induction and maintenance of spinal nociceptive events leading to hyperalgesia following tissue damage, nerve dysfunction and surgery. The ability of antagonists at the numerous modulatory sites on the NMDA receptor complex to reduce hyperalgesia in animal models may provide avenues for the clinical treatment of difficult pains. Two licensed drugs, ketamine, at subanaesthetic doses, and dextromethorphan block the channel and so reduce NMDA-mediated responses in these dorsal horn nociceptive systems and are effective against the hyperalgesia, allodynia and spontaneous pain seen in these neuropathic and inflammatory models.

The NMDA receptor is responsible for the induction and the initiation of the hyperalgesia and for the subsequent maintenance of the neuronal responses in many of these models, so that spinal NMDA receptor antagonism has been shown to be effective against the established central hypersensitivity in most studies (see DICKENSON 1994a; PRICE et al. 1994a) but not all studies (XU et al. 1995). Overall, there is a strong basis for the use of ketamine and dextromethorphan in humans. Neither of these drugs is ideal. Ketamine has a short half-life and produces psychotomimetic side effects whereas dextromethorphan has low potency (DICKENSON et al. 1991).

Wind-up can be demonstrated in elegant psychophysical studies in humans and is inhibited by dextromethorphan (PRICE et al. 1977, 1994b) and recent evidence has shown an NMDA dependency of allodynias and wind-up pains in controlled clinical studies by the use of ketamine (EIDE et al. 1994). In addition, there is evidence, admittedly not always from controlled trials, for effects in post-herpetic neuralgia, post-operative pain and in cancer pain (BACKONJA et al. 1994; EIDE et al. 1995; MATHISEN et al. 1995; MAURSET et al. 1989; ROYTBLAT et al. 1993; STANNARD and PORTER 1993; TVERSKOY et al. 1994). However, there have been negative findings as well, in this case with dextromethorphan (MCQUAY et al. 1994). Increased doses may possibly have been effective. This broad effectiveness of licensed NMDA antagonists against inflammatory and neuropathic pains is in good accord with the conclusions from the animal studies.

However, the NMDA receptor is not exclusive to pain but is implicated in memory, visual plasticity, epilepsy and motor function (BASHIR and COLLINGRIDGE 1992; BLISS and COLLINGRIDGE 1993; COLLINGRIDGE and SINGER 1990; DAW et al. 1993; HEADLEY and GRILLNER 1990). In addition to potential interference with these functions, possible side effects of NMDA antagonists include sedation and psychotomimesis (see RUPNIAK et al. 1993; WILLETTS et al. 1990). Spinal routes of administration would avoid systemic side effects but are not always appropriate. Another licensed drug which shows promise as an acceptable NMDA receptor blocker is memantine. This has been shown to be a channel blocker (BRESINK et al. 1995), and the doses needed to achieve central NMDA block have been established for systemic administration (KORNHUBER and QUACK 1995). The drug is effective against joint inflammation induced hyper-responsiveness of spinal neurones (NEUGEBAUER et al. 1993a) and also in the formalin model (EISENBERG et al. 1993, 1994). The kinetics of the channel block with memantine are such that it is hoped that it will possibly block only highly active neurones (PARSONS et al. 1995). The development of drugs effective at other sites on the NMDA receptor-channel complex may fulfil the promise of NMDA antagonists with acceptable therapeutic indices (BOBELIS and BALSTER 1993; LODGE and JOHNSTONE 1990; LOSCHER et al. 1991; OLNEY 1990; ROGAWSKI 1993; WATKINS et al. 1990; WILLETS et al. 1990).

From attempts to manipulate the receptor, the channel and the glycine site there are a number of pieces of evidence to suggest that antagonists at the latter site may produce reduced NMDA function with low side effect profiles (LEESON and IVERSEN 1994). For example, antagonists at the glycine site, effective against wind-up (DICKENSON and AYDAR 1991) inflammation induced c-*fos* expression (CHAPMAN et al. 1995) and the second phase of the formalin response in animals, are devoid of motor effects, unlike channel blockers and a number of other agents (SEGUIN et al. 1995). LTP also requires glycine site activation for its mainifestation (BASHIR et al. 1990).

II. Peripheral Block of Afferent Activity

Another approach would ignore the spinal NMDA receptors and to attempt to prevent their activation. The basis for this is that not only is spinal NMDA activity needed to maintain these pain states but afferent inputs are required as peripheral local anaesthetic blockade at the site of formalin injection interrupts the spinal NMDA-mediated neuronal responses (DICKENSON and SULLIVAN 1987b). Furthermore, this approach has revealed that a temporary peripheral block of the first phase does not change the second phase (HALEY et al. 1990), demonstrating their independence. A recent clinical study of disordered central processing, indicative of central hypersensitivity, in sympathetic dystrophy has also shown that peripheral local anaesthesia temporarily removes all symptoms (GRACELY et al. 1993). Although one behavioural study indicates that the formalin-induced nociception is partly independent of peripheral activity (CODERRE et al. 1990), a recent study confirms the electrophysiological findings in that peripheral local anaesthesia reduces the cardiovascular manifestations of formalin injection (TAYLOR et al. 1995). Local anaesthetics can also reduce NMDA-mediated wind-up after spinal administration, presumably by their ability to block open channels (FRASER et al. 1992).

III. NMDA Receptor Antagonists in Combination with Opioids

NMDA receptor involvement in pain-related responses can lead to reduced opioid sensitivity. As a consequence a rational approach in difficult pains would be to use low-dose combination therapy, hopefully avoiding side effects, with ketamine or dextromethorphan and morphine. Interestingly, some opioids when given alone may be better than others since pethidine and ketobemidone appear to have both opioid and weaker but still functionally relevant NMDA-blocking actions, as revealed by both binding and electrophysiological approaches (EBERT et al. 1995). There are a number of pathological and physiological events that can lead to poor opioid sensitivity. Many appear to be operative in the neuropathic models, supporting the clinical view that neuropathic pains can be less sensitive to opioids (ARNER and MEYERSON 1988; JADAD et al. 1992; PORTENOY et al. 1990). NMDA receptor activation itself contributes to poor opioid sensitivity because it increases excitation in the pain transmitting systems. Quite simply, in order for analgesia to occur excitation must be balanced by inhibitions. Thus more opioid is needed to control the activity when enhanced by NMDA receptor activation. In neuropathic states not only is there NMDA receptor activation, but a potential loss of opioid receptors and upregulation of the "anti-opioid peptide" chole-cystokinin reduces morphine analgesia to below normal (DICKENSON 1994b; STANFA et al. 1994). Thus the combination of these factors causes particular problems in the control of neuropathic pains.

The neuronal excitations produced by post-synaptic NMDA receptor ac-tivation breaks through the opioid inhibitions, and at moderate doses opioids thus delay the onset of wind-up without inhibiting the process itself (CHAPMAN and DICKENSON 1992; DICKENSON and SULLIVAN 1986). By contrast, as dis-cussed, NMDA antagonists abolish wind-up. Likewise, the hypersensitized reflex requires higher doses of morphine for reduction compared to the baseline responses (WOOLF and WALL 1986).

Marked neuronal inhibitions can be achieved as a result of powerful synergism between the combination of threshold doses of morphine with low doses of NMDA antagonists (CHAPMAN and DICKENSON 1992). In addition, in a model of neuropathic pain in which morphine is inoperative the co-administration of an NMDA antagonist, in this case MK-801, restores the ability of morphine to inhibit the response (YAMAMOTO and YAKSH 1992a). Synergism is also seen with the combination of spinal lignocaine and mor-phine, partly due to the ability of the former to block NMDA-mediated spinal events (ACKERMAN et al. 1988; FRASER et al. 1992).

F. Indirect Influences on NMDA Receptor Activation

In addition to the direct modulation of central NMDA receptors, there are a number of pharmacological events can accompany NMDA receptor activa-tion. Some of these NMDA-induced changes act to enhance excitatory trans-mission whilst others act to control it.

There is now good evidence (see MELLER and GEBHART 1993) that nitric oxide (NO), a diffusible gas transmitter, is produced in response to NMDA receptor activation. Additionally, spinal prostanoids also appear to be gener-ated after NMDA receptor events, and in both cases these mediators seem to further enhance NMDA receptor activation in nociception and may well be at least part of the basis for central actions of non-steroidal anti-inflammatory drugs (MALMBERG and YAKSH 1992a,b, 1993a). By contrast to positive in-fluences on NMDA function, after injection of carrageenan into the paw, although some neurones show enhanced activity many exhibit reduced re-sponses. The evolution of the inflammation elicits spinal mechanisms, them-selves driven by NMDA activity, which act to limit further neuronal responses. Here the greater the NMDA-mediated wind-up exhibited by the neurones, the the greater the chance of the response being inhibited as the inflammation develops (STANFA et al. 1992). Adenosine may be involved in this type of control (REEVE and DICKENSON 1995). Furthermore, the administration of NMDA onto the spinal cord in normal animals has been shown to elicit both nociception and antinociception (KOLHEKAR et al. 1993; RAIGORODSKY and

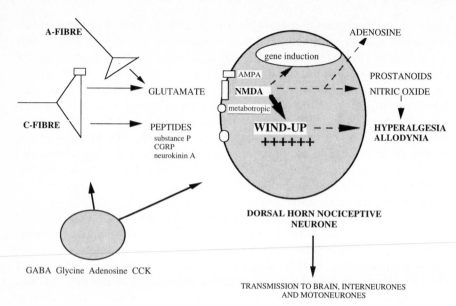

Fig. 2. A schematic diagram showing A fibre (non-noxious) inputs onto a dorsal horn neurone. The post-synaptic receptors for glutamate and peptides interact to induce wind-up and neuronal hyperractivity, which, as described, can lead to hyperalgesia and some forms of allodynia. There may also be functional pre-synaptic receptors on the afferent. The production of NO by spinal neurones appears essential for these events and prostanoids may also contribute to excitability. Inhibitory influences, produced by GABA and adenosine can act to limit the extent of central hypersensitivity. Changes in either the excitatory or the inhibitory system can occur in different pain states, especially neuropathic and inflammatory conditions

URCA 1987), with the latter study showing that as the dose of NMDA is increased so does the hypoalgesia. Thus there is evidence for both positive and negative influences on NMDA receptor function, thus providing potential indirect targets for the control of NMDA events (Fig. 2).

I. Nitric Oxide as a Target

The results of a number of studies demonstrate that NO (EDELMAN and GALLY 1992) plays a role as a transmitter in the central nervous system. Spinal cord neurones have the capacity to produce NO (SAITO et al. 1994), and evidence indicates a role of the gas in the spinal transmission of acute noxious but not innocuous stimuli in normal animals (HALEY et al. 1992; KITTO et al. 1992; MALMBERG and YAKSH 1993b; MELLER et al. 1992a, 1994). NMDA receptors are expressed on spinal neurones with the capacity to produce NO (DOHRN and BEITZ 1994), and, again, calcium influx appears to trigger production of NO by activation of the synthetic enzyme (MELLER and GEBHART 1993). NO plays a role in the spinal transmission of nociceptive information following 3 h of carrageenan inflammation but to no greater extent than in normal animals (STANFA et al. 1996). The results of this study fit with immunocytochemical studies which show no increase in the levels of NO synthase (NOS) immunoreactivity in the spinal cord following carrageenan-induced inflammation (TRAUB et al. 1994). Behavioural studies are generally unable to find a role for spinal NO in nociceptive reflexes in normal animals, whereas NOS inhibitors are highly effective at blocking these same reflexes following the induction of peripheral inflammation (MELLER et al. 1994) or neuropathy (MELLER et al. 1992a) and are effective only on the second phase of the formalin response (MALMBERG and YAKSH 1993b). NO may also play a role in peripheral vascular events during inflammation (DRAY et al. 1994).

The NOS inhibitor 7-nitroindazole (7-NI), selective for neuronal NOS and effective against formalin-induced nociception (MOORE et al. 1991, 1993) produces a greater inhibition of the wind-up and consequent post-discharge of the neurones in normal animals than the modest inhibition of the C fibre evoked response due to direct afferent transmission. This differential inhibition is also seen with specific NMDA receptor antagonists in this model (DICKENSON and AYDAR 1991; DICKENSON and SULLIVAN 1987a, 1990), whereas antinociceptive drugs such as morphine are less effective against the wind-up of the neurones (DICKENSON and SULLIVAN 1986). The preferential inhibition of the NMDA receptor mediated post-discharge and wind-up (DAVIES and LODGE 1987; DICKENSON and SULLIVAN 1987a) of the neurones by 7-NI conforms to the idea that under these circumstances the NO generated in the spinal cord during the transmission of nociceptive information is generated as a consequence of NMDA receptor activation. This agrees well with a number of other studies, including electrophysiological demonstrations, that block of NO production reduces the excitatory effects of NMDA on spinal neurones (RADHAKRISHNAN and HENRY 1993a), and behavioural studies in which block of NO production reduced nociceptive responses or the effects of NMDA (KITTO et al. 1992; MALMBERG and YAKSH 1993b; MELLER et al. 1992a,b, 1994; SEGUIN et al. 1995). However, other studies have shown that block of synthesis of NO reduces spinal neuronal responses but in a complex manner, not necessarily via spinal sites (SEMOS and HEADLEY 1994), has no effect in vitro (THOMPSON et al. 1995) or even increases wind-up (BUDAI et al. 1995).

A reason for these differences, apart from experimental conditions, may be the form of stimulation. The stimuli used as the test must be sufficient to allow activation of NMDA receptor circuits and therefore the generation and involvement of NO in spinal nociceptive transmission. In contrast, the threshold stimulus used to determine spinal nociceptive reflexes in behavioural studies in normal animals does not appear to result in activation of spinal NMDA receptors (MALMBERG and YAKSH 1993b; REN and DUBNER 1993; REN et al. 1992a,b; YAKSH 1989; YAMAMOTO and YAKSH 1992b; YAMAMOTO et al. 1993); therefore it is unlikely that this stimulus is capable of stimulating the generation of NO under these circumstances. Following the development of peripheral inflammation and consequent hyperalgesia, however, the NMDA receptor is able to participate in spinal nociceptive reflexes (MALMBERG and YAKSH 1993b; REN et al. 1992a,b; REN and DUBNER 1993; YAMAMOTO et al. 1993), providing a mechanism whereby NO is generated so that NOS inhibitors do block nociceptive reflexes in behavioural studies in animals with peripheral inflammation. Once NO is generated in the spinal cord, the mechanism by which it produces its effects, such as the role played by NO in the wind-up process, has yet to be confirmed. Although NO can act in the neurone in which it is produced to increase levels of cGMP, NO can also diffuse to other neurones to produce its effects (see MELLER and GEBHART 1993).

It has been shown that activation of NMDA receptors in the cord can produce an NO-mediated release of glutamate (SORKIN 1993), some of which may represent release from primary afferent terminals following the retrograde diffusion of NO. NO can also evoke the release of CGRP and SP from the dorsal horn of the spinal cord (GARRY et al. 1994). More indirect evidence is that glutamate release in both normal animals and after inflammation can be reduced by block of the excitatory amino acid receptors (SLUKA and WESTLUND 1993; SLUKA et al. 1994a,b), indicating that post-synaptic neurones can influence pre-synaptic release sites; some intermediate messenger such as NO would be needed for this link. Any NO-evoked release of glutamate, CGRP and SP may operate as a positive feedback system to further generate wind-up and centrally mediated hyperalgesia. Thus the development of clinically useful neuronal NOS inhibitors could provide a novel approach to indirectly controlling NMDA-mediated transmission. As with agents acting directly at the NMDA receptor-channel complex, side effects may preclude their use.

II. Increasing Inhibitory Controls

NMDA receptor activation, whilst clearly enhancing nociception, can also influence inhibitory interneurones in the spinal cord. Excessive NMDA activation in the CNS is one mechanism behind excitotoxicity so that elevated NMDA activation may trigger inhibitory systems as an auto-limiting device to prevent over-excitation and perhaps even cell death (OLNEY 1990). In fact, there is evidence that nerve section can cause dysfunction and possibly death of interneurones in the rat spinal cord (SUGIMOTO et al. 1989), and this is enhanced by block of the inhibitory glycine receptors. Interestingly, cholecystokinin, upregulated after nerve damage and at least partly responsible for reduced morphine analgesia in neuropathic states (STANFA et al. 1994), can protect against glutamate neurotoxicity in the cortex (AKAIKE et al. 1991).

In the model of carrageenan inflammation there is a clear relationship between the degree of wind-up exhibited by the neurones prior to the induction of inflammation and the effect of the inflammation on the subsequent activity of the neurones. Neurones with a low level of initial wind-up are facilitated by the inflammation whereas those cells with high wind-up prior to the inflammation become inhibited. Since these effects are correlated with NMDA-mediated wind-up, they clearly represent activity-induced inhibitions (STANFA et al. 1992), as also seen in the cortex (BENARDO 1993), but as yet the pharmacological bases are not known. It has been shown that either local or descending controls can be elicited when high levels of NMDA are adminis-tered intrathecally (CHAPMAN et al. 1994; KOLHEKAR et al. 1993; RAIGORODSKY and URCA 1987). Also, NOS is found in GABA neurones in the spinal cord (VALTSCHANOFF et al. 1992). Adenosine may also play a role in these auto-limiting effects since both in the hippocampus and cortex this transmitter has been shown to be released by NMDA receptor activation and then acts to further control activity (CRAIG and WHITE 1992, 1993; MANZONI et al. 1994; DE MENDONCA and RIBEIRO 1993).

III. Adenosine as a Target

There is much evidence for a role of adenosine in the control of nociception at the spinal cord level, with the A_1 receptor playing a key role on these events (see SALTER et al. 1993; SAWYNOK and SWEENEY 1989). A_1 receptor mediated antinociception has been reported with behavioural tests (KARLSTEN et al. 1990; MALMBERG and YAKSH 1993a; SOSNOWSKI et al. 1989; SOSNOWSKI and YAKSH 1989).

Theophylline, an adenosine receptor antagonist, given alone has been reported to enhance the C fibre evoked responses, post-discharge and wind-up of spinal neurones, indicative of an antagonism of tonic or evoked release of endogenous adenosine (REEVE and DICKENSON 1995). However, theophylline can act to produce phosphodiesterase inhibition as well as both A_1 and A_2 receptor antagonism (FREDHOLM et al. 1994; WILLIAMS 1991). Neuronal recordings suggest that A_1 receptor agonists, in particular N^6-cyclopentyladenosine (N^6-CPA), inhibit both phases of the formalin response, but that lower doses tend to be selective for the second phase, the NMDA-dependent component (REEVE and DICKENSON 1995). Other studies have shown that another A_1 agonist, N6-[L-2-phenylisopropl]-adenosine (L-PIA) inhibits the second but not the first phase of the formalin-evoked response (MALMBERG and YAKSH 1993a). Differences between electrophysiological and behavioural studies may be due to the fact that L-PIA is a less potent agonist (FREDHOLM et al. 1994), and that reductions in motor function (KARLSTEN et al. 1990; SOSNOWSKI et al. 1989) have prevented the doses from being increased to reveal first-phase effects.

The overall profile of the adenosine A1 receptor agonists in reducing the NMDA-mediated wind-up, post-discharges and second phase of the formalin response (DICKENSON 1994a; HALEY et al. 1990; HUNTER and SINGH 1994) is suggestive of post-synaptic A_1 receptor locations near or adjacent to the NMDA receptors. Allodynia, touch-evoked nociception, has also been shown to be NMDA receptor mediated (YAKSH 1989) and modulated by L-PIA (SOSNOWSKI and YAKSH 1989). A plausible mechanism for these results is inhibition of excitatory interneurones in NMDA polysynaptic nociceptive pathways by activation of the A_1 receptor. However, the equivalent inhibitions of the non-NMDA-mediated acute C fibre responses and the first early phase of the formalin response indicates further pre-synaptic actions, akin to opioids (Dickenson 1994b). In fact, spinal A_1 receptors are on interneurones (Choca et al. 1988; Geiger et al. 1984; Goodman and Snyder 1982) as well as on pre-synaptic sites (Geiger et al. 1984), in keeping with conclusions from the functional and anatomical studies.

There is evidence for a pre-synaptic release of adenosine (Sweeney et al. 1989) and small neurones in dorsal root ganglia have been shown to contain adenosine deaminase (Nagy and Daddona 1985; Nagy et al. 1984). Stimulation of low-threshold Pacinian afferents causes both excitatory and inhibitory post-synaptic potentials in dorsal horn neurones which are mediated by adenosine (Salter and Henry 1987). This idea of release from primary afferent neurones suggests low-threshold fibres but not nociceptive fibres as the source, and these may therefore be related to mechanisms behind the ability of adenosine to control allodynia (Sosnowski and Yaksh 1989). There is evidence for post-synaptic release mechanisms elsewhere in the CNS; in the cortex adenosine can be released by AMPA and NMDA receptor activation (Craig and White 1992, 1993; Hoehn and White 1990). As mentioned, studies (Craig and White 1992; Manzoni et al. 1994; de Mendonca and Ribeiro 1993) have shown that adenosine may exert a negative feedback causing presynaptic depression in the cortex and hippocampus following postsynaptic NMDA receptor induced release. It also appears that adenosine acting at the A_1 receptor has an important role in indirectly controlling spinal NMDA-dependent nociceptive pathways as well as other antinociceptive influences and could also function as a feedback mechanism in the spinal cord. A possible, relatively selective control of NMDA-mediated events is suggested by the greater inhibitions of wind-up and post-discharge responses of the neurones.

IV. GABA as a Target

The final transmitter to be considered with regard to indirect control of NMDA-mediated events is GABA. GABA has been firmly established as the major inhibitory neurotransmitter in the central nervous system with the extensive distribution and influence of GABAergic terminals indicating that the nervous system operates under a considerable degree of tonic GABA restraint.

In the spinal cord between 24% and 33% of inhibitory interneurones in laminae I–III, the main site of termination of nociceptive afferents, are reported to contain GABA, often found to coexist with either glycine, galanin, met-enkephalin or neuropeptide Y in separate populations (Rowan et al. 1993; Simmons et al. 1995; Todd and Spike 1992; Todd et al. 1996). GABA also is found in synaptic apposition to NO-producing neurones in these areas (Bernardi et al. 1995).

GABA acts at either the ligand-gated chloride channel $GABA_A$ receptor or the G protein linked $GABA_B$ receptor, both of which are found pre- and post-synaptically on $A\delta$ and C fibre afferents (see CLAVIER et al. 1992). $GABA_A$ receptors are the targets of a diverse range of pharmacologically and clinically important drugs, many of which interact with the allosteric binding site for the benzodiazepines (BZs) which enhance the action of GABA (SIEGHART 1992).

The results from much experimental and clinical investigation into BZ modulation of GABA transmission in nociceptive processes and their potential use as analgesics are inconsistent. Several studies have demonstrated BZs to be analgesic, whereas others have found BZs to be ineffective, and there are contradictory reports of BZs both potentiating and antagonizing morphine analgesia (see CLAVIER et al. 1992). This diversity is the product of many different experimental protocols, models of nociception and routes of administration. In addition, the sedative and myorelaxant effects of these compounds must be considered with behavioural and clinical studies in a similar way to the caution that is needed in interpretation of the effects of NMDA antagonists.

A recent study (BERNARDI et al. 1995) provides a morphological basis for selective inhibitory gating of input into the spinal cord as GABAergic terminals contact more $A\delta$ fibre terminals than C fibre terminals. CLAVIER et al. (1992) report that the BZ midazolam causes only a weak depression of C fibre evoked responses but has a marked, dose-dependently depressive effect on the $A\delta$ fibre evoked response. In addition, the GABAA antagonist bicuculline causes a facilitation of C fibre evoked responses which is much less than the profound potentiation seen on the $A\delta$ fibre evoked response (REEVE and DICKENSON 1995). These effects could be pre- or post-synaptic (BESSON and CHAOUCH 1987; CLAVIER et al. 1992) but show that BZs are unlikely to be effective against C fibre evoked responses yet influence $A\delta$ responses.

GABA modulation of nociceptive transmission is seen to alter during inflammatory conditions. Carrageenan-induced unilateral inflammation increases the subsequent number of GABA-immunoreactive cells in the ipsilateral dorsal horn. This increase has been suggested to be caused by increased noxious input (CASTRO-LOPES et al. 1994). Furthermore, the levels of the synthetic enzyme for GABA are also augmented by inflammation (NAHIN and HYLDEN 1991). An increased GABA inhibitory tone may then be suspected in inflammation.

In the formalin model of inflammatory pain intrathecal $GABA_A$ and $GABA_B$ agonists cause a dose-dependent suppression of nociceptive behaviour in both the phase 1 and phase 2 responses (DIRIG and YAKSH 1995). Intrathecally administered antagonists and BZs, however, have been shown to have no effect on nociceptive behaviour in the formalin response (DIRIG and YAKSH 1995). A likely explanation for this lack of antinociceptive effect of BZs is that levels of endogenous GABA in the spinal cord in rapidly induced inflammatory events are too low for an allosteric potentiator such as a BZ, or indeed an antagonist, to cause significant analgesia or hyperalgesia. However, the release of excitatory amino acids induced by longer term inflammation (SORKIN et al. 1992) can be prevented by $GABA_A$ receptor antagonism (SLUKA et al. 1994a,b), suggesting that GABA controls are complex.

Thus there appears to be little ongoing control of noxious evoked activity by GABA. By contrast, the block of $GABA_A$ controls by bicuculline and also the antagonism of glycine causes an induction of tactile-evoked allodynia in normal animals (YAKSH 1989). Here tactile stimuli cause behavioural and cardiovascular responses indicative of nociception which are markedly reduced by NMDA antagonism (YAKSH 1989). In electrophysiological studies the blocking of inhibitory amino acid receptors allows low-threshold inputs to activate nociceptive reflexes (SIVILOTTI and WOOLF 1994). These studies show glycine and $GABA_A$ controls to be exerted on low-threshold mechanoreceptors and $A\beta$ afferents (SIVILOTTI and WOOLF 1994; YAKSH 1989).

Neuropathic pain states also appear to be subject to GABAergic control. In the well known, BENNETT and XIE (1988) model unilateral loose ligatures around the sciatic nerve induces a number of symptoms including an ipsilateral thermal hyperalgesia. Intrathecal bicuculline, administered post-surgery and again on days 1 and 2, has been shown to cause a dose-dependent increase in the magnitude of the hyperalgesia observed 1 week after ligation (YAMAMOTO and YAKSH 1993). However, at later stages there appears to be a loss of GABA control after nerve injury since it has been reported that spinal levels of GABA are reduced 3 weeks after lesion (CASTRO-LOPES et al. 1993). In addition, in a model of deafferentation pain the importance of glycine controls is illustrated by increased NMDA receptor mediated pain behaviour after block by spinal strychnine (SELTZER et al. 1991b). Thus in neuropathic conditions GABA appears to exert important controls on NMDA-mediated hyperalgesia, controls which may be lost with time, thus exacerbating the pain.

$GABA_A$ and $GABA_B$ receptors coexist on nociceptive primary afferents (DESARMENIEN et al. 1984) and are therefore ideally located to modulate spinal nociceptive transmission. The selective $GABA_B$ receptor agonist baclofen has been shown to produce presynaptic inhibition of primary afferent terminals (HENRY 1982), to inhibit the release of both glutamate (JOHNSTON et al. 1980) and SP (MALCANGIO and BOWERY 1994) and to cause a selective inhibition of C fibre evoked responses of rat dorsal horn neurones (DICKENSON et al. 1985). Furthermore, behavioural studies have clearly demonstrated anti-nociceptive effects of baclofen (see SAWYNOK 1987). None of these studies suggests any role of the $GABA_B$ receptor in selectively controlling NMDA-mediated events. However, it has been shown that a profound allodynia-like syndrome can be produced by photochemical lesions of the rat spinal cord (HAO et al. 1991a). In this case baclofen but not a $GABA_A$ receptor agonist or morphine reduces the allodynia. This is interesting since in this model NMDA receptor antagonists are able to reduce the allodynia only at very early stages (HAO et al. 1991b).

From these studies on GABA it can be suggested that the controls exerted by this inhibitory amino acid act to prevent low-threshold afferents from triggering nociception in normal animals (SIVILOTTI and WOOLF 1994; YAKSH 1989). In inflammation there appear to be enhanced GABA controls on noxious transmission, and therefore the extent of NMDA-mediated transmission is held in check. In neuropathic states these inhibitory controls appear to be reduced; excitations thus dominate, and hypersensitivity is no longer balanced by inhibitions. Interestingly, for LTP to occur in the hippocampus GABA-mediated inhibitions must be turned off (BASHIR and COLLINGRIDGE 1992; WATKINS and COLLINGRIDGE 1994). It may well be that in normal circumstances wind-up and other NMDA-mediated events are prevented from becoming persistent by inhibitory controls, whether via GABA, adenosine or other receptor systems.

G. Conclusions

It is clear that the concept of central hypersensitivity is supported by a wealth of data, derived from studies using behavioural, electrophysiological, neurochemical and anatomical techniques. Furthermore, a number of human studies show that the idea is of great importance to clinical pain states and, in some cases common substrates have been demonstrated.

The key factors for central hypersensitivity are activation of peripheral C fibre afferents either by tissue damage or by nerve damage and ectopic activity. Consequently the release of excitatory amino acids and activation of the AMPA, metabotropic and NMDA receptors occur. The AMPA receptor appears to set up a baseline response to the stimulus. Only if the stimulus is of sufficient intensity and frequency does the NMDA receptor become activated because of the need to remove the block of the channel by Mg^{2+}. Once this has occurred, the level of depolarization produced by the receptor-channel complex means that large enhancements of excitatory transmission result, although peripheral activity remains constant. Wind-up appears to be the neuronal manifestation of these events, and NMDA receptor induction and maintenance of hyperalgesia and allodynias has been reported in animal models of inflammation, ischaemia and many forms of neuropathy.

The gas NO can then be generated by spinal neurones subsequent to NMDA receptor activation and seems to further enhance transmission; gene induction can also occur. The processes leading to NMDA receptor activation appear to rely on co-activation of neurokinin receptors in both normal and inflamed states. In neuropathic states changes in the phenotype of peripheral fibres may mean that peptides other than SP etc. play this role (HOKFELT et al. 1994). However, in normal and inflamed states, inhibitory events such as those produced by adenosine and GABA may limit NMDA receptor activation so that any reduction of spinal inhibitions contributes to NMDA receptor activation. The central hypersensitivity seen in neuropathic states may be due as much to failed inhibitions as to excitatory events. This may explain why inflammatory pains, a typical example being post-operative pain, rarely become chronic and resolve themselves as tissue heals. By contrast, neuropathic pains are often severe and chronic despite the fact that there must be relatively low levels of afferent input arriving in the spinal cord from the damaged nerve. Despite similarities with long-term potentiation and depression, the spinal events thus appear to be much less persistent in normal animals and more open to modulation after inflammation; the balance shifts towards excitatory events in neuropathic pains.

There is therefore much potential for the development of NMDA antagonists for the control of both acute and persistent pains when central hypersensitivity occurs. The block of NMDA function does not produce an analgesia in the strict sense of the word, but by preventing or blocking central hypersensitivity it removes hyperalgesia and allodynia. However, there is little evidence that spinal NMDA receptor mediated events occur in the absence of peripheral inputs; they are not self-sustaining and differ from LTP and other forms of plasticity in this regard. In fact, it would make little sense for sensory events to be generated independently of peripheral drives. Consequently, blocking the maintenance stage with NMDA antagonists interrupts the pain, but it is likely to recur as the drug effect wears off. Preventing the induction delays and reduces the subsequent pain but may also have long-term beneficial effects, especially in neuropathic pains where excessive NMDA receptor activation may cause maladaptive changes such as neuronal death, gene induction etc. Less direct ways to control NMDA receptor function could be via neuronal NO synthesis inhibitors, adenosine receptor agonists and by simply increasing inhibitions such as opioid and GABA function. Thus a number of targets are available, both in terms of the clincial control of pain and for the development of novel therapeutic agents (DICKENSON 1995a,b; YAKSH and MALMBERG 1994).

As always the clinical usefulness of drugs is a balance between therapeutic effects and side effects. If the latter limit the use of NMDA receptor or other drugs, combination therapy with local anaesthetics and opioids has great potential.

Acknowledgements. I thank Tina Bashford for her excellent secretarial assistance and Victoria Chapman, Alvaro Diaz, Mark Green, Wahida Rahman, Alison Reeve and Louise Stanfa for their inputs into this review.

References

Aanonsen LM, Wilcox GL (1987) Nociceptive action of excitatory amino acids in the mouse: effects of spinally administered opioids, phencyclidine and sigma agonists. J Pharmacol Exp Ther 243:9–19
Aanonsen LM, Lei S, Wilcox GL (1990) Excitatory amino acid receptors and nociceptive neurotransmission in rat spinal cord. Pain 41:309–321
Abram SE, Yaksh TL (1993) Morphine, but not inhalation anesthesia, blocks post-injury facilitation. Anesthesiology 78:713–721

Ackerman B, Arwestrom E, Post C (1988) Local anesthetics potentiate spinal morphine analgesia. Anesth Analg 67:943–948

Akaike A, Tamura Y, Sato Y, Ozaki K, Matsuoka R, Miura S, Yoshinaga T (1991) Cholecystokinin-induced protection of cultured cortical neurons against glutamate neurotoxicity. Brain Res 557:303–307

Arancio O, Yoshimura M, Murase K, MacDermott AB (1993) The distribution of excitatory amino acid receptors on acutely dissociated dorsal horn neurones from postnatal rats. Neurosci 52:159–167

Arner S, Meyerson BA (1988) Lack of analgesic effect of opioids on neuropathic and idiopathic forms of pain. Pain 33:11–23

Ault B, Hildebrand LM (1993) Activation of nociceptive reflexes by peripheral kainate receptors. J Pharmacol Exp Ther 265:927–932

Backonja M, Arndt G, Gombar KA, Check B, Zimmermann M (1994) Response of chronic neuropathic pain syndromes to ketamine: a preliminary study. Pain 56:51–57

Banos JE, Verdu E, Buti M, Navarro X (1994) Effects of dizocilpine on autonomy behavior after nerve section in mice. Brain Res 636:107–110

Baranauskas G, Traversa U, Rosati AM, Nistri A (1995) An NK1 receptor-dependent component of the slow excitation recorded intracellularly from rat motoneurons following dorsal root stimulation. Eur J Neurosci 7:2409–2417

Barnard E, Henley JM (1990) The non-NMDA receptors: types, protein structure and molecular biology. Trends Pharmacol Sci 11:500–507

Bashir ZI, Collingridge GL (1992) Synaptic plasticity: long-term potentiation in the hippocampus. Curr Opin Neurobiol 2:328–335

Bashir ZI, Tam B, Collingridge GL (1990) Activation of the glycine site in the NMDA receptor is necessary for the induction of LTP. Neurosci Lett 108:261–266

Battaglia G, Rustioni A (1988) Coexistence of glutamate and substance P in dorsal root ganglion cells of the rat and monkey. J Comp Neurol 277:302–312

Benardo LS (1993) Recruitment of inhibition by enhanced activation of synaptic NMDA responses in the rat cerebral cortex. Brain Res 627:314–324

Bennett GJ (1994) Animal models of neuropathic pain. In: Gebhart GF, Hammond DL, Jensen T (eds) Proceedings of the 7th World Congress on Pain, vol 2. International Association for the Study of Pain, Seattle, pp 495–510

Bennett GJ, Xie YK (1988) A peripheral mononeuropathy in rat that produces pain disorders like those seen in man. Pain 33:87–107

Bernardi PS, Valtschanoff JG, Weinberg RJ, Schmidt HHHW, Rustioni A (1995) Synaptic interactions between primary afferent terminals and GABA and nitric oxide-synthesizing neurons in the superficial laminae of the rat spinal cord. J Neurosci 15:1363–1371

Besson J-M, Chaouch A (1987) Peripheral and spinal mechanisms of nociception. Physiol Rev 67:67–186

Birch PJ, Grossman CJ, Hayes AG (1988) 6,7-Dinitro-quinoxaline-2,3-dion and 6-nitro,7-cyano-quinoxaline-2,3-dion antagonise responses to NMDA in the rat spinal cord via an action at the strychnine-insensitive glycine receptor. Eur J Pharmacol 156:177–180

Birch PJ, Beresford IJM, Bowers JS, Harrison SM, Rogers H, Smith GD (1993) Profile of activity of NK1 receptor antagonists in nociceptive tests. Neuropeptides 24:219

Bleakman D, Rusin KI, Card PS, Glaum SR, Miller RJ (1992) Metabotropic glutamate receptors potentiate ionotropic glutamate responses in the rat dorsal horn. Mol Pharmacol 42:192–196

Bliss TVP, Collingridge GL (1993) A synaptic model of memory: long-term potentiation in the hippocampus. Nature 361:31–39

Bobelis DJ, Balster RL (1993) Pharmacological specificity of the discriminative stimulus properties of 2-amino-4,5-(1,2-cyclohexyl)-7-phosphono-heptanoic (NPC 12636), a competitive N-methyl-d-aspartate receptor antagonist. J Pharmacol Exp Ther 264:845–853

Bond A, Lodge D (1995) Pharmacology of metabotropic glutamate receptor-mediated enhancement of responses to excitatory and inhibitory amino acids on rat spinal neurones in vivo. Neuropharmacology 34:1015–1023

Bresink I, Danysz W, Parsons CG, Tiedtke P, Mutschler E (1995) Chronic treatment with the uncompetitive NMDA receptor antagonist memantine influences the polyamine and glycine binding sites of the NMDA receptor complex in aged rats. J Neur Transm 10:11–26

Broman J, Adahl F (1994) Evidence for vesicular storage of glutamate in primary afferent terminals. Neuroreport 5:1801–1804

Broman J, Anderson S, Ottersen OP (1993) Enrichment of glutamate-like immunore-activity in primary afferent terminals throughout the spinal cord dorsal horn. Eur J Neurosci 5:1050–1061

Brugger F, Evans RH, Hawkins NS (1990) Effects of N-methyl-aspartate antagonists and spantide on spinal reflexes and responses to substance P and capsaicin in isolated spinal cord preparations from mouse and rat. Neuroscience 36:611–622

Budai D, Wilcox GL, Larson AA (1992) Enhancement of NMDA-evoked neuronal activity by glycine in the rat spinal cord in vivo. Neurosci Lett 135:265–268

Budai D, Wilcox GL, Larson AA (1995) Effects of nitric oxide availability on responses of spinal wide dynamic range neurones to excitatory amino acids. Eur J Pharmacol 278:39–47

Carlton SM, Hargett GL, Coggeshall RE (1995) Localization and activation of glutamate receptors in unmyelinated axons of rat glabrous skin. Neurosci Lett 197:25–28

Cartmell SM, Mitchell D (1993) Attenuation of reperfusion hyperalgesia in the rat by systemic administration of benzodiazepines. Br J Pharmacol 110:1067–1072

Castro-Lopes JM, Tavares I, Coimbra A (1993) GABA decreases in the spinal cord dorsal horn after peripheral neurectomy. Brain Res 620:287–291

Castro-Lopes JM, Tavares I, Tolle TR, Coimbra A (1994) Carrageenan-induced in-flammation of the hind foot provokes a rise of GABA-immunoreactive cells in the rat spinal cord that is prevented by peripheral neurectomy or neonatal capsaicin treatment. Pain 56:193–201

Cerne R, Randic M (1992) Modulation of AMPA and NMDA responses in rat spinal dorsal horn neurons by trans-1-aminocyclopentane-1-3-dicarboxylate. Neurosci Lett 153:180–184

Chapman V, Dickenson AH (1992) The combination of NMDA antagonism and morphine produces profound antinociception in the rat dorsal horn. Brain Res 573:321–323

Chapman V, Dickenson AH (1993) The effect of intrathecal administration of RP67580, a potent neurokinin 1 antagonist on nociceptive transmission in the rat spinal cord. Neurosci Lett 157:149–152

Chapman V, Dickenson AH (1994) Enhanced responses of rat dorsal horn neurones after UV irradiation of the hindpaw; roles of the NMDA receptor. Neurosci Lett 176:41–44

Chapman V, Dickenson AH, Tjolsen A (1994) Bi-directional effects of intrathecal NMDA and substance P on rat dorsal horn neuronal responses. Neurosci Lett 178:90–94

Chapman V, Honoré P, Buritova J, Besson JM (1995) The contribution of NMDA receptor activation to spinal c-Fos expression in a model of inflammatory pain. Br J Pharmacol 116:1628–1634

Chen L, Huang L-Y M (1992) Protein kinase C reduces Mg^{2+} block of NMDA-receptor channels as a mechanism of modulation. Nature 356:521–523

Chinnery RM, Shaw PJ, Ince PG, Johnson M (1993) Autoradiographic distribution of binding sites for the non-NMDA receptor antagonist [3H]CNQX in human motor cortex, brainstem and spinal cord. Brain Res 630:75–81

Choca JI, Green, RD, Proudfit HK (1988) Adenosine A1 and A2 receptors of the substantia gelatinosa are located predominantly on intrinsic neurons: an autorad-iography study. J Pharmacol Exp Ther 247:757–764

Choi Y, Yoon YW, Na HS, Kim SH, Chung JM (1994) Behavioral signs of ongoing pain and cold allodynia in a rat model of neuropathic pain. Pain 59:369–376

Clavier N, Lombard M-C, Besson J-M (1992) Benzodiazepines and Pain: effects of midazolam on the activities of nociceptive non-specific dorsal horn neurons in the rat spinal cord. Pain 48:61–71

Clements JR, Magnusson KR, Hautman J, Beitz AJ (1991) Rat tooth pulp projections to spinal trigeminal subnucleus caudalis are glutamate-like immunoreactive. J Comp Neurol 309:281–288

Coderre TJ (1993) Potent analgesia induced in rats by combined action at PCP and polyamine recognition sites of the NMDA receptor complex. Eur J Neurosci 5:390–393

Coderre TJ, Melzack R (1992a) The role of NMDA receptor-operated calcium channels in persistent nociception after formalin-induced tissue injury. J Neurosci 12:3671–3675

Coderre TJ, Melzack R (1992b) The contribution of excitatory amino acids to central sensitization and persistent nociception after formalin-induced tissue injury. J Neurosci 12:3665–3670

Coderre TJ, Vaccarino AL, Melzack R (1990) Central nervous system plasticity in tonic pain response to subcutaneous formalin injection. Brain Res 535:155–158

Collingridge G, Singer W (1990) Excitatory amino acid receptors and synaptic plasticity. Trends Pharmacol Sci 11:290–296

Craig CG, White TD (1992) Low-level N-methyl-d-aspartate receptor activation provides a purinergic inhibitory threshold against further N-methyl-D-aspartate-mediated neurotransmission in the cortex. J Pharmacol Exp Ther 260:1278–1284

Craig CG, White TD (1993) N-methyl-d-aspartate- and non-N-methyl-D-aspartate-evoked adenosine release from rat cortical slices: distinct purinergic sources and mechanisms of release. J Neurochem 60:1073–1080

Cumberbatch MJ, Chizh BA, Headley PM (1994) AMPA receptors have an equal role in spinal nociceptive and non-nociceptive transmission. Neuroreport 5:877–880

Cumberbatch MJ, Chizh BA, Headley PM (1995) Modulation of excitatory amino acid responses by tachykinins and selective tachykinin receptor agonists in the rat spinal cord. Br J Pharmacol 115:1005–1012

Curtis DR, Phillis JW, Watkins JC (1959) Chemical excitation of spinal neurones. Nature 183:611–612

Davar G, Hama A, Deykin A, Vos B, Maciewicz R (1991) MK-801 blocks the development of thermal hyperalgesia in a rat model of experimental painful neuropathy. Brain Res 553:327–330

Davies J, Watkins JC (1983) Role of excitatory amino acid receptors in mono- and polysynaptic excitation in the cat spinal cord. Exp Brain Res 49:280–290

Davies SN, Lodge D (1987) Evidence for involvement of N-methylaspartate receptors in "Appletonwind-up" of class 2 neurones in the dorsal horn of the rat. Brain Res 424:402–406

Daw NW, Stein PSG, Fox K (1993) The role of NMDA receptors in information processing. Annu Rev Neurosci 16:207–222

DeBiasi S, Rustioni A (1983) Glutamate and substance P coexist in primary afferent terminals in superficial laminae of spinal cord. Proc Natl Acad Sci USA 85:820–824

De Mendonca A, Ribeiro JA (1993) Adenosine inhibits the NMDA receptor-mediated excitatory postsynaptic potential in the hippocampus. Brain Res 606:351–356

Desarmenien M, Feltz P, Occhipinti G, Santangelo F, Schlichter R (1984) Coexistence of GABAA and GABAB receptors on Aδ and C primary afferents. Br J Pharmacol 81:327–333

Dickenson AH (1990) A cure for wind-up: NMDA receptor antagonists as potential analgesics. Trends Pharmacol Sci 11:307–309

Dickenson AH (1994a) NMDA receptor antagonists as analgesics. In: Fields HL, Liebeskind JC (eds) Progress in pain research and management, vol 1. International Association for the Study of Pain, Seattle, p 173

Dickenson AH (1994b) Where and how opioids act. In: Gebhart GF, Hammond DL, Jensen T (eds) Proceedings of the 7th World Congress on Pain, vol 2. International Association for the Study of Pain, Seattle, pp 525–552

Dickenson AH (1995a) Novel pharmacological targets in the treatment of pain. Pain Rev 2:1–12

Dickenson AH (1995b) Spinal cord pharmacology of pain. Br J Anaesth 75:132–144

Dickenson AH, Aydar E (1991) Antagonism at the glycine site on the NMDA receptor reduces spinal nociception in the rat. Neurosci Lett 121:263–266

Dickenson AH, Sullivan AF (1986) Electrophysiological studies on the effects of the effects of intrathecal morphine on nociceptive neurones in the rat dorsal horn. Pain 24:211–222

Dickenson AH, Sullivan AF (1987a) Evidence for a role of the NMDA receptor in the frequency dependent potentiation of deep rat dorsal horn nociceptive neurones following C-fibre stimulation. Neuropharmacology 26:1235–1238

Dickenson AH, Sullivan AF (1987b) Peripheral and central modulation of subcutaneous formalin induced activity of rat dorsal horn neurones. Neurosci Lett 83:207–211

Dickenson AH, Sullivan AF (1989) Subcutaneous formalin induced activity of dorsal horn neurones in the rat: differential response to an intrathecal opiate administered pre or post formalin. Pain 30:349–360

Dickenson AH, Sullivan AF (1990) Differential effects of excitatory amino acid antagonists on dorsal horn nociceptive neurones in the rat. Brain Res 506:31–39

Dickenson AH, Brewer CM, Hayes NA (1985) Effects of topical baclofen on C fibre-evoked neuronal activity in the rat dorsal horn. Neuroscience 14:557–562

Dickenson AH, Sullivan AF, Stanfa LC, McQuay H (1991) Dextromethorphan and levorphanol on dorsal horn nociceptive neurones in the rat. Neuropharmacology 30:1303–1308

Dirig DM, Yaksh TL (1995) Intrathecal baclofen and muscimol, but not midazolam, are antinociceptive using the rat-formalin model. J Pharmacol Exp Ther 275:219–227

Dohrn CS, Beitz AJ (1994) NMDA receptor mRNA expression in NOS-containing neurons in the spinal trigeminal nucleus of the rat. Neurosci Lett 175:28–32

Dougherty PM, Willis WD (1991a) Enhancement of spinothalamic neuron responses to chemical and mechanical stimuli following combined micro-iontophoretic application of NMDA and substance P. Pain 47:85–93

Dougherty PM, Willis WD (1991b) Modification of the responses of primate spinothalamic neurons to mechanical stimulation by excitatory amino acids and an N-methyl-d-aspartate antagonist. Brain Res 542:15–22

Dougherty M, Palecek J, Paleckova V, Sorkin LS, Willis WD (1992) The role of NMDA and non-NMDA excitatory amino acid receptors in the excitation of primate spinothalamic tract neurons by mechanical, chemical, thermal and electrical stimuli. J Neurosci 12:3025–3041

Dray A (1995) Inflammatory mediators of pain. Br J Anaesth 75:125–131

Dray A, Urban L, Dickenson AH (1994) Pharmacology of chronic pain. Trends Pharmacol Sci 15:190–197

Dubner R, Ruda MA (1992) Activity dependent neuronal plasticity following tissue injury and inflammation. Trends Neurol Sci 15:96–103

Dubuisson, D, Dennis SG (1977) The formalin test: a quantitative study of the analgesic effects of morphine, meperidine and brain stem stimulation in rats and cats. Pain 4:161–174

Dudek SM, Bear MF (1992) Homosynaptic long term depression in area CA1 of the hippocampus and effects of NMDA receptor blockade. Proc Natl Acad Sci USA 89:4363–4367

Duggan AW, Hendrey IA, Morton CR, Hutchinson WD, Zhao ZO (1988) Cutaneous stimuli releasing immunoreactive substance P in the dorsal horn of the cat. Brain Res 451:261–273

Eaton SA, Salt TE (1996) Role of N-methyl-d-aspartate and metabotropic glutamate receptors in corticothalamic excitatory postsynaptic potentials in vivo. Neuroscience 73:1–5

Ebert B, Andersen S, Krogsgaard-Larsen P (1995) Ketobemidone, methadone and pethidine are non-competitive N-methyl-d-aspartate antagonists in the rat cortex and spinal cord. Neurosci Lett 187:165–168

Edelman GM, Gally JA (1992) Nitric oxide: linking space and time in the brain. Proc Natl Acad Sci USA 89:11651–11652

Eide PK, Jorum E, Stubhaug A, Bremnes J, Breivik H (1994) Relief of post-herpetic neuralgia with the N-methyl-d-aspartate receptor antagonist ketamine: a double blind, cross-over comparison with morphine and placebo. Pain 58:347–354

Eide PK, Stubhaug A, Oye I, Breivik H (1995) Continuous subcutaneous administration of the N-methyl-d-aspartic acid (NMDA) receptor antagonist ketamine in the treatment of post-herpetic neuralgia. Pain 61:221–228

Eisenberg E, Vos BP, Strassman AM (1993) The NMDA antagonist memantine blocks pain behavior in a rat model of formalin-induced facial pain. Pain 54:301–307

Eisenberg E, LaCross S, Strassman AM (1994) The effects of the clincially tested NMDA receptor antagonist memantine on carrageenin-induced thermal hyperalgesia in rats. Eur J Pharmacol 255:123–129

Elliot KJ, Brodsky M, Hyansky A, Foley KM, Inturissi CE (1994) Dextromethorphan suppresses the formalin-induced increase in c-fos mRNA. Am Soc Neurosci Abstr 568.15

Ericson A-C, Blomqvist A, Craig AD, Ottersen OP, Broman J (1995) Evidence for glutamate as neurotransmitter in trigemino-and spinothalamic tract terminals in the nucleus submedius of cats. Eur J Neurosci 7:305–317

Fitzgerald M (1990) c-Fos and the changing face of pain. Trends Neurol Sci 13:439–440

Foster AC, Fagg GE (1987) Taking apart NMDA receptors. Nature 329:395–396

Fraser H, Chapman V, Dickenson AH (1992) Spinal local anaesthetic actions on afferent evoked responses and wind-up of nociceptive neurones in the rat spinal cord: combination with morphine produces marked potentiation of antinociception. Pain 49:33–41

Fredholm BB, Abbracchio MP, Burnstock G, Daly JW, Harden TK, Jacobson KA, Leff P, Williams M (1994) VI Nomenclature and classification of purinoceptors. Pharmacol Rev 46:143–156

Garry MG, Richardson JD, Hargreaves KM (1994) Sodium nitroprusside evoked the release of immunoreactive calcitonin gene-related peptide and substance P from dorsal horn slices via nitric-oxide-dependent and nitric oxide-independent mechanisms. J Neurosci 14:4329–4337

Geiger JD, Labella FS, Nagy JI (1984) Characterization and localization of adenosine receptors in rat spinal cord. J Neurosci 4:2303–2310

Gerber G, Randic M (1989a) Excitatory amino acid-mediated components of synaptically evoked input from dorsal roots to deep dorsal horn neurones in the rat spinal cord slice. Neurosci Lett 106:211–219

Gerber G, Randic M (1989b) Participation of excitatory amino acid receptors in the slow excitatory synaptic transmission in the rat spinal cord in vitro. Neurosci Lett 106:220–228

Goodman RR, Snyder SH (1982) Autoradiographic localization of adenosine receptors in rat brain using [3H]cyclohexyladenosine. J Neurosci 2:1230–1241

Gracely R, Lynch SA, Bennett GJ (1993) Painful neuropathy: altered central processing maintained dynamically by peripheral input. Pain 52:251–253

Haley JE, Sullivan AF, Dickenson AH (1990) Evidence for spinal N-methyl-d-aspartate receptor involvement in prolonged chemical nociception in the rat. Brain Res 518:218–226

Haley JE, Dickenson A H, Schachter M (1992) Electrophysiological evidence for a role of nitric oxide in prolonged chemical nociception in the rat. Neuropharmacology 31:51–58

Hao J-X, Xu X-J, Aldskogius, Seiger A, Wiesenfeld-Hallin Z (1991a) Allodynia-like effects in rat after ischaemic spinal cord injury photochemically induced by laser irradiation. Pain 45:175–185

Hao J-X, Xu X-J, Aldskogius, Seiger A, Wiesenfeld-Hallin Z (1991b) The excitatory amino acid receptor antagonist MK-801 prevents the hypersensitivity induced by spinal ischaemia in the rat. Exp Neurol 113:182–191

Headley PM, Grillner S (1990) Excitatory amino-acids and synaptic transmission: the evidence for a physiological function. Trends Pharmacol Sci 11:205–211

Henley JM, Jenkins R, Hunt SP (1993) Localisation of glutamate receptor binding sites and mRNAs to the dorsal horn of the rat spinal cord. Neuropharmacology 32:37–41

Henry JL (1982) Pharmacological studies on the prolonged depressant effects of baclofen on lumbar dorsal horn units in the cat. Neuropharmacology 21:1085–1093

Hoehn K, White TD (1990) Role of excitatory amino acid receptors in K+- and glutamate-evoked release of endogenous adenosine from rat cortical slices. J Neurochem 54:256–265

Hokfelt T, Zhang X, Wiesenfeld-Hallin Z (1994) Messenger plasticity in primary sensory neurones following axotomy and its functional implications. Trends Neurosci 17:22–30

Hunskaar S, Hole K (1987) The formalin test in mice: dissociation between inflammatory and non-inflammatory pain. Pain 30:103–114

Hunter JC, Singh L (1994) Role of excitatory amino acid receptors in the mediation of the nociceptive response to formalin in the rat. Neurosci Lett 174:217–221

Ishida M, Saitoh T, Shimamoto K, Ohfune Y, Shinozaki H (1993) A novel metabotropic glutamate receptor agonist: marked depression of monosynaptic excitation in the newborn rat isolated spinal cord. Br J Pharmacol 109:1169–1177

Jadad AR, Carroll D, Glynn CJ, Moore RA, McQuay HJ (1992) Morphine responsiveness of chronic pain: double-blind randomized crossover study with patient-controlled analgesia. Lancet 339:1367–1371

Jakowec MW, Fox AJ, Martin LJ, Kalb RG (1995) Quantitative and qualitative changes in AMPA receptor expression during spinal cord development. Neuroscience 67:893–907

Jansen KLR, Faull RLM, Dragunow M, Waldvogel H (1990) Autoradiographic localisation of NMDA quasqualate and kainic acid recptors in human spinal cord. Neurosci Lett 108:53–57

Jeftinija S, Jeftinija K, Liu F, Skilling SR, Smullin DH, Larson AA (1991) Excitatory amino acids are released from rat primary afferent neurons in vitro. Neurosci Lett 125:191–194

Jensen TS, Yaksh TL (1992) Brainstem excitatory amino acid receptor in nociception: microinjection mapping and pharmacological characterization of glutamate-sensitive sites in the brainstem associated with algogenic behavior. Neurosci 46:535–547

Johnston GAR, Hailstone MH, Freeman CG (1980) Baclofen; stereoselective inhibition of excitatory amino acid release. J Pharm Pharmacol 32:230–231

Kangra I, Randic M (1991) Outflow of endogenous aspartate and glutamate from the rat spinal dorsal horn in vitro by activation of low- and high-threshold primary afferent fibres Modulation by μ opioids. Brain Res 553:347–352

Karlsten R, Gordh T, Hartvig P, Post C (1990) Effects of intrathecal injection of the adenosine receptor agonists R-phenylisopropyl-adenosine and N-ethylcarboxamide-adenosine on nociception and motor function in the rat. Anesth Analg 71:60–64

Kehl LJ, Gogas KR, Lichtblau L, Pollack CH, Mayes M, Basbaum AI, Wilcox GL (1991) The NMDA antagonist MK801 reduces noxious stimulus-evoked FOS expression in the spinal cord dorsal horn. In: Bond MR, Charlton JR, Woolf CJ (eds) Proceedings of the 4th World Congress on Pain. Elsevier, Amsterdam

Kim SH, Chung JM (1992) An experimental model for peripheral neuropathy produced by segmental spinal nerve ligation in the rat. Pain 50:355–363

King AE, Lopez-Garcia JA (1993) Excitatory amino acid receptor-mediated neurontransmission from cutaneous afferents in rat dorsal horn in vitro. J Physiol (Lond) 472:443–457

King AE, Thompson SWN, Urban L, Woolf CJ (1988) An intracellular analysis of amino acid induced excitations of deep dorsal horn neurones in the rat spinal cord slice. Neurosci Lett 89:286–292

Kitto KF, Haley JE, Wilcox GL (1992) Involvement of nitric oxide in spinally mediated in the mouse. Neurosci Lett 148:1–5

Kolhekar R, Gebhart GF (1994) NMDA and quisqualate modulation of visceral nocieption in the rat. Brain Res 651:215–226

Kolhekar R, Meller ST, Gebhart GF (1993) Characterization of the role of spinal N-methyl-d-aspartate receptors in thermal nociception in the rat. Neuroscience 57:385–395

Kolhekar R, Meller ST, Gebhart GF (1994) N-methyl-d-aspartate receptor-mediated changes in thermal nociception: allosteric modulation at glycine and polyamine recognition sites. Neuroscience 63:925–936

Kombian SB, Malenka RC (1994) Simultaneous LTP on non-NMDA-and LTD of NMDA-receptor-medicated responses in the nucleus accumbens. Nature 368:242–246

Kornhuber J, Quack G (1995) Cerebrospinal fluid and serum concentrations of the N-methyl-d-aspartate (NMDA) receptor antagonist memantine in man. Neurosci Lett 195:137–139

Lambolez B, Curutchet P, Stinnakre J, Bregestovski P, Rossier J, Prado de Carvalho L (1991) Electrophysiological and pharmacological properties of GluR1, a subunit of a glutamate receptor-channel expressed in Xenopus oocytes. Neurosci Lett 123:69–72

Leeson PD, Iversen LL (1994) The glycine site on the NMDA receptor: structure-activity relationships and therapeutic potential. J Med Chem 37:4053–4067

Lodge D, Johnson KM (1990) Noncompetitive excitatory amino acid receptor antagonists. Trends Pharmacol Sci 11:81–86

Long SK, Smith DAS, Siarey RJ, Evans RH (1990) Effect of 6-cyano-2,3-dihydroxy-7-nitro-quinoxaline (CNQX) on dorsal root-, NMDA-, kainate-and quisqualate-mediated depolarization of rat motoneurones in vitro. Br J Pharmacol 100:850–854

Loscher W, Fredow G, Ganter M (1991) Comparison of pharmacodynamic effects of the non-competitive NMDA receptor antagonists MK-801 and ketamine in pigs. Eur J Pharmacol 192:377–382

MacDonald JF, Nowak LM (1990) Mechanisms of blockade of excitatory amino acid receptor channels. Trends Pharmacol Sci 11:167–172

Malcangio M, Bowery N (1994) Spinal cord SP release and hyperalgesia in monoarthritic rats; involvement of the GABAB receptor system. Br J Pharmacol 113:1561–1566

Malmberg AB, Yaksh TL (1992a) Hyperalgesia mediated by spinal glutamate or substance P receptor blocked by spinal cyclooxygenase inhibition. Science 257:1276–1279

Malmberg AB, Yaksh TL (1992b) Antinociceptive actions of spinal non-steroidal anti-inflammatory agents on the formalin test in the rat. J Pharmacol Exp Ther 263:136–146

Malmberg AB, Yaksh TL (1993a) Pharmacology of the spinal action of ketorolac, morphine, ST-91, U50488H, and L-PIA on the formalin test and an isobolographic analysis of the NSAID interaction. Anesthesiology 79:270–281

Malmberg AB, Yaksh TL (1993b) Spinal nitric oxide synthesis inhibition blocks NMDA-induced thermal hyperalgesia and produces antinociception in the formalin test in rats. Pain 54:291–300

Manzoni OJ, Manabe T, Nicoll RA (1994) Release of adenosine by activation of NMDA receptors in the hippocampus. Science 265:2098–2101

Mao J, Price DD, Mayer DJ, Lu J, Hayes RL (1992a) Intrathecal MK801 and local nerve anesthesia synergistically reduce nociceptive behaviors in rats with experimental mononeuropathy. Brain Res 576:254–262

Mao J, Price DD, Hayes RL, Lu J, Mayer DJ (1992b) Differential roles of NMDA and non-NMDA receptor activation in induction and maintenance of thermal hyprealgesia in rats with painful peripheral mononeuropathy. Brain Res 598:271–278

Mao J, Price DD, Hayes RL, Lu J, Mayer DJ, Frank H (1993) Intrathecal treatment with dextrophan or ketamine potently reduces pain-related behaviours in a rat model of peripheral mononeuropathy. Brain Res 605:164–168

Mathisen LC, Skjelbred P, Skoglund LA, Oye I (1995) Effect of ketamine, an NMDA receptor inhibitor, in acute and chronic orofacial pain. Pain 61:215–220

Maurset A, Skoglund LA, Hustveit O, Oye I (1989) Comparison of ketamine and pethidine in experimental and postoperative pain. Pain 36:37–41

Maxwell DJ, Christie WM, Short AD, Storm-Mathison J, Ottersen D (1990) Central boutons of glomeruli in the spinal cord of the cat are enriched with l-glutamate-like immunoreactivity. Neuroscience 36:83–104

Mayer ML, Westbrook GL (1987) Permeation and block of N-methyl-d-aspartic acid receptor channels by divalent cations in mouse cultured central neurones. J Physiol (Lond) 394:501–527

McMahon SB, Lewin GR, Wall PD (1993) Central excitability triggered by noxious inputs. Curr Opin Neurobiol 3:602–610

McMahon SB, Dmitriveva N, Koltzenburg M (1995) Visceral pain. Br J Anaesth 75:132–144

McQuay H, Dickenson AH (1990) Implications of central nervous system plasticity for pain management. Anaesthesia 45:101–102

McQuay H, Carroll D, Jadad AR, Glynn CJ, Jack T, Moore RA, Wiffen PJ (1994) Dextromethorphan for the treatment of neuropathic pain: a double-blind randomized controlled crossover trial with integral n-of-1 design. Pain 59:127–133

Meller ST, Gebhart GF (1993) Nitric oxide (NO) and nociceptive processing in the spinal cord. Pain 52:127–136

Meller ST, Dykstra C, Gebhart GF (1992a) Production of endogenous nitric oxide and activation of soluble guanylate cyclase are required for NMDA-produced facilitation of the nociceptive tail-flick reflex. Eur J Pharmacol 214:93–96

Meller ST, Pechman PS, Gebhart GF, Maves TJ (1992b) Nitric oxide mediates the thermal hyperalgesia produced in a model of neuropathic pain in the rat. Neuroscience 50:7–10

Meller ST, Cummings CP, Traub RJ, Gebhart GF (1994) The role of nitric oxide in the development and maintenance of the hyperalgesia produced by intraplantar injection of carrageenan in the rat. Neuroscience 60:367–374

Mendell LM (1966) Physiological properties of unmyelinated fibre projections to the spinal cord. Exp Neurol 16:316–332

Merighi A, Polak JM, Theodosis DT (1991) Ultrastructural visualisation of glutamate and aspartate immunoreactivities in the rat dorsal horn, with special reference to the co-localisation of glutamate, substance P and calcitonin-gene related peptide. Neuroscience 40:67–80

Millan MJ, Seguin L (1993) (+)-HA 966, a partial agonist at the glycine site coupled to NMDA receptors, blocks formalin-induced pain in mice. Eur J Pharmacol 238:445–447

Millan MJ, Seguin L (1994) Chemically-diverse ligands at the glycine B site coupled to N-methyl-d-aspartate (NMDA) receptors selectively block the late phase of formalin-induced pain in mice. Neurosci Lett 178:139–143

Miller KE, Clements JR, Larson AA, Beitz AJ (1988) Organization of glutamate-like immunoreactivity in the rat superficial dorsal horn: light and electron microscopic observations. J Comp Neurol 2:28–36

Miller KE, Douglas VD, Kaneko T (1993) Glutaminase immunoreactive neurons in the rat dorsal root ganglion contain calcitonin gene-related peptide (CGRP). Neurosci Lett 160:113–116

Mjellem-Joly N, Lund A, Berge O-G, Hole K (1992) Intrathecal co-administration of substance P and NMDA augments nociceptive responses in the formalin. Pain 51:195–198

Momiyama A, Feldmeyer D, Cull-Candy SG (1996) Identification of a low-conductance NMDA channel with reduced sensitivity to Mg^{++} in rat central neurones. J Physiol (Lond) 494:479–492

Moore PK, Oluyomi AO, Babbedge RC, Wallace P, Hart SL (1991) l-N^G-nitro arginine methyl ester exhibits antinociceptive activity in the mouse. Br J Pharmacol 102: 198–202

Moore PK, Babbedge RC, Wallace P, Gaffen ZA, Hart SL (1993) 7-Nitroindazole, an inhibitor of nitric oxide synthase, exhibits anti-nociceptive activity in the mouse without increasing blood pressure. Br J Pharmacol 108:296–297

Morgan JI (1991) Discussions in neuroscience, proto-oncogene expression in the nervous system, vol VII, no 4. Elsevier, Amsterdam

Morris R (1989) Responses of spinal dorsal horn neurones evoked by myelinated primary afferent stimulation are blocked by excitatory amino acid antagonists acting at kainate/quisqualate receptors. Neurosci Lett 105:79–85

Nagy JI, Daddona PE (1985) Anatomical and cytochemical relationships of adenosine deaminase-containing primary afferent neurones in the rat. Neuroscience 15:799–813

Nagy JI, Buss M, Labella LA, Daddona PE (1984) Immunohistochemical localization of adenosine deaminase in primary afferent neurons of the rat. Neurosci Lett 48:133–138

Nagy JI, Maggi CA, Dray A, Woolf CJ, Urban L (1993) The role of neurokinin and N-methyl d-aspartate receptors in synaptic transmission from capsaicin-sensitive primary afferents in the rat spinal cord in vitro. Neuroscience 52:1029–1037

Nahin RL, Hylden JLK (1991) Peripehal inflammation is associated with increased glutamic acid decarboxylase immunoreactivity in the rat spinal cord. Neurosci Lett 128:226–230

Neugebauer V, Kornhuber J, Lucke, Schaible H-G (1993a) The clinically available NMDA receptor antagonist memantine is antinociceptive on rat spinal neurones. Neuroreport 4:1259–1262

Neugebauer V, Lucke T, Schaible H-G (1993b) Differential effects of N-methyl-D-aspartate (NMDA) and non-NMDA receptor antagonists on the responses of rat spinal neurones with joint input. Neurosci Lett 155:29–32

Neugebauer V, Lucke T, Schaible HG (1994) Requirement of metabotropic glutamate receptors for the generation of inflammation-evoked hyperexcitability in rat spinal cord neurons. Eur J Neurosci 6:1179–1186

Olney JW (1990) Excitotoxic amino-acids and neuropsychiatric disorders. Annu Rev Pharmacol Toxicol 30:47–71

Parsons CG, Gruner R, Rozental (1994) Comparative patch clamp studies on the kinetics and selectivity of glutamate receptor antagonism by 2,3-dihydroxy-6-nitro-7-sulfamoyl-benzo(F)quinoxaline (NBQX) and 1-(4-Amino-phenyl)-4-methyl-7,8-methyl-endioxyl-5H-2,3-benzodiazepine (GYKI 52466). Neuropharmacology 33(5):589–604

Parsons CG, Quack G, Bresink I, Baran L, Przegalinski E, Kostowski W, KrzascikP, Hartmann S, Danysz W (1995) Comparison of the potency, kinetics and voltage-dependency of a series of uncompetitive NMDA receptor antagonists in vitro with anticonvulsive and motor impairment activity in vivo. Neuropharmacology 34: 1239–1258

Porro CA, Cavazzuti M (1993) Spatial and temporal aspects of spinal cord and brainstem activation in the formalin pain model. Prog Neurobiol 41:565–607

Portenoy RK, Foley KM, Inturrisi CE (1990) The nature of opioid responsiveness and its implications for neuropathic pain: new hypotheses derived from studies of opioid infusions. Pain 43:273–286

Price DD, Wu JW, Dubner R, Gracely RH (1977) Peripheral suppression of first pain and central summation of second pain evoked by noxious heat pulses. Pain 3:57–68

Price DD, Mao J, Mayer DJ (1994a) Central neural mechanisms of normal and abnormal pain states. In: Fields HL, Liebeskind JC (eds) Pharmacological approaches to the treatment of chronic pain: new concepts and critical issues. Progress in pain research and management, vol 1. International Association for the Study of Pain, Seattle, pp 61–84

Price DD, Mao J, Frenk H, Mayer DJ (1994b) The N-methyl-d-aspartate antagonist dextromethorphan selectively reduces temporal summation of second pain. Pain 59:165–174

Qian J, Brown SD, Carlton SM (1996) Systemic ketamine attenuates nociceptive behaviors in a rat model of peripheral neuropathy. Brain Res 715:51–62

Radhakrishnan V, Henry JL (1993a) l-NAME blocks responses to NMDA, substance P and noxious cutaneous stimuli in cat dorsal horn. Neuroreport 4:323–326

Radhakrishnan V, Henry JL (1993b) Excitatory amino acid receptor mediation of sensory inputs to functionally identified dorsal horn neurons in cat spinal cord. Neuroscience 55:531–544

Raigorodsky G, Urca G (1987) Intrathecal N-methyl-d-aspartate (NMDA) activates both nociceptive and antinociceptive systems. Brain Res 422:158–162

Randic M, Hecimovic H, Ryu PD (1990) Substance P modulates glutamate-induced currents in the acutely isolated rat spinal dorsal horn neurons. Neurosci Lett 117:74–80

Reeve AJ, Dickenson AH (1995) The roles of adenosine in the control of acute and more persistent nociceptive responses of dorsal horn neurones in the anaesthetized rat. Br J Pharmacol 116:2221–2228

Ren K, Dubner R (1993) NMDA receptor antagonists attenuate mechanical hyperalgesia in rats with unilateral inflamation of the hindpaw. Neurosci Lett 163:22–26

Ren K, Hylden JLK, Williams GM, Ruda MA, Dubner R (1992a) The effects of a non-competitive NMDA receptor antagonist, MK-801, on behavioural hyperalgesia and dorsal horn neuronal activity in rats with unilateral inflammation. Pain 50:331–344

Ren K, Williams GM, Hylden JKL, Ruda MA, Dubner R (1992b) The intrathecal administration of excitatory amino acid receptor antagonists selectively attenuated carrageenan-induced behavioral hyperalgesia in rats. Eur J Pharmacol 219:235–243

Rice ASC, McMahon SB (1994) Pre-emptive intrathecal administration of an NMDA receptor antagonist (AP-5) prevents hyper-reflexia in a model of persistent visceral pain. Pain 57:335–340

Rogawski MA (1993) Therapeutic potential of excitatory amino acid antagonists; channel blockers and 2,3-benzodiazepines. Trends Pharmacol Sci 14:325–331

Rowan S, Todd AJ, Spike RC (1993) Evidence that neuropeptide Y is present in GABAergic neurons in the superficial dorsal horn of the rat spinal cord. Neuroscience 53:537–545

Roytblat L, Korotkouchko A, Katz J, Glazer M, Greenberg L, Fisher A (1993) Postoperative pain: the effect of low-dose ketamine in addition to general anaesthesia. Anesth Analg 77:1161–1165

Rupniak NMJ, Boyce S, Tye S, Cook G, Iversen SD (1993) Anxiolytic-like and antinociceptive effects of MK-801 accompanied by sedation and ataxia in primates. Pharmacol Biochem Behav 44:153–156

Rusin KI, Jiang MC, Cerne R, Randic M (1993) Interactions between excitatory amino acids and tachykinins in the rat spinal dorsal horn. Brain Res Bull 30:329–338

Rusin KI, Ryu PD, Randic M (1992) Modulation of excitatory amino acid responses in rat dorsal horn neurons by tachykinins. J Neurophysiol 68:265–286

Saito S, Kidd GJ, Trapp BD, Dawson TM, Bredt DS, Wilson DA, Traystman RJ, Snyder SH, Hanley DF (1994) Rat spinal cord neurons contain nitric oxide synthase. Neuroscience 59:447–456

Salt TE (1987) Excitatory amino-acid receptors and synaptic transmission in the rat ventrobasal thalamus. J Physiol (Lond) 391:499–510

Salt TE, Eaton SA (1991) Sensory excitatory postsynaptic potentials mediated by NMDA and non-NMDA receptors in the thalamus in vivo. Eur J Neurosci 3:296–300

Salter MW, Henry JL (1987) Evidence that adenosine mediates the depression of spinal dorsal horn neurones induced by peripheral vibration in the cat. Neuroscience 22:631–650

Salter MW, De Koninck Y, Henry JL (1993) Physiological roles for adenosine and ATP in synaptic transmission in the spinal dorsal horn. Prog Neurobiol 41:125–156

Sawynok J (1987) GABAergic mechanisms of analgesia; an update. Pharmacol Biochem Behav 26:463–474

Sawynok J, Sweeney MI (1989) The role of purines in nociception. Neuroscience 32:557–569

Schaible HG, Grubb BD, Neugebauer V, Oppmann M (1991) The effects of NMDA antagonists on neuronal activity in cat spinal cord evoked by acute inflammation in the knee joint. Eur J Neurosci 3:981–991

Schaible HG, Hope PJ, Lang CW, Duggan AW (1992) Calcitonin gene related peptide causes intespinal spreading of substance P produced by peripheral stimulation. Eur J Neurosci 4:750–757

Seeburg PH (1993) The molecular biology of mammalian glutamate receptor channels. Trends Pharmacol Sci 14:297–303

Seguin L, Le Marouille-Girardon S, Millan MJ (1995) Antinociceptive profiles of non-peptidergic neurokinin1 and neurokinin2 receptor antagonists: a comparison to other classes of antinociceptive agent. Pain 61:325–343

Seltzer Z, Beilin BZ, Ginzburg R, Paran Y, Shimko T (1991a) The role of injury discharge in the induction of neuropathic pain behavior in rats. Pain 46:327–336

Seltzer Z, Cohn S, Ginzburg R, Beilin BZ (1991b) Modulation of neuropathic pain in rats by spinal disinhibition and NMDA receptor blockade of injury discharge. Pain 45:69–76

Semos ML, Headley PM (1994) The role of nitric oxide in spinal nociceptive reflexes in rats with neurogenic and non-neurogenic peripheral inflammation. Neuropharmacology 33:1487–1497

Shaw PJ, Ince PG, Johnson M, Perry EK, Candy J (1991) The quantitative autoradiographic distribution of [3H] MK-801 binding sites in the normal human spinal spinal cord. Brain Res 539:164–168

Sheardown MJ, Nielsen EO, Hansen AJ, Jacobsen P, Honoré T (1990) 2,3-Dihydroxy-6-nitro-7-sulfamoylbenzo(f)-quinoxaline: a neuroprotectant for cerebral ischaemia. Science 247:571–574

Sher G, Mitchell D (1990a) N-Methyl-d-aspartate receptors mediate responses of rat dorsal horn neurones to hindlimb ischaemia. Brain Res 522:55–62

Sher GD, Mitchell D (1990b) Intrathecal N-methyl-d-aspartate induces hyperexcitability in rat dorsal horn convergent neurones. Neurosci Lett 119:199–202

Shigemoto R, Ohishi H, Nakanishi S, Mizuno N (1992) Expression of the mRNA for the rat NMDA receptor (NMDAR1) in the sensory and autonomic ganglion neurons. Neurosci Letts 144:229–232

Sieghart W (1992) GABAA receptors: ligand-gated Cl⁻ channels modulated by multiple drug-binding sites. Trends Pharmacol Sci 13:446–451

Simmons DR, Spike RC, Todd AJ (1995) Galanin is contained in GABAergic neurons in the rat spinal dorsal horn. Neurosci Lett 187:119–122

Sivilotti L, Woolf CJ (1994) The contribution of GABAA and glycine receptors to central sensitization: disinhibition and touch-evoked allodynia in the spinal cord. J Neurophysiol 72:169–179

Sluka KA, Westlund KN (1993) Spinal cord amino acid release and content in an arthritis model: the effect of pretreatment with non-NMDA, NMDA, and NK1 receptor antagonists. Brain Res 627:89–103

Sluka KA, Jordan HH, Willis WD, Westlund KN (1994a) Differential effects of N-methyl-d-aspartate (NMDA) and non-NMDA receptor antagonists on spinal release of amino acids after development of acute arthritis in rats. Brain Res 664:77–84

Sluka KA, Willis WD, Westlund KN (1994b) Inflammation-induced release of excitatory amino acids is prevented by spinal administration of a GABAA but not by a GABA$_B$ receptor antagonist in rats. J Pharmacol Exp Ther 271:76–82

Smith GD, Wiseman J, Harrison SM, Elliott PJ, Birch PJ (1994) Pre treatment with MK-801, a non-competitive NMDA antagonist, prevents development of mechanical hyperalgesia in a rat model of chronic neuropathy, but not in a model of chronic inflammation. Neurosci Lett 165:79–83

Sorkin LS (1993) NMDA evokes an l-NAME sensitive spinal release of glutamate and citrulline. Neuroreport 4:479–482

Sorkin LS, Westlund KN, Sluka KA, Dougherty PM, Willis WD (1992) Neural changes in acute arthritis in monkeys. IV time-course of amino acid release into the lumbar dorsal horn. Brain Res Rev 17:39–50

Sosnowski M, Yaksh TL (1989) Role of spinal adenosine receptors in modulating the hyperesthesia produced by spinal glycine receptor antagonism. Anesth Analg 69:587–592

Sosnowski M, Stevens CW, Yaksh TL (1989) Assessment of the role of A1/A2 adenosine receptors mediating the purine antinociception, motor and autonomic function in the rat spinal cord. J Pharmacol Exp Ther 250:915–922

Stanfa LC, Dickenson AH (1997) Wind-up in the rat dorsal horn is largely independent of AMPA receptor activation. Eur J Pharmacol (in press)

Stanfa LC, Sullivan AF, Dickenson AH (1992) Alterations in neuronal excitability and the potency of spinal mu, delta and kappa opioids after carrageenan-induced inflammation. Pain 50:345–354

Stanfa LC, Dickenson AH, Xu X-J, Wiesenfeld-Hallin Z (1994) Cholecystokinin and morphine analgesia: variations on a theme. Trends Pharmacol Sci 15:65–66

Stanfa LC, Misra C, Dickenson AH (1996) Amplification of spinal nociceptive transmission depends on the generation of nitric oxide in normal and carrageenan. Brain Res 737:92–98

Stannard CF, Porter GE (1993) Ketamine hydrochloride in the treatment of phantom limb pain. Pain 54:227–230

Sugimoto T, Bennett GJ, Kajander KC (1989) Strychnine-enhanced transsynaptic degeneration of dorsal horn neurons in rats with an experimental painful neuropathy. Neurosci Lett 98:139–143

Sweeney MI, White TD, Sawynok J (1989) Morphine, capsaicin and K+ release purines from capsaicin-sensitive primary afferent nerve terminals in the spinal cord. J Pharmacol Exp Ther 248:447–454

Tal M, Bennett GJ (1993) Dextrophan relieves neuropathic heat-evoked hyperalgesia in the rat. Neurosci Lett 151:107–110

Tallaksen-Greene SJ, Young AB, Penney JB, Beitz AJ (1992) Excitatory amino acid binding sites in the trigeminal principal sensory and spinal trigeminal nuclei of the rat. Neurosci Lett 141:79–83

Taylor BK, Peterson MA, Basbaum AI (1995) Persistent cardiovascular and behavioral responses to subcutaneous formalin require peripheral nerve input. J Neurosci 15:7575–7584

Thompson SWN, King AE, Woolf CJ (1990) Activity-dependent changes in rat ventral horn neurons in vitro; summation of prolonged afferent evoked postsynaptic depolarizations produce a d-2-amino-5-phosphonovaleric acid sensitive windup. Eur J Neurosci 2:638–649

Thompson SWN, Gerber G, Sivilotti LG, Woolf CJ (1992) Long duration ventral root potentials in the neonatal rat spinal cord in vitro: the effects of inonotrophic and metabotropic excitatory amino acid receptor antagonists. Brain Res 595:87–97

Thompson SWN, Urban L, Dray A (1993) A contribution of NK1 and NK$_2$ receptor activation to high threshold afferent fibre evoked ventral root responses in the rat spinal cord. Brain Res 625:100–108

Thompson SWN, Dray A, Urban L (1994) Injury-induced activity of spinal reflex activity: NK1 neurokinin receptor activation and enhanced A- and C-fiber mediated responses in the rat spinal cord in vitro. J Neurosci 14:3672–3687

Thompson SWN, Babbedge R, Levers T, Dray A, Urban L (1995) No evidence for contribution of nitric oxide to spinal reflex activity in the rat spinal cord in vitro. Neurosci Lett 188:121–124

Tjolsen A, Berge OG, Hunskaar S, Rosland JH, Hole K (1988) The formalin test: an evaluation of the method. Pain 51:5–17

Todd AJ, Spike RC (1992) Immunohistochemical evidence that Met-enkephalin and GABA coexist in some neurones in rat dorsal horn. Brain Res 584:149–156

Todd AJ, Watt C, Spike RC, Sieghart W (1996) Colocalization of GABA, glycine, and their receptors at synapses in the rat spinal cord. J Neurosci 16:974–982

Tohyama M, Kiyama H, Satoh K, Araki T, Maeno H, Oyamada H, Kondo E (1994) Glutaminergic neurotransmission, proto-oncogenes and pain. In: Gebhart GF, Hammond DL, Jensen T (eds) Proceedings of the 7th World Congress on Pain, vol 2. International Association for the Study of Pain, Seattle, pp 395–408

Tolle TR, Berthele A, Zieglgansberger W, Seeburg PH, Wisden W (1993) The differential expression of 16 NMDA and non-NMDA receptor subunits in the rat spinal cord and in periaqueductal gray. J Neurosci 13:5009–5028

Tölle TR, Castro-Lopes JM, Evan G, Zieglgänsberger W (1991) C-fos induction in the spinal cord following noxious stimulation: prevention by opiates but not by NMDA antagonists. In: Bond MR, Charlton JR, Woolf CJ (eds) Proceedings of the 4th World Congress on Pain. Elsevier, Amsterdam, p 299

Traub RJ, Solodkin A, Meller, ST, Gebhart GF (1994) Spinal cord NADPH-diaphorase histochemical staining but nitric oxide synthase immunoreactivity increases following carrageenan-produced hindpaw inflammation in the rat. Brain Res 668:204–210

Tverskoy M, Oz Y, Isakson A, Finger J, Bradley EL, Kissin I (1994) Preemptive effect of fentanyl and ketamine on postoperative pain and wound hyperalgesia. Anesth Analg 78:205–209

Urban L, Thompson SWN, Dray A (1994) Modulation of spinal excitability: cooperation between neurokinin and excitatory amino acid neurotransmitters. Trends Neurosci 17:432–438

Vaccarino AL, Marek P, Kest B, Weber E, Keana JFW, Liebeskind JC (1993) NMDA receptor antagonists, MK-801 and ACEA-1011, prevent the development of tonic pain following subsutaneous formalin. Brain Res 615:331–334

Valtschanoff JG, Weinberg RJ, Rustioni A, Schmidt HH (1992) Nitric oxide synthase and GABA colocalize in lamina II of rat spinal cord. Neurosci Lett 148:6–10

Watanabe M, Mishina M, Inoue Y (1994) Distinct spatiotemporal distributions of the N-methyl-d-aspartate receptor channel subunit mRNAs in the mouse cervical spinal cord J Comp Neurol 345:314–319

Watkins J, Collingridge G (1994) Phenylglycine derivative as antagonists of metatotropic glutamate receptors. Trends Pharm Sci 15:333–342

Watkins JC, Krogsgaard-Larsen P, Honore T (1990) Structure-activity relationships in the development of excitatory amino acid agonists and competitive antagonists. Trends Pharmacol Sci 11:25–33

Westlund KN, SunYC, Sluka KA, Dougherty PM, Sorkin LS, Willis WD (1992) Neural changes in acute arthritis in monkeys. II. Increased glutamate immunoreactivity inthe medial articular nerve. Brain Res Rev 17:15–27

Willetts J, Balster RL, Leander D (1990) The behavioral pharmacology of NMDA receptor antagonists. Trends Pharmacol Sci 11:423–428

Williams (1991) Adenosine receptor agonists and antagonists. In: Stone T (ed) Adenosine in the nervous system. Academic, London, pp 137–171

Wisden W, Errington ML, Williams S, Dunnett SB, Waters C, Ditchcock D, Evan G, Bliss TVP, Hunt SP (1990) Differential expression of immediate early genes in the hippocampus and spinal cord. Neuron 4:603–614

Woolf CJ (1983) Evidence for a central component of post-injury pain hypersensitivity. Nature 221:313–328

Woolf CJ (1995) Somatic pain – pathogenesis and prevention. Br J Anaesth 75:169–176

Woolf CJ, Doubell TP (1994) The pathophysiology of chronic pain – increased sensitivity to low threshold $A\beta$-fiber inputs. Curr Opin Neurobiol 4:525–534

Woolf CJ, Thompson SWN (1991) The induction and maintenance of central sensitization is dependent on N-methyl-d-aspartic acid receptor activation; implications for the treatment of post-injury hypersensitivity states. Pain 44:293–299

Woolf CJ, Wall PD (1986) Morphine sensitive and morphine insensitive actions of C-fibre input on the rat spinal cord. Neurosci Lett 64:221–225

Xu X-J, Dalsgaard C-J, Wiesenfeld-Hallin Z (1992) Spinal substance P and N-methyl-d-aspartate receptors are coactivated in the induction of central sensitization of the nociceptive flexor reflex. Neuroscience 51:641–648

Xu X-J, Hoa J-X, Seiger A, Wiesenfeld-Hallin Z (1993) Systemic excitatory amino acid receptor antagonists of the α-amino-3-hydroxy-5-methyl-4-isoxazolepropionic acid (AMPA) receptor and of the N-methyl-d-aspartate (NMDA) receptor relieve mechanical hypersensitivity after transient spinal cord ischemia in rats. J Pharmacol Exp Ther 267:140–144

Xu X-J, Zhang X, Hokfelt T, Wiesenfeld-Hallin Z (1995) Plasticity in spinal nociception after peripheral nerve section: reduced effectiveness of the NMDA receptor antagonist MK-801 in blocking wind-up and central sensitization of the flexor reflex. Brain Res 670:342–346

Yaksh TL (1989) Behavioural and autonomic correlates of the tactile evoked allodynia produced by spinal glycine inhibition: effects of modulatory receptor systems and excitatory amino acid antagonists. Pain 37:111–123

Yaksh TL, Malmberg AB (1994) Interaction of spinal modulatory systems. In: Fields HL, Liebeskind JC (eds) Progress in pain research and management. International Association for the Study of Pain, Seattle, pp 151–171

Yamamoto T, Yaksh TL (1992a) Studies on the spinal interaction of morphine and the NMDA antagonist MK-801 on the hyperesthesia observed in a rat model of sciatic mononeuropathy. Neurosci Lett 1992:135:67–70

Yamamoto T, Yaksh TL (1992b) Spinal pharmacology of thermal hyperesthesia induced by constriction injury of sciatic nerve excitatory amino acid antagonists. Pain 49:121–128

Yamamoto T, Yaksh TL (1993) Effects of intrathecal strychnine and bicuculline on nerve compresion-induced thermal hyperalgesia and selective antagonism by MK-801. Pain 54:79–84

Yamamoto T, Shimoyama N, Mizuguchi T (1993) The effects of morphine, MK-801, an NMDA antagonist, and CP-96,345, an NK1 antagonist, on the hyperesthesia evoked by carrageenan injection in the rat paw. Anesthesiology 78 124–133

Yashpal K, Radhakrishnan V, Henry JL (1991) NMDA receptor antagonist blocks the facilitation of the tail flick relex in the rat induced by intrathecal administration of substance P and by noxious cutaneous stimulation. Neurosci Lett 128:269–272

Yoshimura M, Jessell T (1990) Amino acid-mediated EPSPs at primary afferent synapses with substantia gelatinosa neurones in the rat spinal cord. J Physiol (Lond) 430:315–335

Young, MR, Fleetwood-Walker, M, Mitchell R, Munro FE (1994) Evidence for a role of metabotropic glutamate receptors in sustained nociceptive inputs to rat dorsal horn neurons Neuropharmacology 33:141–144

Young MR, Fleetwood-Walker SM, Mitchell R, Dickenson T (1995) The involvement of metabotropic glutamate receptors and their intracellular signalling pathways in sustained nociceptive transmission in rat dorsal horn neurons. Neuropharmacology 34:1033–1041

CHAPTER 9
Novel Modulators in Nociception

X.-J. Xu and Z. Wiesenfeld-Hallin

A. Introduction

As novel modulators in nociception, the three messengers discussed in this chapter – one gas (nitric oxide) and two peptides (cholecystokinin and galanin) – have a number of characteristics in common. First, the presence of these messengers in the nervous system has been discovered only in the past one or two decades. Second, their roles in nociceptive transmission and modulation have been extensively studied only in recent years. Third, the expression of all three substances becomes greatly increased in sensory neurons after peripheral nerve injury. There is ample evidence that nerve injury or inflammation induces dramatic morphological and functional plasticity in the nervous system, and such plasticity plays a vital part in the development of chronic pain states known to be associated with these pathological states (WILLIS 1994; HÖKFELT et al. 1994). Thus because of the apparent involvement of these messengers in neuronal plasticity they may be important targets for the development of novel analgesics.

B. Nitric Oxide

NO, a simple gas, has emerged as a unique regulatory molecule and has been implicated in diverse physiological functions (see MONCADA et al. 1991; DAWSON and SNYDER 1994 for review). NO was initially identified as the mediator for macrophages by which they exert their tumoricidal and bactericidal effects. NO is a mediator in endothelial cells where it has been identified as the endothelial-derived relaxing factor. NO has also been recognized to have a prominent role in the nervous system, both as an intracellular second messenger and as a neurotransmitter.

As a neuronal messenger NO has interesting features. NO can simply diffuse from nerve terminals, as opposed to classical neurotransmitters which are stored in synaptic vesicles and are released by exocytosis. Consequently the movement of NO after synthesis is interesting as it can diffuse quickly in both aqueous and lipid environments (see illustrations in MELLER and GEBHART 1993). NO can act on intracellular targets (i.e., stay in the same cell where it is produced) or diffuse from nerve terminals where it is produced and act on postsynaptic neurons (i.e., behave more as a classical transmitter). NO can also diffuse form its site of production to influence adjacent neurons or glia. Finally, NO synthesized in postsynaptic neurons upon synaptic activation may diffuse to act on presynaptic terminals (i.e., acting as a retrograde transmitter). The latter property of NO suggests that it may be a suitable mediator for synaptic plasticity and long-term potentiation. NO does not undergo reversible receptor interaction but forms covalent linkages with its potential target including but not confined to enzymes such as guanylyl cyclase (GC). The activation of GC and increased cGMP levels appears to be the major cellular response to NO in the nervous system, although NO may have other targets whose action in independent of the production of cGMP (see Dawson and Snyder 1994 for review).

I. Nitric Oxide Synthase

NO synthase (NOS) is a family of enzymes responsible for the synthesis of NO. Many isoforms of NOS have been suggested to exist, and a number have been identified and cloned (Bredt and Synder 1989; Förstermann et al. 1991; Marleta 1993). Three major isoforms are widely recognized: neuronal NOS (also known as type I), macrophage- and non-macrophage-inducible NOS (type II) and endothelial NOS (type III). The neuronal NOS and endothelial NOS are constitutive in the sense that their activation does not require new protein synthesis, although they are also inducible in response to certain stimuli. On the other hand, macrophage, astrocytes, and microglia do not contain detectable levels of NOS protein under normal conditions but express NOS upon stimulation with cytokines (Dawson and Snyder 1994).

The modulation of NOS activity is complex. All isoforms of NOS use free L-arginine and molecular oxygen as substrates to generate NO and L-citrulline, requiring nicotinamide adenine dinucleotide phosphate (NADPH), flavins, and tetrahydrobiopterin as cofactors. The constitutive forms of NOS are activated by increase in intracellular Ca^{2+} via a calmodulin-sensitive site on the enzyme. The inducible form of NOS does not respond to Ca^{2+} but instead is induced by endotoxins and cytokines via regulation at the level of gene transcription. NOS activity can also be modulated by phosphorylation by protein kinase. Recently NOS was found to contain heme, which reacts with CO and NO to inhibit NOS activity. Thus there appear to exist negative feedback mechanisms whereby NO or cGMP inhibit NOS activity (see Dawson and Snyder 1994 for review).

Numerous approaches have been adapted to pharmacologically alter the NO system. Precursors and donors of NO, such as L-arginine, can be used to increase the amounts of NO. Conversely, a number of NOS inhibitors have been developed to block endogenous synthesis of NO. Compounds which block GC, such as methylene blue, have also been employed to interfere with the NO-cGMP pathway. The first generation of NOS inhibitors, such as N^G-monomethyl-L-arginine, N-iminoethyl-l-ornithine, and N^G-nitro-L-arginine methylester (L-NAME) are L-arginine analogues which are specific and potent, and some are orally active and able to penetrate the blood-brain barrier. However, these compounds do not show selectivity towards various isoforms of NOS. This may lead to confounding results as in some systems NO generated by different NOSs may result in opposite physiological effects. There are some recently developed NOS inhibitors, such as 7-nitroindazole (Babbedge et al. 1993), which are reported to have more selective action on neuronal isoform of NOSs. It is also now possible to generate genetically engineered mutant mice which lack various isoforms of NOS. These new developments should aid the elucidation of the role of NO under physiological and pathophysiological conditions.

II. Distribution of NOS in Pathways Related to Nociception

The purification of NOSs has allowed the generation of antibodies against various isoforms of NOS and the subsequent visualization of NOS-like immunoreactivity (LI) in the nervous system by immunohistochemical methods. This has been accompanied by in situ hybridization which enables the localization of NOS mRNA. The presence of NADPH diaphorase has also been used as a marker for NOS activity, but the specificity of this approach has recently been questioned (Vizzard et al. 1994).

1. Dorsal Root Ganglia

Dorsal root ganglia (DRG) of rats have been shown to contain variable amounts of NADPH diaphorase, with higher proportion of positive neuronal cell bodies detected in the lumbosacral, thoracic, and nodose ganglia than at other levels (Aimi et al. 1991). In contrast, lumbar and trigeminal ganglia contain very few NADPH diaphorase positive cells. This uneven distribution has been confirmed with in situ hybridization and immunohistochemistry using antibodies to neuronal NOS (Zhang et al. 1993a; Verge et al. 1994). In lumbar DRGs of normal rats fewer than 4% of neurons, mainly small and medium sized, contain neuronal NOS-LI, and it usually coexists with calcitonin gene-related peptide (CGRP)- and substance P (SP)-LI. There appears to be some species differences with regard to the presence of NOS, as in the monkey up to 15% of lumbar DRG neurons exhibit NOS-LI (Zhang et al. 1993a).

2. Spinal Cord

Neurons exhibiting NOS-LI are concentrated in three fairly well-defined regions of the spinal cord in a number of species: (a) the intermediolateral column in thoracic and sacral segments, (b) lamina X of all segments, and (c) the superficial layers of the dorsal horn of all segments (Dun et al. 1993; Zhang et al. 1993a). In the superficial laminae of the rat dorsal horn NOS-positive small-sized cells are concentrated in the inner layer of lamina II, where they are likely to coexist with γ-aminobutyric acid (GABA), glycine, and acetylcholine (Spike et al. 1993). In addition, discrete NOS-LI fibers are observed in all regions of the gray matter of the spinal cord. The densest NOS-LI fiber network has been noted in superficial laminae of the dorsal horn, where it forms a dense band at the inner layer of lamina II (Dun et al. 1993; Zhang et al. 1993a).

3. Plasticity of NOS Activity in Nociceptive Pathways After Injury

Peripheral nerve injury (axotomy or nerve ligation of both somatic or visceral nerves) induces a dramatic upregulation of NOS activity in the ipsilateral DRG (Zhang et al. 1993a; Verge et al. 1994; Vizzard et al. 1995). In rat lumbar DRGs the percentage of NOS positive cells can increase to up to 50% of the total DRG cell population. Some NOS-LI coexists with galanin, neuropeptide Y, and peptide-histidine-isoleucine, neuropeptides that are also upregulated in DRG after axotomy (Hökfelt et al. 1994). The increase in NOS apparently results in increased amounts of enzyme which is transported centrifugally since there is an increase in NOS-LI in the dorsal roots as well as in the dorsal horn of the spinal cord (Zhang et al. 1993a). In contrast, peripheral axotomy seems to cause a reduction in NOS positive neurons in lamina II of the ipsilateral dorsal horn (Zhang et al. 1993a).

III. Evidence for the Involvement of NO in Nociception

1. Periphery

Subcutaneous injection of NO in humans induces a brief burning pain sensation (Holthusen and Arndt 1994). In contrast, animal experiments have suggested that generation of NO and subsequent increases in cGMP levels are involved in antinociceptive mechanisms in the periphery, particularly in inflamed tissue. For example, intraplantar injection of L-arginine or other NO donors exerts an antinociceptive effect on paw inflammation-induced hyperalgesia (Duarte et al. 1992; Kawabata et al. 1992). Moreover, NOS inhibitors reduce the peripheral analgesic effect of morphine and acetylcholine under such conditions (Duarte and Ferreira 1992).

2. Spinal Cord

Generation of NO at spinal level has a minor or no role in acute nociception, as evidenced by the lack of effect of systemically or spinally administered NOS inhibitors on behavioral measures of acute nociception, dorsal horn neuronal activity, and magnitude of the flexor reflex (Haley et al. 1992; Kitto et al. 1992; Meller et al. 1992; Malmberg and Yaksh 1993; Verge et al. 1994). On the other hand, NO appears to be an important mediator for spinal sensitization and hyperalgesia after inflammation, nerve injury, and intense activation of C fibers. Intrathecal injection of N-methyl-D-aspartate (NMDA) produces thermal hyperalgesia in behavioral tests, which is blocked by NOS inhibitors (Kitto et al. 1992; Meller and Gebhart 1993; Malmberg and Yaksh 1993).

These behavioral observations are supported by electrophysiological data in which the excitatory effect of NMDA on dorsal horn neurons is substantially reduced by NOS inhibitors (RADHAKRISHNAN and HENRY 1993). Facilitation of the flexor reflex by high-frequency stimulation of C fibers is also blocked by intrathecally administered NOS inhibitors (VERGE et al. 1994). Furthermore, NOS inhibition blocks subcutaneous formalin-induced behavioral and neuronal responses (HAELY et al. 1992; MALMBERG and YAKSH 1993) as well as hyperalgesia observed after carrageenan injection (MELLER et al. 1994).

Most events known to be attenuated by NOS inhibitors are also sensitive to blockade of NMDA receptors and in many cases can be also blocked by GC blockers (MELLER et al. 1992, 1994). Thus in the spinal cord, similarly to other parts of the nervous system, the involvement of NO requires a link between NMDA receptor activation, NO production, and increase in cGMP level. However, there is evidence that the excitatory effect of other compunds, such as SP, also involve the production of NO in the spinal cord (RADHAKRISHNAN and HENRY 1993). Considering the low level of NOS in normal rat lumbar DRG, it is unlikely that the source of NO is from primary afferents under normal conditions. Therefore NO produced in spinal interneurons is likely to account for the effects described above. It has been reported that NMDA-induced thermal hyperalgesia is reversibly blockaded by hemoglobin (KITTO et al. 1992), indicating that intracellularly generated NO, upon activation of NMDA receptors, may have to leave the neuron where it is produced and enter another neuron or glial cell to activate GC-S and to exert its hyperalgesic action (MELLER and GEBHART 1993). There are also some data that suggest that NO acts presynaptically to stimulate the release of neuroactive substances in the spinal cord (GARRY et al. 1994; SORKIN 1993).

Whether NO also has some role in mediating mechanical allodynia, where innocuous stimulation provokes painful sensation, is unclear. While MELLER et al. (1993) maintain that the spinal NMDA-NO-cGMP system is not involved in mechanical allodynia, MINAMI et al. (1995) reported that intrathecal injection of L-arginine produces increased response in mice to innocuous mechanical stimulation and intrathecal L-NAME blocked intrathecal prostaglandin-induced mechanical allodynialike effect in mice. In contrast, ZHUO et al. (1993) found that intrathecal L-arginine increases the mechanical threshold and NOS inhibitors enhanced the allodynialike effect of cholinergic agonists.

3. Supraspinal Sites

Relatively little is known about the role of NO in the mediation of nociception at supraspinal level. There have been some reports that intracerebroventricular injection of L-arginine produces a biphasic effect on nociception, and NOS inhibitors have antinociceptive effects (MOORE et al. 1991; KAWABATA et al. 1993). The antinociceptive effect of L-arginine has been attributed to the generation of kyotorphin, an opioid peptide (KAWABATA et al. 1993). It is interesting to note that sensory stimulation induces the release of L-arginine in the thalamus, which facilitated sensory transmission (Do et al. 1994). Therefore it appears that the physiological role for NO at supraspinal sites is likely to be pronociceptive, although the site(s) and mechanisms for such action remain to be clarified.

IV. NO and Chronic Pain

Peripheral nerve lesion causes an upregulation of NOS-LI in primary sensory neurons and their central terminals. We have presented evidence that NO plays a critical role in maintaining ongoing discharges generated by DRG cells after axotomy (Wiesenfeld-Hallin et al. 1993a). Furthemore, the depressive effect of systemic L-NAME on C fiber conditioning stimulation-induced facilitation of the flexor reflex is also enhanced after nerve section, indicating a possible involvement of upregulated NOS in meditaing C fiber input in axotomized sensory afferents (Verge et al. 1994). In agreement with this notion, it has been reported that intrathecal NOS inhibitors reverses thermal hyperalgesic responses in rats after sciatic nerve ligation (Meller et al. 1992). We have recently developed an animal model of chronic allodynia in rats after spinal cord ischemia (Xu et al. 1994a). With this model we have observed that systemically administered L-NAME and 7-nitroindazole dose-dependently alleviate this chronic allodynialike behavior (Hao et al. 1993; unpublished observations). Taken together, these data indicate a potential role for NO in maintaining chronic painful states in animals after lesions of PNS and CNS tissue.

V. NO and Opioid Analgesia

Differential interaction between NO and opioid analgesia at various levels of the nervous system have been reported. The peripheral analgesic effect of morphine requires production of NO in the periphery whereas intracere-broventricular morphine-induced antinociception is unaffected by NO inhibitors (Duarte and Ferreira 1992). Interestingly, intrathecal L-NAME potentiates morphine's antinociceptive effect (Przewlocki et al. 1993), and recent reports indicate that chronic administration of NOS inhibitors prevents the development of morphine tolerance (Kolesnikov et al. 1993; Elliot et al. 1994). Both effects of NOS inhibitors have been found to be associated with NMDA receptor blockade (Elliot et al. 1994). Therefore the involvement of the NMDA-NO-cGMP pathway in mediating opioid analgesia and tolerance is very likely.

VI. Therapeutic Potentials of NOS Inhibitors

As the generation of NO appears to be involved predominantly in nociceptive events associated with inflammation or nerve injury, inhibitors of NOS may have a therapeutic potential for treating chronic pain. Another advantage of

NOS inhibitors over NMDA receptor antagonists is that the former appear to cause much less motor stimulation associated with NMDA receptor blockade (HAO et al., unpublished). A clinical problem that would be associated with the administration of nonselective NOS inhibitors is hypertension. This can be overcomed by using selective neuronal NOS inhibitors, such as 7-nitroindazole. However, although the indazole derivatives selectively block neuronal NOS and produce analgesia (MOORE et al. 1992; BABBEDGE et al. 1993), they apparently also possess effects unrelated to NOS inhibition (ALLAWI et al. 1994) which lead to sedation and motor impairment in rats (Hao et al., unpublished). Therefore the clinical administration of NOS inhibitors for treating pain may depend on successful development of selective and specific neuronal NOS inhibitors.

C. Cholecystokinin

Cholecystokinin (CCK) was originally purified from intestine and belongs to the gastrin family of peptides. In the nervous system it is present mainly in the form of the C-terminal octapeptide (CCK-8) of the gut hormone CCK (1-33). CCK is widely distributed in the CNS, as revealed by biochemical, immunohistological, and in situ hybridization techniques (WILLIAMS et al. 1987; SCHIFFMANN and VANDERHAEGHEN 1991), and has been shown to be a neurotransmitter mediating many important physiological functions (see BABER et al. 1989 for review).

I. Distribution of CCK in Nociceptive Pathways

1. Dorsal Root Ganglia

It had earlier been reported that CCK-LI is present in a substantial number of small and medium-sized DRG cells in rat (DALSGAARD et al. 1982). The identity of CCK-LI in rat primary sensory neuron has been challenged, however, and it has been suggested that several antisera to CCK described in the literature cross-react with the C-terminal portion of CGRP (JU et al. 1986). Studies using N-terminally directed antibodies or in situ hybridization techniques on rat show no or only a few CCK-LI or CCK mRNA positive neurons in rat DRG (WILLIAMS et al. 1987; SEROOGY et al. 1990; VERGE et al. 1993a). There appear to be considerable species differences in the presence of CCK in sensory neurons. In guinea pig and monkey a large portion of DRG cells, mainly small to medium-sized, contain CCK mRNA (SEROOGY et al. 1990; VERGE et al. 1993a), although the presence of CCK-LI in primate DRG cells has not been confirmed (ZHANG et al. 1993b).

2. Spinal Cord

CCK-LI and mRNA can be visualized in a substantial number of dorsal horn neurons across many species (WILLAMS et al. 1987; VERGE et al. 1993a; ZHANG et al. 1993b, 1995c). CCK positive cells were found mainly in deeper laminae of the dorsal horn and around the central canal (lamina X). In addition, a dense network of CCK-LI fibers and terminals can be identified in dorsal horn, mainly in deeper levels of the substantia gelatinosa and lamina III. It has been suggested that these fibers are derived primarily from local CCK neurons or from descending tracts (Skirboll et al. 1983; Zouaoui et al. 1991; Jacquin et al. 1992; Zhang et al. 1995c).

3. Supraspinal Sites

As one of the most abundant peptides in the CNS, CCK-LI and mRNA have been described in many areas related to nociceptive transmission, such as periaqueductal gray, thalamus, and cortex (Williams et al. 1987; Schiffmann and Vanderhaeghen 1991). Interestingly, some areas in which CCK-LI neurons are located, are involved in the mediation of the supraspinal analgesic effect of morphine. Therefore the anatomical localization of CCK may be related to the documented interaction betweeen the opioid and CCK systems (see below).

II. CCK Receptors

1. Classificiation of CCK Receptor Subtypes

It has long been known that CCK receptors are heterogeneous, with receptors in the periphery differing from those in the CNS (Innis and Snyder 1980). Moran et al. (1986) termed the peripheral type A receptor to distinguish it form classical brain (type B) receptors. However, it is now known that even the peripheral type CCK_A receptor is present to a limited extent in rat CNS (Hill and Woodruff 1990). Moreover, in monkeys the presence of CCK_A receptor in the CNS is even more substantial (Hill et al. 1990). Both CCK_A and CCK_B receptors have been cloned.

2. CCK Receptors in the Spinal Cord

Receptor binding sites for CCK have been visualized in areas throughout the dorsal horn with highest density in the superficial laminae. In the rat these receptors are predominantly the B type whereas in monkey the majority of receptors are of the A type (Hill and Woodruff 1990; Hill et al. 1990; Ghilardi et al. 1992). It has been suggested that a substantial portion of the CCK-binding sites in the superficial dorsal horn arisen from small-diameter primary sensory neurons as neonatal capsaicin treatment reduces CCK binding (Ghilardi et al. 1992). This finding was supported by binding and in situ hybridization studies on DRG (Ghilardi et al. 1992; Zhang et al. 1993c). Although the binding sites in rat DRG have been reported to be of low intensity, and in situ studies indicate that only about 4% of rat DRG neurons synthesize CCK_B receptor mRNA, up to 90% of DRG cells in rabbit and 20% in monkey express CCK binding sites (Ghilardi et al. 1992; Zhang et al.

1993c). Interestingly, in all species examined the receptors in DRG cells appear to be of the B type (GHILARDI et al. 1992).

3. CCK Receptor Antagonists

Several nonpeptide CCK receptor antagonists have been developed. The first generation of CCK antagonists, represented by proglumide and lorglumide, have been extensively used but have the drawback of low potency, poor selectivity towards receptor subtypes, and the presence of effects unrelated to CCK receptor antagonism. However, the efforts of several pharmaceutical companies have resulted in several series of compounds which represent second-generation CCK receptor antagonists. These compounds include the benzodiazepine series, for example, MK-329 (CCK_A) and L365260 (CCK_B), the dipeptoid series, for example, CI-988 and the pyrazolidinones, for example, LY 262691 (see SHOWELL et al. 1994). These compounds are potent and exhibit good selectivity toward CCK receptor subtypes and have been proven to be very valuable experimental tools. However, these compounds also have some limitations in their affinity, selectivity, aqueous solubility and bioavailability. Thus their usefulness as therapeutic agents is limited. There have been further recent developments with compounds such as L740093 (SHOWELL et al. 1994). These third-generation compounds are highly potent and selective and have improved aqueous solubility and bioaviability. Thus they may represent therapeutic agents with several possible CNS indications (SCHIANTARELLI 1993).

III. Plasticity of Spinal CCK Systems After Injury

Peripheral nerve injury induces a dramatic upregulation of CCK-LI and CCK mRNA in rat DRG cells. VERGE et al. (1993a) showed that 3 weeks after sciatic nerve section in the rat up to 30% of ipsilateral DRG cells express CCK mRNA, with a distinct but less apparent increase also in the contralateral DRG. However, less clear changes were observed in monkeys after axotomy, and in fact axotomy seems to reduce CCK-LI fibers in the ipsilateral dorsal horn (VERGE et al. 1993a; ZHANG et al. 1993b).

   Not only CCK-LI is increased after axotomy in DRG neurons in rat. Using in situ hybridization ZHANG et al. (1993c) showed that there is also a dramatic increase in the expression of CCK_B receptor mRNA in rat DRG neurons after peripheral nerve section. Up to 60% of all DRG cells of all sizes express CCK_B receptor mRNA. These changes occur as early as 2 days after axotomy and persist for at least 4 weeks. The CCK_B receptor positive cells in axotomized rats have been found to contain both galanin and neuropeptide Y, but not CCK itself. All three peptides are upregulated after nerve injury.

IV. CCK in Nociception

CCK appears to have an important but complex involvement in nociceptive transmission and modulation. The most well defined and apparently physiological role for CCK is that it is a functional antagonist of opioid-induced analgesia. Recent studies further indicated that the level of endogenous CCK activity controls the degree of opioid responsiveness under a number of chronic pain conditions.

1. CCK and Opioid-Mediated Analgesia

Faris et al. (1983) were the first to demonstrate that systemically administered CCK significantly attenuated morphine-induced antinociception. Since then, a large body of literature has emerged which supports this notion. Thus, CCK has been shown upon systemic, intrathecal or intracerebral injection to reduce the effect of exogenous opioids in behavioral and electrophysiological studies (Han et al. 1985; Wiesenfeld-Hallin and Duranti 1987; Baber et al. 1989; O'Neill et al. 1989; Kellstein et al. 1991; Magnuson et al. 1990; Wang et al. 1990). CCK also blocks the antinociceptive effect of endogenous opioids, such as after electroacupuncture and electric shocks (Watkins et al. 1984; Han et al. 1986). The site of interaction between CCK and opioids are clearly multiple, but the spinal cord is an important site. Among the three subtypes of opioid receptors it appears that μ and κ receptor mediated analgesia is antagonized by CCK whereas δ opioids are less affected (Magnuson et al. 1990; Wang et al. 1990; Noble et al. 1995).

The antagonism by CCK of opioid-induced analgesia is present in normal conditions as blockade of endogenous CCK results in a clearcut enhancement of opioid-induced antinociception (Watkins et al. 1985). This has been confirmed with several newly developed highly potent and specific CCK receptor antagonists as well as CCK receptor antisense oligonucleotides (Dourish et al. 1990a; Wiesenfeld-Hallin et al. 1990; Zhou et al.1993; Vanderah et al. 1994; Chapman et al. 1995; Noble et al. 1995). Comparison of the potency of these drugs indicates that it is the CCK_B receptor which is responsible for the interaction between the CCK and opioid systems in rats. This is supported by the fact that the predominant receptor subtype in rodent CNS is the B receptor. The effectiveness of endogenously released opioids following the administration of inhibitors of endopeptidases or electroacupuncture is also potentiated by CCK_B receptor antagonists (Han et al. 1986; Valverde et al. 1994).

The mechanism by which CCK antagonizes opioid analgesia is not fully understood. It is clear that the blockade of morphine analgesia by CCK is not due to a direct hyperalgesic effect of CCK, as in most experimental settings CCK does not alter baseline pain threshold. The majority of receptor binding studies fail to show an affinity for CCK to opioid receptors (Wang and Han 1989). However, one study does indicate that binding of CCK-8 to the CCK receptor reduces the binding affinity of μ receptor ligands (Wang and Han 1989). There is also evidence that the CCK counteracts intracellular events subsequent to opioid receptor activation (Wang et al. 1992). If such interaction occurs in cells that have both opioid and CCK receptors, it results in decreased opioid-induced analgesia. This hypothesis is supported by the parallel localization of opioid and CCK receptors in a number of CNS areas important for opioid analgesia, such as terminals of primary sensory afferents, spinal cord interneurons, and the periaqueductal gray. Another hypothesis concerning the mechanism of CCK-induced antagonism of opioid analgesia has been suggested by WIERTELAK et al. (1992). They found that CCK is the mediator for conditioned antianalgesia, which is a conditioning procedure related to safety signals with reduced analgesia induced by morphine.

CCK antagonists are not analgesic on their own in most behavioral and electrophysiological studies, indicating that CCK does not markedly tonically inhibit endogenous opioids. However, increased stimulation of opioid receptors by either exogenously administered opioids or by increased endogenous release may stimulate the release of CCK, which in turn reduces and curtails the action of opioids. There is some experimental evidence for this hypothesis. For example, several groups have reported increased release of CCK-LI from the spinal cord after morphine treatment in vivo and in vitro (TANG et al. 1984; BENOLIEL et al. 1991; ZHOU et al. 1993). Acute morphine treatment may also increase the gene expression and tissue content of CCK in several brain regions and spinal cord (DING and BAYER 1993).

2. CCK and Opioid Tolerance

Repeated and chronic administration of opiates gradually reduces their ability to induce analgesia, a condition known as tolerance, which presents great hindrance to the clinical administration of opiates for the relief of chronic pain. Since CCK is a potent antagonist of opiate analgesia and is widely distributed, it is possible that endogenous CCK is involved in the development of tolerance. Studies of tolerance with CCK receptor antagonists have shown that this is indeed the case. Thus both the weak nonspecific antagonist proglumide and the more recently developed potent antagonists L365 260 and CI 988 have been found to both prevent (when antagonists are administered chronically together with morphine) and reverse (when antagonists are administered acutely in already tolerant animals) morphine tolerance (WATKINS et al. 1984; DOURISH et al. 1990a; KELLSTEIN and MAYER 1991; XU et al. 1992; HOFFMANN and WIESENFELD-HALLIN 1995). The receptor responsible for this action of CCK is also the B type in the rat. Interestingly, the symptom of physical dependence induced by chronic morphine is not prevented by CCK receptor antagonists, indicating a separate mechanism for dependence (DOURISH et al. 1990a; XU et al. 1992).

The mechanism for preventing and reversing morphine tolerance by CCK antagonists has also been addressed. Repeated injection of morphine using a paradigm which causes behavioral tolerance induces upregulation of CCK mRNA in the spinal cord and discrete brain areas, which is accompanied by increased CCK content in some spinal and brian areas (ZHOU et al. 1992; DING and BAYER 1993). Thus opiate tolerance may be related to an upregulation of endogenous CCK, which induces greater blockade of opiate analgesia, hence causing tolerance. Blockade of the action of the upregulated CCK system by receptor antagonists restores some of the analgesic effect of opioid, resulting in reversal of morphine tolerance. Upregulation of the CCK system may require chronic stimulation of CCK receptors by repeated opiate administration as CCK antagonists also prevent morphine tolerance.

3. CCK and Opioid Sensitivity

The analgesic effects of morphine vary in different clinical states of pain. For example, neuropathic pain, that is, pain after injury to the nervous system, usually responds poorly to opiates. There is also experimental evidence that morphine is less effective in inducing antinociception at spinal level after peripheral nerve injury in rats (Xu and Wiesenfeld-Hallin 1991; Mao et al. 1995) and does not cause antinociception in a number of animal models of neuropathic pain (Xu et al. 1993).

The mechanism(s) for a lack of (or reduced) effect of morphine on neuropathic pain is unclear, but this phenomenon is similar to the appearance of morphine tolerance, i.e., under both circumstances morphine fails to elicit the expected analgesic effect. Thus it is reasonable to suggest that CCK is also involved in both phenomena. As described above, peripheral axotomy causes a dramatic upregulation of CCK and CCK receptor mRNA in rat DRG cells. Electrophysiological and behavioral experiments have verifed the implications of this plasticity in morphine-induced antinociception (or the lack of it). In the flexor reflex model in spinal rats systemic morphine exhibited reduced antinociceptive effect in axotomized rats compared to normals, and addition of the CCK_B receptor antagonist CI 988 strongly potentiated the effect of morphine (Xu et al. 1994b). Furthermore, chronic intrathecal morphine had no effect on autotomy behavior in rats after peripheral nerve section, which is an animal model of neuropathic pain. However, the combination of CI|988 plus morphine significantly suppressed autotomy (Xu et al. 1993). These data indicate that in the rat opiate insensitivity of painlike symptoms after nerve injury may be related to enhanced activity in the endogneous CCK system.

Control over the degree of opiate sensitivity by CCK is also observed in animal models of inflammation, although it is the mirror image of neuropathic pain. Thus it has been known for some time that inflammation enhances the antinociceptive effect of opiates in animals. It has been shown that during inflammation exogenous CCK is still able to attenuate the antinociceptive effect of morphine, indicating that the mechanism by which CCK reduces the action of morphine is still intact. However, during inflammation CCK receptor antagonists no longer enhance the antinociceptive effect of morphine (Stanfa and Dickenson 1993). Thus a decrease in the availability of CCK within the spinal cord following inflammation, due either to decreased release of CCK or to reduced concentration of this peptide within the dorsal horn, may underlie the lack of effect of the CCK antagonists.

The mechanism by which upregulated CCK causes tolerance and opiate insensitivity in neuropathic pain may explain the mechanism for the development and maintanence of neuropathic pain. In an animal model of chronic allodynialike response in rats after spinal cord lesion we observed that while systemic morphine is quite ineffective, systemic CI 988 is very effective in reducing the allodynialike state (Xu et al. 1994a). More interestingly, the analgesic effect of CI 988 in this model is reversed by the opioid antagonist naloxone. This finding suggests that injury to the nervous system leads to upregulation of the endogenous CCK system, which blocks endogenous opioidergic control, resulting in the development of neuropathic pain-related symptoms and reducing the effects of exogenously administered opiates, resulting in opiate insensitivity.

4. Other Effects of CCK Related to Nociception

In addition to interaction with opioid-induced analgesia, CCK has been reported to have effects related to nociception that may be unrelated to the above mentioned "opioid connection." For example, electrophysiological studies have shown that CCK affects the excitability of dorsal horn neurons in vivo and in vitro. The observed effect, however, is not consistent as excitation; no effect or inhibition has been reported (see KELLSTEIN et al. 1991).

There is considerable evidence that systemic, intrathecal, or intracerebroventricular CCK and its naturally occurring analogue cerulein induce behavioral antinociception in rats and mice in a number of tests (see BABER et al. 1989 for review). The effects are generally observed after high doses of CCK (higher than those required to observe an interaction between CCK and morphine) and are sometimes accompanied by other behavioral side effects such as sedation and ptosis, which makes interpretation difficult. In most cases the alleged antinociceptive effect of CCK is reversed by naloxone, indicating an activation of the endogenous opioid system (BABER et al. 1989). It has recently been suggested that the analgesia result form CCK administration is due to activation of the CCK_A receptor in rat which results in increased release of enkephalin and activation of δ receptors (RATTRAY et al. 1988; DERRIEN et al. 1993). Cerulein has been found to relieve pain in a number of clinical trials, again, usually in a naloxone-reversible fashion (BABER et al. 1989).

V. Therapeutic Potentials for CCK Receptor Related Compounds

The possibility that CCK antagonists enhances opiate analgesia, prevents opioid tolerance, and reverses opiate insensitivity in neuropathic pain represents a interesting target for drug development. This is boosted by the finding that CCK antagonists do not potentiate two major side effects of morphine, respiratory depression and clonus (DOURISH et al. 1990b). The addition of a CCK antagonist in opiate therapy could therefore reduce the amount of opiate required for inducing adequate level of analgeisa, delay or even prevent tolerance development, restore the opioid's efficacy in already tolerant patients, and possibly most importantly, either alone or in combination with opiates, provide relief for patients with neuropathic pain who have not obtained adequate relief otherwise.

It has been reported that proglumide enhances morphine analgesia in both experimental and clinical pain (Baber et al. 1989). The clinical availability of some of the recently developed, highly potent CCK receptor antagonists will hopefully open a new era in exploring the therapeutic potential for CCK receptor antagonists in treating pain. It should be noted that although most experimental studies are conducted with CCK_B selective antagonists, since the primate CNS, including spinal cord, contains both CCK_A and CCK_B receptors, agonists of both receptors should be evaluated.

D. Galanin

Galanin is a neuropeptide consisting of 29 amino acids which is widely distributed in the nervous system and has been implicated in a number of physiological functions. Galanin acts on specific receptors to exert its effect, and at least one human galanin receptor has been cloned and found to belong to the G protein coupled receptor family. There are some indications that galanin receptors are heterogeneous (Bartfai et al. 1993). Galanin occurs in a small population of primary sensory neurons and also in spinal interneurons (Ch'ng et al. 1985; Skofitsch and Jacobowitz 1985). The role of galanin in spinal nociception has been extensively studied in our laboratory in recent years.

I. Distribution of Galanin and Galanin Receptors in Sensory Neurons and Spinal Cord: Response to Injury

1. Dorsal Root Ganglia

Galanin mRNA and galanin-LI in normal rats can be observed in only a fairly small population of small-diameter rat DRG cells which also express SP- and CGRP-LI (Ch'ng et al. 1985; Skofitsch and Jacobowitz 1985). Similarly low figures for galanin-positive neurons in DRG cells have been noted in monkeys (Zhang et al. 1993b). Peripheral nerve injury induces a strong upregulation of galanin synthesis in ipsilateral DRG cells in both rat and monkey, resulting in the detection of galanin-LI in up to 50% of DRG cells (Villar et al. 1989; Zhang et al. 1993b). This increase in galanin mRNA can be observed as early as 1 day after nerve lesion and persists for at least 60 days. In many cases galanin coexists with vasoactive intestinal peptide, another peptide that is upregulated after axotomy (Xu et al. 1990b). The transport of newly synthesized galanin occurs in both central and peripheral branches of sensory neurons (Villar et al. 1991). No galanin binding sites have been noted in rat DRG, whereas some binding sites were seen in monkey DRG, but these are not affected by peripheral axotomy (Zhang et al. 1995a).

2. Spinal Cord

Galanin-LI has been localized in small dorsal horn neurons, mainly in lamina II, where it coexists with GABA, enkephalin, and neuropeptide Y (SIMMONS et al. 1995; ZHANG et al. 1995c). Another population of galanin-LI neurons has been identified in areas around the central canal (laminae X and VII). A dense network of galanin-LI fibers is visualized in the superficial laminae of the dorsal horn. Dorsal rhizotomy or neonatal capsaicin treatment significantly reduces the immunoreactivity, indicating the some of these fibers are terminals of primary sensory afferents (CH'NG et al. 1985; SKOFITSCH and JACOBOWITZ 1985). This has been supported by studies at the ultrastructural level where coexistence of galanin-LI with SP-LI and CGRP-LI has been reported in afferent terminals and varicosities (TUCHSCHERER and SEYBOLD 1989; ZHANG et al. 1995b).

Peripheral nerve injury causes an expansion of the distribution of galanin-LI fibers in the outer layers of the dorsal horn in the rat, where terminal processes are extended from laminae I and II into laminae III and IV (ZHANG et al. 1993b, 1995d). The expansion of galanin-LI fibers, presumably from primary afferents, in the dorsal horn after axotomy is even more dramatic in monkeys (ZHANG et al. 1993a–c). The number of local neurons expressing galanin-LI is not altered after axotomy, although some ultrastructural changes are observed (ZHANG et al. 1995d). In contrast, it has recently been reported that inflammation induces an increase in the number of neurons expressing galanin mRNA in the dorsal horn, although the level in sensory neurons is unchanged (TOGUNAGA et al. 1992; JI et al. 1995).

Very high density galanin binding sites are located in spinal cord laminae I, II, and X of the normal rat and monkey (KAR and QUIRION 1994; ZHANG et al. 1995a). These binding sites are not affected by dorsal rhizotomy or neonatal capsaicin treatment, indicating that they are derived primarily from post-synatic neurons.

II. Involvement of Galanin in Nociception Under Normal Conditions

1. Behavioral Studies

Studies examining the behavioral effect of galanin on acute nociception has revealed conflicting results. While POST et al. (1987) and CRIDLAND and HENRY (1988) reported that intrathecal galanin evokes thermal antinociception, KURAISHI et al. (1991) suggested that intrathecal galanin evokes mechanical hyperalgesia without affecting thermal nociception. In an attempt to resolve this discrepancy we conducted a study on the effect of intrathecal galanin on thermal and mechanical nociception. We found no evidence for a hyperalgesic effect of galanin in either test. However, at a high dose ($10 \mu g$) intrathecal galanin elicited moderate but significant thermal antinociception (WIESENFELD-HALLIN et al. 1993b). Studies on the interaction between galanin and morphine further support an antinociceptive property for galanin. Intrathecal galanin significantly potentiated the spinal analgesic effect of morphine in the hot-plate test (Wiesenfeld-Hallin et al. 1992a), and spinal administration of galanin receptor antagonist blocks intrathecal morphine induced antinociception, indicating that the spinal effect of morphine is mediated in part by the inhibitory action of galanin (Reimann et al. 1994).

2. Electrophysiological Studies

Overwhelming evidence supporting an antinociceptive role for galanin has been obtained from electrophysiological studies. Galanin has been found to hyperpolarize the majority of dorsal horn neurons recorded in vitro (Randic et al. 1987). Similarly, in two in vitro preprations using newborn rats, galanin depressed C fiber mediated ventral root potentials elicited by capsaicin or electrical stimulation of the saphenous nerves at doses which did not affect the excitability of motoneurons (Yanagisawa et al. 1986; Nussbaumer et al. 1989).

Using a spinal nociceptive flexor reflex model in decerebrate, spinalized, unanesthetized rats, we analyzed in detail the effects of exogenously administered galanin on spinal reflex excitabiliy (see Wiesenfeld-Hallin et al. 1992a for review). We found that intrathecal galanin induces a biphasic dose-dependent effect on the flexor reflex with facilitation at low doses and depression at high doses (Wiesenfeld-Hallin et al. 1989). The reflex depression caused by intrathecal galanin is not reversed by naloxone or bicucculine, indicating that the depression probably does not involve endogenous opioid peptides or the GABA system. Moreover, intrathecal galanin does not affect the monosynaptic reflex, again, suggesting that galanin has no effect on motoneuron activity.

It is well established that conditioning stimulation (CS) of a peripheral nerve at an intensity that activates C fibers induces an increase in spinal cord excitability lasting from several minutes to about 1 h, depending on the type of peripheral nerve activated (Wall and Woolf 1984). This effect, known as central sensitization, may be an important mechanism for the development of tissue injury related pain and hyperalgesia. Galanin potently inhibits the increase in spinal cord excitability following CS of both cutaneous and muscle nerves or after sciatic nerve transection (Wiesenfeld-Hallin et al. 1989; Xu et al. 1990b, 1991). Further analysis indicated that this effect of galanin is at least in part due to a postsynaptic blockade of the facilitatory effect of SP and CGRP, excitatory peptides known to be involved in the mediation of such spinal hyperexcitability (Xu et al. 1990b).

A series of chimeric peptides have been developed as highly potent galanin receptor antagonists. Intrathecal injection of M-35 [galanin (1-16)-bradykinin-(2-9)] significantly potentiates the facilitation of the flexor reflex induced by cutaneous C fiber CS, indicating that even under normal conditions galanin is released upon C fiber stimulation and plays an inhibitory role in mediating spinal cord excitability (Wiesenfeld-Hallin et al. 1992b). This is in agreement with the finding in biochemical experiments where basal and evoked release of galanin in the spinal cord was observed in normal animals (KLEIN et al. 1992; HOPE et al. 1994).

3. Pharmacology and Mechanisms of the Spinal Effects of Galanin

The N-terminal fragment of galanin is a full agonists of spinal galanin receptors while the C-terminal exhibits no biological activity in rat spinal cord (XU et al. 1990a). Spinal galanin receptors exhibited differential sensitivity to a number of chimeric galanin receptor antagonists (XU et al. 1995). The order of potency of these drugs in rat spinal cord is different than in the hypothalamus or pancreas (BARTFAI et al. 1994). For example, the spinal galanin receptor appears to be intermediate between brain and peripheral galanin receptors.

The mechanisms of the spinal inhibitory effect of galanin have not been studied in detail. Galanin binds with high affinity to crude synaptosomal fraction preparation of rat lumbar spinal cord, which is blocked by GTP and pertussin toxin, suggesting that the galanin receptor in rat spinal cord is coupled to a G_i or G_o protein. Potassium-stimulated cGMP synthesis is potently inhibited by galanin in slices of rat lumbar spinal cord (BEDECS et al. 1992). Other consequences of galanin receptor activation in other systems include closure of voltage-dependent Ca^{2+} channels, opening of an ATP-sensitive K^+ channel, inhibition of adenylate cyclase activity, and inhibition of inositol trisphosphate production.

III. Involvement of Galanin in Nociception After Peripheral Nerve Injury

Peripheral axotomy strongly increases the expression of galanin in primary sensory neurons, followed by an increase in galanin-LI in the terminals in the dorsal horn. Intrathecal galanin blocks facilitation of the reflex induced by C fiber CS of the axotomized nerve in a similar fashion as with intact nerves (XU et al. 1990b). After nerve section galanin-blocked reflex facilitation induced by vasoactive intestinal polypeptide and CGRP, but not by SP. At the same time, a strong coexistence between galanin and vasoactive intestinal polypeptide is found in deafferented DRG cells. The galanin receptor antagonist M35 strongly potentiates reflex facilitation by C fiber CS in axotomized rats (WIESENFELD-HALLIN et al. 1992b). Interestingly, such potentiation is clearly higher in axotomized rats than in normals. These data indicate that the endogenous inhibitory role of galanin is enhanced in sensory neurons after axotomy. This is further supported by two behavioral experiments in which chronic infusion of M35 or galanin antisense oligonucleotides enhanced autotomy behavior (VERGE et al. 1993b; JI et al. 1994). It is important to note that primates exhibit similar upregulation of galanin after nerve injury (HÖKFELT et al. 1994). If galanin is also inhibitory in humans after nerve injury, it is anticipated that galanin receptor agonists, possibly of nonpeptide nature, may have therapeutic potential in treating pain of neuropathic origin.

References

Aimi Y, Fujimura M, Vincent SR, Kimura H (1991) Localization of NADPH-diapho-rase-containing neurons in sensory ganglia of the rat. J Comp Neurol 306:382–392

Allawi HS, Wallace P, Pitcher A, Gaffen Z, Bland-Ward PA, Moore PK (1994) Effect of 7-nitro indazole on neurotransmission in the rat vas deferens: mechanisms unrelated to inhibition of nitric oxide synthase. Br J Pharmacol 113:282–288

Babbedge RC, Bland-Ward PA, Hart SL, Moore PK (1993) Inhibition of rat cerebellar nitric oxide synthase by 7-nitroindazole and related substituted indazoles. Br J Pharmacol 110:225–228

Baber NS, Dourish CT, Hill DR (1989) The role of CCK, caerulein, and CCK antagonists in nociception. Pain 39:307–328

Bartfai T, Langel Ü, Bedecs K, Andell S, Land T, Gregersen S, Ahrén B, Girotti P, Consolo S, Corvin R, Crawley, J, Xu X-J, Wiesenfeld-Hallin Z, Hökfelt T (1993) Galanin-receptor ligand M40 peptide distinguish between putative galanin-receptor subtypes. Proc Natl Acad Sci USA 90:11287–11291

Bedecs K, Langel Ü, Bartfai T, Wiesenfeld-Hallin Z (1992) Galanin receptors and their second messengers in the lumbar dorsal spinal cord, the effect of GTP and sciatic nerve transection. Acta Physiol Scand 144:213–220

Benoliel JJ, Bourgoin S, Mauborgne A, Legrand JC, Hamon M, Cesselin F (1991) Differential inhibitory/stimulatory modulation of spinal CCK release by mu and delta opioid agonists, and selective blockade of mu-dependent inhibition by kappa receptor stimulation. Neurosci Lett 124:204–207

Bredt DS, Snyder SH (1990) Isolation of nitric oxide synthetase, a calmodulin-requiring enzyme. Proc Natl Acad Sci USA 87:682–685

Chapman V, Honore P, Buritova J, Besson J-M (1995) Cholecystokinin B receptor antagonism enhances the ability of a low dose of morphine to reduce C-fos expression in the spinal cord of the rat. Neuroscience 67:731–739

Ch'ng JLC, Christofides ND, Anand P, Gibson, SJ, Allen YS, Su HC, Tatemoto K, Morrison JFB, Polak JM, Bloom SR (1985) Distribution of galanin immunoreactivity in the central nervous system and the response of galanin-containing neuronal pathways to injury. Neuroscience 16:343–354

Cridland RA, Henry JL (1988) Effects of intrathecal administration of neuropeptides on a spinal nociceptive reflex in the rat: VIP, galanin, CGRP, TRH, somatostatin and angiotensin II. Neuropeptides 11:23–32

Dalsgaard CJ, Vincent SR, Hökfelt T, Lundberg JM, Dahlström A, Schultzberg M, Dockray GJ, Cuello AC (1982) Coexistence of cholecystokinin and substance P-like peptides in the neurons of the dorsal root ganglia of the rat. Neurosci Lett 33:159–163

Dawson TM, Synder SH (1994) Gases as biological messengers: nitric oxide and carbon monoxide in the brain. J Neurosci 14:5147–5159

Derrien M, Noble F, Maldonado R, Rogues BP (1993) Cholecystokinin-A but not cholecystokinin-B receptor stimulation induces endogenous opioid-dependent antinociceptive effects in the hot plate test in mice. Neurosci Lett 160:193–196

Ding XZ, Bayer BM (1993) Increases of CCK mRNA and peptide in different brain areas following acute and chronic administration of morphine. Brain Res 625:139–144

Do KQ, Binns KE, Salt TE (1994) Release of the nitric oxide precursor, arginine, from the thalamus upon sensory afferent stimulation, and its effect on thalamic neurons in vivo. Neuroscience 60:581–586

Dourish CT, O'Neill MF, Coughlan J, Kitchener SJ, Hawley D, Iversen SD (1990a) The selective CCK-B receptor antagonist L-365,260 enhances morphine analgesia and prevents morphine tolerance in the rat. Eur J Pharmacol 176:35–44

Dourish CT, O'Neill MF, Schaffer LW, Siegl PKS, Iversen SD (1990b) The cholecysto-kinin receptor antagonist devazepide enhances morphine-induced analgesia but not morphine-induced respiratory depression in the squirrel monkey. J Pharmacol Exp Ther 255:1158–1165

Duarte IDG, Ferreira SH (1992) The molecular mechanisms of central analgesia induced by morphine or carbachol and the l-arginine-nitric oxide-cGMP pathway. Eur J Pharmacol 221:171–174

Duarte IDG, Santos IR, Lorenzetti BB, Ferreira SH (1992) Analgesia by direct antagonism of nociceptor sensitization involves the arginine-nitric oxide-cGMP pathway. Eur J Pharmacol 217:225–227

Dun NJ, Dun SL, Wu SY, Förstermann U, Schmidt HHHW, Tseng LF (1993) Nitric oxide synthase immunoreactivity in the rat, mouse, cat and squirrel monkey spinal cord. Neuroscience 54:845–857

Elliot K, Minami N, Kolesnikov Y, Pasternak GW, Inturrisi CEI (1994) The NMDA receptor antagonists, LY2764614 and MK-801, and the nitric oxide synthase inhibitor, N^G-nitro-L-arginine, attenuate analgesic tolerance to the mu-opioid morphine but not to kappa opioids. Pain 56:69–75

Faris PL, Komisaruk BR, Watkins LR, Mayer DJ (1983) Evidence for the neuropeptide cholecystokinin as an antagonist of opiate analgesia. Science 219:310–312

Förstermann U, Schmidt HHHW, Pollock JS, Sheng H, Mitchell JA, Warner TD, Nakane M, Murad F (1991) Isoforms of nitric oxide synthase. Characterization and purification from different cell types. Biochem Pharmacol 42:1849–1857

Garry MG, Richardson JD, Hargreaves KM (1994) Sodium nitriprusside evokes the release of immunoreactive calcitonin gene-related peptide and substance P from dorsal horn slices via nitric oxide-dependent and nitric oxide-independent mechanisms. J Neurosci 14:4329–4337

Ghilardi JR, Allen CJ, Vigna SR, McVey DC, Mantyh PW (1992) Trigeminal and dorsal root ganglion neurons express CCK receptor binding sites in the rat, rabbit and monkey: possible site of opiate-CCK analgesic interactions. J Neurosci 12:4854–4866

Haley JE, Dickenson AH, Schachter M (1992) Electrophysiological evidence for a role of nitric oxide in prolonged chemical nociception in the rat. Neuroscience 31:251–258

Han JS, Ding XZ, Fan XG (1985) Is cholecystokinin octapeptide (CCK-8) a candidate for endogenous antiopioid substrates. Neuropeptides 5:399–402

Han JS, Ding XZ, Fan SG (1986) Cholecystokinin octapeptide (CCK-8): antagonism to electroacupuncture analgesia and a possible role in electroacupuncture tolerance. Pain 27:101–115

Hao J-X, Xu, X-J, Wiesenfeld-Hallin Z (1993) Systemic nitro-L-arginine-ester, inhibitor of nitric oxide synthase, relieved chronic allodynia-like phenomenon in rats with chronic spinal lesions. Acta Physiol Scand 150:457–458

Hill DR, Woodruff GN (1990) Differentiation of central cholecystokinin receptor binding sites using the non-peptide antagonists MK-329 and L-365,260. Brain Res 526:276–283

Hill DR, Shaw TM, Graham W, Woodruff GN (1990) Autoradiographical detection of cholecystokinin-A receptors in primate brain using ^{125}I-bolton hunter CCK-8 and ^{3}H-MK-329. J Neurosci 10:1070–1081

Hoffmann O, Wiesenfeld-Hallin Z (1995) The CCK-B receptor antagonist Cl 988 reverses tolerance to morphine in rats. Neuroreport 5:2565–2568

Hökfelt T, Zhang X, Wiesenfeld-Hallin Z (1994) Messenger plasticity in primary sensory neurons following axotomy and its functional implications. Trends Neurosci 17:22–30

Holthusen H, Arndt JO (1994) Nitric oxide evokes pain in humans on intracutaneous injection. Neurosci Lett 165:71–74

Hope PJ, Lang CW, Grubb BD, Duggan AW (1994) Release of immunoreactive galanin in the spinal cord of rats with ankle inflammation: studies with anitbody microprobes. Neuroscience 60:801–807

Innis RB, Snyder SH (1980) Distinct cholecystokinin receptors in brain and pancreas. Proc Natl Acad Sci USA 77:6917–6921

Jacquin MF, Beinfeld MC, Chiaia NL, Zahm DS (1992) Cholecystokinin concentrations and peptide immunoreactivity in the intact and deafferented medullary dorsal horn of the rat. J Comp Neurol 326:22–43

Ji RR, Zhang Q, Bedecs K, Arvidsson J, Zhang X, Xu XJ, Wiesenfeld-Hallin Z, Bartfai T, Hökfelt T (1994) Galanin antisense oligonucleotides reduce galanin levels in dorsal root ganglia and induce autotomy in rats after axotomy. Proc Natl Acad Sci USA 91:12540–12543

Ji RR, Zhang X, Zhang Q, Dagerlind A, Nilsson S, Wiesenfeld-Hallin Z, Hökfelt T (1995) Central and peripheral expression of galanin in response to inflammation. Neuroscience 68:563–576

Ju G, Hökfelt T, Fischer JA, Frey P, Rehfeld JF, Dockray GJ (1986) Does cholecystokinin-like immunoreactivity in rat primary sensory neuorns represent calcitonin gene-related peptide. Neurosci Lett 68:305–310

Kar S, Quirion R (1994) Galanin receptor binding sites in adult rat spinal cord respond differentially to neonatal capsaicin, dorsal rhizotomy and peripheral axotomy. Eur J Neurosci 6:1917–1921

Kawabata A, Fukuzumi Y, Fukushima Y, Takagi H (1992) Antinociceptive effect of l-arginine on the carrageenin-induced hyperalgesia of the rat: possible involvement of central opioidergic systems. Eur J Pharmacol 218:153–158

Kawabata A, Umeda N, Takagi H (1993) L-Arginine exerts a dual role in nociceptive processing in the brain: involvement of the kyotorphin-Met-enkephalin pathway and NO-cyclic GMP pathway. Br J Pharmacol 109:73–79

Kellstein DE, Mayer DJ (1991) Spinal co-administration of cholecystokinin antagonists with morphine prevents the development of opioid tolerance. Pain 47:221–229

Kellstein DE, Price DD, Mayer DJ (1991) Cholecystokinin and its antagonist lorglumide respectively attenuate and facilitate morphine-induced inhibition of c-fiber evoked discharges of dorsal horn nociceptive neurons. Brain Res 540:302–306

Kitto KF, Haley JE, Wilcox GL (1992) Involvement of nitric oxide in spinally mediated hyperalgesia in the mouse. Neurosci Lett 148:1–5

Klein CM, Coggeshall RE, Carlton SM, Sorkin LS (1992) The effects of A- and C-fiber stimulation on patterns of neuropeptide immunostaining in the rat superficial dorsal horn. Brain Res 580:121–128

Kolesnikov Y, Pick CG, Ciszewska G, Pasternak GW (1993) Blockade of tolerance to morphine but not to κ opioids by a nitric oxide synthase inhibitor. Proc Natl Acad Sci USA 90:5162–5166

Kuraishi Y, Kawamura M, Yamaguchi H, Houtani T, Kawabata S, Futaki S, Fujii N, Satoh M (1991) Intrathecal injections of galanin and its antiserum affect nociceptive response of rat to mechanical, but not thermal, stimuli. Pain 44:321–324

Magnuson DS, Sullivan AF, Simonnet G, Roques BP, Dickenson AH (1990) Differential interactions of cholecystokinin and FLFQPQRF-NH2 with mu and delta opioid antinociception in the rat spinal cord. Neuropeptides 16:213–218

Malmberg AB, Yaksh TL (1993) Spinal nitrix oxide synthesis inhibition blocks NMDA-induced thermal hyperalgesia and produces antinociception in the formalin test in rats. Pain 54:291–300

Mao J, Price DD, Mayer DJ (1995) Experimental mononeuropathy reduces the antinociceptive effect of morphine: implications for common intracellular mechanisms involved in morphine tolerance and neuropathic pain. Pain 61:353–364

Marletta MA (1993) Nitric oxide synthase structure and mechanism. J Biol Chem 268:12231–12234

Meller ST, Gebhart GF (1993) NO and nociceptive processing in the spinal cord. Pain 52:127–136

Meller ST, Pechman PS, Gebhart GF, Maves TJ (1992) Nitric oxide mediates the thermal hyperalgesia produced in a model of neuropathic pain in the rat. Neuroscience 50:7–10

Meller ST, Dykstra C, Gebhart GF (1993) Acute mechanical hyperalgesia in the rat is produced by coactivation of ionotropic AMPA and metabotropic glutamate receptors. Neuroreport 4:879–882

Meller ST, Cummings CP, Traub RJ, Gebhart GF (1994) The role of nitric oxide in the development and maintenance of the hyperalgesia produced by intraplantar injection of carrageenan in the rat. Neuroscience 60:367–374

Minami T, Nishihara I, Ito S, Sakamoto K, Hyodo M, Hayaishi O (1995) Nitric oxide mediates allodynia induced by intrathecal administration of prostaglandin E_2 or prostaglandin F_{2a} in conscious mice. Pain 61:285–290

Moncada S, Palmer RMJ, Higgs EA (1991) Nitric oxide: pysiology, pathophysiology, and pharmacology. Pharmacol Rew 43:109–141

Moore PK, Oluyomi AO, Babbedge RC, Wallace P, Hart SL (1991) L-N^G-nitro arginine methyl ester exhibis antinociceptive activity in the mouse. Br J Pharmacol 102:198–202

Moore PK, Wallace P, Gaffen Z, Hart SL, Babbedge RC (1992) Characterization of the novel nitric oxide synthase inhibitor 7-nitro indazole and related indazoles: antinociceptive and cardiovascular effects. Br J Pharmacol 110:219–224

Moran T, Robinson P, Goldrich MS, McHugh P (1986) Two brain cholecystokinin receptors: implications for behavioural actions. Brain Res 362:175–179

Noble F, Blommaert A, Fourniezaluski MC, Roques BP (1995) A selective CCK-B receptor antagonist potentiates mu-, but not delta-opioid receptor-mediated antinociception in the formalin test. Eur J Pharmacol 273:145–151

Nussbaumer J-C, Yanagisawa M, Otsuka M (1989) Pharmacological properties of a C-fibre response evoked by sapheous nerve stimulation in an isolated spinal cord-nerve preparation of the newborn rat. Br J Pharmacol 98:373–382

O'Neill MF, Dourish CT, Iversen SD (1989) Morphine-induced analgesia in the rat paw pressure test is blocked by CCK and enhanced by the CCK antagonist MK-329. Neuropharmacology 28:243–247

Post C, Alari L, Hökfelt T (1988) Intrathecal galanin increases the latency in the tail flick anbd hot plate tests in mouse. Acta Physiol Scand 132:583–584

Przewlocki R, Machelska H, Przewlocka B (1993) Inhibition of nitric oxide synthase enhances morphine antinociception in the rat spinal cord. Life Sci 53:PL1–5

Radhakrishnan V, Henry JL (1993) L-NAME blocks responses to NMDA, substance P and noxious cutaneous stimuli in cat dorsal horn. Neuroreport 4:323–326

Randic M, Gerber G, Ryu PD, Kangrga I (1987) Inhibitory actions of galanin and somatostatin 28 on rat spinal dorsal horn neurons. Abstr Soc Neurosci 17:1308

Rattray M, Jordan CC, DeBelleroche J (1988) The novel CCK antagonist L364,718 abolishes caerulein- but potentiates morphine-induced antinociception. Eur J Pharmacol 152:163–166

Reimann W, Englberger W, Friderichs E, Selve N, Wilffert B (1994) Spinal antinociception by morphine is antagonised by galanin receptor antagonists. Naunyn Schmiedebergs Arch Pharmacol 350:380–386

Schiantarelli P (1993) Theraputic potentials of cholecystokinin receptor antagonists in CNS disorders. Pharmacol Res 28:1–9

Schiffmann SN, Vanderhaeghen JJ (1991) Distribution of cells containing mRNA encoding cholecystokinin in the rat central nervous system. J Comp Neurol 304:219–233

Seroogy KB, Mohapatra NK, Lund PK, Réthelyi M, McGehee DS, Perl ER (1990) Species-sepcific expression of cholecystokinin messenger RNA in rodent dorsal root ganglia. Mol Brain Res 7:171–176

Showell GA, Bourrain S, Neduvelil JG, Fletcher SR, Baker R, Watt AP, Fletcher AE, Freedman SB, Kemp JA, Marshall GR, Patel S, Smith AJ, Matassa VG (1994) High affinity and potent, water-soluable 5-amino-1,4-benzodiazepine CCKB/gastrin receptor antagonists containing a cationic solubilizing group. J Med Chem 37:719–721

Simmons DR, Spike RC, Todd AJ (1995) Galanin is contained in GABAergic neurons in the rat spinal dorsal horn. Neurosci Lett 187:119–122

Skirboll L, Hökfelt T, Dockray G, Gehfeld J, Brownstein M, Cuello AC (1983) Evidence of periaqueductal cholecystokinin-substance P neurons projecting to the spinal cord. J Neurosci 3:1151–1157

Skofitsch G, Jacobowitz D (1985) Galanin-like immunoreactivity in capsaicin sensitive sensory neurons and ganglia. Brain Res Bull 15:191–195

Sorkin LS (1993) NMDA evokes an L-NAME sensitive spinal release of glutamate and citrulline. Neuroreport 4:479–482

Spike RC, Todd AJ, Johnston HM (1993) Coexistence of NADPH disphorase with GABA, glycine, and acetylcholine in rat spinal cord. J Comp Neurol 335:320–333

Stanfa LC, Dickenson AH (1993) Cholecystokinin as a factor in the enhanced potency of spinal morphine following carrageenin inflammation. Br J Pharmacol 108:967–973

Tang J, Chou J, Iadarola M, Yang HY, Costa E (1984) Proglumide prevents and curtails acute tolerance to morphine in rats. Neuropharmacology 23:715–718

Togunaga A, Senba E, Manabe Y, Shida T, Ueda Y, Tohyama M (1992) Orofacial pain increas mRNA level for galanin in the trigeminal nucleus caudalis of the rat. Peptides 13:1067–1072

Tuchscherer MM, Seybold VS (1989) A quantitative study of the coexistence of peptides in varicosities within the superficial laminae of the dorsal horn of the rat spinal cord. J Neurosci 9:195–205

Valverde O, Maldonado R, Fournie-Zaluski MC, Roques BP (1994) Cholecystokinin B antagonists strongly potentiate antinociception mediated by endogenous enkephalins. J Pharmacol Exp Ther 270:77–88

Vanderah TW, Lai J, Yamamura HI, Porreca F (1994) Antisense oligodeoxynucleotide to the CCKB receptor produces naltrindoleand [Leu5]enkephalin antiserum-sensitive enhancement of morphine antinociception. Neuroreport 5:1–5

Verge VMK, Wiesenfeld-Hallin Z, Hökfelt T (1993a) Cholecystokinin in mammalian primary sensory neurons and spinal cord: in situ hybridization studies in rat and monkey. Eur J Neurosci 5:240–250

Verge VM, Xu XJ, Langel U, Hokfelt T, Wiesenfeld-Hallin Z, Bartfai T (1993b) Evidence for endogenous inhibition of autotomy by galanin in the rat after sciatic nerve section: demonstrated by chronic intrathecal infusion of a high affinity galanin receptor antagonist. Neurosci Lett 149:193–197

Verge VMK, Zhang X, Xu X-J, Wiesenfeld-Hallin Z, Hökfelt T (1994) Marked increase in nitric oxide synthase mRNA in rat dorsal root ganglia after peripheral axotomy: in situ hybridization and functional studies. Proc Natl Acad Sci USA 89:11617–11621

Villar MJ, Cortés R, Theodorsson E, Wiesenfeld-Hallin Z, Schalling M, Fahrenkrug J, Emson PC, Hökfelt T (1989) Neuropeptide expression in rat dorsal root ganglion cells and spinal cord after peripheral nerve injury with special reference to galanin. Neuroscience 33:587–604

Villar MJ, Wiesenfeld-Hallin Z, Xu X-J, Theodorsson E, Emson PC, Hökfelt T (1991) Further studies on galanin-, substance P- and CGRP-like immunoreactivities in primary sensory neurons and spinal cord – effects of dorsal rhizotomies and sciatic nerve lesions. Exp Neurol 112:29–39

Vizzard MA, Erdman SL, Roppolo JR, Förstermann U, DeGroat WC (1994) Differential localization of neuronal nitric oxide synthase immunoreactivity and NADPH-diaphorase activity in the cat spinal cord. Cell Tissue Res 278:299–309

Vizzard MA, Erdman SL, DeGroat WC (1995) Increased expression of neuronal nitric oxide synthase (NOS) in visceral neurons after nerve injury. J Neurosci 15:4033–4045

Wall PD, Woolf CJ (1984) Muscle but not cutaneous C-afferent input produces prolonged increases in the excitability of the flexion reflex in the rat. J Physiol (Lond) 356:443–458

Wang XJ, Han JS (1989) Modification by cholecystokinin octapeptide of the binding of μ, δ- and κ-opioid receptors. J Neurochem 55:1379–1382

Wang XJ, Wang XH, Han JS (1990) Cholecystokinin octapeptide antagonized opioid analgesia mediated by μ and κ- but not δ-receptors in the spinal cord of the rat. Brain Res 523:5–10

Wang JF, Ren MF, Han JS (1992) Mobilization of calcium from intracellular stores is one of the mechanisms underlying the antiopioid effect of cholecystokinin octapeptide. Peptides 13:947–951

Watkins LR, Kinscheck IB, Mayer DJ (1984) Potentiation of opiate analgesia and apparent reversal of morphine tolerance by proglumide. Science 224:395–396

Watkins LR, Kinscheck IB, Kaufman EF, Miller J, Frenk H, Mayer DJ (1985) Cholecystokinin antagonists selectively potentiate analgesia induced by endogenous opiates. Brain Res 327:181–190

Wiertelak EP, Maier SF, Watkins LR (1992) Cholecystokinin antianalgesia: safety cues abolish morphine analgesia. Science 256:830–833

Wiesenfeld-Hallin Z, Duranti R (1987) Intrathecal cholecystokinin interacts with morphine but not substance P in modulating the nociceptive flexion reflex in the rat. Peptides 8:153–158

Wiesenfeld-Hallin Z, Villar MJ, Hökfelt T (1989) The effect of intrathecal galanin and C-fiber stimulation on the flexor reflex in the rat. Brain Res 486:205–213

Wiesenfeld-Hallin Z, Xu X-J, Hughes J, Horwell DC, Hökfelt T (1990) PD134308, a selective antagonist of cholecystokinin type-B receptor, enhances the analgesic effect of morphine and synergistically interacts with intrathecal galanin to depress spinal nociceptive reflexes. Proc Natl Acad Sci USA 87:7105–7109

Wiesenfeld-Hallin Z, Bartfai T, Hökfelt T (1992a) Galanin in sensory neurons in the spinal cord. Front Neuroendocrinol 13:319–343

Wiesenfeld-Hallin Z, Xu X-J, Langel Ü, Bedecs K, Hökfelt T, Bartfai T (1992b) Galanin-mediated control of pain: enhanced role after nerve injury. Proc Natl Acad Sci USA 89:3334–3337

Wiesenfeld-Hallin Z, Hao J-X, Xu X-J, Hökfelt T (1993a) Nitric oxide mediates ongoing discharges in dorsal root ganglion cells after peripheral nerve injury. J Neurophysiol 70:2350–2354

Wiesenfeld-Hallin Z, Xu XJ, Hao JX, Hökfelt T (1993b) The behavioural effects of intrathecal galanin on tests of thermal and mechanical nociception in the rat. Acta Physiol Scand 147:457–458

Williams RG, Dimaline R, Varro A, Isetta AM, Trizio D, Dockray GJ (1987) Cholecystokinin octapeptide in rat central nervous system: immunocytochemical studies using a monoclonal antibody that does not react with CGRP. Neurochem Int 11:433–442

Willis DW (1994) Central plastic responses to pain. In: Gebhart GF, Hammond DL, Jensen TS (eds) Proceedings of the 7th World Congress on Pain, vol 2. International Association for the Study of Pain, Seattle, pp 301–324

Xu XJ, Wiesenfeld-Hallin Z (1991) The threshold for the depressive effect of intrathecal morphine on the spinal nociceptive flexor reflex is increased during autotomy after sciatic nerve section in rats. Pain 46:223–229

Xu X-J, Wiesenfeld-Hallin Z, Fisone G, Bartfai T, Hökfelt T (1990a) The N-terminal, but not C-terminal, galanin fragment affects the flexor reflex in rats. Eur J Pharmacol 182:137–141

Xu X-J, Wiesenfeld-Hallin Z, Villar MJ, Fahrenkrug J, Hökfelt T (1990b) On the role of galanin, substance P and other neuropeptides in primary sensory neurons of the rat: studies on spinal reflex excitability and peripheral axotomy. Eur J Neurosci 2:733–743

Xu X-J, Wiesenfeld-Hallin Z, Hökfelt T (1991) Intrathecal galanin blocks the prolonged increase in spinal cord flexor reflex induced by conditioning stimulation of unmyelinated muscle afferents in the rat. Brain Res 541:350–353

Xu X-J, Wiesenfeld-Hallin Z, Hughes J, Horwell DC, Hökfelt T (1992) CI988, a selective antagonist of cholecystokinin type-B receptor, prevents morphine tolerance in the rat. Br J Pharmacol 105:591–596

Xu X-J, Puke MJC, Verge VMK, Wiesenfeld-Hallin Z, Hughes J, Hökfelt T (1993) Up-regulation of cholecystokinin in primary sensory neurons is associated with morphine insensitivity in experimental neuropathic pain. Neurosci Lett 152:129–132

Xu X-J, Hao J-X, Seiger Å, Hughes J, Hökfelt T, Wiesenfeld-Hallin Z (1994a) Chronic pain-related behaviors in spinally injured rats: evidence for functional alterations of the endogenous cholecystokinin and opioid systems. Pain 56:271–278

Xu XJ, Hökfelt T, Hughes J, Wiesenfeld-Hallin Z (1994b) The CCK-B antagonist CI988 enhances the reflex-depressive effect of morphine in axotomized rats. Neuroreport 5:718–720

Xu XJ, Wiesenfeld-Hallin Z, Langel Ü, Bedecs K, Bartfai T (1995) New high affinity peptide antagonists to the spinal galanin receptor. Br J Phamracol 116:2076–2080

Yamamoto T, Shimoyama N (1995) Role of nitric oxide in the development of thermal hyperalgesia induced by sciatic nerve constriction injury in the rat. Anesthesiology 82:1266–1273

Yanagisawa M, Yagi N, Otsuka M, Yanaihara C, Yanaihara N (1986) Inhibitory effects of galanin on the isolated spinal cord of the newborn rat. Neurosci Lett 70:278–282

Zhang X, Verge VMK, Wiesenfeld-Hallin Z, Ju G, Bredt D, Snyder SH, Hökfelt T (1993a) Nitric oxide synthase-like immunoreactivity in lumbar dorsal root ganglia and spinal cord of rat and monkey and effect of peripheral axotomy. J Comp Neurol 335:563–575

Zhang X, Ju G, Elde R, Hökfelt T (1993b) Effect of peripheral nerve cut on neuropeptides in dorsal root ganglia and the spinal cord of monkey with special reference to galanin. J Neurocytol 22:342–381

Zhang X, Dagerlind Å, Elde RP, Castel MN, Broberger C, Wiesenfeld-Hallin Z, Hökfelt T (1993c) Marked increase in cholecystokinin B receptor messenger RNA levels in rat dorsal root ganglia after peripheral axotomy. Neuroscience 57:227–233

Zhang X, Ji RR, Nilsson S, Villar M, Ubink R, Ju G, Wiesenfeld-Hallin Z, Hökfelt T (1995a) Neuropeptide Y and galanin binding sites in rat and monkey lumbar dorsal root ganglia and spinal cord and effect of peripheral axotomy. Eur J Neurosci 7:367–380

Zhang X, Nicholas AP, Hökfelt T (1995b) Ultrastructural studies on peptides in the dorsal horn of the spinal cord. I. Co-existence of galanin with other peptides in primary afferents in normal rats. Neuroscience 57:365–384

Zhang X, Nicholas AP, Hokfelt T (1995c) Ultrastructural studies on peptides in the dorsal horn of the rat spinal cord. II. Coexistence of galanin with other peptides in local neurons. Neuroscience 64:875–891

Zhang X, Bean AJ, Wiesenfeld-Hallin Z, Xu XJ, Hökfelt T (1995d) Ultrastructural studies on peptides in the dorsal horn of the rat spinal cord. III. Effects of peripheral axotomy with special reference to galanin. Neuroscience 64:893–915

Zhou Y, Sun YH, Zhang ZW, Han JS (1992) Accelerated expression of cholecystokinin gene in the brain of rats rendered tolerant to morphine. Neuroreport 3:1121–1123

Zhou Y, Sun YH, Zhang ZW, Han JS (1993) Increased release of immunoreactive cholecystokinin octapeptide by morphine and potentiation of μ-opioid analgesia by CCKB receptor antagonist L365,260 in rat spinal cord. Eur J Pharmacol 234:147–154

Zhuo M, Meller ST, Gebhart GF (1993) Endogenous nitric oxide is required for tonic cholinergic inhibition of spinal mechanical transmission. Pain 54:71–78

Zouaoui D, Benoliel JJ, Cesselin F, Conrath M (1991) Cholecystokinin-like immunoreactivity in the rat spinal cord: effects of thoracic transection. Brain Res Bull 26:543–547

CHAPTER 10

Pharmacological Studies of Nociceptive Systems Using the C-Fos Immunohistochemical Technique: An Indicator of Noxiously Activated Spinal Neurones

V. Chapman and J.-M. Besson

A. Introduction

To date a considerable number of oncogenes have been identified and have had their proto-oncogene counterparts cloned. In general the induction of proto-oncogenes, for example c-*fos*, is rapid, transient, and protein synthesis independent (see references in Hughes and Dragunow 1995; Morgan 1991; Morgan and Curran 1995). There are considered to be at least two different pathways leading to the induction of c-*fos*, as established from cell culture, one involving the activation of the inositol–phosphate–protein kinase C pathway (the serum response element) and the other involving an increase in intracellular calcium. It is considered that the proteins involved in the induction of c-*fos* transcription require only posttranslational modification (phosphorylation) for activation, thus at least partly explaining the rapid induction of c-*fos*. Since protein synthesis inhibition results in a huge induction of c-*fos* mRNA, it is suggested that a de novo synthesized protein is required for the "shut off" of c-*fos* transcription (see references in Hughes and Dragunow 1995). The protein responsible for the transcriptional "shut off" is the c-*fos* protein product, Fos; however, such a negative feedback mechanism (*trans*-repression) influences only c-*fos* serum-inducible promoter elements. In addition to *trans*-repression, the induction of c-*fos* is also transient due to untranslated AT-rich sequences within the transcript which reduce c-*fos* stability (see references in Hughes and Dragunow 1995).

The protein products of proto-ongenes are generated in the cell membrane, cytosol and importantly in the nucleus; thus they are ideally located for the regulation of gene expression. A huge amount of work has demonstrated that c-Fos and c-Jun (protein product from c-*jun*) form a heterodimer, leucine zipper configuration, and bind to the activating protein-1 site of DNA and transactivate gene transcription.

Diverse types of stimulation have been shown to result in an increased expression of immediate-early gene (IEG) mRNA and protein in neuronal and non-neuronal cells in the brain. For example, chemically induced seizures have been shown to induce c-*fos* mRNA and protein initially in the nuclei of the dentate gyrus, pyriform and cingulate cortices and thereafter throughout the cortex, hippocampus and limbic system (see references in Morgan 1991; Hughes and Dragunow 1995). Furthermore, kindling, an animal model of seizure development induced by repetitive subconvulsive focal electrical stimulation in the amydala or hippocampus, has been shown to induce c-*fos* mRNA and protein as well as other IEGs in the dentate granule cells, hippoc-ampus and amydala. Focal brain injury to the hippocampus by needle inser-tion and saline injection has been shown to result in the induction of c-*fos* and other IEGs in the nerve cells of the dentate gyrus. Overall when considering the brain the list of stimuli which activate the induction of the IEGs is exhaus-tive, and most certainly not complete (for further reading see HUGHES and DRAGUNOW 1995). The basal level of c-Fos immunoreactivity varies for differ-ent areas of the brain, and multiple factors can influence the level of this expression. Furthermore, stress such as immobilization, capsaicin administra-tion and earclipping further induces c-Fos expression in the brain. In contrast, at the level of the spinal cord the basal expression of c-Fos is negligible, and animal handling or injection of saline does not induce the expression of the c-Fos protein. Thus since there is virtually no background activity, the immuno-histochemical study of the level of spinal c-Fos protein following various types of noxious stimuli (see below) is ideal. Furthermore, c-*fos* is one of the first IEGs to be induced, the half-life of which is relatively short, and the resultant rapid speed of onset/offset of c-*fos* induction following stimulation means that the level of c-*fos* follows closely the intensity/duration of the noxious stimulation.

This review discusses the findings and implications of numerous different studies on the physiological aspects of noxiously evoked c-Fos expression at the level of the spinal cord. Following this discussion we present a review of the results of various pharmacological investigations which manipulate the excitatory and inhibitory systems involved in nociceptive transmission.

B. Spinal Expression of c-Fos: Physiological Aspects

It is nearly a decade since the original study demonstrating that the basal level of spinal c-Fos is extremely low, and that physiological stimulation of rat peripheral somato-sensory neurones results in the spinal expression of c-Fos immunoreactive protein in post-synaptic dorsal horn neurones (HUNT et al. 1987). Activation of the cutaneous fine primary afferent fibres by both noxious heat and a chemical stimuli (mustard oil) resulted in a rapid appearance of c-Fos immunoreactivity in predominantly the superficial laminae (laminae I–II outer) of the dorsal horn of the spinal cord. [The grey matter of the spinal cord is divided into ten laminae on a cytoarchitectonic basis (REXED 1952). As illustrated throughout this handbook the superficial laminae (I–II, outer) of the dorsal horn of the spinal cord are the main termination sites of fine myelinated ($A\delta$) and unmyelinated (C) nociceptive fibres. The superficial laminae contains a very high density of numerous neurotransmitters, neuromodulators and receptors involved in the modulation of pain.] In con-trast, non-noxious brushing and gentle hindlimb manipulation resulted in the appearance of fewer c-Fos immunoreactive neurones in laminae II–IV but rarely in laminae I of the dorsal horn (HUNT et al. 1987). This initial report was the starting point of a huge amount of scientific investment and hope, using this technique to investigate both physiological and pharmacological aspects of pain processing at the spinal level (see references in FITZGERALD 1990).

Following numerous investigations there is considerable evidence that spinal expression of c-Fos can be evoked by various types of peripheral noxious cutaneous stimuli, including heat (ABBADIE et al. 1994c; BULLITT 1989, 1990; HERDEGEN et al. 1991; HUNT et al. 1987; LIMA et al. 1993; LIMA and AVELINO 1994; NARANJO et al. 1991; TÖLLE et al. 1990, 1991; WILLIAMS et al. 1990a; WISDEN et al. 1990), cold (ABBADIE et al. 1994b), and mechanical stimulation (ABBADIE and BESSON 1993b; BULLITT 1989, 1990, 1991; LEAH et al. 1992; LIMA et al. 1993; LIMA and AVELINO 1994), local application of mustard oil (WILLIAMS et al. 1989) and acute capsaicin treatment (WILLIAMS et al. 1989) and high-intensity peripheral electrical stimulation (BULLITT et al. 1992; HERDEGEN et al. 1991). Furthermore, various models of inflammatory pain have also been shown to evoke an extensive spinal expression of c-Fos, including intraplantar injection of formalin (ABBADIE et al. 1992; CHAPMAN et al. 1995a; ELLIOTT et al. 1995; HERDEGEN et al. 1994; KEHL et al. 1991; LEAH et al. 1992; LIMA et al. 1993; PRESLEY et al. 1990; WILLIAMS et al. 1989), carrageenan (CHAPMAN et al. 1995c; DRAISCI and IADAROLA 1989; HONORÉ et al. 1995a; NOGUCHI et al. 1991, 1992) and complete Freund's adjuvant administration (ABBADIE and BESSON 1992; HYLDEN et al. 1992; MENÉTREY et al. 1989). In addition, numerous types of noxious visceral stimulation also evoke the spinal expression of c-Fos; these include intraperitoneal injection of acetic acid (HAMMOND et al. 1992; MENÉTREY et al. 1989; LANTÉRI-MINET et al. 1993a,b), irritation of the lower urinary tract (BIRDER and DE GROAT 1992a,b), cystitis (LANTÉRI-MINET et al. 1995), electrical stimulation of the pelvic nerve (BIRDER et al. 1991) and colorectal distension (TRAUB et al. 1992, 1993). Although we discuss in particular the noxiously evoked spinal c-Fos expression, it is important to bear in mind that similar findings have been reported at the trigeminal level (BEREITER et al. 1994; CUTRER et al. 1995a,b; LU et al. 1993; STRASSMAN et al. 1993; STRASSMAN and VOS 1993).

One of the main problems of both physiological and pharmacological nociceptive studies using spinal Fos immunohistochemical technique concerns the specificity of the labelling, i.e. are spinal neurones expressing Fos those exclusively involved in nociceptive processes? This has been an issue from the very beginning (HUNT et al. 1987) and has been again brought to light by the recent study demonstrating that continuous walking for 1 h evokes a high level of c-Fos expression in the cervical and lumbar spinal cord (JASMIN et al. 1994a). This expression is observed in laminae that contain neurones which respond to non-noxious stimuli: the inner part of the substantia gelatinosa (laminae IIi), and the nucleus proprius (laminae III–IV). Importantly, an increase in c-Fos expression in laminae I and the outer substantia gelatinosa (laminae IIo), which contains noxiously activated neurones (see references in

Besson and Chaouch 1987) was not observed following walking (Jasmin et al. 1994a). Despite the fact that the study by Jasmin et al. suggests that spinal c-Fos expression is not a specific marker of neurones activated by noxious inputs, this finding should not be overemphasized since an overwhelming number of studies have clearly highlighted the preferential expression of spinal c-Fos by noxious stimulation (see above).

The following section presents the main arguments (since 1987) which in our opinion favour the use of this technique to study spinal nociceptive processes:

I. Acute Noxious Stimulation

1. In the initial report Hunt et al. (1987) observed relatively few spinal Fos-like immunoreactive (Fos-LI) neurones following non-noxious mechanical and proprioceptive stimulation as compared to those produced by noxious stimulation of the rat hindpaw. Thereafter it was demonstrated that non-noxious mechanical and proprioceptive stimulation of the rat hindpaw does not result in the spinal expression of c-Fos (Bullitt 1989, 1990).

2. As mentioned above, several studies have shown that noxious, but not innocuous, thermal stimulation evokes the spinal expression of c-Fos. For example, we have quantitatively shown that the temperature threshold for consistent induction of spinal c-Fos expression in urethane anaesthetized rats is in the order of 44°–46°C (Abbadie et al. 1994c) and thus in good agreement with the nociceptive reaction of freely moving animals to the same stimulation and with the threshold for activation of C polymodal and some mechano-heat nociceptors (see references in Willis and Coggeshall 1991). Increasing temperatures over the 44°–52°C range (Fig. 1) induces a higher number of Fos-LI neurones, and there is a clear relationship between the stimulus intensity and the number of Fos-LI neurones. Moreover, for the same intensity of noxious stimulation we have shown that increasing the duration of the stimulation induces an incremental increase in the number of Fos-LI neurones (Fig. 1). Interestingly, with 52°C a 5-s stimulation period is sufficient to evoke a substantial number of spinal Fos-LI neurones, thus demonstrating at least for heat stimulation that this technique based on immunohistochemistry is very sensitive to changes of spinal neuronal activity (see also Williams et al. 1989). In our study with a post-stimulation perfusion time point of 2 h up to 85% of noxious heat evoked spinal Fos-LI neurones were located in the superficial laminae of the dorsal horn.

3. The relatively preferential noxious, and not innocuous, evoked expression of spinal c-Fos has been exemplified by a study demonstrating that electrical activation of $A\delta$ and C fibres, but not $A\beta$ fibres, activates the induction and subsequent expression of c-Fos protein in the nuclei of dorsal horn neurones of the spinal cord (Herdegen et al. 1991; see also Molander et al. 1992). In addition, following noxious stimulation of the hindpaw Fos-LI neurones are essentially located in the superficial (I–II) and deep (V–VI)

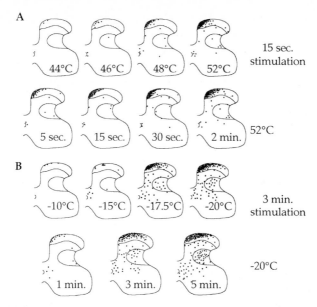

Fig. 1. Comparison of the number of spinal Fos-LI neurones in the lumbar L4–L5 segment of the spinal cord following various intensities of heat (**A**) and intense cold (**B**) stimulation of the hindpaw. Increasing the duration of noxious heat or cold stimulation results in a concomitant increase in the number of Fos-LI neurones in the dorsal horn of the spinal cord. Each image is a computer-aided design of a camera lucida drawing of a 40-μm section of the spinal cord. *Outlined*, the limits of the superficial laminae and the reticular part of the neck; *each point*, one Fos-LI neurone. (From ABBADIE et al. 1994b,c)

laminae of the dorsal horn of the L4–L5 segment of the spinal cord, thus laminae containing noxious specific and wide dynamic range neurones (BESSON and CHAOUCH 1987; WILLIS and COGGESHALL 1991).

4. The number of noxiously evoked Fos-LI neurones in the dorsal horn of the spinal cord can be dramatically reduced by neonatal capsaicin treatment, which selectively destroys a large proportion of C fibres (HYLDEN et al. 1992; ZHANG et al. 1994a).

5. The localization of spinal Fos-LI neurones following noxious heat stimulation closely resembles the well-established spinal projection of afferent fibres innervating the hindpaw. It has been clearly demonstrated that noxious mechanical stimulation of individual digits results in a distinct somatotopic pattern of Fos-LI neurones in laminae I–II and V–IX of the dorsal horn of the spinal cord (BULLITT 1991). Furthermore, spinal c-Fos expression has been used to map the extent of the rostral-caudal projection of a single dorsal root by using various types of rhizotomies (ABBADIE et al. 1992, 1994d). A clear somatotopy of c-Fos expression in the trigeminal complex following noxious facial stimulation which closely matches that previously established by

anatomical and electrophysiological studies has also been demonstrated (Strassman and Vos 1993).

6. Noxiously evoked spinal c-Fos expression has been shown to be reduced by the activation of bulbo-spinal inhibitory descending systems (Jones and Light 1990; Morgan et al. 1994) which have been shown to be strongly involved in the modulation of spinal nociceptive transmission. In addition, formalin-evoked spinal c-Fos expression has been shown to be increased after lesion of the dorsal lateral funiculus, which contains numerous descending bulbo-spinal fibres (Zhang et al. 1994b).

7. Although there have been relatively few studies of spinal c-Fos expression in the neonate rat, it has been illustrated that noxious stimuli evokes the spinal expression of c-Fos as early as the day of birth (Williams et al. 1990b; Yi and Barr 1995). Interestingly, the more recent study demonstrated that the progressive increase in the number of Fos-LI neurones following noxious stimulation was age related, up to postnatal day 14. These results are in agreement with electrophysiological studies demonstrating the gradual postnatal maturation of the fine primary nociceptive afferents (Fitzgerald 1987).

8. As early as 1989 it was demonstrated that inflammatory-evoked spinal expression of c-Fos is followed by an increase of spinal preprodynorphin mRNA, which outlasts the increase of c-fos mRNA (Draisci and Iadarola 1989). Subsequently a number of studies have demonstrated that following inflammation there is a co-localization of Fos- and Fos-related proteins with different upregulated peptide mRNA. For example, during carrageenan inflammation there is a huge upregulation of preproenkephalin mRNA (Noguchi et al. 1992) and dynorphin mRNA and peptide (Noguchi et al. 1991) in dorsal horn neurones. In both cases a large proportion of the upregulated mRNA or peptide was co-localized with Fos protein, in particular in the superficial and deep laminae of the dorsal horn. However, in both studies it was clear that the number of Fos-LI neurones was considerably greater than the subpopulation of double-labelled neurones. Additional co-localization studies have demonstrated that following formalin inflammation up to 20% of Fos-LI neurones in the superficial laminae and up to 35% of Fos-LI neurones in the remaining laminae are GABA immunoreactive and in some cases also glycine immunoreactive (Todd et al. 1994). Thus the majority of the current studies at the spinal level have provided evidence for the co-localization of c-fos mRNA and c-Fos protein with endogenous inhibitory substances. However, it is important to point out that an additional large population of spinal cord neurones expressing the c-Fos protein following noxious stimulation project to the thalamus and the major brainstem targets of the ascending spinal pathways (Menétrey et al. 1989; Jasmin et al. 1994b).

II. Persistent Chronic Nociception

1. The spinal expression of c-Fos evoked during adjuvant-induced polyarthritis, which is induced by intradermal injection of Freund's adjuvant

into the base of the tail and resembles human rheumatoid polyarthritis (ABBADIE and BESSON 1992) has been investigated. In this study we demonstrated that the total number of Fos-LI neurones in the lumbar segment of the spinal cord (basal labelling), which was observed in the absence of any intentional stimulation, is correlated with the development of the adjuvant arthritis. c-Fos expression was absent at week 1, moderate at the 2nd week, dramatically increased by the 3rd week after inoculation, and declined the weeks thereafter (Fig. 2). The peak of polyarthritis-evoked c-Fos expression paralleled the peak of the maximal acute hyperalgesia (CALVINO et al. 1987), at this time point maximal Fos-immunoreactivity was observed in the deep laminae (laminae V–VI) of the dorsal horn of segments L3 and L4 of the spinal cord. Interestingly, such a basal labelling was attenuated by a prior "vaccination" with diluted Freund's adjuvant (ABBADIE et al. 1994a).

Numerous types of chronic pain exhibit not only spontaneous pain but also exaggerated responses to noxious stimulation (hyperalgesia); therefore it was of interest to investigate the phenomenon of hyperalgesia in the polyarthritic rat with the c-Fos technique. We have demonstrated (ABBADIE and BESSON 1993b) that repeated mechanical stimulation of the ankle at week 3 of the polyarthritis is associated with a prominent increase in the number of Fos-LI neurones in the ipsilateral dorsal horn of the spinal cord, significantly higher than in the non-stimulated and stimulated non-arthritic groups (Fig. 3). In both stimulated normal and arthritic rats maximal Fos-LI was present in segments L3 and L4 of the spinal cord, with an intense level of c-Fos expression in the superficial and deep laminae of the dorsal horn of the spinal cord. Overall this study provided evidence for hyperalgesia during arthritis and illustrated that the population of dorsal horn neurones responding during the

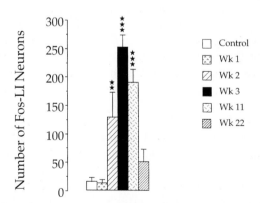

Fig. 2. Expression of spinal c-Fos at various stages following polyarthritis induced by injection of Freund's adjuvant in the base of the tail. The total number of Fos-LI neurones includes all labelled neurones in segments L2–L6 inclusive for the three most labelled sections per segment. Statistical analysis with ANOVA and PLSD Fischer's test as compared to control, **$p < 0.01$, ***$p < 0.001$. (From ABBADIE and BESSON 1992)

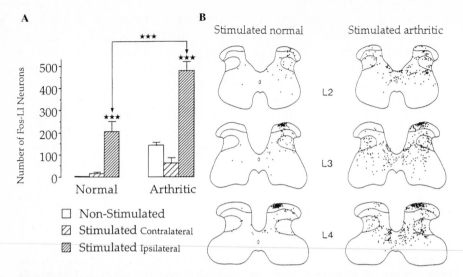

Fig. 3A,B. Effect of mechanical stimulation of the ankle on the number of spinal Fos-LI neurones, ipsilateral versus contralateral to the stimulated ankle, in normal rats and polyarthritic rats. Mechanical stimulation (not exceeding 4 N/cm2) was applied 20 times every 2 min for 30 min, 3 weeks after the induction of the polyarthritis. (From Abbadie and Besson 1993b)

hyperalgesia, evoked by additional stimulation, is different to the population of dorsal horn neurones influenced by the ongoing basal chronic arthritic evoked activity. Thus it appears that the phenomenon of hyperalgesia can be easily detected and visualized with the c-Fos immunohistochemical technique.

These data obtained with chronic polyarthritis differ greatly from those obtained using models of acute arthritis. Indeed after unilateral injection of complete Freund's adjuvant into the hindlimb there is within a day an extensive expression of c-Fos in both the superficial and deep laminae of the dorsal horn of the lumbar spinal cord (Menétrey et al. 1989; Lantéri-Minet et al. 1993a, see also Woolf et al. 1994). The laminar distribution of Fos-LI neurones following acute arthritis resembles that obtained following intraplantar injection of carrageenan, a model of inflammatory pain (Buritova et al. 1995a; Chapman et al. 1995c; Draisci and Iadarola 1989; Honoré et al. 1995a; Noguchi et al. 1991, 1992). The time course of carrageenan-evoked c-Fos expression is considerably faster and shorter in duration (Fig. 4) than that associated with acute arthritis.

2. The are a number of models of neuropathic pain, including "nerve transection", "nerve crush" and "loose nerve ligation" (see Besson and Guilbaud 1991). Studies of spinal c-Fos expression following neuropathy are difficult to compare and interpret, primarily as a result of different methodological paradigms. Thus it is not surprising that there is a controversy concerning the effect of neuropathy on the basal expression of spinal c-Fos,

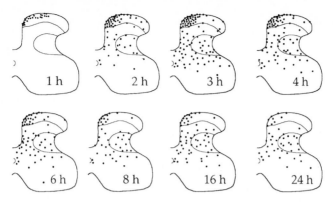

Fig. 4. Time course of the spinal expression of c-Fos in the dorsal horn of the L4–L5 segment of the spinal cord at various time points after the intraplantar injection of carrageenan. Each image is a computer-aided design of a camera lucida drawing of a 40-μm section of the spinal cord. *Outlined*, limits of the superficial laminae and the reticular part of the neck; *each point*, one Fos-LI labelled neurone. (From HONORÉ et al. 1995a, 1996b)

increased (SHARP et al. 1989; CHI et al. 1993; VOS and STRASSMAN 1995) versus not changed (WILLIAMS et al. 1991; HERDEGEN et al. 1992; MOLANDER et al. 1992, 1994). More importantly, changes in evoked spinal c-Fos expression and somatosensory function have been reported in models of neuropathic pain (MOLANDER et al. 1992, 1994; HONGPAISAN and MOLANDER 1993; WILLIAMS et al. 1991). However, these studies have not investigated the relationship between behavioural responses and evoked spinal c-Fos expression by either noxious or innocuous stimuli. A recent study using chronic constriction of the infraorbital nerve as a model of neuropathic pain clearly illustrated that the total increase of evoked Fos-LI neurones in the medullary dorsal horn is positively correlated with the behavioural manifestations of increased trigeminal nociceptive activity (VOS and STRASSMAN 1995). As suggested by the authors, the specific pattern of Fos-LI in models of neuropathy may contribute to the understanding of the associated central pathophysiology. Furthermore, this study, as can be the case with all studies using the c-Fos technique, has the advantage of being combined with behavioural observations. In the future, this dual approach could be extremely useful for the investigation of complex pharmacological aspects of the various neuropathic syndromes.

3. There are several different experimental models which attempt to mimic migraine, including electrical stimulation of the trigeminal ganglion (SHEPHEARD et al. 1995), intracisternal injection of capsaicin (CUTRER et al. 1995a,b) or carrageenan (NOZAKI et al. 1992a) and meningeal irritation by injection of blood into the subarchnoid space (NOZAKI et al. 1992b), which have been shown to evoke c-Fos expression in particular, in the nucleus caudalis of the trigeminal system. All of these studies observed a consistently high level of c-Fos expression in the superficial laminae (laminae I–IIo) of the

nucleus caudalis, which is the main termination site of nociceptive trigeminal afferent fibres. Neonatal capsaicin treatment has been shown to greatly reduce c-Fos expression evoked by chemical stimulation of the meninges (NOZAKI et al. 1992b). Overall the results from the various teams are very homogeneous, and subsequently the c-Fos technique has been used as a tool to perform pharmacological investigations of the possible mechanisms of migraine. In this respect various serotonin 1D and/or 1B receptor agonists (sumatriptan, dihydroergotamine, CP-93 129 and CP-122 288; NOZAKI et al. 1992a; CUTRER et al. 1995b), and the neurokinin 1 receptor antagonist CP-99 994 (SHEPHEARD et al. 1995) and RPR-100 893 (CUTRER et al. 1995a) have been shown to reduce c-Fos expression or c-Fos mRNA associated with the models of migraine described above.

III. c-Fos: The Unknown Factors

Taken together the points listed above strongly support the use of the c-Fos immunohistochemical technique as an indicator of noxiously activated spinal neurones and provide a good basis for the use of this technique for pharmacological investigations of the spinal transmission of nociceptive inputs. However, prior to presenting an overview of the current status of pharmacological investigations using this technique, it is necessary to consider the drawbacks of such an approach.

There are a number of ambiguities concerning the meaning and validity of c-Fos expression as a marker of neuronal activity which should be considered. Such unresolved issues include questions pertaining to the physiological meaning of Fos-LI in a neurone. Furthermore, if the presence of Fos-LI is a marker of intracellular neuronal events, such as calcium entry into a neurone following depolarization, is the intensity of evoked Fos-LI regulated by the basal level of depolarization or hyperpolarization of that individual neurone? What intensity and duration of stimulation are required to reach maximal c-Fos expression, and how does this vary between different neuronal populations? In keeping with these questions it has been suggested that the relative propensity for c-Fos expression may vary for different regions (STRASSMAN and VOS 1993), such as the different laminae of the spinal cord. Thus it could be envisaged that not only the level of neuronal activation but also the tendency of individual neurones to express c-Fos determines which populations express high levels of c-Fos protein.

As discussed above, a relatively large spinal distribution of c-Fos labelling, centred mainly in the superficial and deep laminae of the dorsal horn has been observed following prolonged mechanical stimulation, visceral stimulation including colorectal distension, experimental models of cystitis, intraperitoneal injection of acetic acid and inflammation, and acute arthritis. In contrast following relatively brief noxious thermal stimuli (5–15 s duration) Fos-LI neurones are almost located exclusively in the superficial dorsal horn (WILLIAMS et al. 1989; ABBADIE et al. 1994c; see Fig. 1). Such a selective laminae distribution is remarkable when considering that almost all the laminae I–IIo neurones receive noxious inputs, and that this area corresponds to the main termination site of peripheral nociceptors. However, with an increased duration of noxious heat stimulation Fos-LI neurones are located both in the superficial and deep laminae of the dorsal horn of the spinal cord (Fig. 1). This type of spatiotemporal pattern of c-Fos expression between the superficial and deep laminar indicates that c-Fos expression reflects not only neuronal firing patterns since electrophysiological studies have clearly demonstrated that both superficial and deep laminae neurones respond with short latencies to brief thermal stimulation. Thus it is evident that there is a difference between the ability of noxious inputs to activate c-Fos expression in the deep as compared to the superficial dorsal horn neurones. These differences are not understood and may have various origins related to the firing pattern of the afferent input, the synaptic connectivity (mono- versus polysynaptic relays and the relative number of synaptic boutons per neurone) and transmitter release. Furthermore, the differential contribution and/or intraspinal spreading of neuromodulators, such as nitric oxide (NO) and substance P (SP) with increasing periods of noxious stimulation may contribute to this effect. In line with such a concept it is interesting to note that temporal facilitation is required for the expression of c-Fos in deep laminae nicotinamide-adenine dinucleotide phosphate diaphorase labelled neurones (HERDEGEN et al. 1994). Thus it seems that prolonged repetitive noxious stimulation is a prerequisite for the expression of c-Fos in deep laminae neurones, and that these neurones have a lower propensity for the expression of c-Fos. Alternatively, but not exclusively, it is possible that c-Fos expression in the deep laminae neurones is controlled by an endogenous intracellular braking system.

IV. c-Fos: Experimental and Technical Considerations

There are a number of important experimental and technical considerations when using this technique for the purpose of pharmacological investigations.

1. Since there is an inherent variability of the immunohistochemical labelling between experimental series it is important to perform a control stimulated group for each experiment. In addition, in each experimental series at least five animals per group should be used.

2. For pharmacological investigations, which could consist of a large number of rats, all of the tissue must be immunoreacted at the same time, and the analysis of the number of Fos-LI neurones should be performed by the same person and be double-blind.

3. It is important to bear in mind that the chosen time point of the perfusion after the stimulation can greatly influence the number and laminar distribution of Fos-LI neurones. This is relevant particularly for pharmacological investigations since for example a short delay (in the order of 1.30h) between the stimulation and the perfusion is more appropriate to optimize the analgesic effects on superficial laminae neurones, while a longer delay (in the

order of 3 h) is more suitable to gauge analgesic effects on deep dorsal horn neurones (see below). Furthermore, the duration of drug action versus the perfusion time point can greatly influence the outcome of the observed drug effect, and this may explain some discrepancies within the literature. Thus for putative analgesics with undetermined pharmacokinetic characteristics various perfusion time points should be considered to be sure of the optimal time point for the drug investigation.

4. The duration of the noxious stimulation can also influence the laminar distribution of Fos-LI neurones since with a longer duration of noxious stimulation there is an increased number of Fos-LI neurones in the deep dorsal horn.

5. With all pharmacological studies using the c-Fos technique it is necessary that drugs are given as a pre-treatment since once the c-Fos protein is expressed drug effects are masked, as clearly illustrated with studies of post-administered morphine (Abbadie and Besson 1993a; Tölle et al. 1994b).

6. Since at the present time it is not possible to quantify the intensity of Fos-LI for each individual neurone, only the absolute number of Fos-LI neurones are considered. However, in our experience with higher intensities of noxious stimulation there is a greater intensity of Fos-LI for each neurone.

Thus although there are a number of technical and experimental drawbacks associated with this technique, these are not considerably more than those encountered with other classical methods. Furthermore there are a number of advantages of the c-Fos technique at the level of the spinal cord, including the low level of basal spinal expression. In addition, the presence of c-Fos reveals at the single cell level the neurones preferentially activated by peripheral noxious stimulation, thus allowing the visualization of the rostro-caudal spread of neuronal activation. Furthermore, these studies can be performed with a simultaneous assessment of behavioural responses, and/or clinical signs of the disease such as the extent of the inflammatory aspect. Finally there is a clear relationship between the intensity of the stimulation and the number of neurones expressing c-Fos. Thus we used this technique to pursue a number of pharmacological investigations. The second half of this chapter reviews some of the recent pharmacological studies utilizing this technique.

C. Pharmacological Aspects

I. Opioids

Morphine is a well-established potent analgesic which is efficient when considering all classical nociceptive tests. Therefore it is considered to be a drug of reference when studying various types of nociceptive responses. The depressive effects of morphine upon the transmission of nociceptive messages at the level of the dorsal horn of the spinal cord is well established and documented (see references in Dickenson 1994a; Duggan and North 1984;

ZIEGLGÄNSBERGER and TÖLLE 1993; BASBAUM and BESSON 1991). It has been clearly established that the effect of morphine is selective for noxiously evoked responses of dorsal horn neurones, when administered by either systemic (LEBARS et al. 1975), iontophoretic (DUGGAN et al. 1977) or intrathecal (DICKENSON and SULLIVAN 1986) routes of administration. Thus it is not surprising that numerous studies have shown that pre-administration of opioid receptor agonists, in particular morphine, dose-relatedly reduces spinal c-Fos expression following noxious stimulation. Morphine has been shown to attenuate spinal c-Fos expression following all types of classical noxious stimulation, including noxious heat up to 52°C (ABBADIE et al. 1994c; TÖLLE et al. 1990, 1991, 1994a,b), noxious cold (ABBADIE et al. 1994b), intraplantar injection of formalin (PRESLEY et al. 1990; JASMIN et al. 1994b) or carrageenan (CHAPMAN et al. 1995d), mechanical stimulation in an experimental model of hyperalgesia, the polyarthritic rat (ABBADIE and BESSON 1993a) and intraperitoneal injection of acetic acid (HAMMOND et al. 1992). In general the majority of these studies have demonstrated dose-related effects of morphine (for example see Fig. 5) which are blocked by naloxone.

In addition to the dose-dependent effect of morphine on noxiously evoked spinal c-Fos expression, the effects of morphine have been shown to be more pronounced with high-intensity than low-intensity stimulation (Fig. 6).

Overall there are some discrepancies concerning the degree of effect of morphine on c-Fos expression which may be related to the type, intensity and

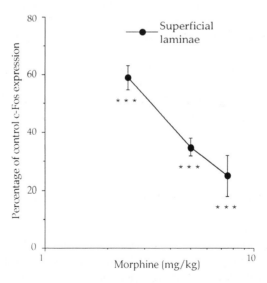

Fig. 5. Effect of systemic morphine on spinal c-Fos expression 2h after noxious heat stimulation (52°C for 15s. Two hours after stimulation c-Fos was located predominantly in the superficial laminae, and strong dose-dependent effects of morphine on this expression were observed, ***$p < 0.001$. (From ABBADIE et al. 1994c)

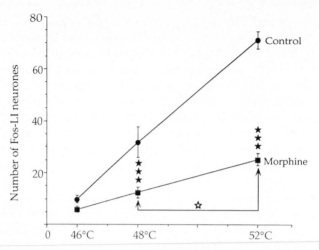

Fig. 6. Effect of 5mg/kg morphine (i.v.) compared to saline on the total number of spinal Fos-LI neurones in segment L4 of the spinal cord following thermal stimulation of the hindpaw during a 15-s period. As clearly illustrated, morphine had a significantly greater attenuating effect on c-Fos expression at 52°C as compared to at 48°C. Results are expressed as mean ± SEM; $*p < 0.05$, $***p < 0.001$. (From Abbadie et al. 1994c)

duration of noxious stimulation used, the route of morphine administration, use or absence of anaesthesia, and the delay between stimulation and perfusion time point. With regards to the latter point we recently demonstrated that consideration of the duration of noxiously evoked c-Fos expression and the relative duration of action of systemic morphine are important (Honoré et al. 1996b). In this study at early time points (up to 1.5h) after intraplantar injection of carrageenan c-Fos expression was located predominantly in the superficial laminae of the dorsal horn of the spinal cord, whereas at later time points (3h) c-Fos expression was located both in the superficial and deep laminae of the dorsal horn of the spinal cord (Honoré et al. 1996b). In the same study preadministered morphine (3mg/kg i.v.) strongly reduced carrageenan-evoked c-Fos expression in the superficial laminae 1.5h after carrageenan (58% ± 3% reduction of control) but was significantly less efficacious 2.5h after carrageenan injection (34% ± 6% reduction of control).

Following formalin stimulation the effect of morphine has been shown to be more pronounced on c-Fos expression in the deep laminae than in superficial laminae (Presley et al. 1990; Jasmin et al. 1994b). In contrast, such a differential effect of morphine on the two populations of neurones has not been observed following noxious heat (Abbadie et al. 1994c), visceral (Hammond et al. 1992), or carrageenan stimulation (Chapman et al. 1995d).

We have recently demonstrated that β-funaltrexamine (βFNA), an extremely long-lasting and selective irreversible antagonist of the μ-opioid receptor, completely blocks the attenuating effect of systemically administered morphine on carrageenan-evoked spinal c-Fos expression (Fig. 7; Honoré et

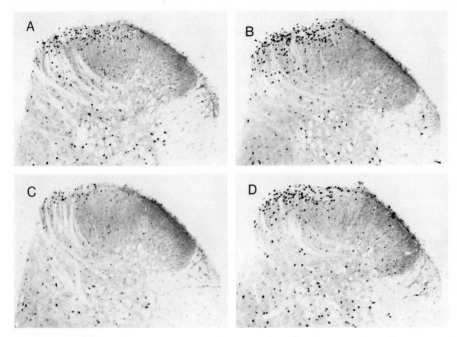

Fig. 7A–D. Ability of a pre-administered bFNA, an irreversible μ-receptor antagonist, to block the effect of morphine on carrageenan-evoked spinal c-Fos expression. Example photomicrographs of 40-μm sections of the L4–L5 segment of the spinal cord. **A** Two hours after the intraplantar injection of carrageenan, with vehicle controls. **B** Two hours after the intraplantar injection of carrageenan in a rat preadministered (24 h earlier) with 10 mg/kg bFNA (i.v.). **C** Two hours after the intraplantar injection of carrageenan in a rat preadministered with morphine (3 mg/kg, i.v.) 10 min before carrageenan administration. **D** Two hours after the intraplantar injection of carrageenan in a rat preadministered (24 h earlier) with 10 mg/kg bFNA (i.v.) and receiving morphine (3 mg/kg i.v.) 10 min before carrageenan administration HONORÉ et al. (1996e). *Bar*, 500 μm

al. 1996e). Following these studies it will be interesting to test the effect of both δ- and κ-opioid receptor agonists after βFNA administration. Selective δ-opioid agonists and irreversible antagonists, which are efficacious when administered systemically, are currently limited. However, studies utilizing βFNA treatment to completely block μ-opioid receptors will be able to assess the level of μ-/δ-opioid receptor overlap of the δ-opioid agonists and the endogenous opioid enkephalin.

The mixed inhibitors of enkephalin-metabolizing enzymes have been shown to reduce (kelatorphan; TÖLLE et al. 1994b) and dose-dependently reduce (N-[(R,S)-2-benzyl-3[(S)(2-amino-4-methyl-thio)butylithiol]-1-oxo-propyl]-L-phenylalanine benzyl ester, RB101; ABBADIE et al. 1994c), noxious heat evoked spinal c-Fos expression, with these effects being blocked by naloxone. These studies suggest that the endogenous opioids, in particular the enkephalins, play a functional role during spinal nociceptive processing. Thus it is perturbing that many studies have not observed an increase in the number of Fos-LI neurones by naloxone alone. However, one study has observed a slight increase in the number of noxious heat evoked Fos-LI neurones by naloxone (Tölle et al. 1994b), and another has observed that naloxone significantly increases the number of Fos-LI neurones evoked by extremely low noxious cold stimulation (Abbadie et al. 1994b). This discrepancy between the effect of the endogenous enkephalinase inhibitors and naloxone is not surprising when considering the comparable complex data obtained from electrophysiological and behavioural studies of opioid antagonists.

There is evidence that the phenomenon of opioid tolerance can be detected by the c-Fos technique. It has previously been shown that the level of noxious heat evoked spinal c-Fos expression in rats rendered tolerant to morphine is not different from the level evoked in naive rats (see however Rohde et al. 1993); nevertheless the ability of systemic morphine to reduce c-Fos expression in tolerant rats is 50% that in naive rats (Abbadie et al. 1994c). However, additional experiments using different types of peripheral stimulation and different doses of morphine are necessary to fully gauge the suitability of this approach for evaluating tolerance.

Overall the ability of systemic morphine to reduce noxiously evoked spinal c-Fos expression is in keeping with the well-established depressive effect of morphine at the spinal level (see references in Dickenson 1994a). Although the direct action of morphine at the dorsal horn level is well documented, there is additional controversial electrophysiological evidence concerning the ability of morphine to increase (for review see Basbaum and Fields 1978; Besson and Le Bars 1978) or not (Bouhassira et al. 1988) the activity of the descending inhibitory controls. In keeping with the former concept it has been shown that intracerebroventricularly administered D-Ala^2, NMe-Phe^4, Gly-ol^5]enkephalin (DAMGO; selective μ-opioid agonist) dose-dependently reduces formalin-evoked spinal c-Fos expression at the lumbar level in a naloxone-reversible manner (Gogas et al. 1991). Furthermore, it has been demonstrated that bilateral lesion of the dorsal lateral funiculus, which relays important descending inhibitory controls to the spinal cord, at the thoracic level completely suppressed the effect of intracerebroventricular DAMGO on spinal c-Fos expression. These findings were interpreted as suggesting that the analgesic action of supraspinally administered opiates results from an increase in descending inhibitory controls that regulate the firing of certain populations of spinal neurones (Gogas et al. 1991). Following these studies it would be interesting to compare the effect of systemic morphine in normal rats and rats with complete spinal cord transection and thus assess the direct spinal effects versus indirect effects at supra-spinal structures of systemically administered morphine.

The sites of action of systemic morphine are probably not limited to the CNS since a peripheral site of action of morphine has been proposed (Stein 1993, 1995). We have addressed this issue by considering the effect of intraplantar injection of morphine on spinal c-Fos expression evoked by intraplantar injection of carrageenan as compared to noxious heat stimulation (HONORÉ et al. 1996a). Intraplantar morphine (10–50 μg in 50 μl) dose-dependently reduced carrageenan, but not noxious heat, evoked spinal c-Fos expression. The effect of morphine on carrageenan-evoked spinal c-Fos expression was blocked by simultaneous intraplantar administration of methiodide naloxone, a μ-opioid antagonist which does not cross the blood-brain barrier. Since systemic administration of the highest concentration of intraplantar morphine studied did not influence c-Fos expression, this indicates a peripheral effect of intraplantar morphine under these conditions. Overall these results suggest that peripheral opioid receptor mediated events play a role during more prolonged inflammatory pain states but not under acute non-inflammatory pain states. Indeed it has previously been proposed that endogenous opioids, β-endorphin and Met-enkephalin, originating from immune cells, T- and B-lymphocytes, monocytes and macrophages infiltrating the inflamed tissue, or originating from the peripheral nervous system contribute to this effect (see references in STEIN 1993).

When considering all of the studies outlined above, it is evident that experimental approaches using the strategy of immunohistochemical analysis of c-Fos protein is valuable particularly for the study of the various sites of action of morphine, as clearly demonstrated at the peripheral, spinal and supra-spinal levels. In the future it will be interesting to compare the effect of various μ-opioid agonists on c-Fos expression according to their clinical potency and the effects of various opioid receptor agonists. In such a respect a selective κ-opioid receptor agonists (U-50488) has been shown to dose-dependently reduce acetic acid induced pain behaviour (abdominal stretches) and spinal c-Fos expression (HAMMOND et al. 1992). Thus it will be possible to clearly analyse the differential contribution of the various types or subtypes of opioid receptors to pain modulation.

It is well established that opioid receptor mediated effects do not occur only in isolation, but that there is considerable interaction with other spinal transmitters. With regards to this aspect we used the c-Fos technique to investigate the possible interactions of the opioidergic systems with the various other transmitter systems implicated in nociceptive processing at the level of the dorsal horn. The following section presents evidence in favour of such interactions which are in agreement with, and extend, previous electrophysiological and behavioural observations.

II. Spinal Transmitter Interactions

1. Morphine and Cholecystokinin

The well established direct antinociceptive effects of morphine at the level of the spinal cord have been shown to be subject to an ongoing modulation by cholecystokinin (CCK), with CCK attenuating the effects of μ-opioid agonists at the spinal level (BARBAZ et al. 1989; FARIS et al. 1984; MAGNUSON et al. 1990;

Wiesenfeld-Hallin and Duranti 1987). Conversely, numerous studies have shown an enhancement of morphine analgesia by selective CCK_B receptor antagonists (Dourish et al. 1990; Wiesenfeld-Hallin et al. 1990; Xu et al. 1994; Zhou et al. 1993) which are essentially without effect when administered alone (Dourish et al. 1990; Zhou et al. 1993). The well-established CCK_B receptor antagonist 3R-(+)-N(2,3-dihydro-1-mthyl-2-oxo-5-phenyl-1H-1,4 benzo-diazepin-3-yl)-N1-(3-methylphenyl urea) (L-365260) has been shown in the rat to be up to 40 times more effective at enhancing the effect of morphine than the CCK_A receptor antagonist devazepide (Zhou et al. 1993).

We have investigated whether an interaction between the effect of morphine and L-365 260 can influence the longer term manifestations of prolonged nociceptive transmission, the spinal expression of c-Fos (Chapman et al. 1995d). This study assessed the effects of two concentrations of systemically administered morphine with and without prior administration of a standard concentration of L-365 260 on carrageenan-evoked spinal c-Fos expression (Table 1).

The lower dose of systemic morphine did not reduce the total number of Fos-LI neurones, whereas the higher dose of morphine significantly reduced the total number of Fos-LI neurones, in a naloxone reversible manner (Table 1). Co-administration of the low dose of morphine and L-365 260, a CCK_B receptor antagonist, significantly reduced the total number of Fos-LI neurones; these effects were significantly different to those of morphine alone and the lack of effect of L-365 260 alone. Co-administration of a higher dose of morphine and L-365 260 significantly reduced the total number of Fos-LI neurones; however, this effect did not differ significantly from the effect of the same dose of morphine alone. Neither systemic morphine nor co-administra-

Table 1. L-365,260, a CCK_B recepter antagonist, augments the attenuating effect of morphine on carrageenan-evoked spinal c-Fos expression (from Chapman et al. 1995d)

Pre-administered drug	% Reduction of the total number of carrageenan-evoked spinal Fos-LI neurons
L,365-260 (0.2 mg/kg)	3% ± 7% Reduction
Morphine (0.3 mg/kg)	4% ± 5% Reduction
Morphine (0.3 mg/kg) and L,365-260 (0.2 mg/kg)	23% ± 6% Reduction*,***,4*
Morphine (3 mg/kg)	26% ± 6% Reduction*,***,4*
Morphine (3 mg/kg) and L,365-260 (0.2 mg/kg)	34% ± 5% Reduction**

Results are presented as percentage reductions in the control carrageenan-evoked spinal c-Fos expression.
Statistical comparisons were performed using ANOVA and PLSD Fisher's test.
Significant differeces as compared to the total numver of Fos-LI neurones, 3 h after intraplantar carrageenan, in the absence of drug administration: $*p \leq 0.05$, $**p \leq 0.001$.
Significant differences as compared to the effect of morphine (0.3 mg/kg): $***p \leq 0.05$.
Significant differences as compared to the effect of L,365-260 (0.2 mg/kg): $^{4*}p \leq 0.05$.

tion of either concentration of morphine and L-365 260 influenced the extent of the peripheral carrageenan-evoked oedema.

These results demonstrating the ability of a normally ineffective dose of morphine to reduce the spinal expression of c-Fos when co-administered with L-365 260 are in agreement with the well-documented potentiation between morphine and CCK_B receptor antagonists as shown by behavioural and electrophysiological studies (DOURISH et al. 1988, 1990; STANFA and DICKENSON 1993; WIESENFELD-HALLIN et al. 1990). However, the effect of a higher concentration of morphine is not enhanced by L-365 260, suggesting that either the effects of the higher dose of morphine are less open to CCK modulation, or that a different dose of L-365 260 is required. It is important to note that none of the various drug administrations influence the peripheral carrageenan-evoked oedema, suggesting spinal and/or supra-spinal sites of action. In conclusion, these results provide evidence that CCK_B receptor antagonism enhances the ability of a low dose of morphine to reduce the longer term intracellular events, the induction and expression of c-Fos, associated with prolonged pain processing.

2. Co-administration of a Full Inhibitor of Enkephalin Catabolizing Enzymes and a CCK_B Receptor Antagonist

The endogenous opioid peptides Met- and Leu-enkephalin are rapidly broken down by various enzymes, and it has been extensively demonstrated that mixed inhibitors of enkephalin degrading enzymes produce profound analgesia (ROQUES et al. 1993, and references therein). More recently the development of RB101, a full inhibitor of enkephalin-catabolizing enzymes, which is systemically active has provided great advances in this aspect of analgesic drug development (NOBLE et al. 1992). Subsequently we showed that RB101 dose-dependently reduces noxious heat evoked (ABBADIE et al. 1994c) and carrageenan-evoked (HONORÉ et al. 1996f) spinal c-Fos expression in a naloxone-reversible manner. These studies clearly demonstrate that the endogenous enkephalins are present during both acute and inflammatory nociceptive processing. Furthermore, it has been shown that CCK_B receptor antagonism enhances the antinociceptive effect of RB101 (MALDONADO et al. 1993; VALVERDE et al. 1994).

We recently investigated the ability of another selective CCK_B receptor antagonist, 4-{[2-[[3-(1H-indol-3-yl)-2-methyl-1-oxo-2-[[tricyclo[3, 3, 1, 137]dec-2-yloxy)carbonyl]amino]propyl]amino]-1-phenylethyl]amin}-4-oxo-[R-(R*,R*)]butanoate-N-methyl-D-glucamine (CI988), to enhance the ability of RB101 to reduce carrageenan-evoked c-Fos expression 1.5h after intraplantar injection of carrageenan. In this study co-administered RB101 and CI988 profoundly reduced carrageenan-evoked spinal c-Fos expression, with these effects being significantly different to the effect of either RB101 alone or CI988 alone (Fig. 8).

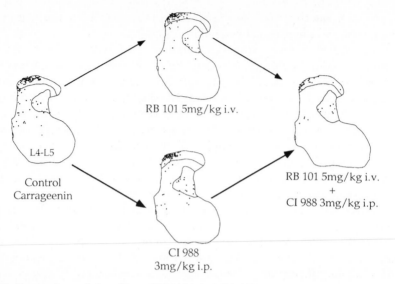

RB 101 5mg/kg i.v.

L4-L5

Control
Carrageenin

RB 101 5mg/kg i.v.
+
CI 988 3mg/kg i.p.

CI 988
3mg/kg i.p.

Fig. 8. Comparison of the effect of RB101 (a full inhibitor of enkephalin-catabolizing enzymes), CI988 (a selective CCK_B receptor antagonist) and co-administered RB101 and CI988 on carrageenan-evoked spinal c-Fos expression. Individual example sections of the spinal cord (L4–L5 segment) are presented. *Each schema*, all Fos-LI neurones in one 40-μm section; *each dot*, one Fos-LI neurone. (From HONORÉ et al. 1996f)

3. Co-administration of an α_2-Adrenoceptor Agonist and Morphine

The modulation of spinal nociceptive transmission by the descending noradrenergic systems (see references in YAKSH 1985) is mediated predominantly by α_2-adrenoceptors (see references in PROUDFIT 1988). The spinal administration of α_2-adrenoceptor agonists, such as clonidine and dexmedetomidine, mimic the descending antinociceptive systems and produce antinociception both in terms of behavioural (FISHER et al. 1991; KALSO et al. 1991; PUKE and WIESENFELD-HALLIN 1993) and neuronal (FLEETWOOD-WALKER et al. 1985; PERTOVAARA 1991; SULLIVAN et al. 1987, 1992) responses. An early study implicated both α_1- and α_2-adrenoceptor subtypes in the attenuating effect of norepinephrine on spinal Fos-LI neurones following noxious heat stimulation (JONES 1992). Subsequently we demonstrated that systemic administration of medetomidine, an α_2-adrenoceptor agonist, dose-dependently reduces carrageenan-evoked spinal c-Fos expression; however, this is associated with a parallel reduction in the peripheral oedema, and thus the site of action of the systemically administered α_2-adrenoceptor agonist cannot be ascertained (HONORÉ et al. 1996c). These effects were blocked by the selective α_2-adrenoceptor antagonist atipamezole. Our results are reminiscent of a previous study in which high doses of intraperitoneal medetomidine (up to 300 μg/kg) reduced formalin-evoked spinal c-Fos expression (PERTOVAARA et al. 1993). Since in our study administration of the α_2-adrenoceptor antagonist atipamezole alone influenced neither c-Fos expression nor the peripheral oedema, this suggests that ongoing tonic activity of the endogenous α_2-adrenoceptor system does not influence the level of carrageenan-evoked spinal c-Fos expression.

In addition to the independent antinociceptive effect of α_2-adrenoceptor agonists, it is well documented that co-administration of an α_2-adrenoceptor agonist with opioids, predominantly morphine, results in dramatically enhanced antinociceptive effects over the individual effect of either drug (LOOMIS et al. 1987; MONASKY et al. 1990; OSSIPOV et al. 1990; PERTOVAARA et al. 1993; SULLIVAN et al. 1987, 1992, and see references in YAKSH 1985). We have recently investigated the effect of co-administration of the selective α_2-adrenoceptor agonist medetomidine and morphine on carrageenan-evoked c-Fos expression and inflammation.

Systemic administration of morphine alone (1.5 mg/kg i.v.) did not influence the number of carrageenan-evoked Fos-LI neurones, and the low concentration of medetomidine studied (12.5 µg/kg) had a limited effect on the number of carrageenan-evoked Fos-LI neurones (Fig. 9). In contrast, co-administration of morphine (1.5 mg/kg) and medetomidine (12.5 µg/kg) signifi-

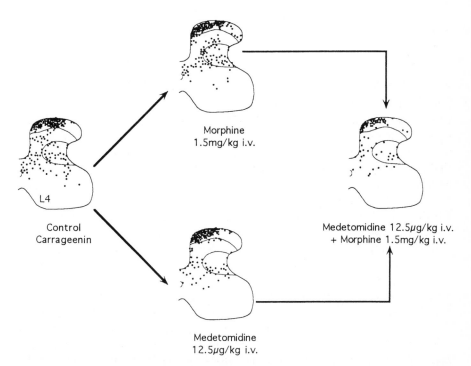

Fig. 9. Comparison of the effect of morphine, medetomidine and morphine plus medetomidine on carrageenan-evoked spinal c-Fos expression. Individual example sections of the spinal cord (L4–L5 segment) are presented. *Each drawing*, all Fos-LI neurones in one 40-µm section; *each dot*, one Fos-LI neurone. (From HONORÉ et al. 1996c)

cantly decreased the total number of Fos-LI neurones (51% ± 8% reduction compared to control carrageenan Fos-LI expression; Fig. 9). The effects of this co-administration were significantly greater than those of medetomidine alone ($p < 0.001$) and morphine alone ($p < 0.0001$). Both atipamezole (75 μg/kg) and the combined injection of atipamezole and naloxone (1 mg/kg) significantly blocked the effects of co-administered medetomidine and morphine on the total number of Fos-LI neurones ($p < 0.05$ and $p < 0.05$ compared to co-administered medetomidine and morphine group, respectively).

Co-administered morphine and medetomidine did not reduce the peripheral carrageenan-evoked oedema to a greater effect than medetomidine alone (Honoré et al. 1996c), thus suggesting that the effects of this co-administration represent a central, and less peripheral site of interaction.

Overall we found that co-administration of low doses of morphine medetomidine greatly reduces the level of carrageenan-evoked c-Fos expression, thus illustrating that the well-established potentiation between opiates and α_2-adrenoceptor systems (see references Dickenson 1994a) influences one of the down-stream consequences of nociceptive transmission, the spinal expression of c-Fos.

4. Co-administration of Morphine and an NMDA Receptor Antagonist

The formalin response is a well-established model of more prolonged inflammatory pain consisting of an acute phase followed by a prolonged inflammatory phase, which is mediated in part by the N-methyl-D-aspartate (NMDA) receptor. It has been shown that NMDA receptor mediated events such as wind-up and the second phase of the formalin response have a reduced sensitivity to intrathecal opioids, which can be overcome by increasing the dose of opioid (Chapman et al. 1994, and see references therein). Since higher doses of opioid are associated with side effect liability, this is not always a suitable alternative. However, co-therapy with subthreshold doses of morphine; μ-opioid agonist and of an antagonist of the glycine site of the NMDA receptor has been shown to considerably reduce electrically evoked wind-up, an NMDA receptor mediated event (Chapman and Dickenson 1992). Although such a drug combination may provide a high level of analgesia, in the absence of side effects, until recently the antagonists at the glycine site of the NMDA receptor such as 7-chlorokynurenate have not been able to cross the blood-brain barrier. However, a relatively new antagonist at the glycine site of the NMDA receptor (+)-(1-hydroxy-3-aminopyrrolidine-2-one) [(+)-HA966], has been extensively investigated (Millan and Seguin 1994), shown to cross the blood-brain barrier and produce analgesic effects in the absence of side effects. We have previously shown that NMDA receptor mediated events contribute to carrageenan-evoked spinal c-Fos expression (see below; Chapman et al. 1995c).

The following results provide strong evidence that co-administration of low doses of morphine and a low dose of the NMDA receptor antagonist, (+)-

HA966, produces a phenomenal supra-additive reduction in the expression of spinal c-Fos evoked by peripheral carrageenan-induced inflammation in unanaesthetized freely moving rats (HONORÉ et al. 1996d). In this series of experiments we studied the effect of co-administration of morphine and (+)-HA966 on carrageenan-evoked c-Fos expression 1.30 and 3 h after carrageenan injection.

Pre-administration of morphine (0.3 mg/kg) or (+)-HA966 (2.5 mg/kg) was ineffective at reducing the number of spinal Fos-LI neurones induced 1.3 or 3 h after intraplantar carrageenan (Table 2). However, co-administered morphine (0.3 mg/kg) and (+)-HA966 (2.5 mg/kg) significantly reduced the total number of spinal Fos-LI neurones at 1h30 after carrageenan (Table 2). Since 1.30 h after carrageenan injection c-Fos expression is located predominantly in the superficial laminae (see above), the effects of co-administered morphine and (+)-HA966 at this time point were observed essentially at the level of the superficial laminae. In contrast, co-administered morphine (0.3 mg/kg) and (+)-HA966 (2.5 mg/kg) did not significantly influence the total number of spinal Fos-LI neurones induced 3 h after intraplantar carrageenan (Table 2).

Since co-administration of the low dose of morphine with (+)-HA966 was ineffective at reducing c-Fos expression 3 h after carrageenan administration, we studied the effect of a higher concentration of morphine. Pre-administered morphine (3 mg/kg i.v.) significantly reduced the total number of spinal Fos-LI neurones 3 h after intraplantar carrageenan (Table 3). Co-administration of morphine (3 mg/kg) with (+)-HA966 (2.5 mg/kg) dramatically reduced the total number of spinal Fos-LI neurones induced at 3 h after carrageenan (Table 3). At 3 hrs after carrageenan injection c-Fos expression is equally located in the superficial and deep laminae of the dorsal horn, and c-Fos expression in both regions was equally reduced by co-administered morphine and (+)-HA966 (Table 3). The effects of morphine and (+)-HA966 on c-Fos expression were significantly different from the effect of morphine alone and the lack of effect of (+)-HA966 alone. The significant reduction in c-Fos

Table 2. The effect of a low dose of morphine or (+)-HA966, and co-administration of morphine plus (+)-HA966 on c-Fos expression induced at 1.5 h and 3 h after intraplantar carrageenan (from HONORÉ et al. 1996d)

Drugs	Dose (mg/kg)	% Reduction of Carrageenan-induced Fos-LI Neurones					
		1.5 h		3 h			
		Total number	Superficial laminae	Total number	Superficial laminae	Deep laminae	
Morphine	0.3	13% ± 11%	4% ± 11%	4% ± 8%	3% ± 8%	0% ± 9%	
(+) HA966	2.5	22% ± 11%	16% ± 14%	9% ± 7%	7% ± 6%	9% ± 12%	
Morphine + (+) HA966	0.3 2.5	60% ± 7%*.**.***	58% ± 7%*.**.***	16% ± 6%	16% ± 8%	16% ± 6%	

Results are expressed as percentage reduction in the control carrageenan group value ± s.e.m. Significance as compared to the control carrageenan group ($*p < 0.01$), to the morphine group ($**p < 0.01$) and the (+)-HA966 group ($***p < 0.01$), was performed using ANOVA and PLSD Fischer's test.

Table 3. The effect of a higher concentration of morphine, (+)-HA966 and co-administration of morphine and (+)-HA966 on c-Fos expression 3 h after intraplantar carrageenan: the reduction in c-Fos expression by co-administered morphine and (+)-HA966 was partially reversed by systemic naloxone, which had no effect when administered alone (from HONORÉ et al. 1996d)

Drugs	Dose (mg/kg)	% Reduction in Carrageenan-induced Fos-LI neurones		
		Total number	Superficial laminae	Deep laminae
Morphine	3	40% ± 7%***	37% ± 9%***	41% ± 11%*
(+) HA966	2.5	11% ± 6%	9% ± 5%	11% ± 11%
Morphine +	3	80% ± 7%***,5*,6*	80% ± 8%***,5*,6*	79% ± 9%***,4*,6*
(+) HA966	2.5			
Naloxone	1 + 1	2% ± 7%	4% ± 3%	4% ± 14%
Morphine +	3			
(+) HA966 +	2.5	26% ± 8%*	9% ± 7%	39% ± 12%*
Naloxone	1 + 1			

Significance as compared to the control carrageenan group ($*p < 0.05$, $**p < 0.01$, $***p < 0.001$), to the morphine group ($**p < 0.05$, $5*p < 0.001$) and the (+)-HA966 group ($6*p < 0.001$), was performed using ANOVA and PLSD Fishcher's test.

expression by co-administered morphine and (+)-HA966 was partially blocked by a co-administration of naloxone (Table 3), which injected alone had no effect.

The peripheral oedema 3 h after carrageenan was extensive; however, none of the drugs studied influenced the extent of the oedema.

The major finding of this study is that co-administration of a low ineffective dose of systemic morphine plus subcutaneous (+)-HA966 decreases the number of Fos-LI neurones induced 1.5 h but not at 3 h after intraplantar carrageenan, whereas co-administration of a higher dose of morphine plus (+)-HA966 strongly reduces spinal c-Fos expression induced 3 h after carrageenan. These results suggest that the interaction between these two drugs is not based on a modification of the pharmacokinetic parameters of the action of morphine (i.e. increasing the duration of action) but supports the presence of pharmacodynamic interactions. The peripheral oedema was not influenced by the co-administration of morphine and (+)-HA966, suggesting that the location of the potentiation is at the spinal cord level or higher brain centres.

Our results suggesting at least supra-additive reductory effects of co-administered morphine and (+)-HA966 on carrageenan-induced spinal c-Fos expression are in good agreement with those of previous studies showing a potentiation between the effects of intrathecal morphine and an NMDA antagonist on wind-up (CHAPMAN and DICKENSON 1992) and on the thermal hyperalgesia in a model of neuropathic pain (YAMAMOTO and YAKSH 1992).

Considering the differences between the μ-opioid receptor (G protein linked) and the NMDA receptor (ion channel linked) systems, and the location of the two types of receptors, it is likely that the supra-additive effect of morphine and NMDA receptor antagonism is due to a functional potentiation between the separate effects of the two receptor systems. Lower concentrations of morphine reduce the steady-state response of dorsal horn neurones to C fibre activation but are less efficacious at reducing the wind-up response of these neurones; however, higher concentrations of morphine are able to reduce the wind-up component of the response (CHAPMAN et al. 1994). In contrast NMDA receptor antagonism reduces wind-up responses but not the steady-state C fibre evoked response (see references in DICKENSON 1994b). Thus it could be envisaged, as previously suggested (CHAPMAN and DICKENSON 1992), that co-administered morphine and an NMDA receptor antagonist target two separate receptor systems which are both pre- and post-synaptic to the C fibre terminal, with morphine reducing the neurotransmitter release from C fibres, thus decreasing the steady-state response of the post-synaptic neurones and NMDA receptor antagonists acting post-synaptically to reduce wind-up responses to the repetitive C fibre input. From our study it appears that such a type of interaction results in a dramatic reduction in nociceptive transmission at the level of the spinal cord, as illustrated by the vast reduction in carrageenan-evoked c-Fos expression.

Overall enhanced antinociceptive effects of morphine co-administered with either α_2-receptor agonists, CCK_B receptor antagonists or NMDA antagonists have important therapeutic implications for reduction in or prevention of the long-term manifestations associated with sustained nociceptive processing, with a reduced side effect liability.

III. Manipulation of Spinal Excitatory Transmitter Systems

1. The Contribution of NMDA Receptor Mediated Events to Spinal c-Fos Expression

There is strong evidence for a contribution of NMDA receptor mediated events to the generation of central hypersensitivity associated with sustained nociceptive inputs in animal models of inflammatory pain, in particular the second phase of the formalin response (HALEY et al. 1990; DICKENSON and AYDAR 1991; CODERRE and MELZACK 1992; YAMAMOTO and YAKSH 1992; VACCARINO et al. 1993; HUNTER and SINGH 1994; MILLAN and SEGUIN 1993, 1994). In addition, previous studies have provided evidence for a contribution of the NMDA receptor to the central hyperalgesia associated with the carrageenan model of inflammatory pain (REN et al. 1992; EISENBERG et al. 1994; LAIRD et al. 1994).

One of the intracellular changes associated with NMDA receptor activation is the influx of calcium into neurones (MAYER and WESTBROOK 1987). Furthermore, increased levels of intracellular calcium are known to stimulate the expression of the IEG c-*fos* (see references in MORGAN 1991) and many of the circumstances under which c-*fos* is induced in the nervous system involves glutamate receptors, including NMDA receptor, activation (see references in MORGAN 1991). However, from the view point of spinal nociceptive transmission the effect of NMDA receptor antagonism on c-Fos expression is not clear. Intrathecal administration of (+)-5-methyl-10,11-dihydro-5H-dibenzo[a.d]cyclo-hepten-5,-10-imine maleate (MK801; Kehl et al. 1991) and subcutaneous administration of dextromethorphan (Elliott et al. 1995), both NMDA receptor antagonists, have been shown to reduce spinal c-Fos expression evoked by peripheral injection of formalin. In contrast, systemic ketamine, also an NMDA receptor antagonist, has been shown not to reduce noxious heat evoked c-Fos expression (Tölle et al. 1991).

We have assessed the effect of subcutaneous (+)-HA966, a partial agonist at the modulatory strychnine insensitive glycine site of the NMDA receptor complex (see references in Kemp and Leeson 1993), on carrageenan-evoked spinal c-Fos expression (Chapman et al. 1995c). Pre-administration of the lower doses of (+)-HA966 did not significantly influence the number of Fos-LI neurones; however, the highest dose of (+)-HA966 did significantly reduce the total number of Fos-LI neurones. Laminar analysis revealed that the number of Fos-LI neurones in the deep but not superficial laminae was significantly reduced by 10 mg/kg of (+)-HA966 (Fig. 10).

Due to the longer time course of the carrageenan inflammation than the duration of action of (+)-HA966 and the importance of the NMDA receptor to the induction and maintenance of central hypersensitivity, we studied the effect of pre- plus post-administered (+)-HA966 on carrageenan-evoked spinal c-Fos expression. Pre- plus post-administration of the lowest dose of (+)-HA966 did not significantly influence the total number of Fos-LI neurones. However pre- plus post-administered of the higher dose of (+)-HA966 did significantly reduce the total number of Fos-LI neurones. With the highest dose of pre- plus post-administered (+)-HA966 the number of both superficial and deep Fos-LI neurones was significantly reduced (Fig. 10). Post-administered (+)-HA966 (10 mg/kg) 45 min after intraplantar injection of carrageenan significantly reduced the total number of Fos-LI neurones; however, this effect was significantly less than the effect of pre- plus post-administration of the same concentration of (+)-HA966 ($p \leq 0.05$).

Our results illustrate that NMDA receptor blockade at early time points of the carrageenan response during the 1 h (pre-administration) significantly reduces c-Fos expression in the deep laminae. However, with a longer blockade of the NMDA receptor for at least the first 2 h of the response (pre- plus post-administration) c-Fos expression in both the superficial and deep laminae is significantly reduced. Simplistically, our results suggest that NMDA receptor activation during the early stages of the carrageenan response contributes to c-Fos expression predominantly in the deep laminae of the dorsal horn; whereas NMDA receptor activation throughout the carrageenan response contributes to c-Fos expression in the superficial and deep laminae of the dorsal horn. However, such an interpretation is further complicated when considering the time course of carrageenan-evoked expression of c-Fos (see Fig. 4). It is important to note that the peripheral oedema associated with intraplantar carrageenan is not influenced by NMDA receptor antagonism, thus suggesting a spinal or supra-spinal site of action. These findings illustrat-

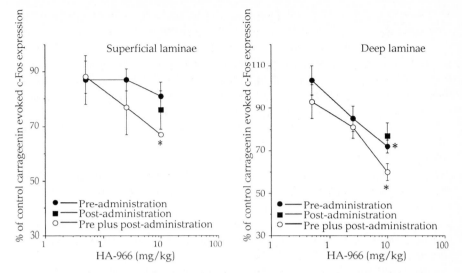

Fig. 10. Effect of pre-, post- and pre- plus post-administered (+)-HA966 on carrag-eenan-evoked c-Fos expression in the superficial and deep laminae of the dorsal horn of the spinal cord. Results are expressed as percentages of the control carrageenan-evoked number of Fos-LI neurones ± SEM; statistical analysis was performed with ANOVA: *$p \leq 0.05$. (From CHAPMAN et al. 1995c)

ing the contribution of NMDA receptor activation to the spinal expression of c-Fos following peripheral inflammation, are in agreement and extent previ-ous studies (KEHL et al. 1991; ELLIOTT et al. 1995). This study clearly demon-strates that continual NMDA receptor blockade has a greater effect on c-Fos expression than blockade during the initial time points, therefore illustrating the contribution of the NMDA receptor to both the induction and mainte-nance of carrageenan-evoked spinal c-Fos expression

2. The Contribution of Substance P to Spinal c-Fos Expression

There is considerable evidence implicating a role of SP in spinal nociceptive processing (see references in HENRY 1994; OTSUKA and YOSHIOKA 1993; and Birch, this volume). Noxious peripheral stimuli have been shown to evoke SP release into the dorsal horn of the lumbar spinal cord (DUGGAN et al. 1995, and see references therein). Previous studies have shown that NK1 receptor an-tagonism reduces facilitated, but less so baseline, nociceptive responses (LAIRD et al. 1993), as well as formalin (CHAPMAN and DICKENSON 1993; SAKURADA et al. 1995; SEGUIN et al. 1995; SMITH et al. 1994) and kaolin plus carrageenan (NEUGEBAUER et al. 1995) evoked nociceptive responses. In addition, neurokinin (NK) 1 receptor antagonism has been shown to reduce intradermal capsaicin-evoked sensitization of spinothalamic tract neurones (DOUGHERTY et al. 1994), neurogenic inflammation of the meninges (LEE et al. 1994;

MOUSSAOUI et al. 1993) and sciatic nerve section evoked spinal cord hyperexcitability (LUO and WIESENFELD-HALLIN 1995).

We compared the ability of systemically administered (3aR,7aR)-7,7-diphenyl-2-[1-immino-2 (2-methoxyphenyl) ethyl] perhydroisindol-4-one (RP67580) and its 3aS,7aS inactive enantiomer RP68651, to reduce formalin-evoked c-Fos expression in the dorsal horn of the spinal cord (CHAPMAN et al. 1995b). Prior administration of systemic RP67580 (0.05, 0.5, 1.5 mg/kg) dose-relatedly reduced the total number of Fos-LI neurones at 3 h after intraplantar injection of formalin; however, in contrast prior administration of 1.5 mg/kg of RP68651, the inactive isomer of RP67580, produced only a small reduction in the total number of Fos-LI neurones, which was significantly smaller than the effect of the equivalent concentration of the active isomer RP67580 ($p < 0.05$).

RP67580 dose-relatedly reduced the number of formalin-evoked Fos-LI neurones in both the superficial and deep laminae of the dorsal horn of the spinal cord (Fig. 11). Since the level of spinal c-Fos expression is an indicator of the level of spinal nociceptive processing, our results suggest that spinal SP contributes to inflammatory-evoked spinal nociceptive processing.

The overall effect of NK1 receptor antagonism on the spinal expression of c-Fos did not exceed 40% reduction; this may represent the use of an insuffi-

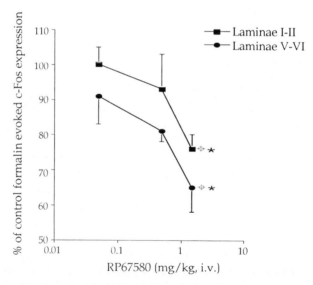

Fig. 11. Dose-response relationship of the effect of RP67580 on the number of Fos-LI neurones in the superficial (laminae I–II) and deep (V–VI) laminae of the dorsal horn of the spinal cord 3 h after the intraplantar injection of formalin (5%, 100 µl). Results are expressed as percentages (± SEM) of the control number of formalin-evoked Fos-LI neurones for the two regions. Statistical analysis was performed with ANOVA and Fischer's PLSD test; *$p < 0.05$ as compared to control; $\oplus p < 0.05$ as compared to 0.05 mg/kg RP67580. (From CHAPMAN et al. 1996)

ciently high dose of RP67580 or be a consequence of the neuromodulatory role of SP (URBAN et al. 1994). Our results with RP67580 are in keeping with those of previous behavioural (SEGUIN et al. 1995) and electrophysiological studies (CHAPMAN and DICKENSON 1993) demonstrating the contribution of spinal SP to formalin-evoked nociceptive responses. It is well established that SP also plays a role in the development of inflammation (see references in DRAY 1994). However, in our study RP67580 did not influence the peripheral oedema, thus suggesting a spinal or supra-spinal site of action of RP67580 at these concentrations.

3. Do Interactions Between NMDA Receptor and Substance P Receptor Mediated Events Influence Spinal c-Fos Expression?

There is an intimate co-operation between tachykinins and excitatory amino acids (EAAs) which is thought to be responsible for maintaining prolonged pain (hyperalgesic) responses. It has been suggested that tachykinins co-released with EAAs from C but not from Aβ fibres can alter the post-synaptic response to EAAs, in particular NMDA receptor mediated events (see references in URBAN et al. 1994) which are associated under normal conditions with repetitive C but not Aβ fibre activation. SP has been shown to modulate NMDA receptor activity in acutely isolated dorsal horn cells (RUSIN et al. 1994) and enhance NMDA and quisqualate-evoked ventral root depolarizations in the neonatal rat spinal cord (see references in URBAN et al. 1994). In vivo studies have shown that spinal co-administration of SP and EAAs results in sustained sensitized spinothalamic tract neuronal responses to mechanical peripheral stimuli (DOUGHERTY et al. 1995) and augmented behavioural responses to peripherally administered formalin (MJELLEM-JOLY et al. 1992). Conversely, co-administration of a low dose of a NMDA receptor antagonist and NK1 receptor antagonist has been shown profoundly to reduce the facilitated flexor reflex (XU et al. 1992) and the formalin response (SEGUIN and MILLAN 1994).

We investigated the effect of co-administration of an ineffective dose of (+)-HA966, an NMDA receptor antagonist (see above), with a low dose of RP67580 on formalin-evoked spinal c-Fos expression (CHAPMAN et al. 1996). In this study, as reported above, prior administration of (+)-HA966 (2.5 mg/kg) or the intermediate dose of RP67580 (0.5 mg/kg) had limited effects on the number of formalin-evoked Fos-LI neurones. However co-administration of RP67580 (0.5 mg/kg) and (+)-HA966 (2.5 mg/kg) significantly reduced the total number of formalin-evoked Fos-LI neurones compared to control; this effect was observed at both the level of the superficial (Fig. 12) and deep laminae. The attenuating effect of co-administered RP67580 and (+)-HA966 was significantly different from the effect of RP67580 alone and the effect of (+)-HA966 alone (Fig. 12).

These results showing positive interactions between NMDA receptor and SP receptor mediated events during more prolonged nociceptive processing

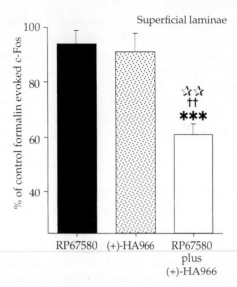

Fig. 12. Co-administered RP67580 (0.5 mg/kg, i.v.) and (+)-HA966 (2.5 mg/kg, s.c.) significantly reduces the number of formalin-evoked spinal Fos-LI neurones compared to the control level of formalin-evoked expression of c-Fos (*asterisks*, $p < 0.001$) and as compared to the lack of effect of either RP67580 (0.5 mg/kg, i.v.) alone (*stars*, $p < 0.01$) or (+)-HA966 (2.5 mg/kg, s.c.) alone (*crosses*, $p < 0.01$). (From Chapman et al. 1996)

are in agreement with previous studies (Seguin and Millan 1994; see references in Urban et al. 1994; Xu et al. 1992). A wide variety of studies have contributed to our further understanding of the mechanisms underlying the co-operativity between NK1 and NMDA receptor mediated events. Overall it has been hypothesized that activation of NK1 receptors has an important pro-activating effect on the NMDA receptor, as demonstrated by studies showing that SP enhances NMDA receptor mediated currents, and that NK1 receptor antagonism blocks this effect (see references in Rusin et al. 1994). Our results demonstrating that co-administration of a NK1 receptor antagonist with an NMDA receptor antagonist results in an enhanced attenuation of formalin-evoked spinal c-Fos expression may be interpreted from a short-term perspective in that reduced spinal expression of c-Fos indicates that dual blockade of the co-operativity of the NK1/NMDA receptor mediated events reduces the level of spinal nociceptive processing and possibly the transition from acute pain processing to more prolonged spinal hyperalgesia.

4. The Nitric Oxide System

There is mounting evidence for a spinal contribution of NO during nociceptive transmission of more prolonged pain states (Haley et al. 1992; Moore et al. 1993; Malmberg and Yaksh 1993; see references Meller and Gebhart 1993; Meller et al. 1994). Furthermore, during hyperalgesia interactions between

NO and NMDA receptor mediated events have been demonstrated (see references MELLER and GEBHART 1993). Previous behavioural and electrophysiological studies have indirectly evaluated the role of NO during nociception using NO synthase (NOS) inhibitors such as N^G-nitro-L-arginine methylester hydrochloride (L-NAME).

L-NAME has been shown dose-dependently to reduce the number of mechanically evoked Fos-LI neurones at the level of the spinal cord (LEE et al. 1992). We recently demonstrated that pre-administered intravenous L-NAME dose-dependently reduces the level of carrageenan-evoked spinal c-Fos expression (HONORÉ et al. 1995c). In addition, L-NAME dose-relatedly reduced the carrageenan-evoked paw and ankle oedema. Furthermore a later post-administration of L-NAME 30min after carrageenan injection also significantly reduced the level of carrageenan-evoked spinal c-Fos expression and both the paw and ankle oedema. To assess the selectivity of the effect of L-NAME we also studied the effect of pre-administered D-NAME, the inactive isomer of L-NAME. In our hands D-NAME produced only a weak reduction in the number of superficial laminae Fos-LI neurones, without influencing the deep Fos-LI neurones or the peripheral oedema. The limited effect of D-NAME compared to L-NAME suggests that the ability of L-NAME to reduce carrageenan-evoked c-Fos expression is as a consequence of NOS inhibition. However, the effects of L-NAME were not blocked by a high concentration of systemic L-arginine, which competes with L-NAME for NOS, which did not reverse the reduction in spinal c-Fos expression or paw and ankle oedema by L-NAME.

Overall we found that there is a strong correlation between the reduction in the number of Fos-LI neurones and the oedema by L-NAME, clearly demonstrating a predominant role of peripheral NO in the development of one of the signs of carrageenan inflammation.

Since it is well established that high concentrations of L-NAME can induce increases of blood pressure and a reduction in blood flow in various organs, the development of the neuronal NOS inhibitors, in particular 7-nitroindazole (7NI) which produces dose-related antinociceptive effects in the absence of changes in blood pressure (MOORE et al. 1993) is of considerable interest. We studied the effect of pre-administered 7NI on intraplantar injection of formalin-evoked spinal c-Fos expression (CHAPMAN et al. 1995a). In this study pre-administered 7NI (5, 10mg/kg) was shown dose-relatedly to reduce the level of formalin-evoked c-Fos expression in the deep but not superficial laminae of the dorsal horn of the spinal cord. 7NI did not influence to any extent the paw or ankle oedema 3h after formalin.

Although direct comparisons between the studies of L-NAME and 7NI cannot be made due to the two different types of inflammatory models used, the findings of the two studies are markedly different. The results clearly demonstrate the contribution of NO derived from neuronal NOS, thus in the absence of the cardiovascular side effects associated with non-selective NOS inhibitors, to inflammatory-evoked c-Fos expression at the spinal level. The lack of effect of 7NI on the inflammatory aspect, contrasts with our previous results showing that L-NAME reduces the peripheral oedema and suggests a central effect of this NOS inhibitor, as would be expected in view of its selectivity for neuronal NOS. Furthermore, it is interesting to contrast the attenuating effect of L-NAME on the level of c-Fos expression in both the superficial and the deep laminae of the dorsal horn with the selective effect of 7NI on c-Fos expression in the deep laminae of the dorsal horn. Since there is considerable evidence for a relationship between spinal NMDA receptor me-diated events and NO at the level of the spinal cord (see references in MELLER and GEBHART 1993), it is intriguing to note that the selective effect of 7NI on the deep laminae neurones is reminiscent of the selective effect of pre-admin-istered (+)-HA966, an NMDA receptor antagonist, on c-Fos expression at the level of the deep laminae following carrageenan inflammation.

IV. Nonsteroidal Anti-inflammatory Drugs and Paracetamol

Following such a diverse range of spinal pharmacology it was important to determine whether such a technique is suitable to study the most commonly used clinical analgesic drugs, paracetamol and aspirin. The analgesic proper-ties of these drugs are classically attributed to their peripheral site of action, but in recent years evidence has been accumulating that there are additional central sites of action. Classically both prostaglandins and bradykinin play a pivotal role during acute inflammation, with bradykinin stimulating the generation of prostaglandins and prostaglandins sensitizing peripheral nociceptors to noxious stimulation by bradykinin (see references in DRAY 1994). Such a contribution of the prostaglandins to inflammatory processing is reflected by the anti-inflammatory and analgesic effectiveness of non-steroidal anti-inflammatory drugs (NSAIDs), which inhibit cyclo-oxygenase enzymes, thus preventing the generation of the prostaglandins.

Generally speaking, neuropharmacological studies of the NSAIDs are limited, probably as a result of the experimental difficulties of recording from thin primary afferent fibres. Behavioural studies have shown NSAIDs to be antinociceptive in the arthritic rat (KAYSER 1983; ATTAL et al. 1988) and electrophysiological studies have demonstrated that aspirin decreases the on-going activity of joint mechanoreceptors, innervating the capsule of the ankle in the polyarthritic rat (GUILBAUD and IGGO 1985).

However, since the peripheral effect of NSAIDs is presumably reflected by an effect on the spinal neurones, it is possible that such a peripheral effect can therefore be detected by the c-Fos immunohistochemical technique. In initial studies of the polyarthritic rat we demonstrated that 3 weeks after inoculation with Freund's adjuvant there is a basal expression of c-Fos in laminae V–VI, central canal and ventral horn of the spinal cord. The spinal expression of c-Fos was not influenced by a chronic treatment during 14 days, starting at 3 weeks after the inoculation, of aspirin (300 mg/kg per day) or paracetamol (500 mg/kg per day; ABBADIE and BESSON 1994). The same chronic treatment started at 1 week after inoculation significantly decreased the number of Fos-LI neurones by about 50% (ABBADIE and BESSON 1994). However, both chronic treatment 3 weeks and 1 week after inoculation signifi- cantly decreased the inflammatory signs associated with the disease. Thus there is a difference between the effect of aspirin and that of paracetamol on inflammatory signs and basal spinal c-Fos expression. This difference may be a consequence of the high level of c-Fos expressed 3 weeks after inoculation and, as discussed above, the insensitivity of established spinal c-Fos expression to post-administered drugs.

The influence of the experimental conditions is also well illustrated when considering the effect of both aspirin and paracetamol on spinal c-Fos expres- sion induced by peripheral stimulation. Indeed neither evoked spinal c-Fos expression following mechanical stimulation of the ankle of the polyarthritic rat (ABBADIE and BESSON 1994) nor c-Fos expression following noxious heat stimulation (ABBADIE et al. 1994c) is sensitive to acute or chronic treatment with aspirin or paracetamol.

More recently we assessed the effects of the NSAIDs (BURITOVA et al. 1995a,b, 1996a–c; HONORÉ et al. 1995a,b), and paracetamol (HONORÉ et al. 1995b) on spinal c-Fos expression following a more acute inflammatory insult, the intraplantar injection of carrageenan. We compared the effect of systemic paracetamol versus aspirin (75 and 150 mg/kg, i.v. for both drugs) on carrageenan-evoked spinal c-Fos expression and inflammation (HONORÉ et al. 1995b). Both paracetamol (150 mg/kg) and aspirin (150 mg/kg) reduced spinal c-Fos expression (43% ± 1% reduction, $p < 0.001$ and 45% ± 1% reduction, $p < 0.001$, respectively). Again, for both compounds the reduction in spinal expression of c-Fos was correlated with a reduction in peripheral inflam- mation. Furthermore, systemic administration of various NSAIDs – indomethacin, ketoprofen, diclofenac, piroxicam, niflumic acid and piroxicam – dose-relatedly reduced carrageenan-evoked spinal c-Fos expression (Fig. 13). Comparison of the dose-response curves, studying similar concentrations of the various compounds, demonstrates that under our conditions ketoprofen is particularly potent when considering c-Fos expression, and this is also the case for its anti-inflammatory effect. All of the NSAIDs tested produced greater than 50% reductions in spinal c-Fos expression, and the degree of c- Fos reduction was correlated with a reduction in inflammatory oedema.

Two isoforms of cyclo-oxygenase (COX), 1 and 2, have been described, with COX-2 being induced at the site of inflammation and contributing to the pathophysiological production of prostaglandins involved in inflammation and pain (MITCHELL et al. 1993; SEIBERT et al. 1994). Non-selective NSAIDs, which inhibit both subtypes of COX enzyme, are associated with gastric side effects. There is evidence that this side effect of non-selective NSAIDs is a conse- quence of COX-1 inhibition at the gastro-intestinal level. Thus we investigated the effect of the selective COX-2 inhibitor NS-398 at concentrations which have previously been shown to be non-ulcerogenic in the rat on carrageenan- evoked spinal c-Fos expression and peripheral oedema. NS-398 dose-relatedly

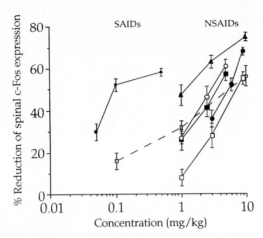

Fig. 13. Comparison of the effect of various NSAIDs and a steroid (*SAID*) on carrageenan-evoked spinal c-Fos expression. All of the tested compounds produced a dose-related reduction in the total number of carrageenan-evoked Fos-LI neurones. NSAIDs and steroid tested were: —□—, NS-398, a selective COX-2 inhibitor, p.o.; —◆—, dexamethasone, steroid, i.v.; —■—, piroxicam, oxicam family of NSAIDs, p.o.; —○—, indomethacin, acetic acid subgroup of carboxylic acid family of NSAIDs, i.v.; —□—, niflumic acid, fenate subgroup of carboxylic acid family of NSAIDs, p.o.; —●—, diclofenac, acetic acid subgroup of carboxylic acid family of NSAIDs, i.v.; —▲—, ketoprofen, propionic acid subgroup of carboxylic acid family of NSAIDs, i.v. L-365 260, a CCKB receptor antagonist, augments the attenuating effect of morphine on carrageenan-evoked spinal c-Fos expression. (Data from Buritova et al. 1995a,b, 1996a–c)

reduced both spinal c-Fos expression and peripheral oedema following carrageenan, with these effects being positively correlated (Buritova et al. 1996b). Comparison of the effect of NS-938 and the other NSAIDs (Fig. 13) clearly illustrates that this COX-2 inhibitor is less potent than the other NSAIDs, although it should be noted that NA-938 was administered orally and not intravenously.

Finally, we compared the effect of systemic administration of the steroid dexamethasone (Buritova et al. 1996c) with the effect of the NSAIDs under the same conditions. Deamethasone dose-relatedly reduced both the spinal expression of c-Fos and the peripheral oedema (Fig. 13); again, these effects were positively correlated.

Overall these studies with the NSAIDs, paracetamol and dexamethasone illustrate that pre-administration before the peripheral injection of carrageenan results in a strong reduction in peripheral oedema and therefore presumably the level of nociceptive inputs to the spinal cord. Subsequently the level of spinal c-Fos expression is reduced in line with the reduction in the inflammatory aspect. However, there is evidence for a central effect of the NSAIDs (Malmberg 1994; Malmberg and Yaksh 1992), and it is important to bear in mind that NSAIDs may also reduce the spinal expression of c-Fos via a direct spinal site of action.

D. Conclusion

Overall the studies highlighted in this chapter, originating from our laboratory and numerous others around the world, demonstrate that the c-Fos technique provides additional information on spinal nociceptive processing to that obtained by behavioural and electrophysiological methods. This technique can be considered as a high-resolution photographic image of the level of neuronal activity of different populations of neurones at a given time point. It is possible to observe drug effects on different neuronal populations simultaneously (superficial versus deep laminae neurones), and therefore this technique is complimentary to electrophysiological methods applied at the spinal level. In comparison with other markers of cellular activity, 2-deoxyglucose and cytochrome oxidase, the c-Fos technique has a number of advantages. The c-Fos technique indirectly provides a cellular resolution of neuronal activity, and the basal expression of c-Fos at the level of the spinal cord is low. In contrast, the 2-deoxyglucose technique, although suitable for spinal analysis, does not provide cellular resolution. However the cytochrome oxidase technique provides adequate cellular resolution at the spinal level of metabolic responses following noxious stimulation, but the basal level of cytochrome oxidase activity is relatively high, and therefore quantification of the evoked activity is not easy. Importantly, the level of noxiously evoked spinal c-Fos expression is highly reproducible, both within and between experimental groups.

To date the pharmacological studies using the c-Fos technique, in combination with either measurements of the behaviour or the extent of the inflammatory aspect, have provided important additional information. Our studies clearly demonstrate the roles of multiple peripheral and spinal transmitter systems and the descending controls during nociceptive processing. With consideration of the multitude of transmitter systems involved we have been interested in the effects of co-administration of various drugs via the systemic route in freely moving animals. Of particular interest we have found extremely strong antinociceptive effects of low doses of systemically co-administered morphine and an α_2-adrenoceptor agonist and low doses of systemically co-administered morphine and an NMDA receptor antagonist. In both cases these effects seem to be centrally mediated since the inflammatory aspect was not greatly influenced by the co-administered drugs.

In conclusion, future pharmacological studies of nociceptive processing, combining multiple experimental approaches, will continue to further our understanding of the various systems and their differential roles during various pain states and may ultimately have important therapeutic implications.

Acknowledgements. We thank Dr. Catherine Abbadie, Prisca Honoré and Jaroslava Buritova, who greatly participated in these studies. These studies were supported by l'Institut National de la Santé et de la Recherche Médicale (INSERM) and an unrestricted grant from Bristol-Myers Squibb. V.C. was supported by fellowships from the Royal Society and the Medical Research Council.

References

Abbadie A, Besson JM (1992) c-fos expression in rat lumbar spinal cord during the development of adjuvant-induced arthritis. Neuroscience 48:985–993

Abbadie C, Besson JM (1993a) Effects of morphine and naloxone on basal and evoked Fos-like immunoreactivity in lumbar spinal cord neurones of arthritic rats. Pain 52:29–39

Abbadie C, Besson JM (1993b) C-fos expression in rat lumbar spinal cord following peripheral stimulation in adjuvant-induced arthritic and normal rats. Brain Research 607:195–204

Abbadie C, Besson JM (1994) Chronic treatments with aspirin or acetaminophen reduce both the development of polyarthritis and Fos-like immunoreactivity in rat lumbar spinal cord. Pain 57:45–54

Abbadie C, Lombard MC, Morain F, Besson JM (1992) Fos-like immunoreactivity in the rat superficial dorsal horn induced by formalin injection in the forepaw: effects of dorsal rhizotomies. Brain Res 578:17–25

Abbadie C, Besson JM, Calvino B (1994a) C-Fos expression in the spinal cord and pain-related symptoms induced by chronic arthritis in the rat are prevented by pretreatment with Freund's adjuvant. J Neurosci 14:5865–5871

Abbadie C, Honoré P, Besson JM (1994b) Intense cold noxious stimulation of the rat hindpaw induces c-fos expression in lumbar spinal cord neurones. Neuroscience 59:457–468

Abbadie C, Honoré P, Fournié-Zaluski MC, Roques BP, Besson JM (1994c) Effects of opioids and non-opioids on c-Fos-like immunoreactivity induced in rat lumbar spinal cord neurones by noxious heat stimulation. Eur J Pharmacol 258:215–227

Abbadie C, Lombard MC, Morain F, Besson JM (1994d) Fos-like immunoreactivity in the rat spinal cord induced by formalin injection in the forelimb to gauge possible plasticity of primary afferent fibres following partial deafferentation. Restor Neurol Neurosci 6:195–207

Attal N, Kayser V, Eschalier E, Benoist JM, Guilbaud G (1988) Behavioural and electrophysiological evidence for an analgesic effect of non-steroidal anti-inflammatory agent, sodium diclofenac. Pain 35:341–348

Barbaz BS, Hall NR, Liebman JM (1989) Antagonism of morphine analgesia by CCK-8-S does not extend to all assays nor all opiate analgesics. Peptides 9:1295–1300

Basbaum AI, Besson JM (1991) Towards a new pharmacotherapy of pain. In: Basbaum AI, Besson JM (eds) Dahlem workshop reports. Wiley, Chichester (Life sciences research report, vol 49)

Basbaum AI, Fields HL (1978) Endogenous pain control mechanisms: review and hypothesis. Ann Neurol 4:451–462

Bereiter D, Hathaway CB, Benetti AP (1994) Caudal portions of the spinal trigeminal complex are necessary for autonomic responses and display Fos-like immunoreactivity after corneal stimulation in the cat. Brain Res 657:73–82

Besson J-M, Chaouch A (1987) Peripheral and spinal mechanisms of nociception. Physiol Rev 67:67–186

Besson JM, Guilbaud G (1991) Lesions of primary afferent fibres as a tool for the study of clinical pain. In: Besson JM, Guilbaud G (eds) Excerpta medica. Elsevier, Amsterdam

Besson JM, Le Bars D (1978) Effect of morphine on the transmission of painful messages at the spinal level. In: Adler ML, Manara L, Samanin B (eds) Factors affecting the actions of narcotics. Raven, New York, p 103

Birder LA, de Groat WC (1992a) Increases co-fos expression in spinal neurones after irritation of the lower urinary tract in the rat. J Neurosci 12(12):4878–4889

Birder LA, de Groat WC (1992b) The effect of glutamate antagonists on c-fos expression induced in spinal neurones by irritation of the lower urinary tract. Brain Res 580:115–120

Birder LA, Roppolo JR, Iadarola MJ, de Groat WC (1991) Electrical stimulation of visceral afferent pathways in the pelvic nerve increases c-fos in the rat lumbosacral spinal cord. Neurosci Lett 129:193–196

Bouhassira D, Villanueva L, Le Bars D (1988) Intracerebroventricular morphine decreases descending inhibitions acting on lumbar dorsal horn neuronal activities related to pain in the rat. J Pharmacol Exp Ther 247:332–342

Bullitt E (1989) Induction of c-fos like protein within the lumbar spinal cord and thalamus of the rat following peripheral stimulation. Brain Res 493:391–397

Bullitt E (1990) Expression of C-fos-like protein as a marker for neuronal activity following noxious stimulation in the rat. J Comp Neurol 296:517–530

Bullitt E (1991) Somatotopy of spinal nociceptive processing. J Comp Neurol 312:279–290

Bullitt E, Lee CL, Light AR, Willcockson H (1992) The effect of stimulus duration on noxious-stimulus induced c-fos expression in the rodent spinal cord. Brain Res 580:172–179

Buritova J, Honoré P, Chapman V, Besson JM (1995a) Concurrent reduction of inflammation and spinal Fos-LI neurones by systemic diclofenac. Neurosci Lett 188:175–178

Buritova J, Honoré P, Chapman V, Besson JM (1995b) Carrageenan oedema and spinal Fos-LI neurones are reduced by piroxicam in the rat. Neuroreport 6:1385–1388

Buritova J, Chapman V, Honoré P, Besson JM (1996a) Interactions between NMDA and prostaglandin receptor mediated events in a model of inflammatory nociception. Eur J Pharmacol 303:91–100

Buritova J, Chapman V, Honoré P, Besson JM (1996b) Selective cyclooxygenase-2 inhibition reduces carrageenin oedema and the associated c-Fos expression in the rat. Brain Res 715:217–220

Buritova J, Honoré P, Chapman V, Besson JM (1996c) Enhanced effects of co-administered dexamethasone and diclofenac on inflammatory pain processing and associated spinal c-Fos expression in the rat. Pain (in press)

Calvino B, Crepon-Bernard MO, Le Bars D (1987) Parallel clinical and behavioural studies of adjuvant-induced arthritis in the rat: possible relationship with chronic pain. Behav Brain Res 24:11–29

Chapman V, Dickenson AH (1992) The combination of NMDA antagonism and morphine produces profound antinociception in the rat dorsal horn. Brain Res 573:321–323

Chapman V, Dickenson AH (1993) The effect of intrathecal administration of RP67580, a potent neurokinin 1 antagonist on nociceptive transmission in the rat spinal cord. Neurosci Lett 157:149–152

Chapman V, Haley JE, Dickenson AH (1994) Electrophysiologic analysis of preemptive effects of spinal opioids on N-methyl-D-aspartate receptor-mediated events. Anaesthesiology 81:1429–1435

Chapman V, Buritova J, Honoré P, Besson JM (1995a) 7-Nitro-indazole, a selective inhibitor of neuronal nitric oxide synthase, reduced formalin evoked c-Fos expression in dorsal horn neurones of the rat spinal cord. Brain Res 697:258–261

Chapman V, Buritova J, Honoré P, Besson JM (1995b) The contribution of nitric oxide and substance P receptor activation to formalin evoked spinal c-Fos expression. 25th Annual Meeting of the Society for Neuroscience (abstract 645.13)

Chapman V, Honoré P, Buritova J, Besson JM (1995c) The contribution of NMDA receptor activation to spinal c-Fos expression in a model of inflammatory pain. Br J Pharmacol 116:1628–1634

Chapman V, Honoré P, Buritova J, Besson JM (1995d) Cholecystokinin B receptor antagonism enhances the ability of a low dose of morphine to reduce c-Fos expression in the spinal cord of the rat. Neuroscience 67:731–739

Chapman V, Buritova J, Honoré P, Besson JM (1996) Physiological contributions of neurokinin 1 receptor activation, and interactions with NMDA receptors, to inflammatory evoked spinal c-Fos expression. J Neurophysiology (in press)

Chi SI, Levine JD, Basbaum AI (1993) Peripheral and central contributions to the persistent expression of spinal cord-like immunoreactivity produced by sciatic nerve transection in the rat. Brain Res 617:225–237

Coderre TJ, Melzack R (1992) The contribution of excitatory amino acids to central sensitization and persistent nociception after formalin-induced tissue injury. J Neurosci 12:3665–3670

Cutrer FM, Moussaoui S, Garrett C, Moskowitz MA (1995a) The non-peptide neurokinin-1 antagonist, RPR 100893, decreases c-fos expression in trigeminal nucleus caudalis following noxious chemical meningeal stimulation. Neuroscience 64:741–750

Cutrer FM, Schoenfeld D, Limmroth V, Pranahian N, Moskowitz MA (1995b) Suppression by the sumatriptan analogue, CP-122,288 of c-fos immunoreactivity in trigeminal nucleus caudalis induced by intracisternal capsaicin. Br J Pharmacol 114:987–992

Dickenson AH (1994a) Where and how do opioids act? In: Gebhart GF, Hammond DL, Jensen TS (eds) Progress in pain research management. International Association for the Study of Pain, Seattle, p 525

Dickenson AH (1994b) NMDA receptor antagonists as analgesics. In: Fields HL, Liebeskind JC (eds) Progress in pain research management. International Association for the Study of Pain, Seattle, p 173

Dickenson AH, Aydar E (1991) Antagonism at the glycine site on the NMDA receptor reduces spinal nociception in the rat. Neurosci Lett 121:263–266

Dickenson AH, Sullivan AF (1986) Electrophysiological studies on the effects of intrathecal morphine on nociceptive neurones in the rat dorsal horn. Pain 24:211–222

Dougherty PM, Paleckova J, Paleckova V, Willis WD (1994) Neurokinin 1 and 2 Antagonists attenuate the responses and NK1 antagonists prevent the sensitization of primate spinothalamic tract neurones after intradermal capsaicin. J Neurophys 72:1464–1475

Dougherty PM, Paleckova V, Willis WD (1995) Infusion of substance P or neurokinin A by microdialysis alters responses of primate spinothalamic tract neurones to cutaneous stimuli and to iontophoretically released excitatory amino acids. Pain 61:411–425

Dourish CT, Hawley D, Iversen SD (1988) Enhancement of morphine and prevention of morphine tolerance in the rat by the cholecystokinin antagonist L-364,718. Eur J Pharmacol 147:469–472

Dourish CT, O'Neill MF, Coughlan J, Kitchener SJ, Hawley D, Iversen SD (1990) The selective CCK-B receptor antagonist L-365,260 enhances morphine analgesia and prevents morphine tolerance in the rat. Eur J Pharmacol 176:35–44

Draisci G, Iadarola MJ (1989) Temporal analysis of increases in c-fos, preprodynorphin and preproenkephalin mRNAs in rat spinal cord. Mol Brain Res 6:31–37

Dray A (1994) Chemical activation and sensitisation of nociceptors. In: Besson J-M, Guilbaud G, Ollat H (eds) Peripheral neurones in nociception, frontiers in pain research. Libbey, Paris, p 49

Duggan AW, North RA (1984) Electrophysiology of opioids. Pharmacol Rev 35:219

Duggan AW, Hall JG, Headley PM (1977) Suppression of transmission of nociceptive impulses by morphine: selective effects of morphine administered in the region of the substantia gelatinosa. Br J Pharmacol 61:65–76

Duggan AW, Riley RC, Mark MA, MacMillan SJA, Schaible H-G (1995) Afferent volley patterns and the spinal release of immunoreactive substance P in the dorsal horn of the anaesthetised spinal cat. Neuroscience 65:849–858

Eisenberg E, LaCross S, Strassman AM (1994) The effects of the clinically tested NMDA receptor antagonist memantine on carrageenin-induced thermal hyperalgesia in rats. Eur J Pharmacol 255:123–129

Elliott KJ, Brodsky M, Hynansky A, Foley KM, Inturrisi CE (1995) Dextromethorphan suppresses both formalin-induced nociceptive behaviour and the formalin-induced increase in spinal c-fos mRNA. Pain 61:401–409

Faris PL, McLaughlin CL, Baile CA, Olney JW (1984) Morphine analgesia potentiated but tolerance not affected by active immunisation against cholecystokinin. Science 226:1215–1217

Fisher B, Zornow MH, Yaksh TL, Peterson BM (1991) Antinociceptive properties of intrathecal dexmedetomidine in rats. Eur J Pharmacol 192:221–225

Fitzgerald M (1987) Cutaneous primary afferent properties in the hindlimb of the neonatal rat. J Physiol (Lond) 383:79–92

Fitzgerald M (1990) c-Fos and the changing face of pain. Trends Neurosci 13:439–440

Fleetwood-Walker SM, Mitchell R, Hope PJ, Molony V, Iggo A (1985) An $\alpha 2$ receptor mediates the selective inhibition by noradrenaline of nociceptive responses of identified dorsal horn neurones. Brain Res 334:243–254

Gogas KR, Presley R W, Levine JD, Basbaum AI (1991) The antinociceptive action of supraspinal opioids results from an increase in descending inhibitory control: correlation of nociceptive behaviour and c-Fos expression. Neuroscience 42:617–628

Guilbaud G, Iggo A (1985) The effect of lysine acetylsalicylate on joint capsule mechanoreceptors in rats with polyarthritis. Exp Brain Res 61:164–168

Haley JE, Sullivan AF, Dickenson AH (1990) Evidence for spinal N-methy-D-aspartate receptor involvement in prolonged chemical nociception in the rat. Brain Res 518:218–226

Haley JE, Dickenson AH, Schachter M (1992) Electrophysiological evidence for a role of nitric oxide in prolonged chemical nociception in the rat. Neuropharmacology 31:251–258

Hammond DL, Presley RW, Gogas KR, Basbaum AI (1992) Morphine or U-50,488 suppresses Fos protein-like immunoreactivity in the spinal cord and nucleus tractus solitarii evoked by a noxious visceral stimulus in the rat. J Comp Neurol 315:244–253

Henry JL (1994) Roles of substance P in spinal nociceptive pathways. In: Hökfelt T, Schaible H-G, Schimdt RF (eds) Neuropeptides, nociception and pain. Chapman and Hall, Weinheim, p 209

Herdegen T, Kovary K, Leah J, Bravo R (1991) Specific temporal and spatial distribution of JUN, FOS and KROX-24 proteins in spinal neurones following noxious transsynaptic stimulation. J Comp Neurol 313:178–191

Herdegen T, Fiallos-Estrada CE, Schmid W, Bravo R, Zimmermann M (1992) The transcription factors c-JUN, JUN D and CREB, but not FOS and KROX-24, are differentially regulated in axotomized neurones following transection of rat sciatic nerve. Mol Brain Res 14:155–165

Herdegen T, Rÿdiger S, Mayer B, Bravo R, Zimmermann M (1994) Expression of nitric oxide synthase and colocalisation with Jun, Fos and Krox transcription factors in spinal cord neurones following noxious stimulation of the rat hindpaw. Mol Brain Res 22:245–258

Hongpaisan J, Molander C (1993) The distribution of C-Fos protein immunolabeled cells in the spinal cord of the rat after electrical and noxious thermal stimulation following sciatic nerve crush, or transection and repair. Rest Neurol Neurosci 5:249–261

Honoré P, Buritova J, Besson JM (1995a) Carrageenin-evoked c-Fos expression in rat lumbar spinal cord: the effects of indomethacin. Eur J Pharmacol 272:249–259

Honoré P, Buritova J, Besson JM (1995b) Aspirin and paracetamol reduced both fos expression in rat lumbar spinal cord and clinical changes occurring during carrageenin inflammation. Pain 63:365–377

Honoré P, Chapman V, Buritova J, Besson JM (1995c) Reduction of carrageenin oedema and the associated c-Fos expression in the rat lumbar cord by nitric oxide synthase inhibitor. Br J Pharmacol 114:77–84

Honoré P, Buritova J, Besson JM (1996a) Intraplantar morphine depresses spinal c-Fos expression induced by carrageenin inflammation but not by noxious heat. Br J Pharmacol 118:671–680

Honoré P, Chapman V, Buritova J, Besson JM (1996b) When is the maximal effect of pre-administered systemic morphine on carrageenin evoked spinal c-Fos expression in the rat. Brain Res 705:91–96

Honoré P, Chapman V, Buritova J, Besson JM (1996c) To what extent do spinal interactions between $\alpha2$-adrenoceptor and μ opioid agonists influence noxiously evoked c-Fos expression in the rat? A pharmacological study. JPET 278:393–403

Honoré P, Chapman V, Buritova J, Besson JM (1996d) Concomitant administration of morphine and an N-methyl-D-aspartate receptor antagonist profoundly reduced inflammatory evoked spinal c-Fos expression. Anesthesiology 85:150–160

Honoré P, Buritova J, Besson JM (1996e) The effects of morphine on carrageenin-induced spinal c-Fos expression are completely blocked by β-funaltrexamine, a selective μ-opioid receptor antagonist. Brain Res (in press)

Honoré P, Buritova J, Fournie-Zaluski MC, Roques BP, Besson JM (1996f) Antinociceptive effects of RB101, a complete inhibitor of enkephalin-catabolizing enzymes, are enhanced by a CCK-B receptor antagonist as revealed by noxiously-evoked spinal c-Fos expression in the rat. JPET (submitted)

Hughes P, Dragunow M (1995) Induction of immediate-early genes and the control of neurotransmitter-regulated expression within the nervous system. Pharmacol Rev 47(1):133–178

Hunt SP, Pini A, Evan G (1987) Induction of c-fos-like protein in spinal cord neurones following sensory stimulation. Nature 328:632–634

Hunter JC, Singh L (1994) Role of excitatory amino acid receptors in the mediation of the nociceptive responses to formalin in the rat. Neurosci Lett 174:217–221

Hylden JLK, Noguchi K, Rude MA (1992) Neonatal capsaicin treatment attenuated spinal fos activation and dynorphin gene expression following peripheral tissue inflammation and hyperalgesia. J Neurosci 12(5):1716–1725

Jasmin L, Gogas KR, Ahlgren SC, Levine JD, Basbaum AI (1994a) Walking evokes a distinctive pattern of Fos-like immunoreactivity in the caudal brainstem and spinal cord of the rat. Neuroscience 58:275–286

Jasmin L, Wang H, Tarcy-Hornoch K, Levine JD, Basbaum AI (1994b) Differential effects of morphine on noxious stimulus-evoked Fos-like immunoreactivity in subpopulations of spinoparabrachial neurones. J Neurosci 14:7252–7260

Jones SL (1992) Noradrenergic modulation of noxious heat-evoked fos-like immunore-activity in the dorsal horn of the rat sacral spinal cord. J Comp Neurol 325:435–445

Jones SL, Light AR (1990) Electrical stimulation in the medullary nucleus raphe magnus inhibits noxious-heat-evoked c-fos protein-like-immunoreactivity in the rat lumbar spinal cord. Brain Res 530:335–338

Kalso EA, Poyhia R, Rosenberg PH (1991) Spinal antinociception by dexme-detomidine, a highly selective α-2-adrenergic agonist. Pharmacol Toxicol 168:140–143

Kayser V (1983) Effects de certaines substances analgésiques sur la réaction de vocalisation et les activités de certains neurones thalamiques, induites chez le rat par des stimulations nociceptives, thèse 3ème cycle. Thesis, Université Pierre et Marie Curie, Paris (VI)

Kehl LJ, Gogas KR, Lichtblau L, Pollack CH, Mayes M, Basbaum AI, Wilcox GL (1991) The NMDA antagonist MK801 reduces noxious stimulus-evoked FOS expression in the spinal cord dorsal horn. In: Bond MR, Charlton JE, Woolf CJ (eds) Proceedings of the 4th World Congress on Pain. Elsevier, Amsterdam, p 307

Kemp JA, Leeson PD (1993) The glycine site of the NMDA receptor-five years on. Trends Pharmacol Sci 14:20–25

Laird JMA, Hargreaves RJ, Hill RG (1993) Effect of RP67580, a non-peptide neurokinin 1 receptor antagonist, on facilitation of a nociceptive spinal flexion reflex in the rat. Br J Pharmacol 109:713–718

Laird JMA, Mason GS, Hargreaves RJ, Hill RG (1994) Antagonists at the glycine modulatory site of the NMDA receptor complex reverse inflammatory-induced mechanical hyperalgesia in the rat. Am Soc Neurosci Abstr 568.10

Lantéri-Minet M, de Pommery J, Herdegen T, Weil-Fugazza J, Bravo R, Menétrey D (1993a) Differential time course and spatial expression of Fos, Jun and Krox-24 proteins in spinal cord of rats undergoing subacute or chronic somatic inflammation. J Comp Neurol 333:223–235
Lantéri-Minet M, Isnardon P, de Pommery J, Menétrey D (1993b) Spinal and hindbrain structures involved in visceroception and visceronociception as revealed by the expression of Fos, Jun and Krox-24 proteins. Neuroscience 55:737–753
Lantéri-Minet M, Bon K, de Pommery J, Michels JF, Menétrey D (1995) Cyclophosphamide cystitis as a model of visceral pain in rats: model elaboration and spinal structures involved as revealed by the expression of c-Fos and Krox-24 proteins. Exp Brain Res 105:220–232
Leah JD, Sandkuhler J, Herdegen T, Murashov A, Zimmermann M (1992) Potentiated expression of fos protein in the rat spinal cord following bilateral noxious cutaneous stimulation. Neuroscience 48:525–532
LeBars D, Menetrey D, Conseiller C, Besson JM (1975) Depressive effects of morphine upon lamina V cells activities in the dorsal horn of the spinal cat. Brain Res 98:261–277
Lee JH, Wilcox GL, Beitz AJ (1992) Nitric oxide mediates Fos expression in the spinal cord induced by mechanical noxious stimulation. Neuroreport 3:841–844
Lee WS, Moussaoui SM, Moskowitz MA (1994) Blockade by oral or parenteral RPR 100893 (a non-peptide NK1 receptor antagonist) of neurogenic plasma protein extravasation within guinea-pig dura mater and conjunctiva. Br J Pharmacol 112:920–924
Lima D, Avelino A (1994) Spinal c-fos expression is differentially induced by brief or persistent noxious stimulation, somatosensory systems. Pain 5:1853–1856
Lima D, Avelino A, Coimbra A (1993) Differential activation of c-fos in spinal neurones by distinct classes of noxious stimuli. Neuroreport 4:747–750
Loomis CW, Jhamandas K, Milne B, Cervenko F (1987) Monoamine and opioid interactions in spinal analgesia and tolerance. Pharmacol Biochem Behav 26:445–451
Lu J, Hathaway CB, Bereiter DA (1993) Adrenalectomy enhances Fos-like immunoreactivity within the spinal trigeminal nucleus induced by noxious thermal stimulation of the cornea. Neuroscience 54:809–818
Luo L, Wiensenfeld-Hallin Z (1995) The effects of pretreatment with tachykinin antagonists and galanin on the development of spinal cord hyperexcitability following sciatic nerve section in the rat. Neuropeptides 28:161–166
Magnuson DSK, Sullivan AF, Simonnet G, Roques BP, Dickenson AH (1990) Differential interactions of cholecystokinin and FLFQPQRF-NH2 with μ and δ opioid antinociception in the rat spinal cord. Neuropeptides 16:213–218
Maldonado R, Derrien M, Noble F, Roques BP (1993) Association of the peptidase inhibitor RB 101 and a CCK-B antagonist strongly enhances antinociceptive responses. Neuroreport 4:947–950
Malmberg AB (1994) Central effects of non-steroidal anti-inflammatory drugs: a role of prostanoids in spinal nociceptive processing, thesis, Göteborg, Sweden
Malmberg AB, Yaksh TL (1992) Anti-nociceptive actions of spinal nonsteroidal anti-inflammatory agents on the formalin test in the rat. JPET 263:136–146
Malmberg AB, Yaksh TL (1993) Spinal nitric oxide synthesis inhibition blocks NMDA-induced thermal hyperalgesia and produces antinociception in the formalin test in rats. Pain 54:291–300
Mayer ML, Westbrook GL (1987) Permeation and block of N-methyl-D-aspartic acid receptor channels by divalent cations in mouse cultured central neurones. J Physiol (Lond) 394:501–527
Meller ST, Gebhart GF (1993) Nitric oxide and nociceptive processing in the spinal cord. Pain 52:127–136
Meller ST, Cummings CP, Traub RJ, Gebhart GF (1994) The role of nitric oxide in the development and maintenance of the hyperalgesia produced by intraplantar injection of carrageenin in the rat. Neuroscience 60:367–374

Menétrey D, Gannon A, Levine JD, Basbaum AI (1989) Expression of c-fos protein in interneurones and projection neurones of the rat spinal cord in response to noxious somatic, articular, and visceral stimulation. J Comp Neurol 285:177–195

Millan MJ, Seguin L (1993) (+)-HA966, a partial agonist at the glycine site coupled to NMDA receptors, blocks formalin-induced pain in mice. Eur J Pharmacol 238:445–447

Millan MJ, Seguin L (1994) Chemically-diverse ligands at the glycine B site coupled to N-methyl-D-aspartate (NMDA) receptors selectively block the late phase of the formalin-induced pain in mice. Neurosci Lett 178:139–143

Mitchell JA, Akarasereenont P, Thielermann C, Flower RJ, Vane JR (1993) Selectivity of nonstereroidal antiinflammatory drugs as inhibitors of constitutive and inducible cyclooxygenase. Proc Natl Acad Sci USA 90:11693–11697

Mjellem-Joly N, Lund A, Berge O-G, Hole K (1992) Intrathecal co-administration of substance P and NMDA augments nociceptive responses in the formalin test. Pain 51:195–198

Molander C, Hongpaisan J, Grant G (1992) Changing pattern of c-fos expression in spinal cord neurones after electrical stimulation of the chronically injured sciatic nerve in the rat. Neuroscience 50:223–236

Molander C, Hongpaisan J, Persson JKE (1994) Distribution of c-fos expressing dorsal horn neurones after electrical stimulation of low threshold sensory fibres in the chronically injured sciatic nerve. Brain Res 644:74–82

Monasky MS, Zinsmeister AR, Stevens CW, Yaksh TL (1990) Interaction of intrathecal morphine and ST91 on antinociception in the rat: dose-response analysis, antagonism and clearance. J Pharmacol Exp Ther 234:383–392

Moore PK, Babbedge RC, Wallace P, Gaffen ZA, Hart SL (1993) 7-nitro indazole, an inhibitor of nitric oxide synthase, exhibits anti-nociceptive activity in the mouse without increasing blood pressure. Br J Pharmacol 108:296–297

Morgan JI (1991) Discussions in neuroscience, proto-oncogene expression in the nervous system, vol VII, no 4. Elsevier, Amsterdam

Morgan JI, Curran T (1995) Immediate-early genes: ten years on. Trends Neurosci 18:66–67

Morgan MM, Gogas KR, Basbaum AI (1994) Diffuse noxious inhibitory controls reduce the expression of noxious stimulus-evoked Fos-like immunoreactivity in the superficial and deep laminae of the rat spinal cord. Pain 56:347–352

Moussaoui SM, Philippe L, Le Prado N, Garrett C (1993) Inhibition of neurogenic inflammation in the meninges by a non-peptide NK1 receptor antagonist, RP67580. Eur J Pharmacol 238:421–424

Naranjo JR, Meelstrsm, Achaval M, Sassone-Corsi P (1991) Molecular pathways of pain: fos/jun-mediated activation of a noncanonical AP-1 site in the prodynorphin gene. Neuron 6:607–617

Neugebauer V, Weiretter F, Schaible H-G (1995) Involvement of substance P and neurokinin-1 receptors in the hyperexcitability of dorsal horn neurones during development of acute arthritis in rat's knee joint. J Neurophysiol 73:1574–1583

Noble F, Soleilhac JM, Soroca-Lucas E, Turcaud S, Fournie-Zaluski MC, Roques BP (1992) Inhibition of the enkephalin-metabolising enzymes by the first systematically active mixed inhibitor prodrug RP 101 induced potent analgesic responses in mice and rats. J Pharmacol Exp Ther 261:181–190

Noguchi K, Kowalski K, Traub R, Solodkin A, Iadarola MJ, Ruda MA (1991) Dynorphin expression and Fos-like immunoreactivity following inflammation induced hyperalgesia are colocalised in spinal cord neurones. Mol Brain Res 10:227–233

Noguchi K, Dubner R, Ruda MA (1992) Preproenkephalin mRNA in spinal dorsal horn neurones is induced by peripheral inflammation and is co-localised with Fos and Fos-related proteins. Neuroscience 46:561–570

Nozaki K, Moskovitz MA, Boccalini P (1992a) CP-93129, sumatriptan, dihydroergotamine block c-fos expression within rat trigeminal nucleus caudalis caused by chemical stimulation of the meninges. Br J Pharmacol 106:409–415

Nozaki K, Moskovitz MA, Boccalini P (1992b) Expression of c-Fos immunoreactivity in brainstem after meningeal irritation by blood in the subarachnoid space. Neuroscience 49:669–680

Ossipov MH, Harris S, Lloyd P, Messineo E, Lin BS, Bagley J (1990) Antinociceptive interaction between opioids and medetomidine: systemic additivity and spinal synergy. Anesthesiology 73:1227–1235

Otsuka M, Yoshioka K (1993) Neurotransmitter functions of mammalian tachykinins. Physiol Rev 73:229–308

Pertovaara A (1991) Antinociception in bulboreticular neurones of the rat produced by spinally administered medetomidine, an α2-adrenoceptor agonist. Eur J Pharmacol 204:9–14

Pertovaara A, Bravo R, Herdegen T (1993) Induction and suppression of immediate-early-genes in the rat brain by a selective alpha-2-adrenoceptor agonist and antagonist following noxious peripheral stimulation. Neuroscience 44:705–714

Presley RW, Menétrey D, Levine JD, Basbaum AI (1990) Systemic morphine suppresses noxious stimulus-evoked Fos protein-like immunoreactivity in the rat spinal cord. J Neurosci 10:323–335

Proudfit HK (1988) Pharmacologic evidence for the modulation of nociception by noradrenergic neurones. In: Fields HL, Besson JM (eds) Progress in brain research. Elsevier Science, Amsterdam, p 357

Puke MJC, Wiesenfeld-Hallin Z (1993) The differential effects of morphine and the α2-adrenoceptor agonists clonidine and dexmedetomidine on the prevention and treatment of experimental neuropathic pain. Anesth Analg 77:104–109

Ren K, Williams GM, Hylden JKL, Ruda MA, Dubner R (1992) The intrathecal administration of excitatory amino acid receptor antagonists selectively attenuated carrageenin-induced behavioural hyperalgesia in rats. Eur J Pharmacol 219:235–243

Rexed B (1952) The cytoarchitectonic organization of the spinal cord in the cat. J Comp Neurol 96:415–495

Rohde DS, Detweiler DJ, Basbaum AI (1993) Spinal cord fos-like immunoreactivity (FLI) during precipitated abstinence: comparison with patterns evoked by noxious stimulation. Neurosci Abstr 19:1247

Roques BP, Noble F, Daugé V, Fournié-Zaluski MC, Beaumont A (1993) Neutral endopeptidase 24.11: structure, inhibition and experimental and clinical pharmacology. Pharmacol Rev 45:87–146

Rusin KI, Jiang MC, Cerne R, Kolaj M, Randic M (1994) Interactions between excitatory amino acids and tachykinins and long term changes of synaptic responses in the rat spinal cord. In: Hökfelt T, Schaible H-G, Schimdt RF (eds) Neuropeptides, nociception and pain. Chapman and Hall, Weinheim, p 163

Sakurada T, Katsumata K, Yogo H, Tan-NO K, Sakurada S, Ohba M, Kisera K (1995) The neurokinin-1 receptor antagonist, sendide, exhibits anti-nociceptive activity in the formalin test. Pain 60:175–180

Seguin L, Millan MJ (1994) The glycine B receptor partial agonist, (+)-HA966, enhances induction of anti-nociception by RP67580 and CP-99,994. Eur J Pharmacol 253:R1–R3

Seguin L, Le Marouille-Girardon S, Millan MJ (1995) Antinociceptive profiles of non-peptidergic neurokinin 1 and neurokinin 2 receptor antagonists: a comparison to other classes of antinociceptive agent. Pain 61:325–343

Seibert K, Zhang Y, Leahy K, Hauser S, Masferrer J, Perkins W, Lee L, Isakon P (1994) Pharmacological and biochemical demonstration of the role of cyclooxygenase 2 in inflammation and pain. Proc Natl Acad Sci USA 91:12013–12017

Sharp FR, Griffith J, Gonzalez MF, Sagar M (1989) Trigeminal nerve section induces Fos-like immunoreactivity (FLI) in brainstem and decreases FLI in sensory cortex. Mol Brain Res 6:217–220

Shepheard SL, Williamson DJ, Williams J, Hill RG, Hargreaves RJ (1995) Comparison of the effects of sumatriptan and the NK1 antagonist CP-99,994 on plasma extravasation in dura matter and c-fos mRNA expression in trigeminal nucleus caudalis of rats. Neuropharmacology 34:255–261

Smith G, Harrison S, Bowers J, Wisemen J, Birch P (1994) Non-specific effects of the tachykinin NK1 receptor antagonist, CP-99,994, in antinociceptive test in rat, mouse and gerbil. Eur J Pharmacol 271:481–487

Stanfa L, Dickenson AH (1993) Cholecystokinin as a factor in the enhanced potency of spinal morphine following carrageenin inflammation. Br J Pharmacol 108:967–973

Stein C (1993) Peripheral mechanisms of opioid analgesia. Anest Analg 76:182–191

Stein C (1995) Peripheral opioid analgesia: mechanisms and therapeutic applications. In: Besson JM, Guilbaud G, Ollat H (eds) Peripheral neurons in nociception. Libbey Eurotext, Paris, p 157

Strassman AM, Vos BV (1993) Somatotopic and laminar organisation of fos-like immunoreactivity in the medullary and upper cervical dorsal horn induced by noxious facial stimulation in the rat. J Comp Neurol 331:495–516

Strassman AM, Vos BP, Mineta Y, Naderi S, Borsook D, Burstein R (1993) Fos-like immunoreactivity in the superficial medullary dorsal horn induced by noxious and innocuous thermal stimulation of facial skin in the rat. J Neurophysiol 70:1811–1821

Sullivan AF, Dashwood MR, Dickenson AH (1987) α-2-Adrenoceptor modulation of nociception in rat spinal cord: location, effects and interactions with morphine. Eur J Pharmacol 138:169–177

Sullivan AF, Kalso EA, McQuay HJ, Dickenson AH (1992) The antinociceptive actions of dexmedetomidine on dorsal horn neuronal responses in the anaesthetised rat. Eur J Pharmacol 215:127–133

Todd AJ, Spike RC, Brodbelt AR, Price RF, Shehab SAS (1994) Some inhibitory neurones in the spinal cord develop c-fos-immunoreactivity after noxious stimulation. Neuroscience 63:805–816

Tölle TR, Castro-Lopes JM, Coimbra A, Zieglänsberger W (1990) Opiates modify induction of c-fos proto-oncogene in the spinal cord of the rat following noxious stimulation. Neurosci Lett 111:46–51

Tölle TR, Castro-Lopes JM, Evan G Zieglgänsberger W (1991) C-fos induction in the spinal cord following noxious stimulation: prevention by opiates but not by NMDA antagonists. In: Bond MR, Charlton JE, Woolf CJ (eds) Proceedings of the 4th World Congress on Pain. Elsevier, Amsterdam, p 299

Tölle TR, Herdegen T, Schadrack J, Bravo R, Zimmermann M, Zieglgänsberger W (1994a) Application of morphine prior to noxious stimulation differentially modulates expression of Fos, Jun and Krox-24 proteins in rat spinal cord neurones. Neuroscience 58:305–321

Tölle TR, Schadrack J, Castro-Lopes JM, Evan G, Roques BP, Zieglgänsberger W (1994b) Effects of Kelatorphan and morphine before and after noxious stimulation on immediate-early gene expression in rat spinal cord neurones. Pain 56:103–112

Traub RJ, Pechman P, Iadorola MJ, Gebhart GF (1992) Fos-like proteins in the lumbosacral spinal cord following noxious and non-noxious colorectal distension in the rat. Pain 49:393–403

Traub RJ, Herdegen T, Gebhart GF (1993) Differential expression of c-fos and c-jun in two regions of the rat spinal cord following noxious colorectal distension. Neurosci Lett 160:121–125

Urban L, Thompson SWN, Dray A (1994) Modulation of spinal excitability: co-operation between neurokinin and excitatory amino acid neurotransmitters. Trends Neurosci 17:432–438

Vaccarino AL, Marek P, Kest B, Weber E, Keana JFW, Liebeskind JC (1993) NMDA receptor antagonists, MK-801 and ACE-1011, prevent the development of tonic pain following subcutaneous formalin. Brain Res 615:331–334

Valverde O, Maldonado R, Fournie-Zaluski MC, Roques BP (1994) Cholecystokinin B antagonists strongly potentiate antinociception mediates by endogenous enkephalins. J Pharmacol Exp Ther 270:77–88

Vos BP, Strassman AM (1995) Fos expression in the medullary dorsal horn of the rat after chronic constriction injury to the infraorbital nerve. J Comp Neurol 357:362–375

Wiesenfeld-Hallin Z, Duranti R (1987) Intrathecal cholecystokinin interacts with morphine but not substance P in modulating the nociceptive flexion reflex in the rat. Peptides 8:153–158

Wiesenfeld-Hallin Z, Xu X-J, Hughes J, Horwell DC, Hskfelt T (1990) PD134308, a selective antagonist of cholecystokinin type B receptor, enhances the analgesic effect of morphine and synergistically interacts with intrathecal galanin to depress spinal nociceptive reflexes. Proc Natl Acad Sci USA 87:7105–7109

Williams S, Pini A, Evan G, Hunt SP (1989) Molecular events in the spinal cord following sensory stimulation. In: Cervero F, Bennett GF, Headley PM (eds) Processing of sensory information in the superficial dorsal horn of the spinal cord. Plenum, New York, pp 273–283

Williams S, Evan GI, Hunt SP (1990a) Changing patterns of c-fos induction in spinal neurones following thermal cutaneous stimulation in the rat. Neuroscience 36:73–81

Williams S, Evan G, Hunt SP (1990b) Spinal c-fos induction by sensory stimulation in neonatal rats. Neurosci Lett 109:309–314

Williams S, Evan G, Hunt SP (1991) C-fos induction in the spinal cord after peripheral nerve lesion. Eur J Pharmacol 3:887–894

Willis WD, Coggeshall RE (1991) Sensory mechanisms of the spinal cord. Plenum, New York

Wisden W, Errington ML, Williams S, Dunnett SB, Waters C, Hitchcock S, Evan G, Bliss TVP, Hunt SP (1990) Differential expression of immediate early genes in the hippocampus and spinal cord. Neuron 4:603–614

Woolf CJ, Safieh-Garabedian B, Ma QP, Crilly P, Winters J (1994) Nerve growth factor contributes to the generation of inflammatory sensory hypersensitivity (letter). Neuroscience 62:327–331

Xu X-J, Dalsgaard C-J, Wiesenfeld-Hallin Z (1992) Spinal substance P and N-methyl-D-aspartate receptors are coactivated in the induction of central sensitisation of the nociceptive flexor reflex. Neuroscience 51:641–648

Xu X-J, Hskfelt T, Hughes J, Wiesenfeld-Hallin Z (1994) The CCK-B antagonist C1988 enhances the effect of the reflex-depressive effect of morphine in axotomized rats. Neuroreport 5:718–720

Yaksh TL (1985) Pharmacology of spinal adrenergic systems which modulate spinal nociceptive processing. Pharmacol Biochem Behav 22:845–858

Yamamoto T, Yaksh TL (1992) Comparison of the antinociceptive effects of pre- and post-treatment with morphine and MK-801, an NMDA antagonist, on the formalin test in the rat. Anesthesiology 77:757–763

Yi DK, Barr GA (1995) The induction of Fos-like immunoreactivity by noxious thermal, mechanical and chemical stimuli in the lumbar spinal cord of infant rats. Pain 60:257–265

Zhang M, Ru-Rong JI, Fang Y, Han JS (1994a) Topical capsaicin treatment suppresses formalin-induced fos expression in rat spinal cord. Acta Pharmacol Sin 15:43–46

Zhang RX, Wang R, Chen JY, Qiao JT (1994b) Effects of descending inhibitory systems on the c-Fos expression in the rat spinal cord during formalin-induced noxious stimulation. Neuroscience 58:299–304

Zhou Y, Sun Y-H, Zhang Z-W, Han J-S (1993) Increased release of immunoreactive cholecystokinin octapeptide by morphine and potentiation of μ-opioid analgesia by CCKB receptor antagonist L-365,260 in the rat spinal cord. Eur J Pharmacol 234:147–154

Zieglgänsberger W, Tölle TR (1993) The pharmacology of pain signalling. Curr Opin Neurobiol 3:611–618

CHAPTER 11

Molecular Aspect of Opioid Receptors

B.L. Kieffer

A. Introduction

Opiates, the prototype of which is morphine, are the most potent available analgesic compounds. They also are strong addictive drugs. Opiates act by mimicking endogenous opioid peptides and specifically activate membrane receptors of the nervous system. The receptors, named opioid receptors, were first discovered in 1973 with the demonstration of stereospecific and saturable binding of radiolabelled opiates to brain membrane preparations (Pert and Snyder 1973; Simon et al. 1973; Terenius 1973). Study of the pharmacological activity of a wide variety of alkaloid compounds and the discovery of enkephalins (Hughes et al. 1975) led to the classification of opioid binding sites into three classes referred to as μ, δ and κ (see Goldstein and Naidu 1989). Autoradiography showed a distinct distribution for each receptor class in brain (Mansour et al. 1987) and evidence has accumulated for a differential role of the three receptors in pain modulation (see Dickenson 1991). μ, δ and κ specific agonists have also been associated with variable abuse liability and distinct mood-altering, autonomic and neuroendocrine effects have been shown mediated by each receptor type (Millan 1990). More recently the availability of novel synthetic opiates and their use in biological assays have highlighted a possible heterogeneity within each receptor class. Thus, the existence of δ_1- and δ_2-, μ_1- and μ_2-, and κ_{1a}-, κ_{1b}-, κ_2- and κ_3-opioid receptors has been proposed (for reviews see Traynor 1989; Traynor and Elliot 1993; Pasternak 1993). Elucidating the molecular structure of opioid receptors appears a crucial issue toward the understanding of pain control and drug addiction. It may also represent an important step for the development of new analgesic compounds devoid of morphine adverse side effects.

Although opioid receptors have been most extensively studied at the pharmacological, biochemichal and physiological levels, their molecular characterization has lagged behind that of most other known receptors of the nervous system. Numerous cloning attempts have failed, presumably due to low abundancy and unstable properties of these proteins or their mRNA. The isolation of a cDNA encoding an opioid-binding protein (OBCAM) was reported following receptor purification and microsequencing (Schofield et al. 1989), but no putative transmembrane domain was found in the deduced protein sequence, and the role of this protein is presently unknown. Homology cloning using probes derived from other G protein coupled receptors did not allow the identification of any opioid receptor cDNA. The *Xenopus* oocyte expression system, which proved useful for the expression cloning of ionic channels and G protein coupled receptors of the nervous system, seemed unappropriate for the cloning of opioid receptors since no physiological response to morphine is observed when brain mRNA is injected. Expression cloning in mammalian cells led to the isolation of a cDNA encoding a putative κ receptor (Xie et al. 1992) with a deduced protein sequence highly homologous to that of tachykinin receptors. However, the affinity of opioid ligands for the recombinant receptor expressed in Cos cells was two orders of magnitude below the expected value, and no κ selectivity has been shown. The first cloning of an opioid receptor of δ subtype was finally achieved by the end of 1992 (Evans et al. 1992; Kieffer et al. 1992). The identification of this cDNA has opened the way to the use of DNA recombinant technology at the receptor level and to the identification of an opioid receptor gene family.

This chapter focuses at the molecular characterization of opioid receptors. The cloning of opioid receptor encoding cDNAs is reviewed, the pharmacological and functional properties of the cloned μ-, δ- and κ-opioid receptors are summarized and related to our knowledge of endogenous receptors found in neurons. Also, structural properties of the receptor proteins as deduced from sequence analysis of the cloned cDNAs and initial structure-fonction studies are discussed. Finally, first insights into the study of opioid receptor genes are provided.

B. cDNA Cloning of Opioid Receptors

I. The δ-Opioid Receptor: First Receptor Cloned by Expression Cloning

Two laboratories simultaneously and independently isolated a cDNA encoding the mouse δ-opioid receptor using expression cloning in mammalian cells (Evans et al. 1992; Kieffer et al. 1992). Both groups constructed a random-primed expression library in the vector pCDM8 (Aruffo and Seed 1987) from the rat/mouse glioma × neuroblastoma NG 108-15 hybrid cell line (Klee and Nirenberg 1974) known to express high levels of δ receptor. The library was transfected into Cos cells which were further screened for opioid peptide binding at their cell surface – mono-(^{125}I)-labelled [D-Ala^2, D-Leu^5]enkephalin (DADLE; see Evans et al. 1992) or [^{3}H]Tyr-D-Thr-Gly-Phe-Leu-Thr (DTLET; see Kieffer et al. 1992). Identification of positive cells led to the isolation of a cDNA containing an open reading frame of 1116 bp with short 5′ and long 3′ non-coding flanking regions. Analysis of both mouse and rat genomic DNA indicated that the isolated cDNA originates from the mouse genome. This cDNA is therefore called mDOR (mouse δ-opioid receptor). Sequence analysis of the 372 amino acid residues mDOR-encoded protein

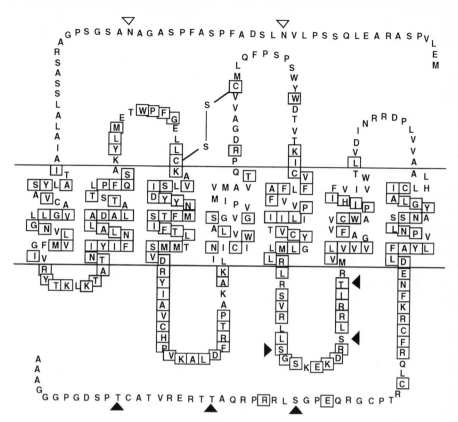

Fig. 1. Primary sequence and putative transmembrane topology of mDOR. The deduced protein sequence of the mDOR cDNA is presented (from EVANS et al. 1992; KIEFFER et al. 1992); *above*, extracellular domains. *Boxes*, amino acid residues strictly conserved across opioid receptor subtypes and species. A putative disulfide bridge is represented. *White arrows*, potential N-glycosylation sites; *black arrows*, phosphorylation sites; these sites differ between subtypes and species

indicated that the cloned receptor is a member of the G protein coupled receptor superfamily (PROBST et al. 1992) with a typical seven transmembrane topology (Fig. 1). This observation appeared to confirm previous biochemical studies showing the G protein-mediated action of opioid compounds (for a review see COX 1993). The human (KNAPP et al. 1994; SIMONIN et al. 1994) and rat (FUKUDA et al. 1993; ABOOD et al. 1994) counterparts of mDOR, termed hDOR and rDOR, respectively, were further cloned from brain or neuroblastoma cells using polymerase chain reaction (PCR) technology with primers based on mDOR nucleotide sequence and/or low-stringency hybridization procedures with the mDOR cDNA probe.

```
opioid receptor consensus
  mDOR         ...............MELVPSARAELQSSPL......VNLSDAFPSAFPSAGANASGSPG.
  rDOR         ...............MEPVPSARAELQFSLL......ANVSDTFPSAFPSASANASGSPG.
  hDOR         ...............MEPAPSAGAELQPPLF......ANASDAYPSACPSAGANASGPPG.
  mMOR         MDSSAGPGNISDCSDPLAPASCSPA..PGSWLNLSHVDGNQSDPCGPNRTGLGGSHSLCPQ.
  rMOR         MDSSTGPGNTSDCSDPLAQASCSPA..PGSWLNLSHVDGNQSDPCGLNRTGLGGNDSLCPQ.
  hMOR         MDSSAAPTNASNCTDALAYSSCSPAPSPGSWVNLSHLDGNLSDPCGPNRTNLGGRDSLCPP.
  mKOR         ...............MESPIQIFRGDPGPTCSPSACLLPNSSSWFPNWAESDSNGSVGSED
  rKOR         ...............MESPIQIFRGEPGPTCAPSACLLPNSSSWFPNWAESDSNGSVGSED
  hKOR         ...............MDSPIQIFRGEPGPTCAPSACLPPNSSAWFPGWAEPDSNGSAGSED
  gpKOR        ...............MGRRRQGPAQPASELPARNACLLPNGSAWLPGWAEPDGNGSAGPQD
  morphan      ....................MESLFPAPFWEVLYGSHFQGNLSLL...NETVPHH
  rorphan      ....................MESLFPAPYWEVLYGSHFQGNLSLL...NETVPHH
  horphan      ....................MEPLFPAPFWEVIYGSHLQGNLSLLSPNHSLLPPH


                                            ***
consensus  LM--WPFG--LCK-V-SIDYYNMFTSIFTL--MSVDRYIAVCHPVKALDFRTP--AK--N-C
  mDOR     LMETWPFGELLCKAVLSIDYYNMFTSIFTLTMMSVDRYIAVCHPVKALDFRTPAKAKLINIC
  rDOR     LMETWPFGELLCKAVLSIDYYNMFTSIFTLTMMSVDRYIAVCHPVKALDFRTPAKAKLINIC
  hDOR     LMETWPFGELLCKAVLSIDYYNMFTSIFTLTMMSVDRYIAVCHPVKALDFRTPAKAKLINIC
  mMOR     LMGTWPFGNILCKIVISIDYYNMFTSIFTLCTMSVDRYIAVCHPVKALDFRTPRNAKIVNVC
  rMOR     LMGTWPFGTILCKIVISIDYYNMFTSIFTLCTMSVDRYIAVCHPVKALDFRTPRNAKIVNVC
  hMOR     LMGTWPFGTILCKIVISIDYYNMFTSIFTLCTMSVDRYIAVCHPVKALDFRTPRNAKIINVC
  mKOR     LMNSWPFGDVLCKIVISIDYYNMFTSIFTLTMMSVDRYIAVCHPVKALDFRTPLKAKIINIC
  rKOR     LMNSWPFGDVLCKIVISIDYYNMFTSIFTLTMMSVDRYIAVCHPVKALDFRTPLKAKIINIC
  hKOR     LMNSWPFGDVLCKIVISIDYYNMFTSIFTLTMMSVDRYIAVCHPVKALDFRTPLKAKIINIC
  gpKOR    LMNSWPFGDVLCKIVISIDYYNMFTSIFTLTMMSVDRYIAVCHPVKALDFRTPLKAKIINIC
  morphan  LLGFWPFGNALCKTVIAIDYYNMFTSTFTLTAMSVDRYVAICHPIRALDVRTSSKAQAVNVA
  rorphan  LLGFWPFGNALCKTVIAIDYYNMFTSTFTLTAMSVDRYVAICHPIRALDVRTSSKAQAVNVA
  horphan  LLGFWPFGNALCKTVIAIDYYNMFTSTFTLTAMSVDRYVAICHPIRALDVRTSSKAQAVNVA
                 ----------TM3---------                           -----


                                    ** *
consensus  -LSGS-EKDR-LRRIT--VLVVV--F--CW-PIHI------L----------------CIAL
  mDOR     LLSGSKEKDRSLRRITRMVLVVVGAFVVCWAPIHIFVIVWTLVDINRRDPLVVAALHLCIAL
  rDOR     LLSGSKEKDRSLRRITRMVLVVVGAFVVCWAPIHIFVIVWTLVDINRRDPLVVAALHLCIAL
  hDOR     LLSGSKEKDRSLRRITRMVLVVVGAFVVCWAPIHIFVIVWTLVDIDRRDPLVVAALHLCIAL
  mMOR     MLSGSKEKDRNLRRITRMVLVVVAVFIVCWTPIHIYVIIKALITI.PETTFQTVSWHFCIAL
  rMOR     MLSGSKEKDRNLRRITRMVLVVVAVFIVCWTPIHIYVIIKALITI.PETTFQTVSWHFCIAL
  hMOR     MLSGSKEKDRNLRRITRMVLVVVAVFIVCWTPIHIYVIIKALVTI.PETTFQTVSWHFCIAL
  mKOR     LLSGSREKDRNLRRITKLVLVVVAVFIICWTPIHIFILVEALGSTSHSTA.ALSSYYFCIAL
  rKOR     LLSGSREKDRNLRRITKLVLVVVAVFIICWTPIHIFILVEALGSTSHSTA.VLSSYYFCIAL
  hKOR     LLSGSREKDRNLRRITRLVLVVVAVFVVCWTPIHIFILVEALGSTSHSTA.ALSSYYFCIAL
  gpKOR    LLSGSREKDRNLRRITRLVLVVVAVFIICWTPIHIFILVEALGSTSHSTA.ALSSYYFCIAL
  morphan  LLSGSREKDRNLRRITRLVLVVVAVFVGCWTPVQVFVLVQGLG.VQPGSETAVAILRFCTAL
  rorphan  LLSGSREKDRNLRRITRLVLVVVAVFVGCWTPVQVFVLVQGLG.VQPGSETAVAILRFCTAL
  horphan  LLSGSREKDRNLRRITRLVLVVVAVFVGCWTPVQVFVLAQGLG.VQPSSETAVAILRFCTAL
                 -----------TM6-----------                        -----
```

Fig. 2. Deduced protein sequences of opioid and opioid-like orphan receptors. Sequences of δ-(DOR), μ-(MOR), κ-(KOR) and opioid-like orphan (orphan) receptors from mouse (m), rat (r), guinea pig (gp) and human (h) are aligned. *Above*, a consensus sequence for conserved residues is shown. *, Amino acid residues found in all G protein coupled receptors; §, localization of conserved splice junctions. Putative transmembrane domains are indicated below. Sequences are from Kieffer et al. 1992 (mDOR), Fukuda et al. 1993 (rDOR and rMOR), Simonin et al. 1994 (hDOR), Kaufman et al. 1995 (mMOR), Wang et al. 1994 (hMOR), Yasuda et al. 1993 (mKOR), Nishi et al. 1993 (rKOR), Xie et al. 1994 (gpKOR), Simonin et al. 1995 (hKOR), Pan et al. 1995 (morphan), Bunzow et al. 1994 (rorphan) and Mollereau et al. 1994 (horphan)

```
                             **   *        §              **  **
           I-A-YS----VGL-GN-LVM--I-RYTK-KTATNIYIFNLALADAL-T-T-PFQS--Y
..ARSAS...SLALAIAITALYSAVCAVGLLGNVLVMFGIVRYTKLKTATNIYIFNLALADALATSTLPFQSAKY
..ARSAS...SLALAIAITALYSAVCAVGLLGNVLVMFGIVRYTKLKTATNIYIFNLALADALATSTLPFQSAKY
..ARSAS...SLALAIAITALYSAVCAVGLLGNVLVMFGIVRYTKMKTATNIYIFNLALADALATSTLPFQSAKY
..TGSPS....MVTAITIMALYSIVCVVGLFGNFLVMYVIVRYTKMKTATNIYIFNLALADALATSTLPFQSVNY
..TGSPS....MVTAITIMALYSIVCVVGLFGNFLVMYVIVRYTKMKTATNIYIFNLALADALATSTLPFQSVNY
..TGSPS....MITAITIMALYSICVVGLFGNFLVMYVIVRYTKMKTATNIYIFNLALADALATSTLPFQSVNY
)QLESAHI...SPAIPVIITAVYSVVFVVGLVGNSLVMFVIIRYTKMKTATNIYIFNLALADALVTTTMPFQSAVY
)QLEPAHI...SPAIPVIITAVYSVVFVVGLVGNSLVMFVIIRYTKMKTATNIYIFNLALADALVTTTMPFQSAVY
\QLEPAHI...SPAIPVIITAVYSVVFVVGLVGNSLVMFVIIRYTKMKTATNIYIFNLALADALVTTTMPFQSTVY
CQLEPAHI...SPAIPVIITAVYSVVFVVGLVGNSLVMFVIIRYTKMKTATNIYIFNLALADALVTTTMPFQSTVY
JLLNASHSAFLPLGLKVTIVGLYLAVCIGGLLGNCLVMYVILRHTKMKTATNIYIFNLALADTLVLLTLPFQGTDI
JLLNASHSAFLPLGLKVTIVGLYLAVCIGGLLGNCLVMYVILRHTKMKTATNIYIFNLALADTLVLLTLPFQGTDI
JLLNASHGAFLPLGLKVTIVGLYLAVCVGGLLGNCLVMYVILRHTKMKTATNIYIFNLALADTLVLLTLPFQGTDI
           ---------TM1------------              -----------TM2----------

        *              §                                 *    *        *
-W-L-S--G--------T--R-------C-L-F-------W----KICVF-FAF--P-LII-VCY-LM-LRL-SVR
:WVLASGVGVPIMVMAVTQPRDGA..VVCMLQFPSPSW.YWDTVTKICVFLFAFVVPILIITVCYGLMLLRLRSVR
:WVLASGVGVPIMVMAVTQPRDGA..VVCTLQFPSPSW.YWDTVTKICVFLFAFVVPILIITVCYGLMLLRLRSVR
:WVLASGVGVPIMVMAVTRPRDGA..VVCMLQFPSPSW.YWDTVTKICVFLFAFVVPILIITVCYGLMLLRLRSVR
JWILSSAIGLPVMFMATTKYRQGS..IDCTLTFSHPTW.YWENLLKICVFIFAFIMPVLIITVCYGLMILRLKSVR
JWILSSAIGLPVMFMATTKYRQGS..IDCTLTFSHPTW.YWENLLKICVFIFAFIMPVLIITVCYGLMILRLKSVR
JWILSSAIGLPVMFMATTKYRQGS..IDCTLTFSHPTW.YWENLVKICVFIFAFIMPVLIITVCYGLMILRLKSVR
:WLLASSVGISAIVLGGTKVREDVDVIECSLQFPDDEYSWWDLFMKICVFVFAFVIPVLIIIVCYTLMILRLKSVR
:WLLASSVGISAIVLGGTKVREDVDVIECSLQFPDDEYSWWDLFMKICVFVFAFVIPVLIIIVCYTLMILRLKSVR
:WLLSSSVGISAIVLGGTKVREDVDVIECSLQFPDDDYSWWDLFMKICVFVFAFVIPVLIIIVCYTLMILRLKSVR
:WLLSSSVGISAIILGGTKVREDVDIIECSLQFPDDDYSWWDLFMKICVFVFAFVIPVLIIIVCYTLMILRLKSVR
:WALASVVGVPVAIMGSAQVEDEE..IECLVEIPAPQ.DYWGPVFAICIFLFSFIIPVLIISVCYSLMIRRLRGVR
:WALASVVGVPVAIMGSAQVEDEE..IECLVEIPAPQ.DYWGPVFAICIFLFSFIIPVLIISVCYSLMIRRLRGVR
:WALASVVGVPVAIMGSAQVEDEE..IECLVEIPTPQ.DYWGPVFAICIFLFSFIVPVLVISVCYSLMIRRLRGVR
-----TM4-----------                         ---------TM5---------

        **  *
;Y-NS-LNP-LYAFLDENFKRCFR--C-------E-----R
;YANSSLNPVLYAFLDENFKRCFRQLCRTPCGRQEPGSLRRPRQATTRERVTACTPS......DGPGGGAAA
;YANSSLNPVLYAFLDENFKRCFRQLCRAPCGGQEPGSLRRPRQATARERVTACTPS......DGPGGGAAA
;YANSSLNPVLYAFLDENFKRCFRQLCRKPCGRPDPSSFSRPREATARERVTACTPS......DGPGGGAAA
;YTNSCLNPVLYAFLDENFKRCFREFCIPTSSTIEQQNSARIRQNTREHPSTANTVDRTNHQLENLEAETAPLP
;YTNSCLNPVLYAFLDENFKRCFREFCIPTSSTIEQQNSTRVRQNTREHPSTANTVDRTNHQLENLEAETAPLP
;YTNSCLNPVLYAFLDENFKRCFREFCIPTSSNIEQQNSTRIRQNTRDHPSTANTVDRTNHQLENLEAETAPLP
;YTNSSLNPVLYAFLDENFKRCFRDFCFPIKMRMERQSTNRVR.NTVQDPASMRDVGGMNKPV
;YTNSSLNPVLYAFLDENFKRCFRDFCFPIKMRMERQSTNRVR.NTVQDPASMRDVGGMNKPV
;YTNSSLNPILYAFLDENFKRCFRDFCFPLKMRMERQSTSRVR.NTVQDPAYLRDIDGMNKPV
;YTNSSLNPILYAFLDENFKRCFRDFCFPIKMRMERQSTSRVR.NTVQDPAYMRNVDGVNKPV
;YVNSCLNPILYAFLDENFKACFRKCCASALHREMQVSDRVRSIAKDVGLGCKTSETVPRPA
;YVNSCLNPILYAFLDENFKACFRKCCASSLHREMQVSDRVRAIAKDVGLGCKTSETVPRPA
;YVNSCLNPILYAFLDENFKACFRKCCASALRRDVQVSDRVRSIAKDVALACKTSETVPRPA
----TM7--------
```

Fig. 2. *Continued*

II. The μ- and κ-Opioid Receptors: Cloning by Homology with the δ-Opioid Receptor

Various homology cloning strategies allowed the identification of two mDOR related cDNAs with 60%–65% sequence similarity at the protein level. CHEN and coworkers used a PCR-generated mDOR probe to screen a rat brain cDNA library in low-stringency conditions and isolated a novel cDNA which was further characterized as a rat μ-opioid receptor clone (rMOR see Chen et al. 1993a). Employing essentially identical cloning approaches, other groups isolated the same cDNA (Fukuda et al. 1993; Thompson et al. 1993; Wang et al. 1993; Bunzow et al. 1995) as well as the human (hMOR see Wang et al. 1994a; Mestek et al. 1995) and mouse (mMOR see Kaufman et al. 1995) homologues. Similarly, a κ-opioid receptor-encoding cDNA was isolated from rat (rKOR see Chen et al. 1993b; Li et al. 1993; Meng et al. 1993; Minami et

Table 1. cDNA cloning of opioid receptors and an opioid-like orphan receptor

Receptor class	Species	cDNA clone	Genbank accession numbers	Chromosomal localization	mRNA size
δ					8–9 kb
	Mouse	mDOR	LO6322 (a), L07271(b), L11064 (c)	4D1–D3	
	Rat	rDOR	D16348 (d), U00475 (e)		
	Human	hDOR	U07882 (f), U10504 (g)	1p34.3–36.1	
μ					10–16 kb
	Mouse	mMOR	U19380 (h)	10	
	Rat	rMOR	D16349 (d), L13069 (i), L20684 (j), L22455 (k), U02083 (l)		
	Human	hMOR	L25119 (m), L29301 (n)	6q24–25	
κ					5–6 kb
	Mouse	mKOR	L11065 (c)	1A2–A3	
	Rat	rKOR	D16534 (o), L22001 (p), L22536 (q), U00442 (r)		
	Guinea pig	gpKOR	U04092 (s)		
	Human	hKOR	L37362 (t), U17298 (u)	8q11–12	
Opioid-like orphan					3–4 kb
	Mouse	mOrphan	U09421 (v)	2H2–H4	
	Rat	rOrphan	D16438 (w), L28144 (x), L29419 (y), L33916 (z), U01913 (za)		
	Human	hOrphan	X77130 (zb)	20q13.2–13.3	

Accession numbers are from references: (a) Kieffer et al. 1992; (b) Evans et al. 1992; (c) Yasuda et al. 1993; (d) Fukuda et al. 1993; (e) Abood et al. 1994; (f) Knapp et al. 1994; (g) Simonin et al. 1994; (h) Kaufman et al. 1995; (i) Chen et al. 1993a; (j) Wang et al. 1993; (k) Thompson et al. 1993; (l) Bunzow et al. 1995; (m) Wang et al. 1994a; (n) Mestek et al. 1995; (o) Nishi et al. 1993; (p) Chen et al. 1993b; (q) Li et al. 1993; (r) Meng et al. 1993; (s), Xie et al. 1994; (t) Zhu et al. 1995; (u) Simonin et al. 1995; (v) Pan et al. 1995; (w) Fukuda et al. 1994; (x) Chen et al. 1994; (y) Wick et al. 1994; (z) Wang et al. 1994b; (za) Bunzow et al. 1994; (zb) Mollereau et al. 1994. Chromosomal assignements are available for mouse and human genes (see references in the text). The approximate size of the major transcript, as determined by northern analysis of brain tissues, is indicated. The size of opioid receptor-encoding mRNAs appears similar accross species.

al. 1993; Nishi et al. 1993), guinea pig (gpKOR see Xie et al. 1994) and human (hKOR see Zhu et al. 1995) brain cDNA libraries. The hKOR cDNA was also obtained by PCR amplification from human placental RNA (hKOR see Mansson et al. 1994; Simonin et al. 1995) using primers based on partial human genomic sequence and rodent cDNA sequences. Independently, Yasuda and coworkers (1993) isolated mouse brain cDNAs using degenerate PCR primers based on the nucleotide sequence of somatostatin receptor subtypes. One of them appeared to be identical to mDOR and the other clone was found to encode a κ-opioid receptor (mKOR). cDNA cloning of opioid receptors is summarized in Table 1 and deduced protein sequences are shown in Fig. 2.

III. Pharmacological Properties of the Cloned DOR, MOR and KOR Receptors

Success in isolating the mDOR clone by expression cloning relied on the ability of the cDNA to encode a high-affinity opioid binding site (Evans et al. 1992; Kieffer et al. 1992). Scatchard analysis further showed that the mDOR-encoded receptor transiently expressed in Cos cells bound [^{3}H]diprenorphine and [^{3}H]DTLET with nanomolar affinities. Detailed analysis of the pharmacological profile of the recombinant receptor demonstrated a typical δ profile, identical to that of the native receptor endogenously expressed by NG 108-15 cells. Similarly, the further cloned MOR- and KOR-encoded receptors were expressed in Cos cells, tested for opioid binding and clearly identified as μ and κ receptor clones. Pharmacological properties of the cloned receptors fit the usual criteria for an opioid binding site: (a) alkaloid binding is stereoselective, (b) the N-terminal Tyr residue of endogenous peptides is needed for high affinity, (c) dissociation constants of prototypal opioid ligands are in the nanomolar range, (d) DOR, MOR and KOR exhibit a ligand selectivity profile in good correspondence with the δ-, μ- and κ-opioid receptor classes described in nervous tissues (Leslie 1987; Goldstein and Naidu 1989).

Binding affinities of representative opioids at the cloned DOR, MOR and KOR receptors are summarized in Fig. 3. Thus, proopiomelanocortin- and preproenkephalin-derived opioid peptides exhibit strong binding potency at DOR and MOR but not at KOR while prodynorphin peptides show KOR preference. Non-selective high-affinity alkaloids, including diprenorphine and bremazocine, display high affinity toward all three cloned receptors, with K_i values in the nanomolar range. Morphine, which has been associated with high abuse potential, clearly demonstrates MOR selectivity. The binding profile of other synthetic opioids is as expected from their previous characterization in membrane preparations: naloxone and levorphanol are poorly MOR selective whereas [D-Ala^2, MePhe^4, Gly-ol^5] enkephalin (DAGO), as with morphine, binds to MOR with a several orders of magnitude greater potency relative to DOR and KOR; [D-Ser^2, Leu^5]enkephalin-Thr (DSLET) and cyclic [D-penicillamine^2, D-penicillamine^5]enkephalin (DPDPE) display high DOR se-

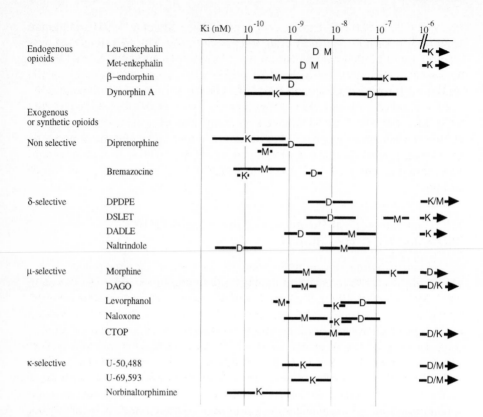

Fig. 3. Binding potency of opioid ligands at the cloned receptors transiently expressed in Cos cells. Affinities of representative ligands for DOR (*D*), MOR (*M*) and KOR (*K*) are from references indicated in Table 1 and RAYNOR et al. 1993. Ranges of K_i values rather than discrete dissociation constants are represented to account for variations in data reported by several investigators (see comment in text) and across species. *Arrows*, dissociation constants above micromolar. *CTOP*, Cyclic D-Phe-Cys-Tyr-D-Trp-Orn-Thr-Pen-Thr amide

lectivity while DADLE poorly discriminates between the cloned MOR and DOR receptors; the κ-specific compounds U-50488, U-69 593 and norbinaltorphimine bind strongly to KOR, with no detectable binding at DOR and MOR receptors. It should be noted that reported dissociation constants of opioid compounds differ markedly between authors (see WOLLEMAN 1994 for comment), presumably depending on the physiological state of the host cell (membrane components, G protein content and intracellular effectors) or receptor density at the cell surface. Consequently the comparison of K_i values of a specific ligand for different receptor subtypes or across species should be performed under strictly identical experimental conditions when heterologous expression is used.

In conclusion, the availability of the cloned DOR, MOR and KOR receptors and their unambiguous assignment to the previously defined δ, μ and κ receptors have opened the way to the study of each receptor type independently. Homogenous sources of recombinant receptors are now produced in host cell lines for further structure-function and signalling studies. An interesting application of heterologous expression is now the possible examination of molecular properties of human receptors from unlimited source of receptor protein. Recently SIMONIN and colleagues (1994) reported ligand binding potencies of a set of representative opioids at mDOR and hDOR receptors expressed in Cos cells and demonstrated a good correspondence between rodent and human δ receptor pharmacology. It is expected in the future that more detailed comparative binding studies will be performed to validate rodent models, and that cloned human receptors will be widely used as screening tools in the search for novel therapeutic agents.

IV. Signalling Properties of the Cloned DOR, MOR and KOR Receptors

Ability of the cloned opioid receptors to couple to a number of signalling pathways is summarized in Table 2. Initial studies reporting the cloning of opioid receptors have shown that DOR, MOR and KOR transiently expressed in Cos cells inhibit the cAMP pathway. Cyclase inhibition by all three opioid receptor types has since been confirmed for the recombinant receptors stably expressed in various host cell lines, including epithelial (CHO, HEK 293), secretory (GH3), pheochromocytoma (PC12) and neuroblastoma (Neuro$_{2A}$, CosNG 108-15) cells. Analysis of opioid-induced incorporation of α-azidoanilido [^{32}P]-GTP into G protein α subunits showed that DOR (PRATHER et al. 1994), MOR (CHAKRABARTI et al. 1995a) and KOR (PRATHER et al. 1995) expressed in CHO cells are coupled to four distinct G protein α subunits. Three of them were identified as $Gi_{2\alpha}$, $Gi_{3\alpha}$ and $Go_{2\alpha}$ while the fourth α subunit is unknown. Their activation occurs simultaneously, with poor receptor/$G\alpha$ selectivity and regardless of receptor density (PRATHER et al. 1995). Heterologous expression in excitable cells was achieved to investigate coupling of cloned opioid receptors to endogenous voltage-dependent Ca^{2+} channels using electrophysiological methods. Agonist-induced inhibition of Ca^{2+} channels was shown for both MOR and KOR in four different cells types. Coupling to L-type Ca^{2+} channel in GH3 cells (PIROS et al. 1995) or N-type Ca^{2+} channel in PC12 cells (TALLENT et al. 1994) indicates that opioid receptors may interact with several types of voltage-gated Ca^{2+} channels. In the two latter studies blockade of opioid-evoked Ca^{2+} currents by pertussis toxin suggests that signalling is mediated through Gi or Go proteins. Coupling of the cloned opioid receptors to inwardly rectifying K^+ channels was shown to occur in the *Xenopus* oocyte expression system when both the receptor and the channel are coexpressed. Agonist activation of all three cloned receptor types evokes large inward K^+ currents in a pertussis toxin insensitive manner, an effect which is mediated by an unknown endogenous G protein. Coexpression of a mammalian $Gi_{2\alpha}$ subunit renders channel activation pertussis toxin sensitive

Table 2. Signalling properties of cloned opioid receptors expressed in heterologous cells

Transduction pathway	Host cell	Cloned receptor	References
Inhibition of adenylate cyclase	Cos	All cloned receptors	See Table 1
	CHO	mDOR	LAW et al. 1994
		mDOR	PRATHER et al. 1994
		hDOR	MALATYNSKA et al. 1995
		rMOR	JOHNSON et al. 1994
		rMOR	CHAKRABARTI et al. 1995a
		rKOR	PRATHER et al. 1995
	HEK 293	mDOR	TSU et al. 1995
		rKOR	LAI et al. 1995
	GH3	rMOR	PIROS et al. 1995
	PC12	mKOR	TALLENT et al. 1994
	Neuro$_{2A}$	rMOR	CHAKRABARTI et al. 1995b
	Cos × NG 108–15	gpKOR	XIE et al. 1994
Activation of adenylate cyclase	*Xenopus* oocytes	rKOR	KANEKO et al. 1994a
Inhibition of voltage-gated Ca^{2+} channels	GH3	rMOR	PIROS et al. 1995
	PC12	mKOR	TALLENT et al. 1994
	Cos × NG 108–15	gpKOR	XIE et al. 1994
	Xenopus occytes	rKOR	KANEKO et al. 1994b
Activation of inwardly rectifying K$^+$ channels	*Xenopus* oocytes	mDOR	DASCAL et al. 1993
		rMOR	CHEN and YU 1994
		rMOR	KOVOOR et al. 1995
		hMOR	MESTEK et al. 1995
		mKOR	MA et al. 1995
		rKOR	HENRY et al. 1995
Activation of phospholipase C	Ltk-	mDOR	TSU et al. 1995
	Xenopus oocytes	mDOR	MIYAMAE et al. 1993
		rMOR	UEDA et al. 1995
		rKOR	UEDA et al. 1995
		rKOR	KANEKO et al. 1994a
Inhibition of phospholipase C	Cos	rMOR	JOHNSON et al. 1994

(DASCAL et al. 1993) and potentiates opioid stimulatory effects (HENRY et al. 1995), suggesting preferential coupling of the mDOR and rKOR receptors to the exogenous Gα subunit. Finally, mDOR-, rMOR, and rKOR-mediated activation of the phosphatidylinositol turnover was also observed in *Xenopus* oocytes, by measurement of opioid agonist evoked Ca^{2+}-dependent chloride currents. Interestingly, these phospholipase C-related currents were observed only in the presence of staurosporine, a protein kinase C inhibitor (KANEKO et al. 1994a) or when the Gi$_{1\alpha}$ subunit – but not Go or Gq generally considered as the classical phospholipase C activator – was coexpressed (MIYAMAE et al. 1993; UEDA et al. 1995).

Altogether these results correlate well with the signalling profile of endogenous opioid receptors in physiological systems: studies performed on various neuronal or non-neuronal tissues, primary neuron cultures or neuroblastoma cell lines have shown that all three δ, μ and κ receptor classes may inhibit the cAMP pathway, decrease voltage-gated Ca^{2+} conductance or activate inwardly rectifying K^+ channels, depending on the cell under study (for reviews see NORTH 1986, 1993; CHILDERS 1991, 1993). From the study of functional properties of the cloned receptors, it is clear also that agonist-induced modification of cellular activity relies on available G proteins and downstream effectors in the host cell. An intriguing observation comes from two reports demonstrating coupling mechanisms in contradiction with other studies. rKOR-mediated cyclase activation (KANEKO et al. 1994a) and rMOR-mediated phospholipase C inhibition (JOHNSON et al. 1994) were observed when the receptors were expressed in *Xenopus* oocytes and Cos cells, respectively. These effects might well result from the absence of effectors generally found in neurons or other host cells. The choice of a host cell to investigate signalling properties of cloned opioid receptors may therefore be critical in our interpretation of experimental results.

It is interesting to note that coexpression of a G protein α subunit, which is absent in the host cell, has been shown to modify receptor/G protein interactions and switch receptor coupling from endogenous to heterologous α subunit (DASCAL et al. 1993; LAI et al. 1995), suggesting preferential interaction of the receptors with specific G proteins. Functional studies have also demonstrated that a single receptor may activate multiple G protein α subunits (PRATHER et al. 1994, 1995; CHAKRABARTI et al. 1995a) and multiple effector pathways (PIROS et al. 1995; XIE et al. 1994; TALLENT et al. 1994; TSU et al. 1995) in the same cell.

In summary, signalling studies validate the use of recombinant receptors expressed in heterologous host cells and model systems have now been established to dessicate transduction pathways associated with opioid receptors. Mutant receptors may now be introduced in these model cell lines. Structural determinants for G protein coupling and modulation of receptor activity should be identified in the future.

C. cDNA Cloning of an Opioid-like Orphan Receptor

Another mDOR-related cDNA was isolated from a human brainstem cDNA library (MOLLEREAU et al. 1994; KEITH et al. 1994), as well as rat brain (BUNZOW et al. 1994; CHEN et al. 1994; FUKUDA et al. 1994; WANG et al. 1994b; WICK et al. 1994; LACHOWICZ et al. 1995) and mouse brain (PAN et al. 1995) cDNA libraries. Sequence comparison shows a high similarity of this clone with the three cloned opioid receptors (55%–60% at the protein level). Particularly, some sequences typically found in opioid receptors, but not in other G protein coupled receptors, are also present in the deduced protein sequence of this cDNA (see consensus sequence in Fig. 2). This structural ressemblance strongly suggests that the cDNA encodes a novel opioid receptor subtype. Surprisingly, attempts to measure specific opioid binding to the putative receptor expressed in Cos cells repeatedly failed, and this cDNA was further refered as to the opioid-like orphan receptor. The close molecular structure and possibly related anatomical and functional properties of this putative receptor (Mollereau et al. 1994; Bunzow et al. 1994) has prompted the search for a novel endogenous peptide related to opioid peptides. Recently two groups have reported the isolation of a neuropeptide which may represent the endogenous activator of the orphan opioid-like receptor (Meunier et al. 1995; Reinscheid et al. 1995). First results indicate a role for this new receptor-ligand system in pain perception and locomotion. A new field of investigation is now opened in pain research with the advent of a novel neurotransmitter system which is distinct from the opioid system but was discovered on the basis of structural similarity of the receptors.

D. Structural Features of the Opioid Receptor Family

I. Homology Pattern

An opioid receptor family has been characterized at the molecular level. At present this receptor family consists of four homologous genes. Three of them encode μ-, δ- and κ-opioid receptors and the fourth gene encodes an orphan receptor whose endogenous ligand is being presently characterized. For each receptor class rodent and human homologues have been cloned (Table 1, Fig. 2). Generally the cloning of each opioid receptor cDNA has been reported by several groups, and sequence comparison indicates that minor differences may be found between otherwise identical nucleotide sequences. In some cases divergence in the DNA sequence modifies the deduced protein sequence (Bunzow et al. 1995; Li et al. 1993), but no apparent change in receptor pharmacology related to such single amino acid substitution has been reported. Whether these differences should be considered as technical or do arise from real polymorphism is not known.

Alignment of the opioid and orphan receptor sequences with other G protein coupled receptors shows that the four sequences display best similarity with somatostatin, angiotensin and chemoattractant receptors. Considering the opioid receptor subfamily itself, comparison of DOR, MOR, KOR and orphan sequences highlights a specific similarity pattern: the putative transmembrane domains – with the exception of Tm IV – the three intracellular loops, the first extracellular loop and a small region of the C-terminal tail prolongating Tm VII are almost identical across subtypes and species whereas no homology is found in the second and third extracellular loops or the N- and C-terminal domains (Fig. 1).

II. Ligand Binding and Transduction

The analysis of sequence homology between opioid receptors, in conjunction with conclusions from extensive structure-function studies performed on previously cloned G protein coupled receptors (for a review see STRADER et al. 1994), allows speculation on molecular determinants of opioid receptor function.

The extremely high sequence conservation in hydrophobic regions suggests that the putative binding pocket delimited by the seven α-helixes is structurally similar across the three opioid receptor subtypes, while the strong sequence divergence of N-terminal tail, second and third extracellular loops supports a role of extracellular regions in selecting μ, δ and κ ligands. Three-dimensional modelling (see UHL et al. 1994; KNAPP et al. 1995) and initial structure-function studies propose an involvement of both transmembrane and extracellular residues in ligand binding and signal transduction. A role for charged transmembrane residues, including an aspartate residue in Tm II (KONG et al. 1993; SURRATT et al. 1994), an aspartate residue in Tm III and a histidine residue in Tm VI (SURRATT et al. 1994), has been postulated from single amino acid replacement experiments. Domain swapping between opioid receptor subtypes, which seems not to induce major changes in receptor conformation, was used to identify molecular determinants underlying opioid receptor selectivity. Analysis of μ/κ (XUE et al. 1994; WANG et al. 1994c) and δ/κ (MENG et al. 1995) chimeric receptors demonstrates a specific interaction of dibasic dynorphin peptides with the strongly negatively charged second extracellular loop of the κ receptor. Chimeric studies have also revealed diverse interaction modes of ligands with the receptors that may rely on the chemical nature of the ligands, their functional properties or the receptor type (KONG et al. 1994; MENG et al. 1995; MINAMI et al. 1995; XUE et al. 1994, 1995). We may anticipate from the presently available data that their is no unique opioid binding pocket but rather a network of multiple interactions which may be specific for each ligand-receptor complex and span transmembrane as well as extracellular regions. More extensive modelling studies and site-directed mutagenesis experiments are required to determine the implication of conserved or subtype-specific amino acid residues in selecting and stabilizing prototypic opioid ligands.

The striking sequence similarity of intracellular regions across opioid receptor subtypes suggests that they may activate the same intracellular effectors. Indeed, functional studies (see above) have suggested that the ability of DOR, MOR and KOR to modulate specific downstream cellular effectors is superimposable. There clearly are common structural determinants within the intracellular domains of these receptors which underly their coupling to specific G proteins. The identification of amino acid residues that interact with G proteins has not been reported yet.

III. Posttranslational Modification Signals

Sequence analysis indicates the presence of posttranslational modification signals typically found in G protein-coupled receptors. A variable number of putative N-glycosylation sites is found in the extracellular N-terminal region (two sites for DOR and KOR and five sites for MOR). Since removal of the N-terminal region does not seem to affect the pharmacological properties of MOR (WANG et al. 1993) or KOR (KONG et al. 1994) but was found to slightly decrease expression levels of MOR (SURRATT et al. 1994), it has been proposed that glycosylation plays a role in protein targeting at the membrane, as previously reported for other G protein-coupled receptors (see PROBST et al. 1992).

Putative phosphorylation sites are present in the third cytoplamic loop and in the C-terminal tail of every opioid receptor clone. Such sites have been extensively studied in the β-adrenergic receptor and shown implicated in the regulation of receptor activity by intracellular kinases, a mechanism involved in receptor desensitization (for a review see LEFKOWITZ et al. 1990). Decreased activity of cloned opioid receptors following prolonged exposure to an agonist has been evidenced in various host cell lines (LAW et al. 1994; CHEN and YU 1994b; KOVOOR et al. 1995; MESTEK et al. 1995; RAYNOR et al. 1994), and the potential implication of phosphorylation steps in loss of cellular function has been suggested (CHEN and YU 1994; RAYNOR et al. 1994; MESTEK et al. 1995). Phosphorylation at receptor sites, however, remains to be demonstrated. Putative phosphorylation sites are poorly conserved between subtypes and species, as a consequence of high sequence variability in the C-terminal region. These differences raise the possibility of a specific regulation pattern for each distinct opioid receptor protein by cellular kinases.

IV. Conservation Across Species

The deduced protein sequence of human opioid receptors are classically 85%–90% identical to their rodent counterparts. The most divergent regions between subtypes, particularly the N- and C-terminal domains, display also highest variability across species. The most striking species variation concerns the first 20 amino acid residues in the KOR sequence which are conserved in rat, mouse and human receptors but totally different in the guinea pig receptor (XIE et al. 1994). At present ligand binding and functional studies reported by the various investigators have not evidenced species-specific features for the cloned opioid receptors, but the possibility remains open that differences in primary structures are related to changes in pharmacology.

E. Opioid Receptor Genes

I. Chromosomal Assignment

In situ hybridization of DOR, MOR, KOR and orphan cDNA probes to metaphase chromosome spread preparations resulted in specific labelling at a single locus for each gene. In humans these experiments have allowed assignment of the DOR gene to chromosome 1 at position p34.3–p36.1 (BEFORT et al.

1994), the MOR gene to chromosome 6 at position q24–25 (WANG et al. 1994a), the KOR gene to chromosome 8 at position q11–12 (SIMONIN et al. 1995; YASUDA et al. 1994) and the orphan gene to chromosome 20 at position q13.2–13.3 (Matthes and Mattéi, unpublished). By use of a similar technique with mouse probes the DOR gene was mapped to the D1–D3 region of mouse chromosome 4 (BEFORT et al. 1994), the KOR gene to the A2–A3 region of chromosome 1 and the orphan gene to the H2–H4 region of mouse chromosome 2 (NISHI et al. 1994). Genetic crossing studies in mouse have confirmed the localization of the mouse DOR gene to chromosome 4 (BZDEGA et al. 1993), the KOR gene to mouse chromosome 1 and assigned the MOR gene to mouse chromosome 10 (GIROS et al. 1995; KOZAK et al. 1994). Mapping of DOR and orphan genes is consistent with comparative mapping studies of the mouse and human genomes which indicate that the determined loci are found in synthenic regions. Genes encoding opioid peptide precursors have also been mapped in mouse (GIROS et al. 1995), and we may note that the proenkephalin gene and the DOR receptor gene are located on the same mouse chromosome (chromosome 4) as do the prodynorphin gene and the orphan receptor gene (chromosome 2).

II. Genomic Organization

The genomic organization of DOR, MOR, KOR and orphan receptor genes has been examined most extensively in mouse (Fig. 4). Initial analysis by SIMONIN and colleagues (1994) indicated that the coding region of the DOR gene is distributed over three exons. Exon-intron junctions are found after putative Tm I and Tm IV of the deduced protein sequence at codons for amino acid residues Arg 76 and Asp 193. A large genomic DNA fragment encompassing the three coding exons has been mapped by AUGUSTIN and colleagues (1995) and intron size estimated to 26kb between first and second coding exons and 3kb between second and third coding exons. Sequencing of the mouse KOR (NISHI et al. 1994; LIU et al. 1995) and orphan (NISHI et al. 1994) genes demonstrates an organization superimposable to that of the DOR gene, with the presence of three coding exons and splice boundaries located at homologous positions. The coding exons of these two genes, however, span shorter genomic regions, and it is notheworthy that the intron located between second and third coding exons is almost nonexistent in the orphan gene (81 bp). The mouse MOR receptor gene appears the largest among this gene family, with coding exons spanning more than 53kb (MIN et al. 1994). Also, the organization of the MOR gene differs slightly from the DOR, KOR and orphan genes, since exon 3 terminates before the stop codon and twelve C-terminal amino acids are encoded by a fourth exon. The first two coding exons are otherwise homologous to those of DOR, KOR and orphan genes. The size and number of putative additionnal non-coding exons, presumed to participate in encoding the large opioid receptor transcripts (see Table 1), is not known. Comparison of genomic and cDNA sequences has nevertheless al-

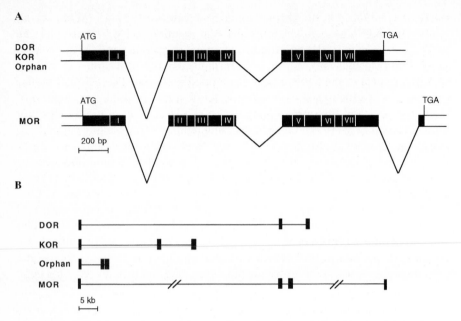

Fig. 4A,B. Organization of opioid receptor and opioid-like orphan receptor genes in mouse. **A** Localization of intron-exon junctions in coding region of the receptors. *Black boxes,* coding regions of DOR, KOR, orphan and MOR genes; *roman numbers,* putative transmembrane domains of the deduced protein sequence. Splice junctions found after domains I and IV are conserved among the four related genes and their exact localization is shown in Fig. 2. An additional 3′ junction is found in the coding region of the MOR gene. **B** Distribution of coding exons in the mouse genome. Coding exons span 8 kb (orphan) to more than 53 kb (MOR). The total size of the genes, including 5′ and 3′ non-coding exons, is presently unknown

lowed demonstration of the existence of a 5′ untranslated exon in the KOR gene (Liu et al. 1995; Yakovlev et al. 1995).

In summary, mouse opioid receptor genes constitute a group of genes with highly similar organization. An identical genomic structure has been reported for human DOR, MOR and KOR counterparts (Simonin et al. 1995). The conserved localization of splice sites after putative transmembrane regions I and IV strongly suggests that opioid receptor genes derive from a common ancestor, and that the orphan gene is evolutionary related to opioid receptors.

III. Initiation of Transcription

Transcription initiation sites have been proposed for DOR (Augustin et al. 1995), MOR (Min et al. 1994; Liang et al. 1995) and KOR (Liu et al. 1995; Yakovlev et al. 1995) genes. Liang and coworkers have identified a single transcription start site in the mouse MOR gene located 793 bp upstream ATG and have assessed the transcriptional activity of a 555-bp region upstream from this putative transcription initiation site using transfection of luciferase reporter genes in SK-N-SH neuroblastoma cells. A 210-bp portion of this DNA fragment was shown to have promoter activity and analysis of the nucleotide sequence indicates the absence of consensus TATA or CAAT boxes but the presence of putative AP1 and AP2 sites (LIANG et al. 1995). In their analysis of the mouse KOR gene YAKOVLEV and coworkers (1995) have identified a cluster of four putative transcription start sites (–932 to –907) preceded by two TATA boxes and a group of two more 3′ putative sites (–565 and –569) preceded by a CAAT box. The authors show the existence of two distinct mRNAs, which may derive from these two clusters of transcription initiation sites, and which exhibit a different tissue distribution, opening the possibility of two distinct operational promoters in the KOR gene (YAKOVLEV et al. 1995).

IV. Genomic Cloning and Perpectives

Characterization of opioid receptor gene promoters is presently under investigation by several groups. The identification of regulatory elements and characterization of transcription factors that bind to these putative promoters should help in understanding how the expression of opioid receptor genes is controlled both spatially and temporally in various physiological and pathological situations. The availability of large gene fragments will also permit manipulation of the mouse genome in vitro and generate transgenic animal with altered opioid receptor genes, thus opening *in vivo* studies of opioid receptor gene function. Finally, mapping linkage studies and the analysis of human polymorphism in opioid receptor genes might in the future allow to establish correlations between specific structural properties of opioid receptor genes and pain perception defects or addictive behaviour.

F. Conclusion: Reconciling Pharmacology and Gene Cloning?

Twenty years of pharmacology have provided a complex picture of opioid receptors and the existence of multiple receptor subtypes within each μ, δ and κ receptor class has been proposed on the basis of numerous *in vivo* and *in vitro* assays. Until now only one receptor has been cloned for each receptor class. Hence the molecular characterization of opioid receptors does not seem to correpate with their apparent heterogeneity in tissues. Several authors have tentatively assigned the cloned receptors to a particular μ, δ or κ subtype. The higher binding potency (RAYNOR et al. 1993) and stronger efficacy (LAW et al. 1994) of NTB compared to BNTX (SOFUOGLU et al. 1991; PORTOGHESE et al. 1992) at the mDOR receptor have led to the hypothesis that DOR encodes a δ receptor of δ_2 subtype. The high affinity of naloxonazine for the MOR receptor is consistent with MOR representing the μ_1 subtype (PAUL et al. 1989) and the high binding potency of U-50488 to the KOR receptor suggests that

KOR encodes a receptor of κ_1 subtype (see Pasternak 1993 for a review). There is, however, no other DOR-, MOR- or KOR-encoding cDNA available for comparison, and these putative assignements remain elusive.

The search for novel opioid receptor subtypes using methods that rely on sequence homology to DOR, MOR, KOR and orphan receptors remains unsuccessful. Another possibility is the existence of opioid receptors structurally unrelated to the presently available clones, which may be cloned using expression cloning approaches. Multiple receptor isoforms may also arise from the three identified DOR, MOR and KOR genes. The presence of introns in the coding region of these genes allows the possibility of alternative splicing and the existence of MOR splice variants with distinct C-terminal tails has been reported (Bare et al. 1994; Zimprich et al. 1995). Alternative initiation of transcription leading to multiple KOR transcripts has also been described (Yakovlev et al. 1995). However none of these variant seems to account for the yet uncharacterized μ-, δ- or κ-opioid receptor subtypes, and isoforms that would arise from alternative splicing at the conserved exon-intron junctions have not been reported. In conclusion the existence of opioid receptor subtypes that are molecular entities distinct from the DOR, MOR and KOR receptors remains to be demonstrated. Therefore another reasonnable hypothesis is to assume that the well-documented heterogeneity of μ-, δ- or κ-opioid receptors may also rely on the direct cellular environnement of the three known receptor protein.

Acknowledgements. I am grateful to Claire Gavériaux-Ruff, Katia Befort, Frédéric Simonin and Hans Matthes for the recent years of productive and stimulating collaboration and friendship. I am also particularly thankful to Pr.P. Chambon for his constant support of our work. I pay homage to C.G. Hirth for having participated in creating our research.

References

Abood ME, Noel MA, Farnworth JS, Tao Q (1994) Molecular cloning and expression of a δ-opioid receptor from rat brain. J Neurosci Res 37:714–719
Aruffo A, Seed B (1987) Molecular cloning of a CD28 cDNA by a high-efficiency COS cells expression system. Proc Natl Acad Sci USA 84:8573–8577
Augustin LB, Flesheim RF, Min BH, Fuchs SM, Fuchs JA, Loh HH (1995) Genomic structure of the mouse δ-opioid receptor gene. Biochem Biophys Res Commun 207:111–119
Bare LA, Mansson E, Yang DM (1994) Expression of two variants of the human μ-opioid receptor mRNA in SK-N-SH cells and human brain. FEBS 354:213–216
Befort K, Mattei M-G, Roeckel N, Kieffer B (1994) Chromosomal localization of the δ-opioid receptor gene to human 1p34.3–p36.1 and mouse 4D bands by in situ hybridization. Genomics 20:143–145
Bunzow JR, Saez C, Mortrud M, Bouvier C, Williams JT, Low M, Grandy DK (1994) Molecular cloning and tissue distribution of a putative member of the rat opioid receptor gene family that is not a μ, δ or κ opioid receptor type. FEBS 347:284–288
Bunzow JR, Zhang G, Bouvier C, Saez C, Ronnekleiv OK, Kelly MJ, Grandy DK (1995) Characterization and distribution of a cloned rat μ-opioid receptor. J Neurochem 64:14–24

Bzdega T, Chin H, Kim H, Jung HH, Kozak CA, Klee WA (1993) Regional expression and chromosomal localization of the δ opiate receptor gene. Proc Natl Acad Sci USA 90:9305–9309

Chakrabarti S, Prather PL, Yu L, Law P-Y, Loh HH (1995a) Expression of the μ-opioid receptor in CHO cells: ability of μ-opioid ligands to promote alpha-azidoanilido [32P]GTP labeling of multiple G protein alpha subunits. J Neurochem 64:2534–2543

Chakrabarti S, Law P-Y, Loh HH (1995b) Neuroblastoma neuro 2A cells stably expressing a cloned mu-opioid receptor: a specific cellular model to study acute and chronic effects of morphine. Mol Brain Res 30:269–278

Chen Y, Mestek A, Liu J, Hurley JA, Yu L (1993a) Molecular cloning and functional expression of a μ-opioid receptor from rat brain. Mol Pharmacol 44:8–12

Chen Y, Mestek A, Lui J, Yu L (1993b) Molecular cloning of a rat κ opioid receptor reveals sequence similarities to the μ and δ opioid receptors. Biochem J 295:625–628

Chen Y, Yu L (1994) Differential regulation by cAMP-dependent protein kinase and protein kinase C of the μ-opioid receptor coupling to a G protein-activated K^+ channel. J Biol Chem 269:7839–7842

Chen Y, Fan Y, Liu J, Mestek A, Tian MT, Kozak CA, Yu L (1994) Molecular cloning, tissue distribution and chromosomal localization of a novel member of the opioid receptor gene family. FEBS 347:279–283

Childers SR (1991) Opioid receptor-coupled second messenger systems. Life Sci 48:1991–2003

Childers SR (1993) Opioid receptor-coupled second messenger systems. In: Herz A (ed) Opioids I. Springer, Berlin Heidelberg New York, pp 189–208 (Handbook of experimental pharmacology, vol 104/I)

Cox BM (1993) Opioid receptor-G protein interactions: acute and chronic effects of opioids. In: Herz A (ed) Opioids I. Springer, Berlin Heidelberg New York, pp 145–180 (Handbook of experimental pharmacology, vol 104/I)

Dascal N, Schreibmayer W, Lim NF, Wang W, Chavkin C, Di ML, Labarca C, Kieffer BL, Gaveriaux-Ruff C, Trollinger D, Lester HA, Davidson N (1993) Atrial G protein-activated K^+ channel: expression cloning and molecular properties. Proc Natl Acad Sci USA 90:10235–10239

Dickenson AH (1991) Mechanisms of the analgesic actions of opiates and opioids. Br Med Bull 47:690–702

Evans CJ, Keith DE, Morrison H, Magendzo K, Edwards RH (1992) Cloning of a δ-opioid receptor by functional expression. Science 258:1952–1955

Fukuda K, Kato S, Mori K, Nishi M, Takeshima H (1993) Primary structures and expression from cDNAs of rat opioid receptor δ- and μ-subtypes. FEBS 327:311–314

Fukuda K, Kato S, Mori K, Nishi M, Takeshima H, Iwabe N, Miyata T, Houtani T, Sugimoto T (1994) cDNA cloning and regional distribution of a novel member of the opioid receptor family. FEBS 343:42–46

Giros B, Pohl M, Rochelle JM, Seldin MF (1995) Chromosomal localization of opioid peptide and receptor genes in the mouse. Life Sci 56:PL369–PL375

Goldstein A, Naidu A (1989) Multiple opioid receptors: ligand selectivity profiles and binding signatures. Mol Pharmacol 36:265–272

Henry DJ, Grandy DK, Lester HA, Davidson N, Chavkin C (1995) K-opioid receptors couple to inwardly rectifying potassium channels when coexpressed by Xenopus oocytes. Mol Pharmacol 47:551–557

Hughes J, Smith TW, Kosterlitz HW, Fothergill LA, Morgan BA, Morris HR (1975) Identification of two related pentapeptides from the brain with potent opiate agonist activity. Nature 258:577–579

Johnson P S, Wang JB, Wang WF, Uhl GR (1994) Expressed μ opiate receptor couples to adenylate cyclase and phosphatidyl inositol turnover. Neuroreport 5:507–509

Kaneko S, Nakamura S, Adachi K, Akaike A, Satoh M (1994a) Mobilization of intracellular Ca^{2+} and stimulation of cyclic AMP production by κ-opioid receptors expressed in Xenopus oocytes. Mol Brain Res 27:258–264

Kaneko S, Fukuda K, Yada N, Akaike A, Mori Y, Satoh M (1994b) Ca^{2+} channel inhibition by κ-opioid receptors expressed in Xenopus oocytes. Neuroreport 5:2506–2508

Kaufman DL, Keith DE, Anton B, Tian J, Magendzo K, Newman D, Tran TH, Lee DS, Wen C, Xia Y-R, Lusis AJ, Evans CJ (1995) Characterization of the murine μ-opioid receptor gene. J Biol Chem 270:15877–15883

Keith D, Maung T, Anton B, Evans CJ (1994) Isolation of cDNA clones homologous to opioid receptors. Regul Pept 54:143–144

Kieffer BL, Befort K, Gaveriaux-Ruff C, Hirth CG (1992) The δ-opioid receptor: isolation of a cDNA by expression cloning and pharmacological characterization. Proc Natl Acad Sci USA 89:12048–12052

Klee WA, Nirenberg M (1974) A neuroblastoma × glioma hybrid cell line with morphine receptors. Proc Natl Acad Sci USA 71:3474–3477

Knapp RJ, Malatynska E, Fang L, Li XP, Babin E, Nguyen M, Santoro G, Varga EV, Hruby VJ, Roeske WR, Yamamura HI (1994) Identification of a human δ-opioid receptor: cloning and expression. Life Sci 54:PL463–PL469

Knapp RJ, Malatynska E, Collins N, Fang L, Wang J-Y, Hruby VJ, Roeske WR, Yamamura HI (1995) Molecular biology and pharmacology of cloned opioid receptors. FASEB J 9:516–525

Kong H, Raynor K, Yasuda K, Moe ST, Porthoghese PS, Bell GI, Reisine T (1993) A single residue, aspartic acid 95, in the δ-opioid receptor specifies selective high affinity agonist binding. J Biol Chem 31:23055–23058

Kong HY, Raynor K, Yano H, Takeda J, Bell GI, Reisine T (1994) Agonists and antagonists bind to different domains of the cloned κ-opioid receptor. Proc Natl Acad Sci USA 91:8042–8046

Kovoor A, Henry D, Chavkin C (1995) Agonist-induced desensitization of the μ-opioid receptor-coupled potassium channel (GIRK1). J Biol Chem 270:589–595

Kozak CA, Filie J, Adamson MC, Chen Y, Yu L (1994) Murine chromosomal location of the μ- and κ-opioid receptor genes. Genomics 21:659–661

Lachowicz JE, ShenY, Monsma FJ Jr, Sibley DR (1995) Molecular cloning of a novel G protein-coupled receptor related to the opiate receptor family. J Neurochem 64:34–40

Lai HWL, Minami M, Satoh M, Wong YH (1995). Gz coupling to the rat κ-opioid receptor. FEBS 360:97–99

Law PY, Mcginn TM, Wick MJ, Erickson LJ, Evans CJ, Loh HH (1994) Analysis of δ-opioid receptor activities stably expressed in CHO cell lines: function of receptor density? J Pharmacol Exp Ther 271:1686–1694

Lefkowitz RJ, Hausdorff WP, Caron MG (1990) Role of phosphorylation in desensitization of β-adrenoceptor. Trends Pharmacol Sci 11:190–194

Leslie FM (1987) Methods used for the study of opioid receptors. Pharmacol Rev 39:197–249

Li S, Zhu J, Chen C, Chen Y-W, Deriel JK, Ashby B, Lui-Chen L-Y (1993) Molecular cloning and expression of a rat κ opioid receptor. Biochem J 295:629–633

Liang Y, Mestek A, Yu L, Carr LG (1995) Cloning and characterization of the promoter region of the mouse μ-opioid receptor gene. Brain Res 679:82–88

Liu H-C, Lu S, Augustin LB, Felsheim RF, Chen H-C, Loh HH, Wei L-N (1995) Cloning and promoter mapping of mouse κ-opioid receptor gene. Biochem Biophys Res Commun 209:639–647

Ma GH, Miller RJ, Kuznetsov A, Philipson LH (1995) K-opioid receptor activates an inwardly rectifying K^+ channel by a G protein-linked mechanism: coexpression in Xenopus oocytes. Mol Pharmacol 47:1035–1040

Malatynska E, Wang Y, Knapp RJ, Santoro G, Li X, Waite S, Roeske WR, Yamamura HI (1995) Human δ-opioid receptor: a stable cell line for functional studies of opioids. Neuroreport 6:613–616

Mansour A, Khachaturian H, Lewis ME, Akil H, Watson SJ (1987) Autoradiographic differentiation of μ, δ and κ receptors in the rat forebrain and midbrain. J Neurosci 7:2445–2464

Mansson E, Bare L, Yang DM (1994) Isolation of a human κ-opioid receptor cDNA from placenta. Biochem Biophys Res Commun 202:1431–1437

Meng F, Xie G-X, Thompson RC, Mansour A, Goldstein A, Watson SJ, Akil H (1993) Cloning and pharmacological characterization of a rat κ opioid receptor. Proc Natl Acad Sci USA 90:9954–9958

Meng F, Hoversten MT, Thompson RC, Taylor L, Watson SJ, Akil H (1995) A chimeric study of the molecular basis of affinity and selectivity of the κ- and the δ-opioid receptors: potential role of extracellular domains. J Biol Chem 270:12730–12736

Mestek A, Hurley JH, Bye LS, Campbell AD, Chen Y, Tian M, Liu J, Schulman H, Yu L (1995) The human μ-opioid receptor: modulation of functional desensitization by calcium/calmodulin-dependent protein kinase and protein kinase C. J Neurosci 15:501–527

Meunier JC, Mollereau C, Toll L, Suaudeau C, Moisand C, Alvinerie P, Butour J-L, Guillemeau J-C, Ferrara P, Monsarrat B, Mazargull H, Parmentier M, Vassart G, Costentin J (1995) Isolation and structure of the endogenous agonist of opioid receptor-like ORL1 receptor. Nature 377:532–535

Millan MJ (1990) κ-Opioid receptors and analgesia. Trends Pharmacol Sci 11:70–76

Min B H, Augustin LB, Felsheim RF, Fuchs JA, Loh HH (1994) Genomic structure and analysis of promoter sequence of a mouse μ-opioid receptor gene. Proc Natl Acad Sci USA 91:9081–9085

Minami M, Toya T, Katao Y, Maekawa K, Nakumura S, Onogi T, Kaneko S, Satoh M (1993) Cloning and expression of a cDNA for the rat κ-opioid receptor. FEBS 329:291–295

Minami M, Onogi T, Nakagawa T, Katao Y, Aoki Y, Katsumata S, Satoh M (1995) DAMGO, a μ-opioid receptor selective ligand, distinguishes between μ- and κ-opioid receptors at a different region from that for the distinction between μ- and δ-opioid receptors. FEBS 364:23–27

Miyamae T, Fukushima N, Misu Y, Ueda H (1993) δ-Opioid receptor mediated phospholipase C activation via Gi in Xenopus oocytes. FEBS 333:311–314

Mollereau C, Parmentier M, Mailleux P, Butour JL, Moisand C, Chalon P, Caput D, Vassart G, Meunier JC (1994) ORL 1, a novel member of the opioid receptor family. Cloning, functional expression and localization. FEBS 341:33–38

Nishi M, Takeshima H, Fukuda K, Kato S, Mori K (1993) cDNA cloning and pharmacological characterization of an opioid receptor with high affinities for κ-subtype-selective ligands. FEBS 330:77–80

Nishi M. Takeshima H, Mori M, Nakagawara K, Takeuchi T (1994) Structure and chromosomal mapping of genes for the mouse κ-opioid receptor and opioid receptor homologue (MOR-C). Biochem Biophys Res Commun 205:1353–1357

North RA (1986) Opioid receptor types and membrane ion channels. Trends Neurosci 9:114–117

North RA (1993) Opioid action on membrane ion channels. In: Herz A (ed) Opioids I. Springer, Berlin Heidelberg New York, pp 773–793 (Handbook of experimental pharmacology, vol 104/I)

Pan Y-X, Cheng J, Xu J, Rossi G, Jacobson E, Ryan-Moro J, Brooks AI, Dean GE, Standifer KM, Pasternak GW (1995) Cloning and functional characterization through antisense mapping of a k3-related opioid receptor. Mol Pharmacol 47: 1180–1188

Pasternak GW (1993) Pharmacological mechanisms of opioid analgesics. Clin Pharmacol 16:1–18

Paul D, Bodnar RJ, Gistrak MA, Pasternak GW (1989) Different μ receptor subtypes mediate spinal and supraspinal analgesia in mice. Eur J Pharmacol 168:307–314

Pert CB, Snyder SH (1973) Opiate receptor: demonstration in nervous tissue. Science 179:1011–1014

Piros ET, Prather PL, Loh HH, Law P-Y, Evans CJ, Hales TG (1995) Ca^{2+} channel and adenylyl cyclase modulation by cloned μ-opioid receptors in GH3 cells. Mol Pharmacol 47:1041–1049

Portoghese PS, Sultana M, Nagase H, Takemori AE (1992) A highly selective d_1 opioid receptor antagonist: 7-benzylidenenaltrexone (BNTX). Eur J Pharmacol 218:195–196

Prather PL, McGinn TM, Erickson LJ, Evans CJ, Loh HH, Law P-Y (1994) Ability of δ-opioid receptors to interact with multiple G-proteins is independent of receptor density. J Biol Chem 269:21293–21302

Prather PL, McGinn TM, Claude PA, Liu-Chen LY, Loh HH, Law P-Y (1995) Properties of a κ-opioid receptor expressed in CHO cells: interaction with multiple G-proteins is not specific for any individual G a subunit and is similar to that of other opioid receptors. Mol Brain Res 29:336–346

Probst WC, Snyder LA, Schuster DI, Brosius J, Sealfon SC (1992) Sequence alignment of the G-protein-coupled receptor superfamily. DNA and cell biol 11:1–20

Raynor K, Kong H, Chen Y, Yasuda K, Yu L, Bell GI, Reisine T (1993) Pharmacological characterization of the cloned κ-, δ- and μ-opioid receptors. Mol Pharmacol 45:330–334

Raynor K, Kong HY, Hines J, Kong GH, Benovic J, Yasuda K, Bell GI, Reisine T (1994) Molecular mechanisms of agonist-induced desensitization of the cloned mouse κ-opioid receptor. J Pharmacol Exp Ther 270:1381–1386

Reinsheid RK, Nothacker HP, Bourson A, Arbati A, Henningsen RA, Bunzow JR, Grandy DK, Langen H, Monsme FJ, Civelli O (1995) Orphanin FQ: a neuropeptide that activates an opioid-like G protein-coupled receptor. Science 270:792–794

Schofield PR, McFarland KC, Hayflick JS, Wilcox JN, Cho TM, Roy S, Lee NM, Loh HH, Seeburg PH (1989) Molecular characterization of a new immunoglobulin superfamily protein with potential roles in opioid binding and cell contact. EMBO J 8:489–495

Simon EJ, Hiller JM, Edelman I (1973) Stereospecific binding of the potent narcotic analgesic ^{3}H etorphine to rat brain homogenate. Proc Natl Acad Sci USA 70:1947–1949

Simonin F, Befort K, Gaveriaux-Ruff C, Matthes H, Nappey V, Lannes B, Micheletti G, Kieffer B (1994) The human δ-opioid receptor: genomic organization, cDNA cloning, functional expression and distribution in human brain. Mol Pharmacol 46:1015–1021

Simonin F, Gavériaux-Ruff C, Befort K, Matthes H, Lannes B, Micheletti G, Mattei M-G, Charron G, Bloch B, Kieffer B (1995) κ-Opioid receptor in humans: cDNA and genomic cloning, chromosomal assignment, functional expression, pharmacology and expression pattern in the central nervous system. Proc Natl Acad Sci USA 92:7006–7010

Sofuoglu M, Portoghese PS, Takemori AE (1991) Differential antagonism of δ opioid agonists by naltrindole and its benzofuran analog (NTB) in mice: evidence for δ-opioid receptor subtypes. J Pharmacol Exp Ther 257:676–680

Strader CD, Fong TM, Tota MR, Underwood D (1994) Structure and function of G protein-coupled receptors. Annu Rev Biochem 63:101–132

Surratt CK, Johnson PS, Moriwaki A, Seidleck BK, Blaschak CJ, Wang JB, Uhl GR (1994) μ-Opiate receptor-charged transmembrane domain amino acids are critical for agonist recognition and intrinsic activity. J Biol Chem 269:20548–2055

Tallent M, Dichter MA, Bell GI, Reisine T (1994) The cloned κ-opioid receptor couples to an N-type calcium current in undifferentiated PC-12 cells. Neuroscience 63:1033–1040

Terenius L (1973) Stereospecific interaction between narcotic analgesics and a synaptic plasma membrane fraction of rat cerebral cortex. Acta Pharmacol Toxicol 32:317–319

Thompson RC, Mansour A, Akil A, Watson SJ (1993) Cloning and pharmacological characterization of a rat μ-opioid receptor. Neuron 11:903–913

Traynor J (1989) Subtypes of the κ-opioid receptor: fact or fiction? Trends Pharmacol Sci 10:52–53

Traynor JR, Elliot J (1993) δ-Opioid receptor subtypes and cross talk with μ-receptors. Trends Pharmacol Sci 14:84–85

Tsu RC, Chan JSC, Wong YH (1995) Regulation of multiple effectors by the cloned δ-opioid receptor: stimulation of phospholipase C and type II adenylyl cyclase. J Neurochem 64:2700–2707

Ueda H, Miyamae T, Fukushima N, Takeshima H, Fukuda K, Sasaki Y, Misu Y (1995) Opioid μ- and κ-receptor mediate phospholipase C activation through Gi_1 in Xenopus oocytes. Mol Brain Res 32:166–170

Uhl GR, Childers S, Pasternak GW (1994) An opiate-receptor gene family reunion. Trends Neurosci 17:89–92

Wang J B, Imai Y, Eppler CM, Gregor P, Spivak CE, Uhl GR (1993) μ Opiate receptor: cDNA cloning and expression. Proc Natl Acad Sci USA 90:10230–10234

Wang JB, Johnson PS, Persico AM, Hawkins AL, Griffin CA, Uhl GR (1994a) Human μ-opiate receptor–cDNA and genomic clones, pharmacological characterization and chromosomal assignment. FEBS 338:217–222

Wang JB, Johnson PS, Imai Y, Persico AM, Ozenberger BA, Eppler CM, Uhl GR (1994b) cDNA cloning of an orphan opiate receptor gene family member and its splice variant. FEBS 348:75–79

Wang JB, Johnson PS, Wu JM, Wang WF, Uhl GR (1994c) Human κ-opiate receptor second extracellular loop elevates dynorphin's affinity for human μ/κ chimeras. J Biol Chem 269:25966–25969

Wick MJ, Minnerath SR, Lin, XQ, Elde R, Law PY, Loh HH (1994) Isolation of a novel cDNA encoding a putative membrane receptor with high homology to the cloned μ, δ and κ opioid receptors. Mol Brain Res 27:37–44

Wollemann M (1994) Discrepancies between identical amino acid sequences of cloned opioid-receptor subtypes and their binding data. Trends Neurosci 17:337

Xie G-X, Miyajima A, Goldstein A (1992) Expression cloning of a cDNA encoding a seven-helix receptor from human placenta with affinity for opioid ligands. Proc Natl Acad Sci USA 89:4124–4128

Xie G-X, Meng F, Mansour A, Thompson RC, Hoversten MT, Goldstein A, Watson SJ, Akil H (1994) Primary structure and functional expression of a guinea pig κ-opioid (dynorphin) receptor. Proc Natl Acad Sci USA 91:3779–3783

Xue JC, Chen CG, Zhu JM, Kunapuli S, Deriel JK, Yu L, Liuchen LY (1994) Differential binding domains of peptide and non-peptide ligands in the cloned rat κ-opioid receptor. J Biol Chem 269:30195–30199

Xue JC, Chen C, Zhu J, Kunapuli SP, Kim de Riel J, Yu L, Liu-Chen L-Y (1995) The third extracellular loop of the mu opioid receptors is important for agonist selectivity. J Biol Chem 270:12977–12979

Yakovlev AG, Krueger KE, Faden AI (1995) Structure and expression of a rat κ-opioid receptor gene. J Biol Chem 270:6421–6424

Yasuda K, Raynor K, Kong H, Breder CD, Takeda J, Reisine T, Bell GI (1993) Cloning and functional comparision of κ- and δ-opioid receptors from mouse brain. Proc Natl Acad Sci USA 90:6736–6740

Yasuda K, Espinosa R, Takeda J, Lebeau MM, Bell GI (1994) Localization of the κ-opioid receptor gene to human chromosome band 8Q11.2. Genomics 19:596–597

Zhu J, Chen C, Xue J-C, Kunapuli S, DeRiel JK, Liu-Chen L-Y (1995) Cloning of a human κ-opioid receptor from the brain. Life Sci 56:201–207

Zimprich A, Simon T, Höllt V (1995) Cloning and expression of an isoform of the rat μ-opioid receptor (rMOR1B) which differs in agonist-induced desensitization from rMOR1. FEBS 359:142–146

CHAPTER 12

Opioid Pharmacology of Acute and Chronic Pain

M.H. Ossipov, T.P. Malan Jr., J. Lai, and F. Porreca

A. Introduction

Although it is well established that exogenously administered opiates attenuate nocifensive responses to nociceptive stimuli of various modalities, it has only recently been demonstrated that endogenous opioids exert tonic activities which can either inhibit nociceptive sensory input under normal conditions, or perhaps increase the sensitivity to sensory input in pathological states. Conditions of chronic pain are known to induce a variety of changes in spinal levels and activities of endogenous peptides including enkephalins and dynorphin, in other regulatory neuropeptides such as cholecystokinin (CCK), and in the receptors for these substances. These changes in neuropeptide levels and activity have strong implications in the etiology of chronic pain states and, critically, are likely to be a major factor in determining the outcome of analgesic therapy. For example, reduced spinal CCK content associated with peripheral inflammation has been suggested to result in an increase in the antinociceptive potency of morphine. Conversely, neuropathic pain states are thought to be associated with increased spinal CCK content and, accordingly, reduced antinociceptive potency and efficacy of morphine. Spinal levels of dynorphin are also thought to be increased in conditions of chronic pain. Whereas dynorphin may serve a physiological role in reducing nociception associated with inflammatory pain, recent evidence suggests that increased spinal content of dynorphin also plays an important part in pathological states, contributing to the maintenance and perhaps the development of neuropathic pain states. As with CCK, changes in the levels and sites of action of endogenous dynorphins may markedly affect the response to proposed analgesic therapy.

B. Pharmacological Characterization

I. Opioids and CCK in Nociception

The sulfated octapeptide variant of CCK is distributed throughout the CNS, with high concentrations in the cerebral cortex and the caudate nucleus. CCK has been found in soma and terminals of neurons in several regions of the CNS, including the cerebral cortex, amygdala, periaqueductal gray, raphe nuclei, and dorsal horns of the spinal cord (see review by SUBERG and WATKINS 1987). Interestingly, the distributions of CCK and of CCK receptors in the CNS overlap considerably with the distributions of endogenous opioid peptides (STENGAARD-PEDERSON and LARSON 1981) and of opioid receptors (GHILARDI et al. 1992). Many of these sites are involved in the modulation of nociception by opiates. These observations suggest the possibility of a modulatory interaction between opioid-induced antinociception and CCK activity.

Based on a number of observations in which CCK appeared to produce physiological responses contradictory to those of opioids, it was suggested that CCK may act as an endogenous antiopioid (FARIS et al. 1983). This hypothesis was further supported by observations that CCK attenuated the antinociceptive effects of morphine and endogenously released opioids (FARIS et al. 1983). It has also been postulated that CCK may act as a modulator of tonic spinal antinociceptive activity, as suggested by observations that morphine administration increases the release of CCK in the spinal cord of the rat (ZHOU et al. 1993; NOBLE et al. 1993; STANFA et al. 1994). Increases or decreases in CCK levels may be elicited by conditions of safety cues or aversive events which lower or raise nociceptive thresholds, respectively, representing an adaptive response to environmental conditions (LAVIGNE et al. 1992; WIERTELAK et al. 1992).

Initial behavioral (SUH and TSENG 1990; WATKINS et al. 1985a,b) and electrophysiological studies had shown that the nonspecific CCK antagonists proglumide and lorglumide elicit enhancement of morphine-induced antinociception while producing no antinociceptive activity when administered alone. Later studies showed that the CCK_B specific antagonists L365260 (DOURISH et al. 1990) and CI-988 (PD134308; HUGHES et al. 1991) enhance the antinociceptive effects of morphine in rats. More detailed pharmacological investigations have recently identified a probable mechanism by which antagonism of CCK activity enhances the antinociceptive activity of morphine (VANDERAH et al. 1994, 1996a; OSSIPOV et al. 1994).

These studies present evidence that CCK tonically reduces the release and/or availability of endogenous substance(s) acting at the δ-opioid receptor. Consequently, blockade of the CCK receptor may result in an increase in the release or activity of substances acting via δ-opioid receptors, resulting in the well-known positive modulation of morphine antinociceptive potency and efficacy (e.g., VAUGHT and TAKEMORI 1979; HEYMAN et al. 1989a,b). OSSIPOV and coworkers (1994) demonstrated that the antinociceptive effect of systemic or intrathecal morphine in the hot-plate or tail-flick tests is significantly enhanced by the selective CCK_B antagonist L365260 in rats. This modulatory effect but not the direct antinociceptive actions of morphine is blocked by doses of naltrindole (NTI) that were selective for δ-opioid, rather than μ- or κ-opioid receptors. These findings were extended by VANDERAH et al. (1996a) who showed NTI-sensitive enhancement of morphine potency by L365260, in the mouse tail-flick test following administration of these compounds by systemic, intrathecal, or intracerebroventricular routes of administration. The same study also showed that antisera to [Leu^5]enkephalin, but not to [Met^5]enkephalin, given intracerebroventricularly blocks the enhanced antinociceptive effect of intracerebroventricular morphine by L365260. Taken together these data suggest that the availability or action of [Leu^5]enkephalin is tonically regulated by CCK, and that activity of this substance, at δ-opioid receptors, modulates the observed antinociceptive effect of morphine. This view is supported by a variety of pharmacological observations. Repeated intracerebroventricular injections of L365260 to mice results in decreased antinociceptive potency of δ-opioid agonists such as [D-Ala^2, Glu^4]deltorphin, suggesting the unlikely observation of 'cross-tolerance' between a CCK$_B$ antagonist and an δ-opioid agonist. Likewise, repeated intracerebroventricular administration of [Leu^5]enkephalin or [D-Ala^2, Glu^4]deltorphin produces antinociceptive cross-tolerance not only to δ-opioid agonists but also to L365260, as shown by the loss of the enhancement of morphine antinociception elicited by the CCK$_B$ antagonist. This finding completed the demonstration of two-way antinociceptive cross-tolerance between δ-opioid agonists and a CCK$_B$ antagonist. If CCK tonically inhibits the release, and/or availability of endogenous opioids such as [Leu^5]enkephalin, direct antinociceptive actions of CCK antagonists should be observed.

While administration of a CCK antagonist does not generally elicit antinociception, WEISENFELD-HALLIN and colleagues (1990) showed that PD134308 (CI-988), a selective CCK$_B$ antagonist, produces an antinociceptive effect when evaluated in depression of the rat flexor reflex. Particularly noteworthy is that this antinociceptive effect was blocked by naloxone, suggesting the involvement of endogenous opioids in the action of the CCK$_B$ antagonist. Given the brief half-life of [Leu^5]enkephalin (HAMBROOK et al. 1976), VANDERAH and colleagues (1996a) administered L365260 alone or together with the neutral endopeptidase inhibitor thiorphan and monitored antinociceptive activity in the mouse tail-flick assay. While neither L365260 or thiorphan produced any antinociceptive effect when given alone by the intracerebroventricular, route, the combination of these compounds produced a robust antinociception which was readily blocked by either NTI or antisera to [Leu^5]enkephalin (but not by antisera to [Met^5]enkephalin; VANDERAH et al. 1996a). As seen with L365260 and morphine, the antinociceptive effect of the combination of thiorphan plus L365260 was lost in mice made tolerant to δ-opioid agonists such as [D-Ala^2, Glu^4]deltorphin.

Additional evidence for the involvement of the CCK$_B$ receptor in the CCK modulation of morphine antinociception comes from application of antisense strategies. Intracerebroventricular treatment of mice with an antisense oligodeoxynucleotide to the CCK$_B$ receptor also resulted in an NTI-sensitive augmentation of the antinociceptive potency of morphine; mismatch oligodeoxynucleotide did not alter the activity of morphine. The enhancement of morphine potency seen in animals treated with antisense oligodeoxynucleotides to the CCK$_B$ receptor was also blocked by antisera to

[Leu[5]]enkephalin, but not by antisera to [Met[5]]enkephalin (Vanderah et al. 1994).

Collectively these data lend support to the conclusion that CCK acts to tonically reduce the release and/or availability of endogenous [Leu[5]]enkephalin (or a [Leu[5]]enkephalin-like substance) acting at the δ-opioid receptor, and that blockade of the CCK_B receptor results in increased availability of this endogenous δ-opioid agonist, which is then available to enhance both the potency and efficacy of morphine at μ-opioid receptors (Ossipov et al. 1994; Vanderah et al. 1994, 1996a). The importance of activity of endogenous δ-opioid agonists on morphine activity has been repeatedly demonstrated by several laboratories in mice (Vaught and Takemori 1979; Heyman et al. 1989a,b) and rats (Larson et al. 1980). This proposed mechanism of enhancement of morphine antinociception by CCK antagonists is also supported by the observations that CCK antagonists increase the antinociceptive effect of endogenously released enkephalin, presumably elicited by footshock (Watkins et al. 1985b) and the antinociceptive effects of the "enkephalinase inhibitor" RB 101 (Maldonado et al. 1993; Noble et al. 1993).

These observations are of particular interest as CCK antagonists move towards possible clinical use as antianxiety agents. It is important to note that CCK_B receptors predominate in the dorsal horn of the spinal cord of rodents whereas the CCK_A receptor subtype predominates in that of the primate (Hill et al. 1988; Ghilardi et al. 1992). Therefore the so-called "balanced" CCK_A/ CCK_B antagonists (Singh et al. 1996) may become of significant utility as adjuncts in the treatment of pain states.

II. Modulation of Opioid Activity by κ Agonists

In contrast to the positive antinociceptive interaction observed between agonists of μ- and δ-opioid receptors, a substantial number of reports indicate that an antagonistic interaction exists between agonists acting at μ- and κ-opioid receptors. Studies employing the electrically stimulated rat isolated vas deferens demonstrate that the κ agonists ethylketocyclazocine and MR2034 antagonize the effects of the μ agonists [D-Ala[2], MePhe[4], Gly-ol[5]]enkephalin (DAMGO) and [D-Ala[2], D-Leu[5]]enkephalin (DADLE; Gillan et al. 1981). Likewise, the κ-opioid agonists U50488H, tifluadom, bremazocine, and ketazocine demonstrated antagonistic activity against μ-opioid agonists in the same preparation (Miller et al. 1986). It was demonstrated that centrally administered U50488H, ethylketocyclazocine, and tifluadom antagonized the inhibitory effects of morphine on spontaneous urinary bladder contractions (Sheldon et al. 1989) in a nor-binaltorphimine sensitive fashion. In the same assay only U50488H, and not ethylketocyclazocine or tifluadom, antagonized the inhibitory effects of DAMGO. Derivatives of putative endogenous κ-opioid agonist dynorphin [e.g., dynorphin A(1-13)] antagonized the antinociceptive effect of DADLE in a mouse tail-flick assay (Tulunay et al.

1981). Antagonism of morphine antinociception by κ-opioid agonists such as bremazocine and U50488H in the rat tail-flick test has been observed (RAMARAO et al. 1988), supporting the view that activation of κ-opioid receptors may act to limit observed actions of μ-opioid agonists.

C. Physiological Roles

I. Opioids, CCK, and Inflammation

Unilateral paw inflammation induced by a subcutaneous injection of carrageenan (KOCHER et al. 1987) elicits changes in the transcription of opioid and other peptides in the spinal cord. Increases in preprodynorphin mRNA and preproenkephalin mRNA have been observed during inflammation (DUBNER and RUDA 1992). Moreover, it has clearly been shown that morphine and other opioid agonists are more efficacious as antinociceptive agents in animals with inflammatory conditions than in normal animals (KAYSER and GUILBAUD 1983; NEIL et al. 1986). STANFA and DICKENSON (1993) demonstrated that the potency of morphine to inhibit evoked C fiber activity is increased 30-fold in the carrageenan-inflamed rat. Increases in sensitivity to the antinociceptive effect of morphine following inflammation have also been shown using behavioral assays (STANFA et al. 1994). The basis for the increase in morphine potency has been speculated to be related to decreases in levels of spinal CCK (STANFA et al. 1994), a peptide which has been demonstrated to reduce the antinociceptive activity of morphine (see above for discussion).

In accordance with earlier observations, carrageenan-induced inflammation of the rat hindpaw has been shown to increase the antinociceptive effect of morphine (OSSIPOV et al. 1995a). As it has been suggested that the antiopioid effect of CCK involves decreased availability of [Leu⁵]enkephalin, either through decreased transmitter release or increased biodegradation (OSSIPOV et al. 1994), the proposal of an increase in morphine antinociceptive potency resulting from inflammation suggests an increase in endogenous enkephalins as a result of decreased CCK activity. Consistent with this interpretation, the administration of δ-receptor selective doses of NTI clearly block the augmented response to morphine seen in the carrageenan-treated rat; in fact, the combined effect of morphine plus NTI in the carrageenan-inflamed rat is nearly identical to that of morphine administered alone to nonpretreated rats (OSSIPOV et al. 1995a). That the attenuated enhancement of morphine antinociception by NTI is not an artifact caused by NTI acting directly to diminish the effect of morphine at the μ-opioid receptor was well demonstrated by the observation that in noncarrageenan-pretreated rats the antinociceptive effect of morphine plus NTI is identical to that of morphine alone (OSSIPOV et al. 1995a). These results support the hypothesis that decreases in levels or activity of CCK activity during inflammation increase the actions of endogenous opioids, perhaps [Leu⁵]enkephalin or a similar substance, acting at δ-opioid receptors, thereby increasing the potency of morphine via a previously proposed interaction (Larson et al. 1980; Vaught and Takemori 1979).

II. Opioids and Inhibitory Tone

1. Role of Endogenous Opioids in Modulation of Tonic Nociceptive Input

A condition of tonic nociception is modeled by a subcutaneous injection of dilute formalin (usually ranging from 2% to 5% solution) into the plantar side of a hindpaw of a rat (Dubuisson and Dennis 1977). This procedure results in a biphasic flinching behavior indicative of a nocifensive response (Wheeler-Aceto et al. 1990). The initial short phase is generally interpreted as reflecting the response to the initial insult, which is the result of activation of nociceptors in the periphery without significant immediate tissue damage, whereas the longer lasting second phase is generally interpreted as representing the development of a state of sensitized dorsal horn neurons (i.e., "central sensitization") consequent to the arrival of the initial afferent barrage and a subsequently enhanced response to continuing, and presumably low-level, peripheral input arising from the developing inflammatory process (Wheeler-Aceto et al. 1990; Hunskaar and Hole 1987; Heapy et al. 1991). Electrophysiological studies have similarly demonstrated a biphasic response of dorsal horn convergent cells after peripheral formalin injection, with similar timecourse as the observed nocifensive behavior (Dickenson and Sullivan 1987). Additionally, since dorsal horn units responsive only to innocuous stimuli do not respond to formalin administration, it has been further concluded that the response to formalin is mediated by primary afferent C fibers (Dickenson and Sullivan 1987).

Tonic noxious stimulation in the periphery may also elicit changes in the activity or levels of endogenous opioids. Bourgoin and colleagues (1990) demonstrated transient increases in spinal [Met^5]enkephalin levels in response to subcutaneous injections of 10% formalin. In contrast, Hunter et al. (1996) measured no increase in spinal preproenkephalin mRNA after formalin injection. Millan and coworkers (1988) demonstrated increased spinal dynorphin levels with no change in either [Met^5]enkephalin or [Leu^5]enkephalin levels after inflammation caused by administration of *Mycobacterium butyricum* in the right hindpaw. Recent studies have also suggested that noxious stimulation induced by subcutaneous injection of mustard oil induces a nociception that can be rekindled by the administration of naloxone (Hu et al. 1993), suggesting tonic activity of endogenous opioids in inflammatory pain. The existence of an inhibitory modulation of tonic peripheral nociception that is mediated by endogenous opioids had been initially suggested by studies indicating enhancement of the formalin-induced flinch response by naloxone (Wheeler-Aceto and Cowan 1993). Recent studies have extended this initial observation and suggested that this endogenous inhibitory tone is mediated through agents acting at κ- and δ-, but not μ-, opioid receptors (OSSIPOV et al. 1996). Pretreatment, but not posttreatment, with systemic naloxone produces a dramatic increase in both the first and the second phase of the flinch response elicited by 2% formalin. Likewise, systemically injected receptor-selective doses of NTI (δ antagonist) and nor-binaltorphimine (κ antagonist), but not β-funaltrexamine (μ antagonist), also significantly increased the magnitude of the formalin response, suggesting the involvement of endogenous opioids acting at δ and κ receptors. These results strongly suggest that endogenous opioids are tonically active to dampen the nociceptive signal which may be elicited by a nociceptive stimulus such as formalin.

Given the involvement of specific opioid receptors, likely candidates are substances such [Leu[5]]enkephalin and dynorphin A(1-17). The observation that intrathecal injections of μ-, δ-, and κ-opioid selective doses of DAMGO, CI-977, or [D-Ala[2], D-Leu[5]]enkephalin significantly attenuate the flinching response compared to that in control groups further confirms that opioid receptor activation attenuates this behavior. Additionally, each antagonist employed blocked the antinociceptive effect only of the agonist acting at the corresponding receptor subtype, and not of agonists acting at other receptor subtypes, confirming the selectivity of the antagonists at the doses employed. In an effort to identify the endogenous ligands acting to tonically inhibit nociception, antisera raised to [Leu[5]]enkephalin, [Met[5]]enkephalin, or dynorphin A(1-13) were given intrathecally prior to formalin administration. The antisera to [Leu[5]]enkephalin or dynorphin A(1-13) both produced significant increases in flinching. In contrast, antisera to [Met[5]]enkephalin produced no change in flinching responses. These studies provide of one of the clearest demonstrations of opioid inhibitory tone and provide strong evidence that nociceptive signals undergo spinal processing which presumably dampens the intensity of the rostrally transmitted pain message.

2. Involvement of Immediate-Early Onset Genes in Opioid Modulation of Tonic Nociception

Nociceptive input has been shown to induce the expression of immediate-early onset gene products, notably that of c-*fos*. The measurement of Fos protein expression has come to be interpreted as a reliable marker for neuronal activity in response to nociceptive stimuli (BULLITT 1990). A complex formed from Fos and Jun is believed ultimately to promote the expression of the gene products of late-onset genes (NARANJO et al. 1991; MORGAN and CURRAN 1989), including preprodynorphin and possibly preproenkephalin (DUBNER 1991). The mRNA levels for c-*fos* and c-*jun* are increased in the spinal cord in response to noxious (heat) stimulation of the hindpaw (WISDEN et al. 1990) and Fos protein levels are increased after formalin (HUNTER et al. 1996) or carrageenan (DUBNER and RUDA 1992) administration in the rat. It is reasonable to propose that tonic peripheral nociception, as induced by formalin injection in the hindpaw of the rat, would lead to increased spinal c-Fos expression, activating a cascade possibly leading to elevated spinal levels of enkephalins and dynorphin.

The use in vivo of antisense oligodeoxynucleotides (ODNs) to prevent the translation of specific gene products has become a valuable pharmacological tool (WAHLESTEDT 1994). Antisense probes of c-*fos* mRNA have successfully been used to inhibit translation of the mRNA into the Fos protein (CHIASSON et al. 1992), which would prevent induction of later-onset gene products dependent on Fos protein. Experiments were recently conducted in our laboratories to investigate the contribution of c-*fos* expression of behavioral nociceptive activity in response to formalin and to investigate the possible importance of endogenous opioid substances involved in the possible modulation of the nociceptive response. Intrathecal pretreatment of rats with a single injection of an antisense, but not mismatch, ODN to c-*fos* 2 h prior to formalin resulted in a dose-dependent increase in flinching behavior compared to control animals (Ossipov, Malan, and Porreca, unpublished observations). The same result was obtained by using a second, nonoverlapping antisense sequence to c-*fos* mRNA (Malan and Porreca, unpublished observations). That the administration of antisense, but not mismatch, ODN to c-*fos* produced an inhibition of the expression of the Fos protein in the spinal cord was confirmed by immunohistochemistry. The greatest concentrations of cells staining for Fos protein were in laminae 1 and 2, with progressively fewer labeled neurons in the deeper laminae. The number of Fos-reactive neurons in laminae 1–4 of rats receiving intrathecal administration of c-*fos* antisense ODN was significantly less than those receiving either mismatch ODN or vehicle. The intrathecal administration of c-*fos* mismatch ODN had no significant effect on Fos immunoreactivity in laminae 1–4. These results demonstrate a correlation between inhibition c-*fos* expression and increased nociceptive activity. Interestingly, the increase in flinching response was not as great as that observed in animals that were pretreated with systemic naloxone or NTI (Ossipov et al. 1996). Administration of naloxone to animals pretreated with intrathecal antisense, but not mismatch, ODN to c-*fos* further enhanced the flinching response elicited by formalin, although the response did not differ from that observed with naloxone or NTI alone. These data suggested that some but possibly not all inhibitory substances which tonically limit the intensity of the pain signal might be regulated by c-*fos*.

Earlier studies clearly demonstrated that superfusion of the spinal cord with c-*fos* antisense ODN results in decreased Fos protein production in response to nociception but does not affect the synthesis of other members of the Fos and Jun protein families (GILLARDON et al. 1994). These findings therefore support the observations of HUNTER et al. (1996), and further advance the hypothesis that the inflammatory process elicits c-*fos* induction, resulting in increased spinal endogenous antinociceptive agents (DUBNER and RUDA 1992; HUNT et al. 1987; NARANJO et al. 1991). However, prevention of c-*fos* induction alone does not result in a maximal increase in the response to a nociceptive stimulus. As the increased nociceptive behavior induced by c-*fos* antisense ODN is significantly augmented by naloxone, it seems clear that other factors not regulated by c-*fos* cascade are involved in endogenous tonic inhibitory modulation of nociception.

D. Pathological Roles: Opioids and Neuropathic Pain

I. Clinical Significance of Neuropathic Pain States

Neuropathic pain refers to abnormal pain syndromes arising from damage to peripheral nerves. Causes of neuropathic pain may include diabetic neuropathy, herpes zoster, nerve traction or compression, radiation therapy for lung and other cancers, reflex sympathetic dystrophy/sympathetically maintained pain, and complications from the acquired immune-deficiency syndrome. It may also arise from idiopathic causes, without evidence of noticeable nerve injury. Neuropathic pain may be long-lasting and continue for long periods after the initial injury has healed. Individuals afflicted with neuropathic pain often show an exaggerated sensitivity to nociceptive stimuli (hyperalgesia) or perceive normally innocuous stimuli as painful (allodynia; PAYNE 1986). Neuropathic dysesthesias are frequently characterized by burning or shooting pains along with tingling, crawling, or electrical sensations. Painful neuropathy represents a seriously debilitating syndrome that affects millions of persons, and their quality of life suffers significantly. In spite of recent progress in pain research our understanding of this pain syndrome is limited, as are the available treatments which allow one to lead a normal and productive life.

II. Proposed Mechanisms of Neuropathic Pain

A number of neuroanatomical and neurochemical changes occurring after nerve injury may underlie the dysesthesias associated with neuropathic states. It has been proposed that the large-diameter myelinated neurons undergo phenotypic changes in response to nerve injury, resulting in inappropriate synaptic connections. For example, either ligation or section of the sciatic nerve (WOOLF et al. 1992) or tight ligation of the L5 and L6 nerve roots (LEKAN et al. 1995) results in a significant sprouting of large-diameter, myelinated ($A\beta$) fibers into the superficial laminae of the dorsal horn of the spinal cord, presumably forming anomalous synapses with rostrally projecting dorsal horn units which normally transmit nociceptive information. By such physiopathic synapses, fibers normally transmitting innocuous stimuli might cause the same to be interpreted as nociceptive, thus producing allodynia (WOOLF et al. 1992; WOOLF and DOUBELL 1994). Damaged peripheral nerves may form peripheral collateral sprouts and ectopic foci, resulting in spontaneous discharges that are perceived as nociceptive (KAJANDER and BENNETT 1992), and there is a correlation between ectopic discharge and behavioral signs of neuropathic pain (HAN et al. 1995). Continuous afferent barrage may elicit hypersensitivity ('wind-up') of wide dynamic range neurons, which respond to both low- (innocuous) and high-threshold (nociceptive) stimuli so that normally innocuous mechanical touch may excessively activate these neurons, thus producing allodynia (Laird and Bennett 1993). Considerable evidence demonstrates that the activity of glutamate released from primary afferent terminals in the dorsal horn of the spinal cord and acting at NMDA receptors mediates wind-up (Davies and Lodge 1987; Dickenson and Sullivan 1987). Thus nerve injury with its spontaneous afferent discharge may evoke NMDA-mediated central sensitization manifested as allodynia and hyperalgesia (Mao et al. 1992; Wilcox 1991).

A sympathetic component of some cases of neuropathic pain has been proposed. Sympathetic efferent fibers may stimulate peripheral mechanoreceptor nerve endings, resulting in a continuous feedback loop of sympathetically maintained pain (Roberts 1986). Fluorescence studies have shown that after sciatic nerve section there is a dramatic sympathetic innervation of the neuroma and sensory nerves (Small et al. 1990) which is inhibited by sympathectomy (Goldstein et al. 1988). Likewise, nerve injury also results in sprouting of postganglionic sympathetic fibers into the dorsal root ganglion and spinal nerves; such innervation is virtually absent in normal rats (Chung et al. 1993; McLachlan et al. 1993). Clonidine given intrathecally to rats produces an antiallodynic effect hypothesized to occur by diminished sympathetic outflow (Yaksh et al. 1995). Surgical sympathectomy prevents signs of mechanical allodynia and heat hyperalgesia in rats with ligations of the L5 and L6 roots of the sciatic nerve, and chemical sympathectomy with phentolamine or guanethidine reversibly relieves signs of mechanical allodynia (Kim et al. 1993). A sympathetic component of neuropathic pain is also suggested by the observations that chemical sympathectomy, by administration of clonidine (Byas-Smith et al. 1995) or phentolamine (Shir et al. 1993) effectively diminishes painful neuropathy in some clinical situations.

There is compelling evidence that neuropathy results in increased spinal CCK levels (Stanfa et al. 1994). In situ hybridization studies have demonstrated increased prepro-CCK mRNA levels in the rat dorsal root ganglia and monkey dorsal horn after nerve transection (Verge et al. 1993), further suggesting a role for CCK in augmenting sensory input subsequent to nerve damage. The importance of elevated spinal CCK levels and its relation to decreased efficacy of opioids is discussed in greater detail below.

Peripheral nerve injury has also been associated with elevated spinal quantities of the endogenous opioid peptides, including enkephalins and dynorphin (Dubner and Ruda 1992). Whereas enkephalins in the spinal cord may provide some degree of endogenous antinociceptive activity, some evidence suggests that high levels of endogenous spinal dynorphin present a pathological, rather than physiological, role. For example, levels of endogenous dynorphin are elevated after traumatic injury of the spinal cord (Cox et al. 1985), and that behavioral sequelae of spinal cord trauma are diminished by the intrathecal administration of antisera to dynorphin (Shukla and Lemaire

1994; FADEN 1990). Likewise, spinal dynorphin levels are increased after spinal nerve injury, and dynorphin antisera given intrathecally reduce neurological impairment after such injuries (Cox et al. 1985; FADEN 1990). Further evidence for a nonopioid, neuropathological role of spinal dynorphin has been obtained with studies employing intrathecal injections of exogenous dynorphins. LONG and coworkers (1988) demonstrated a dose-dependent, nonopioid development of behavioral signs of neurological impairment produced by intrathecal dynorphins, which was accompanied by a depletion of populations of neuronal soma in the lumbosacral cord. Additionally, large doses of dynorphin fragments that do not interact with opioid receptors [e.g., dynorphin A(2-17), dynorphin A(2-13), or dynorphin A(3-13)] given intrathecally also produce hindlimb paralysis (STEVENS and YAKSH 1986; FADEN and JACOBS 1984). The possible pathological role of dynorphin with regard to neuropathic pain and opioid activity is further explored below.

III. Opioids in Neuropathic Pain

The utility of opioid analgesics in the clinical treatment of neuropathic pain is a matter of considerable controversy. The view is held by a number of investigators that clinical neuropathic pain is resistant to amelioration by opioids. For example, neuropathic pains of several origins were shown to be resistant to treatment with morphine infusions (ARNER and MEYERSON 1988), and postherpetic neuralgia was shown to be resistant to codeine (MAX et al. 1988). In contrast, other studies demonstrate efficacy of opioids in controlling neuropathic pain, but at greater than normally administered doses (PORTENOY and FOLEY 1986; JADAD et al. 1992). Spontaneous pain and allodynia caused by postherpetic neuralgia has been controlled by intravenous infusions of morphine (ROWBOTHAM et al. 1991). Hydromorphone infusions have achieved adequate analgesia in neuropathic pain patients (PORTENOY et al. 1990), but the dose-effect curve appears to be shifted to the right. Thus it has been suggested that the reported failure of morphine and other opioid analgesics to relieve neuropathic pain is due to underdosing of the patient (PORTENOY et al. 1990). Clearly, additional investigations into the clinical utility of opioids, taking into consideration the pain modality, route of administration, dosage, and opioid compound need to be performed to fully evaluate opioid treatment protocols for neuropathic pain.

The interpretation of data collected with various animal models of neuropathic pain with regard to the efficacy of opioids is likewise unclear. For example, it has been reported that intrathecal infusions (WIESENFELD-HALLIN 1984) but not bolus intrathecal injections (XU et al. 1993) of morphine reduce autotomy after sciatic nerve section. Morphine given by intrathecal injection produces dose-dependent antihyperalgesic and antinociceptive effect after chronic constriction injury but with a six-fold loss of potency (MAO et al. 1995a). The loss of potency of morphine in inhibiting radiant-heat induced foot-flick was evident even when the underlying hyperalgesia of the paw was eliminated by pretreatment with MK-801. Similar observations were recently made after ligation injury of the L5 and L6 spinal nerve roots (Wegert et al. 1996). In this model morphine given intrathecally produced dose-dependent antinociception when measured in radiant heat-induced foot-flick response in nerve-ligated rats but with a fivefold loss of potency compared to sham-operated rats. Elimination of underlying hyperalgesia by MK-801 pretreatment did not restore the antinociceptive potency of intrathecal morphine in the foot-flick assay.

Interestingly, intrathecal morphine demonstrates a considerable loss of antinociceptive potency to suppress the tail-flick response in animals with L5-L6 nerve ligation injury (Ossipov et al. 1995b). The loss of antinociceptive potency and efficacy of intrathecal morphine determined in the tail-flick test in animals with nerve injury was a surprising finding which was corroborated by a loss of potency, but not efficacy, of intrathecal DAMGO (Ossipov et al. 1995, unpublished observations). In this study there was a fourfold loss of the antinociceptive potency of intrathecal morphine, and, additionally, the maximal effect of morphine was reduced by 40% in the nerve injured rats. Baseline tail-flick latencies did not differ between the sham-operated and nerve-ligated groups of rats when evaluated at a variety of stimulus intensities, indicating that, unlike the hyperalgesia evident in the foot of the nerve-injured rat, no similar hyperalgesia could be demonstrated in the tail, and therefore the loss of potency and efficacy of morphine to suppress a nociceptive stimulus applied to the tail could not be attributed to this factor (Wegert et al. 1996). Additionally, there was a loss of potency and efficacy of intrathecal clonidine to suppress the tail-flick response in animals with nerve injury, suggesting that the observed changes were generalized beyond the activity of opioids acting via μ receptors (Ossipov et al. 1997). The results suggest that nerve ligation injury elicits such changes that the effect of opioid and adrenergic agonists, even at sites remote from the site of nerve injury (e.g., sacral spinal levels), may be attenuated. Several factors might have an influence on these observations (discussed below).

The intrathecal injection of up to 100 μg morphine failed to produce any change in the responses of rats with ligation injury of the L5 and L6 nerve roots to probing with von Frey filaments, indicating a lack of efficacy against tactile allodynia (Bian et al. 1995). In contrast, however, the high-efficacy, selective μ-opioid agonist DAMGO demonstrated a clear dose-dependent antiallodynic effect after intrathecal injection to nerve-injured rats (Nichols et al. 1995). Additionally, morphine administered either systemically or intracerebroventricularly produced a dose-dependent antiallodynic effect at doses close to the normally expected antinociceptive range (Bian et al. 1995; Lee et al. 1995). These studies suggest that loss of opioid activity in animal models of neuropathic pain is influenced by the route of administration, parameter chosen (e.g., hyperalgesia vs. allodynia), and efficacy of the opioid employed. The observed failure of spinal morphine, but not DAMGO, to suppress tactile allodynia in nerve-injured rats, may be explained by a variety of factors which are presumably important in determining the outcome of proposed analgesic therapy in patients with neuropathic pain.

1. Development of Tolerance

It has been suggested on the basis of experiments employing the chronic constriction injury model that the reduced efficacy of intrathecal morphine against thermal hyperalgesia results from processes similar to those of development of tolerance to opioids (MAO et al. 1995b). This possibility remains to be explored more fully. In initial experiments in our laboratory, evaluation of the opioid-transduction pathway using a $[^{35}S]GTP-\gamma-S$ binding assay in lumbar spinal cord of sham-operated and nerve-injured animals showed no differences for morphine in these tissues, suggesting that the initial step in the transduction pathway is not altered (unpublished observations). Perhaps more revealing is the observation in nerve-injured rats of a loss of antinociceptive potency and efficacy of intrathecal clonidine, an α-adrenergic agonist which does not show antinociceptive cross-tolerance to opioids (OSSIPOV et al. 1989; COOMBS et al. 1985). This observation suggests that the changes which may occur after nerve injury induce a state similar to that seen in opioid tolerance, but that these changes are more generalized in the case of nerve injury.

NMDA antagonists have been shown to prevent or delay the onset of opioid tolerance when evaluated with morphine (TRUJILLO and AKIL 1991; MAO et al. 1995a). On the other hand, MK-801 blocks the hyperalgesia of the foot associated with the chronic constriction injury but does not restore the loss of potency of morphine to suppress the foot-flick response in either the constriction injury or the ligation injury models (MAO et al. 1995a; WEGERT et al. 1997). NMDA antagonists have also been shown to delay the onset of (SMITH et al. 1995) or to attenuate mechanical allodynia after partial ligation of the sciatic nerve (SELTZER et al. 1991). Recent work has raised the possibility that blockade of the NMDA receptor complex with MK-801 can block the allodynia seen in animals with the nerve-ligation injury (LEE and YAKSH 1995). Unfortunately, this observation involves the use of intrathecal doses of MK-801, which produce severe behavioral toxicity that makes interpretation of the data difficult. Administration of intrathecal doses of MK-801 which do not elicit behavioral toxicity does not result in a blockade of allodynia in nerve-injured rats (BIAN et al. 1995) in spite of the fact that these doses do block thermal hyperalgesia without producing analgesia of the paw ipsilateral to the ligation the L5 and L6 nerve roots (WEGERT et al. 1997). For these reasons the possibility that an 'opioid' tolerance develops after nerve injury remains an intriguing hypothesis which will require further exploration before firm conclusions can be drawn.

2. Location of Opioid Receptors

It is generally accepted that the spinal action of morphine in acute pain is in large part mediated through opioid receptors residing on central terminals of small-diameter afferent fibers (see Lombard and Besson 1989; Yaksh et al. 1995). Both peripheral nerve section and dorsal rhizotomies have been associated with decreased opioid binding sites in the superficial layers of the dorsal horn, and appear to be correlated with the degree of peripheral nerve damage (Besse et al. 1992). Additionally, it has been demonstrated that chronic constriction injury of the sciatic nerve may be associated with decreased levels of substance P and calcitonin gene-related peptide in the cells of the dorsal root ganglia and in laminae I and II of the dorsal horn, implying proximal degeneration of small-diameter fibers after peripheral nerve injury (Bennett et al. 1989). Based on these observations it has been presumed that ligation of the L5 and L6 sciatic nerve roots would likewise result in a degeneration of small-diameter primary afferent neurons and the accompanying opioid receptors, thus leading to the observed loss of efficacy and potency of intrathecal morphine in the nerve-injured animal (Yaksh et al. 1995). However, alterations in spinal opioid receptor populations following nerve injury appear complex. For example, it has been shown that although unilateral dorsal rhizotomy of T13 to S2 produces reductions in μ- and δ-opioid binding sites of approximately 60% and 70%, respectively (Besse et al. 1990), chronic constriction injury of the sciatic nerve results in permanent increases in μ-opioid binding sites of 30%–50% both ipsilaterally and contralaterally, but only transient increases after sciatic nerve section. Interestingly, the ipsilateral/contralateral ratio of μ-opioid binding sites was significantly decreased only at 2 weeks after nerve injury (Besse et al. 1992).

Similar trends have been observed with regard to spinal δ-opioid binding sites. These results demonstrate that it is important to consider the type and extent of nerve injury result in complex and unpredictable changes in spinal opioid binding sites. Recent studies (Mayfield and Porreca, unpublished observations) demonstrate that 3 weeks after ligation of the L5 and L6 nerve roots the number of binding sites (B_{max}) or affinity (K_D) for [³H]DAMGO observed in dorsal quadrants of the lumbar cord from sham-operated and nerve-ligated rats were not significantly different; there were no differences either between the sections ipsilateral and contralateral to the ligation nor between the ligated and sham-operated groups. Immunohistochemical studies also suggest, however, the possibility of a loss of opioid μ receptors in the superficial lamina of the spinal dorsal horn which is highly restricted in its rostrocaudal distribution after nerve ligation injury (Elde, Reidl, and Porreca, unpublished observations). The results of these studies strongly suggest that nerve ligation injury, while producing allodynia, does not significantly change μ-opioid receptor content of the spinal cord, either ipsi- or contralaterally to the nerve ligation injury, and therefore the loss of opioid μ receptors is an unlikely explanation for the loss of intrathecal μ-opioid antiallodynic and antinociceptive activity after nerve injury.

3. Change in Relevant Receptors/Afferent Fibers

As noted above, an important component in the spinal action of morphine is mediated in large part through μ-opioid receptors residing on small-diameter afferent fibers (Lombard and Besson 1989). However, it is entirely possible that tactile allodynia is not transmitted by C fiber nociceptors but by low-threshold mechanoreceptors. Neuroanatomical studies have provided ample evidence that after peripheral nerve injury, large-diameter, low-threshold, myelinated primary afferent (e.g., Aβ) fibers form novel anomalous synapses with the ascending nociceptive neurons in the superficial lamina of the spinal dorsal horn following transection of the nerve (e.g., see Woolf and Doubell 1994). Similar anomalous connections may also occur after the L5/L6 nerve ligation procedure (Lekan et al. 1995). Through these connections are normally innocuous, input transmitted by low-threshold mechanoreceptors may be conveyed to projection neurons coding for nociception, perhaps producing the sensation interpreted as allodynia. Evidence for the existence of opioid receptors on the central terminals of large-diameter myelinated neurons is not strong. Mansour and colleagues (1994, 1995) have described a differential distribution of mRNA for opioid receptors in cells of the DRG.

Expression of mRNA for the μ-opioid receptor has been found in medium- and large-diameter DRG cells, that for the δ receptor predominantly in large-diameter neurons and that for the κ receptor in smaller diameter neurons. However, other than noting neuronal diameter, these DRG cells have not been fully characterized. Additionally, cell diameter of medium-sized neurons is a poor predictor of conduction velocity (Taddese et al. 1995); therefore it is difficult to characterize mRNA expressed in such cells as occurring in myelinated or unmyelinated neurons. Opioid receptor binding distributions are predominant in the DRG and the superficial layers of the dorsal horn (Mansour et al. 1995), corresponding with terminals of C fibers rather than the terminal region of larger diameter fibers (e.g., laminae 3 and 4). Finally, Taddese and colleagues (1995), using patch-clamp techniques on isolated nociceptors, found that activation of μ-opioid receptors predictably inhibited Ca^{2+} channels of small-diameter nociceptors and not of large-diameter cells, and suggest that μ-receptor activation selectively inhibits the activity of C fibers.

Based on these observations and the hypothesis that tactile allodynia is not transmitted through C fibers, the remaining opioid receptor population that may be relevant to attenuation of transmission of allodynia is that existing "postsynaptic" to the afferent neurons or on cell bodies of projection neurons. This population may represent only 30%–40% of the total spinal μ- and δ-opioid receptor population (see above). Evaluation of the actions of spinal opiates to block tactile allodynia would in this case be similar to the situation in which the receptor reserve has been greatly decreased by a pharmacological manipulation, such as treatment with an irreversible antagonist (e.g., β-funaltrexamine for μ-opioid receptors). Such a manipulation would be expected to displace the agonist dose-effect curve to the right, and for an agonist of limited efficacy, produce a decrease in the maximal response, a pattern typical of partial, irreversible blockade of a fraction of the relevant receptor population. This is precisely the pattern seen for spinal μ-opioids and suppression of tactile allodynia in nerve-injured rats. For morphine, an agonist with

limited efficacy, the dose-effect curve is displaced to the right such that virtually no agonist effect is elicited (YAKSH et al. 1995; NICHOLS et al. 1995). On the
other hand, a high-efficacy μ-opioid agonist such as DAMGO should elicit a
significant antiallodynic action following spinal administration, although with
somewhat reduced potency, a prediction which is supported by the experimental data (NICHOLS et al. 1995).

4. Loss of Spinal/Supraspinal Morphine Synergy

A number of studies have clearly demonstrated that there is a significant
antinociceptive synergistic interaction between supraspinal and spinal sites, as
shown by coadministration of opiates such as morphine by the intrathecal and
intracerebroventricular routes. A 1:1 fixed ratio of morphine administered
intrathecally and intracerebroventricularly produced an approximately 30-
fold increase in potency compared to intracerebroventricular morphine alone
when evaluated in the tail-flick test (YEUNG and RUDY 1980). Isobolographic
analyses clearly demonstrate multiplicative interactions between intrathecal
and intracerebroventricular morphine in mice (ROERIG et al. 1991; SUH et al.
1995) and in rats (MIYAMOTO et al. 1991). Likewise, the μ-selective opioid
agonist DAMGO also demonstrates a synergistic antinociceptive effect when
given spinally and supraspinally (ROERIG and FUJIMOTO 1989).

The finding of reasonable antiallodynic actions of systemic and
supraspinal morphine (BIAN et al. 1995) was puzzling in that the clinical
perception of morphine activity in neuropathic pain states was one of poor
activity. For this reason we hypothesized that the normally present spinal/
supraspinal synergy known to exist with μ-opiates, such as morphine, is lost or
substantially diminished in neuropathic pain states. In order to test this hypothesis dose-response curves for intracerebroventricular morphine and a 1:1
fixed ratio of intrathecal to intracerebroventricular morphine were constructed using tactile allodynia as the pharmacological endpoint. Isobolographic analysis of this interaction using the procedure described by PORRECA
and colleagues (1990) for the instance where one compound is inactive determined the observed potency ratio of 2.3 to be an additive rather than a
synergistic interaction. The potency ratio determined in this situation contrasts sharply with the robust synergistic antinociceptive effect of morphine
(i.e., approximately 30-fold potency increase) shown by YEUNG and RUDY
(1980) in the rat tail-flick test. These data suggest that opiates such as morphine should theoretically be effective in suppressing allodynia, although at
much higher than normally analgesic doses. Without the expected synergy
which occurs in acute pain settings, however, morphine would not achieve the
necessary potency to make it a clinically comfortable choice as a useful analgesic drug. For this reason our study, demonstrating an additive rather than a
synergistic spinal/supraspinal interaction for suppression of tactile allodynia in
nerve-ligated animals, implies that the loss of synergy underlies the clinically
perceived "resistance of neuropathic pain to opiates."

A possible mechanism underlying this observed loss of spinal/supraspinal synergy may occur at the supraspinal level. Facilitatory ("ON") and inhibitory ('OFF') cells of the rostral ventromedial medulla promote and inhibit nocifensive responses to acute nociceptive stimuli. These neurons are differentially affected by morphine administered either systemically or into the periaqueductal gray, with the inhibitory OFF cells being disinhibited and the facilitatory ON cells being inhibited (CHENG et al. 1986; HEINRICHER et al. 1994). Interestingly, it has also been found that intrathecal morphine produced similar effects on these neurons in the rostral ventromedial medulla (HEINRICHER and DRASNER 1991). It was suggested that these changes in ON and OFF cell activity mediated by morphine given either spinally or supraspinally underlie the observed synergistic action. In light of this suggestion, it is interesting that recent observations show prolonged thermal noxious stimuli to result in increased ON cell activity and decreased OFF cell activity (MORGAN and FIELDS 1994). These observations suggest that supraspinal mechanisms contribute to enhanced sensitivity to tonic nociceptive input. It is plausible to speculate that these alterations in neuronal activity in the rostral ventromedial medulla consequent to prolonged nociceptive input lead to decreased sensitivity of the ON and OFF neurons to morphine and perhaps result in a loss of the spinal/supraspinal synergistic interaction.

5. Afferent Drive

It is known that injury in peripheral nerves is associated with the development of ectopic foci resulting in repetitive afferent input to the spinal dorsal horn which may underlie the maintained state of central hyperexcitability (DEVOR et al. 1990). On this basis, attenuation of the presumed constant afferent input which may be associated with peripheral nerve injury may underlie the sustained allodynia and possibly affect the observed potency and efficacy of spinal opioids to block allodynia or acute nociception. This hypothesis was tested by attempting to block the presumed sustained afferent drive by local application of an anesthetic agent at the site of the nerve injury by a previously placed cannula (OSSIPOV et al. 1995c). Application of bupivacaine at the site of the injury produced a complete block of afferent information as demonstrated by a failure to respond to von Frey stimulation. Additionally, however, following application of local bupivacaine, the intrathecal dose-effect curve for morphine inhibition of the tail-flick response in the nerve-injured animals was displaced to the left, achieving a maximal response. The data show that the antinociceptive potency and efficacy of intrathecal morphine is restored by application of a local anesthetic at the site of the injury, suggesting the importance of afferent drive in limiting the activity of potential pain-relieving drugs in pathological states (OSSIPOV et al. 1995c). The presumed afferent drive resulting from nerve injury may involve excitatory amino acid transmission. This possibility was tested by intrathecal administration of MK-801. As noted, pretreatment with intrathecal MK-801 at nonbehaviorally toxic doses did not directly block allodynia associated with nerve-ligation injury. However, as with blockade of the injury site with local bupivacaine, intrathecal pretreatment with MK-801 resulted in a full antiallodynic and antinociceptive efficacy of intrathecal morphine in nerve-injured rats (Ossipov et al. 1995c).

6. Upregulation of Endogenous Antiopioid Substances

Endogenous CCK has been demonstrated to exhibit antiopioid effects particularly in the spinal cord (Faris et al. 1983; Kellstein et al. 1991; Watkins et al. 1985a,b). CCK attenuates morphine antinociception in several assays whereas CCK antagonists potentiate morphine-induced antinociception in vivo and electrophysiologically (Baber et al. 1989; Stanfa and Dickenson 1993; Stanfa et al. 1994). As noted above, it has been suggested that the antiopioid effects of CCK are due to a reduction in enkephalin availability, through either increased metabolism or decreased release (Ossipov et al. 1994; Vanderah et al. 1994, 1996a; see Sect. B).

There is compelling evidence that neuropathy results in increased spinal CCK levels (Stanfa et al. 1994). In situ hybridization studies have demonstrated increased CCK mRNA levels in the rat dorsal root ganglia or monkey dorsal horn after nerve transection (Verge et al. 1993), further suggesting a role for CCK in augmenting sensory input subsequent to nerve damage. Sciatic nerve section has been found to produce autotomy, along with an upregulation of CCK mRNA in the rat dorsal root ganglia (Xu et al. 1993). Neither morphine nor CI 988, a CCK_B antagonist, given intrathecally alone had any significant effect on autotomy. However, the coadministration of these substances did produce a significant reduction in autotomy scores in rats after sciatic nerve section, further demonstrating that CCK affects responsiveness to morphine in a neuropathic pain model (Xu et al. 1993). Administration of the CCK_B antagonist alone did not block nerve-injury induced allodynia. A recent study found that although intrathecal morphine does not modify tactile allodynia in rats with ligation injury of the L5 and L6 nerve roots, the coadministration of intrathecal morphine and L365260, a CCK_B antagonist produces a significant antiallodynic action (Nichols et al. 1995). Interestingly, this enhancement of the effect of morphine is blocked by NTI, again suggesting that CCK functions to inhibit the availability of an endogenous δ-opioid agonist, perhaps such as [Leu⁵]enkephalin, as suggested by studies with acute nociceptive stimuli. In support of this hypothesis, it has also been demonstrated that an inactive dose of the δ-opioid agonist [D-Ala², Glu⁴]deltorphin also produces an NTI-sensitive enhancement of intrathecal morphine (Nichols et al. 1995). Interestingly, while the CCK antagonist alone does not elicit an antiallodynic action, coadministration of the CCK antagonist with thiorphan elicits a significant antiallodynic action, which is readily antagonized by NTI or by antisera to [Leu⁵]enkephalin (Nichols and Porreca, unpublished observations). Thus CCK_B receptor blockade may enhance endogenous enkephalin actions resulting in enhancement of morphine efficacy through a μ-δ receptor interaction. It appears that the upregulation of anti-μ substances (notably CCK) act to limit observed efficacy of morphine, and that antagonists at CCK receptors may be useful adjuncts for the treatment of neuropathic pain.

Exploration of the possible role of endogenous spinal CCK in the nerve-injured animal was extended to include modulation of the activity of morphine against an acute nociceptive stimulus. If nerve ligation injury produced elevated spinal CCK levels, blockade of the CCK_B receptor should also enhance morphine potency and efficacy in the tail-flick test. It was found that L365260 given intrathecally, although inactive alone, significantly increased the antinociceptive effect of intrathecal morphine in the warm water (55°C) tail-flick assay in a naltrindole-sensitive fashion. These data further strengthen the suggestion that the reduced antinociceptive potency and efficacy observed in the nerve-injured animal is influenced at least in part by changes in spinal CCK activity. Clearly the outcome of proposed analgesic therapy in cases of neuropathic pain is markedly affected by the multiple changes that occur in such states, including the upregulation of substances such as CCK.

IV. Pathological Role of Dynorphin

1. Allodynic Effects of Exogenous Administration of a Single Intrathecal Injection of Dynorphin or Its des-Tyr Fragments: Blockade by MK-801 and Not Naloxone

The involvement of endogenous dynorphin in the development of some neuropathologies is suggested by observations that intrathecal administration of dynorphin produces neurological dysfunctions in rats (LONG et al. 1988). It has also been demonstrated that spinal dynorphin levels are increased after spinal nerve injury, and that the intrathecal administration of antibodies to dynorphin reduces neurological impairment after such injuries (COX et al. 1985; FADEN 1990). Depletion of neuronal cell bodies appears to be correlated with the degree of behavioral deficit and dose of dynorphin (LONG et al. 1988). It is therefore reasonable to speculate that subparalytic doses of intrathecal dynorphin produce sufficient spinal neuronal necrosis to induce a hyperesthetic condition.

Dynorphin may interact with NMDA receptors (MASSARDIER and HUNT 1989) and produce 'nonopioid' effects, including neurological deficits, motor dysfunctions, and flaccid hindlimb paralysis (WALKER et al. 1982). Dynorphin fragments that do not bind to opioid receptors [e.g., dynorphin A(2-17), dynorphin A(2-13), and dynorphin A(3-13); Lai and Porreca, unpublished observations] also produce hindlimb paralysis through nonopioid mechanisms (STEVENS and YAKSH 1986; FADEN and JACOBS 1984). It has also been suggested that dynorphin facilitates C fiber evoked reflexes (KNOX and DICKENSON

1987). Both the paralytic and nociceptive effects of dynorphin are inhibited by NMDA antagonists (Caudle and Isaac 1988; Shukla and Lemaire 1994). Since spinal dynorphin levels are elevated after peripheral nerve injury, and since dynorphin or its fragments may act via NMDA receptors, endogenous dynorphins may perhaps play an important role in the etiology of neuropathic pain states. The possible involvement of dynorphins in the development of dysesthesias resulting from nerve injury may be related to the fact that excitation of the NMDA receptor complex is clearly a significant factor in the development of central hypersensitivity due to tonic afferent input. Therefore the effect of nonparalytic doses of dynorphin A(1-17) on the development of allodynias in the rat was explored and related to NMDA- or opioid-receptor mediated effects.

It has recently been demonstrated that a single intrathecal injection of a subparalytic dose (15 nmol) of dynorphin A(1-17) in rats produces a significant tactile allodynia, determined by probing with von Frey filaments, by the second day after administration and lasting for at least 60 days (Vanderah et al. 1996b). Similarly, intrathecal treatment with dynorphin A(1-13), dynorphin A(2-17), or dynorphin A(2-13) also produce a significant reduction in paw withdrawal threshold by the second day after administration (Vanderah et al. 1996b). No adverse behavioral effects, such as flaccid paralysis and loss of locomotor activity, were observed in these studies. Intrathecal pretreatment with MK-801 prevents dynorphin A(1-17) induced development of allodynia, whereas intrathecal administration of MK-801 alone has no effect on responses to tactile stimuli. In contrast, intrathecal pretreatment with doses of naloxone sufficient to block opioid receptors does not affect the dynorphin A(1-17) induced development of tactile allodynia in rats. These results demonstrate that a single dose of dynorphin A, or its des-Tyr fragments, produces long-lasting allodynia which may be irreversible in the rat. Further, this effect appears to be mediated through activation of NMDA, rather than opioid, receptors. This conclusion is supported by the observations made with MK-801 and naloxone, and the fact that the des-Tyr dynorphin fragments, which do not possess opioid activity, also produced tactile allodynia.

While the precise mechanisms underlying the development and maintenance of the allodynia is unclear, it seems possible that dynorphin produces a degree of spinal neuronal degeneration which contributes to the development of signs reminiscent of a "neuropathic" state. The neuronal degeneration resulting from dynorphin administration may involve among other possibilities: (a) damage to intrinsic spinal nerves induced by localized ischemia and reperfusion injury (Schmelzer et al. 1989), (b) release of excitatory amino acids which may lead to central sensitization and excitotoxicity (Skilling et al. 1992), and (c) direct agonist activity of dynorphin on NMDA receptors, causing spinal neuronal hyperexcitability (Massardier and Hunt 1989). Given that levels of dynorphin are elevated following nerve injury, it seems reasonable to speculate that dynorphin has a pathologically relevant role in neuropathic pain states.

2. Antisera to (Intrathecal) Dynorphin Restores the Antiallodynic and Enhances the Antinociceptive Efficacy of Intrathecal Morphine

Peripheral nerve injury is known to increase spinal dynorphin content. Additionally, spinal trauma to the spinal cord also results in elevated dynorphin levels, and dynorphins given exogenously produce signs that mimic neuropathology, including hindlimb flaccidity and paralysis, urinary bladder atonia and urinary incontinence (see Sect. D.II). Interestingly, the intrathecal administration of antisera to dynorphin has been shown to diminish the behavioral sequelae of spinal cord trauma, suggesting a role of this endogenous peptide in the development of spinal neurological dysfunctions (SHUKLA and LEMAIRE 1994; FADEN 1990). Based on the hypothesis that pathological levels of dynorphin interact with the NMDA receptor complex (MASSARDIER and HUNT 1989) and the observation that intrathecal MK-801 restores the antinociceptive efficacy of morphine in animals with nerve injury (OSSIPOV et al. 1995c), it has been proposed that elevated spinal dynorphin contributes to maintenance or initiation of some aspects of nerve-injury related pain. Recent observations have shown that the intrathecal administration of antisera to dynorphin A(1-17), as with MK-801, does not block allodynia associated with nerve injury. As MK-801, however, intrathecal pretreatment with antisera to dynorphin A(1-17) results in a highly significant antiallodynic action of intrathecal morphine in the nerve-injured rat (NICHOLS et al. 1997). Interestingly, intrathecal infusion of antisense ODN to c-*fos* mRNA prevents resistance to the antiallodynic effect of morphine in nerve-injured rats (Malan and Porreca, unpublished observations). Since c-*fos* expression increases dynorphin expression (see above), antisense ODN to c-*fos* mRNA may act to prevent the increase in spinal dynorphin after nerve injury. Additionally, intrathecal administration of antisera to dynorphin also significantly increases the antinociceptive efficacy of intrathecal morphine in the 55°C warm-water tail-flick test in nerve-ligated but not in sham-operated rats (NICHOLS et al. 1997). These data suggest that the reduced antinociceptive efficacy and lack of antiallodynic efficacy of intrathecal morphine are due in part to the activity of pathological levels of spinal dynorphin in the nerve-ligated rat. The data suggest that activation of the NMDA receptor complex either by sustained afferent drive involving excitatory amino acids, or perhaps sustained activity of elevated levels of endogenous dynorphin, or both, is critical in determining the outcome of proposed analgesic therapy.

E. Conclusions

The pharmacology of opioids and other endogenous neuromediators involved in pain is complex. In states of acute nociception, endogenous dynorphins and enkephalins may be activated to act as modulators of nociception acting as an "analgesic brake." It is also suggested that CCK attenuates opioid activity by limiting the availability of endogenous enkephalins acting at δ-opioid sites.

Likewise, states of tonic nociception may elicit the production of endogenous dynorphins and enkephalins through activation of immediate-early onset genes, such as the c-*fos* cascade. In conditions of inflammatory pain it appears that CCK activity is diminished, and consequently the effect of exogenously administered opioids such as morphine is increased. At the same time initiation of the c-*fos* cascade may upregulate endogenous opioids, such as dynorphin, which can act through opioid receptors to dampen the intensity of the pain signal. These physiological actions of endogenous transmitters are clearly active under such acute pain states and differ markedly from the actions of the same transmitters under conditions involving chronic pain such as those associated with peripheral nerve injury.

Neuropathic pain involves multiple neuroanatomical and neurochemical alterations. It appears that in states of nerve injury there is an upregulation of CCK and dynorphin, among other substances; such substances may be active to perhaps maintain the pathological state of abnormal sensitivity to sensory stimuli. Further, neuroanatomical changes, such as sprouting of $A\beta$ fibers onto nociceptive projection neurons result in unnatural responses to normally innocuous stimuli. Together such changes and adaptations by a nervous system dealing with pain over a long time scale may be very important in determining the success of any clinical attempt to manage such abnormal pain. Several points are clear from the current data which can influence attempts for the development of rational therapy in such pain states. First, it is clear that the activity of opioids at the spinal level in animals with nerve injury depends upon the nature of the stimulus modality being evaluated. Thus, in animals with nerve-ligation injury, intrathecal morphine is completely ineffective against tactile allodynia but is fully active (although with reduced potency) in suppressing the radiant heat foot-flick response. This observation argues that the involvement of C fibers is a clearly important component of determination of the 'activity' of morphine against "neuropathic pain."

Second, the activity of intrathecal morphine against tactile allodynia in the nerve-injured animal depends on a variety of factors which includes the presence of sustained afferent input as indicated by our experiments with application of bupivacaine at the site of the nerve injury or pretreatment with intrathecal MK-801 (OSSIPOV et al. 1995c).

Third, the activity of intrathecal morphine also depends on the changes in the activity of endogenous transmitters which occur following nerve injury such as dynorphin and CCK, suggesting the possibility of development of adjunctive therapies (e.g., CCK antagonists, or use of high-efficacy μ-opioids). It is important to note that the activity of some of these substances, such as dynorphin, occur through different mechanisms in abnormal pain states (i.e., through NMDA, rather than opioid, receptors) so that the same transmitter may serve in both physiological and pathological roles to either limit or increase the response to sensory stimuli (through different receptor mechanisms), respectively.

Fourth, the proposed resistance of "neuropathic pain" to opioids may be related to a loss or significant decrease in the supraspinal/spinal antiallodynic synergy for morphine which normally occurs against acute pain, and which ultimately makes morphine a clinically useful pain-relieving drug. It is unclear whether such loss of supraspinal/spinal synergy is true for opioids acting at other types of opioid receptors or in other endpoints (e.g., foot-flick). All of these changes serve to limit the efficacy of opioids in the treatment of neuropathic pain and form a part of our understanding of the background state against which rational therapies can be developed.

References

Arner S, Meyerson BA (1988) Lack of analgesic effect on neuropathic and idiopathic forms of pain. Pain 33:11–23

Baber NS, Dourish CT, Hill DR (1989) The role of CCK caerulein and CCK antagonists in nociception. Pain 39:307–328

Bennett GJ, Kajander KC, Sahara Y, Iadorola MJ, Sugimoto T (1989) Neurochemical and anatomical changes in the dorsal horn of rats with an experimental painful peripheral neuropathy. In: Cervero F, Bennett GJ, Headley PM (eds) Processing of sensory information in the superficial dorsal horn of the spinal cord. Plenum, New York, pp 463–471

Besse D, Lombard MC, Zajac JM, Roques BP, Besson JM (1990) Pre- and postsynaptic distribution of μ δ and κ opioid receptors in the superficial layers of the cervical dorsal horn of the rat spinal cord. Brain Res 521:15–22

Besse D, Lombard MC, Perrot S, Besson JM (1992) Regulation of opioid binding sites in the superficial dorsal horn of the rat spinal cord following loose ligation of the sciatic nerve: comparison with sciatic nerve section and lumbar dorsal rhizotomy. Neuroscience 50:921–933

Bian D, Nichols ML, Ossipov MH, Lai J, Porreca F (1995) Characterization of the antiallodynic efficacy of morphine in a model of neuropathic pain in rats. Neuroreport 6:1981–1984

Bourgoin S, LeBars D, Clot AM, Hamon M, Cesselin F (1990) Subcutaneous formalin induces a segmental release of Met-enkephalin-like material from the rat spinal cord. Pain 41:323–329

Bullitt E (1990) Expression of C-fos-like protein as a marker for neuronal activity following noxious stimulation in the rat. J Comp Neurol 296:517–530

Byas-Smith MG, Max MB, Muir J, Kingman A (1995) Transdermal clonidine compared to placebo on painful diabetic neuropathy using a two-stage "enriched enrollment" design. Pain 60:267–274

Caudle RM, Isaac L (1988) A novel interaction between dynorphin(1-13) and N-methyl-D-aspartate. Brain Res 443:329–332

Cheng ZF, Fields HL, Heinricher MM (1986) Morphine microinjected into the periaqueductal gray has differential effects on 3 classes of medullary neurons. Brain Res 375:57–65

Chiasson BJ, Hooper ML, Murohy PR, Robertson HA (1992) Antisense oligonucleotide eliminates in vivo expression of c-fos in mammalian brain. Eur J Pharmacol 227:451–453

Chung K, Kim HJ, Na HS, Park MJ, Chung M (1993) Abnormalities of sympathetic innervation in the area of an injured peripheral nerve in a rat model of neuropathic pain. Neurosci Lett 162:85–88

Coombs DW, Saunders RL, LaChance D, Savage S, Ragnarsson TS, Jensen LE (1985) Intrathecal morphine tolerance: use of intrathecal clonidine DADLE and intraventricular morphine. Anesthesiology 62:358–363

Cox BM, Molineaux CJ, Jacobs TP, Rossenberger JG, Faden AI (1985) Effects of traumatic injury on dynorphin immunoreactivity in spinal cord Neuropeptides 5:571–574

Davies SN, Lodge D (1987) Evidence for involvement of N-methylaspartate receptors in "wind-up" of class 2 neurons in the dorsal horn of the rat. Brain Res 424:402–406

Devor M, Keller CH, Ellisman MH (1990) Spontaneous discharge of afferents in a neuroma reflects original receptor tuning. Brain Res 517:245–250

Dickenson AH, Sullivan AF (1987) Subcutaneous formalin-induced activity of dorsal horn neurones in the rat: differential response to an intrathecal opiate administered pre or post formalin. Pain 30:349–360

Dourish CT, O'Neill MF, Coughlan J, Kitchener SJ, Iversen SD (1990) The selective CCK-B receptor antagonist L-365260 enhances morphine analgesia and prevents morphine tolerance in the rat. Eur J Pharmacol 176:35–44

Dubner R (1991) Neuronal plasticity and pain following peripheral tissue inflammation or nerve injury. In: Bond MR, Charlton JE, Woolf CJ (eds) Proceedings of the 6th World Congress on Pain. Elsevier Science, Amsterdam, pp 263–276

Dubner R, Ruda MA (1992) Activity-dependent neuronal plasticity following tissue injury and inflammation. Trends Neurosci 15:96–103

Dubuisson D, Dennis SG (1977) The formalin test: a quantitative study of the analgesic effects of morphine, meperidine, and brain stem stimulation in rats and cats. Pain 4:161–174

Faden AI (1990) Opioid and nonopioid mechanisms may contribute to dynorphin's pathophysiological actions in spinal cord injury. Ann Neurol 27:67–74

Faden AI, Jacobs TP (1984) Dynorphin-related peptides cause motor dysfunction in the rat through a non-opiate action. Br J Pharmacol 81:271–276

Faris PL, Komisaruk BR, Watkins LR, Mayer DJ (1983) Evidence for the neuropeptide cholecystokinin as an antagonist of opiate analgesia. Science 219:310–312

Ghilardi JR, Allen CJ, Vigna SR, McVey DC, Mantyh PW (1992) Trigeminal and dorsal root ganglion neurons express CCK receptor binding sites in the rat rabbit and monkey: Possible site of opiate-CCK analgesic interactions. J Neurosci 12: 4854–4866

Gillan MG, Kosterlitz HW, Magnan J (1981) Unexpected antagonism in the rat vas deferens by benzomorphans which are agonists in other pharmacological tests. Br J Pharmacol 72:13–15

Gillardon F, Beck H, Uhlmann E, Herdegen T, Sandkuhler J, Peyman A, Zimmermann M (1994) Inhibition of c-Fos protein expression in rat spinal cord by antisense oligodeoxynucleotide superfusion. Eur J Pharmacol 6:880–884

Goldstein RS, Raber P, Govrin-Lippmann R, Devor M (1988) Contrasting time course of catecholamine accumulation and of spontaneous discharge in experimental neuromas in the rat. Neurosci Lett 94:58–63

Hambrook JM, Morgan BA, Rance MJ, Smith CFC (1976) Mode of deactivation of the enkephalins by rat and human plasma and rat brain homogenates. Nature 262:782–783

Han HC, Lee DH, Chung JM (1995) Correlation between pain behaviors and ectopic discharges in a rat neuropathic pain model. Soc Neurosci Abstr 21:896

Heapy CG, Farmer SC, Shaw JS (1991) The inhibitory effects of HOE 140 in the mouse abdominal constriction assays. Br J Pharmacol 101 [Suppl]:455P

Heinricher MM, Drasner K (1991) Lumbar intrathecal morphine alters activity of putative nociceptive modulatory neurons in rostral ventromedial medulla. Brain Res 549:338–341

Heinricher MM, Morgan M, Tortorici V, Fields HL (1994) Disinhibition of off-cells and antinociception producd by an opioid action within the rostral ventromedial medulla. Neurosci 63:279–288

Heyman JS, Vaught JL, Mosberg HI, Haaseth RC, Porreca F (1989a) Modulation of mu-mediated antinociception by delta agonists in the mouse: selective potentiation of morphine and normorphine by [D-Pen^2, D-Pen^5]enkephalin. Eur J Pharmacol 165:1–10

Heyman JS, Jiang Q, Rothman RB, Mosberg HI, Porreca F (1989b) Modulation of mu-mediated antinociception by delta agonists: characterization with antagonists. Eur J Pharmacol 169:43–52

Hill DR, Shaw TM, Woodruff GN (1988) Binding sites for 125I-cholecystokinin in primate spinal cord are of the CCK-A subclass. Neurosci Lett 89:133-139

Hu X-M, Hu JW, Haas DA, Vernon H, Sessle BJ (1993) Opioid involvement in jaw electromyographic (EMG) responses induced by injection of inflammatory irritant into temporomandibular joint (TMJ). Pain [Suppl]:544

Hughes J, Hunter JC, Woodruff GN (1991) Neurochemical actions of CCK underlying the therapeuticpotential of CCK-B antagonists. Neuropeptides 19:85–89

Hunskaar S, Hole K (1987) The formalin test in mice: dissociation between inflammatory and non-inflammatory pain. Pain 30:103–114

Hunt SP, Pini A, Evan G (1987) Induction of c-fos-like protein in spinal cord neurons following sensory stimulation. Nature 328:632–634

Hunter JC, Woodburn VL, Durieux C, Pettersson EKE, Poat JA, Hughes J (1996) C-fos antisense oligodeoxynucleotide increases formalin-induced nociception and regulates preprodynorphin expression. Neuroscience 65:485–492

Jadad AR, Carroll D, Glynn CJ, Moore RA, McQuay HJ (1992) Morphine responsiveness of chronic pain: double blind randomized cross-over study with patient-controlled analgesia. Lancet 339:1367–1371

Kajander KC, Bennett GJ (1992) Onset of a painful peripheral neuropathy in rat: a partial and differential deafferentation and spontaneous discharge in $A\beta$ and $A\delta$ primary afferent neurons. J Neurophysiol 68:734–744

Kayser V, Guilbaud G (1983) The analgesic effects of morphine but not those of the enkephalinase inhibitor thiorphan are enhanced in the arthritic rat Brain Res 267:131–138

Kellstein DE, Price DD, Mayer DJ (1991) Cholecystokinin and its antagonists lorglumide respectively attenuate and facilitate morphine-induced inhibition of C-fiber evoked discharges of dorsal horn nociceptive neurons. Brain Res 540:302–306

Kim SH, Na HS, Sheen K, Chung JM (1993) Effects of sympathectomy on a rat model of peripheral neuropathy. Pain 55:85–92

Knox RJ, Dickenson AH (1987) Effects of selective and non-selective kappa-opioid receptor agonists on cutaneous C-fibre-evoked responses of rat dorsal horn neurones. Brain Res 415:21–29

Kocher L, Anton F, Reeh PW, Handwerker HO (1987) The effect of carageenan-induced inflammation on the sensitivity of unmyelinated skin nociceptors in the rat. Pain 29:363–373

Laird JMA, Bennett GJ (1993) An electrophysiological study of dorsal horn neurons in the spinal cord of rats with an experimental peripheral neuropathy. J Neurophysiol 69:2072–2085

Larson AA, Vaught JL, Takemori AE (1980) The potentiation of spinal analgesia by leucine enkephalin. Eur J Pharmacol 61:381–383

Lavigne GJ, Millington WR, Mueller GP (1992) The CCK-A and CCK-B receptor antagonists devazepide and L365260 enhance morphine antinociception only in non-acclimated rats exposed to a novel environment. Neuropeptides 21:119–129

Lee Y-W, Yaksh TL (1995) Analysis of drug interaction between intrathecal clonidine and MK-801 in peripheral neuropathic pain rat model. Anesthesiology 82:741–748

Lee Y-W, Chaplan SR, Yaksh TL (1995) Systemic and supraspinal but not spinal opiates suppress allodynia in a rat neuropathic pain model. Neurosci Lett 199:111–114

Lekan HA, Carlton SM, Coggeshall RE (1995) Sprouting of B-HRP filled fibers of the L5 spinal nerve following L5 and L6 spinal nerve ligation in the rat. Soc Neurosci Abstr 21:895

Lombard MC, Besson J-M (1989) Attempts to gauge the relative importance of pre- and postsynaptic effects of morphine on the transmission of noxious messages in the dorsal horn of the rat spinal cord. Pain 37:335–345

Long JB, Petras JM, Mobley WC, Holaday JW (1988) Neurological dysfunction after intrathecal injection of dynorphin A(1-13) in the rat II Nonopioid mechanisms mediate loss of motor sensory and autonomic function. J Pharmacol Exp Ther 246:1167–1174

Maldonado R, Derrien M, Noble F, Roques BP (1993) Association of the peptidase inhibitor RB 101 and a CCK-B antagonist strongly enhances antinociceptive responses. Neuroreport 4:947–950

Mansour A, Fox CA, Thompson RC, Akil H, Watson SJ (1994) μ-Opioid receptor mRNA expression in the rat CNS: comparison to μ-receptor binding. Brain Res 643:245–265

Mansour A, Fox CA, Akil H, Watson SJ (1995) Opioid-receptor mRNA expression in the rat CNS: anatomical and functional implications. Trends Neurosci 18:22–29

Mao J, Price DD, Hayes RL, Lu J, Mayer DJ (1992) Differential roles of NMDA and non-NMDA receptor activation in induction and maintenance of thermal hyperalgesia in rats with painful peripheral mononeuropathy. Brain Res 598:271–278

Mao J, Price DD, Mayer DJ (1995a) Experimental mononeuropathy reduces the antinociceptive effects of morphine: implications for common intracellular mechanisms involved in morphine tolerance and neuropathic pain. Pain 61:353–364

Mao J, Price DD, Mayer DJ (1995b) Mechanisms of hyperalgesia and morphine tolerance: a current view of their possible interactions. Pain 62:259–274

Massardier D, Hunt PF (1989) A direct non-opiate interaction of dynorphin-(1-13) with the N-methyl-D-aspartate (NMDA) receptor. Eur J Pharmacol 170:125–126

Max MB, Schafer SC, Culnane M (1988) Association of pain relief with drug side-effects in postherpetic neuralgia: a single dose study of clonidine codeine ibuprofen and placebo. Clin Pharmacol Ther 43:363–371

McLachlan EM, Janig W, Devor M, Michaelis M (1993) Peripheral nerve injury triggers noradrenergic sprouting within dorsal root ganglia. Nature 363:543–546

Millan MJ, Czlonkowski A, Morris B, Stein C, Arendt R, Huber A, Hollt V, Herz A (1988) Inflammation of the hind limb as a model of unilateral, localized pain: influence on multiple opioid systems in the spinal cord of the rat. Pain 35:299–312

Miller L, Shaw JS, Whiting EM (1986) The contribution of intrinsic activity to the action of opioids in vitro. Br J Pharmacol 87:595–601

Miyamoto Y, Morita N, Kitabata Y, Yamanishi T, Kishioka S, Ozaki M, Yamamoto H (1991) Antinociceptive synergism between supraspinal and spinal sites after subcutaneous morphine evidenced by CNS morphine content. Brain Res 552:136–140

Morgan JI, Curran T (1989) Stimulus-transcription coupling in neurons: role of cellular immediate-early genes. Trends Neurosci 12:459–462

Morgan MM, Fields HL (1994) Pronounced changes in the activity of nociceptive modulatory neurons in the rostral ventromedial medulla in response to prolonged thermal noxious stimuli. J Neurophysiol 72:1161–1170

Naranjo JR, Mellstrom B, Achaval M, Sassone-Corsi P (1991) Molecular pathways of pain: Fos/Jun-mediated activation of a noncanonical AP-1 site in the prodynorphin gene. Neuron 6:607–617

Neil A, Kayser V, Gacel G, Besson JM, Guilbaud G (1986) Opioid receptor types and antinociceptive activity in chronic inflammation: both κ- and μ-opiate agonistic effects are enhanced in arthritic rats. Eur J Pharmacol 130:203–208

Nichols ML, Bian D, Ossipov MH, Lai J, Porreca F (1995) Regulation of opioid antiallodynic efficacy by cholecystokinin in a model of neuropathic pain in rats. J Pharmacol Exp Ther 275:1339–1345

Nichols ML, Lopez Y, Bian D, Ossipov MH, Porreca F (1997) Enhancement of the antiallodynic and antinociceptive activity of intrathecal morphine by antisera to dynorphin. Pain 69:317–322

Noble F, Derrien M, Roques BP (1993) Modulation of opioid antinociception by CCK at the supraspinal level: evidence of regulatory mechanisms between CCK and enkephalin systems in the control of pain. Br J Pharmacol 109:1064–1070

Ossipov MH, Suarez LJ, Spaulding TC (1989) Antinociceptive interactions between alpha-2 adrenergic and opiate agonists at the spinal level in rodents. Anesth Analg 68:194–200

Ossipov MH, Kovelowski CJ, Vanderah T, Porreca F (1994) Naltrindole an opioid delta antagonist blocks the enhancement of morphine-antinociception induced by a CCK_B antagonist in the rat. Neurosci Lett 181:9–12

Ossipov MH, Kovelowski CJ, Porreca F (1995a) The increase in morphine antinociceptive potency produced by carrageenan-induced hindpaw inflammation is blocked by NTI a selective δ-opioid antagonist. Neurosci Lett 184:173–176

Ossipov MH, Nichols ML, Bian D, Porreca F (1995b) Inhibition by spinal morphine of the tail-flick response is attenuated in rats with nerve ligation injury. Neurosci Lett 199:83–86

Ossipov MH, Lopez Y, Nichols ML, Bian D, Porreca F (1995c) The loss of antinociceptive efficacy of spinal morphine in rats with nerve ligation injury is prevented by reducing spinal afferent drive. Neurosci Lett 199:87–90

Ossipov MH, Kovelowski CJ, Wheeler-Aceto H, Cowan A, Hunter JC, Lai J, Malan TP, Porreca F (1996) c-fos Antisense increases the nociceptive response to formalin: demonstration of a tonic opioid κ and δ but not μ inhibitory tone. J Pharmacol Exp Ther 227:784–788

Ossipov MH, Lopez Y, Bian D, Nichols ML, Porreca F (1997) Synergistic antinociceptive interactions of morphine and clonidine in rats with nerve-ligation injury. Anesthesiology 86:196–204

Payne R (1986) Neuropathic pain syndromes with special reference to causalgia and reflex sympathetic dystrophy. Clin J Pain 2:59–73

Porreca F, Jiang Q, Tallarida RJ (1990) Modulation of morphine antinociception by peripheral [Leu^5]enkephalin: a synergistic interaction. Eur J Pharmacol 179:463–468

Portenoy RK, Foley KM (1986) Chronic use of opioid analgesics in non-malignant pain: report of 38 cases. Pain 25:171–186

Portenoy RK, Foley KM, Inturrisi CE (1990) The nature of opioid responsiveness and its implications for neuropathic pain: new hypotheses derived from studies of opioid infusions. Pain 43:273–286

Ramarao P, Jablonski HI Jr, Rehder KR, Bhargava HN (1988) Effect of kappa-opioid receptor agonists on morphine analgesia in morphine-naive and morphine-tolerant rats. Eur J Pharmacol 156:239–246

Roberts WJ (1986) A hypothesis on the physiological basis for causalgia and related pains. Pain 24:297–311

Roerig SC, Fujimoto JM (1989) Multiplicative interaction between intrathecally and intracerebroventricularly administered mu opioid agonists but limited interactions between delta and kappa agonists for antinociception in mice. J Pharmacol Exp Ther 249:762–768

Roerig SC, Hoffman RG, Takemori AE, Wilcox GL, Fujimoto JM (1991) Isobolographic analysis of analgesic interactions between intrathecally and intracerebroventricularly administered fentanyl, morphine and D-Ala2-D-Leu5-enkephalin in morphine-tolerant and nontolerant mice. J Pharmacol Exp Ther 257:1091–1099

Rowbotham MC, Reisner-Keller LA, Fields HL (1991) Both intravenous lidocaine and morphine reduce the pain of postherpetic neuralgia. Neurology 41:1024–1028

Schmelzer JD, Zochodne DW, Low PA (1989) Ischemic and reperfusion injury of rat peripheral nerve. Proc Natl Acad Sci USA 86:1639–1642

Seltzer Z, Cohn S, Ginzburg R, Beilin BZ (1991) Modulation of neuropathic pain behavior in rats by spinal disinhibition and NMDA receptor blockade of injury discharge. Pain 45:69–75

Sheldon RJ, Nunan L, Porreca F (1989) Differential modulation by [D-Pen^2 D-Pen^5]enkephalin and dynorphin A-(1-17) of the inhibitory bladder motility effects of selected mu agonists in vivo. J Pharmacol Exp Ther 249:462–469

Shir Y, Cameron LB, Srinivasa NJ, Bourke DL (1993) The safety of intravenous phentolamine administration in patients with neuropathic pain. Anesth Analg 76:1008–1111

Shukla VK, Lemaire S (1994) Non-opioid effects of dynorphins: possible role of the NMDA receptor. Trends Pharmacol Sci 15:420–424

Singh L, Oles RJ, Field MJ, Atwal P, Woodruff GN, Hunter JC (1996) Effect of CCK receptor antagonists on the antinociceptive reinforcing and gut motility properties of morphine. Br J Pharmacol 118:1317–1325

Skilling SR, Sun X, Kurtz HJ, Larson AA (1992) Selective potentiation of NMDA-induced activity and release of excitatory emino acids by dynorphin: possible roles in paralysis and neurotoxicity. Brain Res 575:272–278

Small JR, Scadding JW, Landon DN (1990) A fluorescence study of changes in norad-renergic sympathetic fibres in experimental peripheral nerve neuromas. J Neurol Sci 100:98–107

Smith GD, Harrison SM, Birch PJ (1995) Peri-administration of clonidine or MK801 delays but does not prevent the development of mechanical hyperalgesia in a model of mononeuropathy in the rat. Neurosci Lett 192:33–36

Stanfa LC, Dickenson AH (1993) Cholecystokinin as a factor in the enhanced potency of spinal morphine following carrageenan inflammation. Br J Pharmacol 108:967–973

Stanfa L, Dickenson A, Xu X-J, Weisenfeld-Hallin Z (1994) Cholecystokinin and morphine analgesia: variations on a theme. Trends Pharmacol Sci 15:65–66

Stengaard-Pedersen K, Larsson L-I (1981) Localization and opiate receptor binding of enkephalin CCK and ACTH/β-endorphin in the rat central nervous system. Peptides 2:3–19

Stevens CW, Yaksh TL (1986) Dynorphin A and related peptides administered intrathecally in the rat: a search for putative kappa opiate receptor activity. J Pharmacol Exp Ther 238:833–838

Suberg, SN, Watkins LR (1987) Interaction of cholecystokinin and opioids in pain modulation. Pain Headache 9:247–265

Suh HH, Tseng LF (1990) Differential effects of sulfated cholecystokinin octapeptide and proglumide injected intrathecally on antinociception induced by β-endorphin and morphine administered intracerebroventricularly in mice. Eur J Pharmacol 179:329–338

Suh HW, Song DK, Choi YS, Kim YH (1995) Multiplicative interaction between intrathecally and intracerebroventricularly administered morphine for antinociception in the mouse: involvement of supraspinal NMDA but not non-NMDA receptors. Life Sci 56:PL181–185

Taddese A, Nah S-Y, McCleskey EW (1995) Selective opioid inhibition of small nociceptive neurons. Science 270:1366–1369

Trujillo KA, Akil H (1991) Inhibition of morphine tolerance and dependence by the NMDA receptor antagonist MK-801. Science 251:85–87

Tulunay FC, Jen M, Chang JK, Loh HH, Lee NM (1981) Possible regulatory role of dynorphin on morphine-and beta-endorphin analgesia. J Pharmacol Exp Ther 210:296–298

Vanderah TW, Lai J, Yamamura HI, Porreca F (1994) Antisense oligodeoxyneucleotide to the CCK$_B$ receptor produces naltrindole- and [Leu^5]enkephalin antiserum-sensitive enhancement of morphine antinociception. Neuroreport 5:2601–2605

Vanderah TW, Bernstein RN, Yamamura HI, Hruby VJ, Porreca F (1996) Enhancement of morphine antinociception by a CCK$_B$ antagonist in mice is mediated via opioid delta receptors. J Pharmacol Exp Therap 278:212–219

Vanderah T, Laughlin T, Lashbrook JM, Nichols ML, Wilcox GL, Ossipov MH, Malan, TP Porreca F (1996b) Single intrathecal injections of dynorphin A Or des-tyr-dynorphins produce long-lasting allodynia in rats: blockade by MK-801 but not naloxone. Pain 68:275–281

Vaught JL, Takemori AE (1979) Differential effects of leucine and methionine en-
    kephalin on morphine-induced analgesia acute tolerance and dependence. J
    Pharmacol Exp Ther 208:86–90
Verge VMK, Wiesenfeld-Hallin Z, Hokfelt T (1993) Cholecystokinin in mammalian
    primary sensory neurons and spinal cord: in situ hybridization studies in rat and
    monkey. Eur J Neurosci 5:040–250
Wahlestedt C (1994) Antisense oligonucleotide strategies in neuropharmacology.
    Trends Pharmacol Sci 15:42–46
Walker JM, Moises HC, Coy DH, Baldrighi G, Akil H (1982) Nonopiate effects of
    dynorphin and des-Tyr-dynorphin. Science 218:1136–1138
Watkins LR, Kinschek IB, Mayer DJ (1985a) Potentiation of morphine analgesia by
    the cholecystokinin antagonist proglumide. Brain Res 327:169–180
Watkins LR, Kinschek IB, Kaufman EFS, Miller J, Frenk H, Mayer DJ (1985b)
    Cholecystokinin antagonists selectively potentiate analgesia induced by en-
    dogenous opiates. Brain Res 327:181–190
Wegert S, Ossipov MH, Nichols ML, Bian D, Vanderah TW, Porreca F (1997)
    Hyperalgesia produced by nerve ligation injury is reversed by intrathecal MK-801
    or morphine. Pain (in press)
Wheeler-Aceto H, Cowan A (1993) Naloxone causes apparent antinociception and
    pronociception simultaneously in the rat paw test. Eur J Pharmacol 236:193–199
Wheeler-Aceto H, Porreca F, Cowan A (1990) The rat paw formalin test: comparison
    of noxious agents. Pain 40:229–238
Wiertelak EP, Maier SF, Watkins LR (1992) Cholecystokinin antianalgesia: safety cues
    abolish morphine analgesia. Science 256:830–833
Wiesenfeld-Hallin Z (1984) The effects of intrathecal morphine and naltrexone on
    autotomy in sciatic nerve sectioned rats. Pain 18:267–278
Wiesenfeld-Hallin Z, Xu X-J, Hughes J, Horwell DC, Hokfelt T (1990) PD134308 a
    selective antagonist of cholecystokinin type B receptor enhances the analgesic
    effect of morphine and synergistically interacts with intrathecal galanin to depress
    spinal nociceptive reflexes. Proc Natl Acad Sci USA 87:7105–7109
Wilcox GL (1991) Excitatory neurotransmitters and pain. In: Bond MR, Woolf CJ
    (eds) Proceedings of the 6th World Congress on Pain. Elsevier, Amsterdam, pp
    97–117
Wisden W, Errington ML, Williams S, Dunnett SB, Waters C, Hitchcock D, Evan G,
    Bliss TVP, Hunt SP (1990) Differential expression of immediate early genes in the
    hippocampus and spinal cord. Neuron 4:603–614
Woolf CJ, Doubell TP (1994) The pathophysiology of chronic pain-increased sensitiv-
    ity to low threshold Aβ-fibre inputs. Curr Opin Neurobiol 4:525–534
Woolf CJ, Shortland P, Coggeshall RE (1992) Peripheral nerve injury triggers central
    sprouting of myelinated afferents. Nature 355:75–78
Xu X-J, Puke MJC, Verge VMK, Wiesenfeld-Hallin ZW, Hughes J, Hokfelt T (1993)
    Up-regulation of cholecystokinin in primary sensory neurons is associated with
    morphine insensitivity in experimental neuropathic pain in the rat. Neurosci Lett
    152:129–132
Yaksh TL, Pogrel JW, Lee YW, Chaplan SR (1995) Reversal of nerve ligation-induced
    allodynia by spinal alpha-2 adrenoceptor agonists. J Pharmacol Exp Ther 272:207–
    214
Yeung JC, Rudy TA (1980) Multiplicative interaction between narcotic agonisms
    expressed at spinal and supraspinal sites of antinociceptive action as revealed by
    concurrent intrathecal and intracerebroventricular injections of morphine. J
    Pharmacol Exp Ther 215:633–642
Zhou Y, Sun Y-H, Zhang Z-W, Han J-S (1993) Increased release of immunoreactive
    cholecystokinin octapeptide by morphine and potentiation of μ-opioid analgesia
    by CCK_B receptor antagonist L-365260 in rat spinal cord. Eur J Pharmacol
    234:147–154

Opioid Problems, and Morphine Metabolism and Excretion

H.J. McQuay and R.A. Moore

The fact that most patients do achieve at least some degree of pain relief from opioids is a tribute to the efficacy of the drugs. The choice of drug and the prescription regimens remain largely empirical because there are still large gaps in knowledge of the clinical pharmacology of these drugs. These gaps are a function of the variety of chemical structures among opioids and the fact that they are often used in patients whose renal or hepatic function is compromised. Above all, most of these drugs are potent, and doses and concentrations in body fluids are therefore low. Detailed knowledge requires specific and sensitive analytical methods for measuring both parent drugs and metabolites.

Identification of a toxic metabolite of pethidine and an active metabolite of morphine (the two most commonly used opioids) is important for both physician and patient. It shows the importance of knowledge of both metabolism and excretion for rational prescribing.

This chapter discusses first some of the problem areas in opioid clinical pharmacology and then the metabolic pharmacology of morphine. A previous review (Moore et al. 1987) covered the chemistry, pharmacology of metabolites, analysis, metabolites in body fluids, enzymology and pathophysiology of other drugs in the morphine family, buprenorphine, pethidine, methadone, and fentanyl (Table 1).

A. Clinical Aspects

Opioids are often prescribed on the basis of opinion rather than on the basis of evidence. In part this is because opioid use in chronic non-cancer pain is an orphan area, in part because trial design and conduct are not easy in this patient group (McQuay and Moore 1994), and in part it is historic – many opioids are old drugs, and the registration trials required for new drugs have therefore not been carried out. It is remarkable how little new evidence on oral and intramuscular opioid use has emerged since earlier reviews (McQuay 1989, 1991; Nagle and McQuay 1990). An added complication is that there are many routes by which these drugs can be given. The fact that 'it can be done' very often preempts the more important question of 'should it be done?' Enthusiasts for the new route carry it into practice without adequate comparison of risk and benefit with 'established' routes. Again, these arguments have

Table 1. Metabolism and excretion

Drug	Metabolic paths	Faeces (% of dose)	Urine (% of dose)
Morphine	Glucuronidation Sulphation N-Dealkylation	Trace	90% in 24h of which: 10% morphine 70% glucuronides 10% 3-sulphate 1% normorphine 3% normorphine glucuronide
Codeine	O-Demethylation Glucuronidation	Trace	86% in 24h of which: 5%–10% codeine 60% codeine glucuronide 5%–15% morphine (mainly conjugated) trace normorphine
Heroin	O-deacetylation Glucuronidation	Trace	80% in 24h of which: 5%–7% morphine 90% morphine glucuronides 1% 6-acetylmorphine 0.1% heroin
Buprenorphine	Glucuronidation N-Dealkylation	70% mainly unchanged	2%–13% in 7 days of which mainly: N-dealkylbuprenorphine (and glucuronide), buprenorphine-3-glucuronide
Pethidine	N-demethylation Hydrolysis		70% in 24h of which (plus small amounts of other metabolites): 10% pethidine 10% norpethidine 20% pethidinic acid 16% pethidinic acid glucuronide 8% norpethidinic acid 10% norpethidinic acid glucuronide
Methadone	N-Dealkylation	30%	60% in 24h of which (plus small amounts of other metabolites): 33% methadone 43% EDDP 10% EMDP
Fentanyl	N-Dealkylation Hydroxylation	9%	70% in 4 days of which (plus other metabolites): 5%–25% fentanyl 50%-4-N-(N-proprionylanilino-piperidine)

been well rehearsed (McQuay 1990). Much of the 'new' evidence for spinal or transdermal opioids does not answer the real clinical questions.

I. Effectiveness

Just how effective are opioids in managing chronic pain, whether cancer or non-cancer? The usual claim from audits of the World Health Organisation guidelines for oral opioids in cancer pain is that two-thirds of patients achieve good or moderate pain relief. Why does the pain of the other one-third of patients respond poorly to opioids? The commonest explanation of pain which is poorly responsive is that it is neuropathic in character.

1. Neuropathic Pain

There are two extreme positions on opioid responsiveness or sensitivity. One suggests that opioid sensitivity is a relative phenomenon, and therefore that any pain can be controlled by opioids provided that there is an adequate dose escalation and control of adverse effects (Portenoy et al. 1990). The other extreme insists that some pains are intrinsically insensitive to opioids, and that this insensitivity can be predicted from the clinical characteristics of the pain (Arner and Meyerson 1988). Nociceptive pain is thought to be sensitive to opioids while neuropathic pain is regarded as insensitive. When neuropathic pain shows an analgesic response with opioid, this is often attributed to mood improvement rather than to a direct effect on pain pathways (Kupers et al. 1991).

Both extremes of this controversy are supported by a very small number of controlled trials, each of which has methodological limitations. These studies have used either single doses (Kupers et al. 1991; Tasker et al. 1983), infusions of various opioids (Arner and Meyerson 1988; Portenoy et al. 1990) or measurements of pain without simultaneous assessment of adverse effects (Arner and Meyerson 1988; Kupers et al. 1991; Tasker et al. 1983; Rowbotham et al. 1991). The flaw in studies which use a single (fixed) dose or infusion rate is that they may underestimate responses in patients with previous opioid exposure. These patients may need more opioid to achieve analgesic effect than the opioid naive.

Using patient-controlled analgesia with simultaneous nurse observer measurement of analgesia and adverse effects, we administered two concentrations of morphine in a double-blind randomised cross-over fashion and compared their respective clinical responses (Jadad et al. 1992). The results did not support the assumption that neuropathic pains are always opioid insensitive. Half of the pains judged as neuropathic achieved a good response. Nociceptive pains collectively showed a better analgesic response because all of them achieved a good response in at least one of the sessions. No nociceptive pain had a poor response in this study.

It has been suggested that the analgesic response of neuropathic pains to opioids can be explained by the changes in mood induced by the opioids

(Kupers et al. 1991). When the results of patients with consistent responses were compared, changes in mood reflected changes in pain intensity and relief regardless of the clinical character of the pain, nociceptive or neuropathic. Mood improved when pain intensity decreased or pain relief increased. No patient had a change in mood in the absence of a change in pain intensity or pain relief, and patients with nociceptive pains in fact showed a greater change in mood than those with neuropathic pain. Therefore the theory that relief of neuropathic pains by opioids is due to changes in mood was not supported by our findings.

II. Red Herrings

1. Tolerance

Clinicians argue that tolerance to opioids, if it occurs, is driven by disease rather than by pharmacological tolerance. The first problem is that tolerance is defined by some to mean any increase in dose, whereas others use it in the more technical sense of an increased dose required to produce the same effect.

It is ingenuous to argue that opioid tolerance does not occur in humans – fleeting glimpses have been seen which echo the solid findings of both acute and chronic opioid tolerance in animal models (Colpaert et al. 1980). The classic Houde experiments showed chronic tolerance when patients' analgesic response to a test dose was measured before and after chronic dosing (Houde 1985; Houde et al. 1966). The pragmatic issues are whether the dose escalation required by some patients, but which produces difficult adverse effects, could be avoided (safely) by blocking a tolerance-induced need for dose escalation, or (more simply) by changing opioid or indeed route of administration. The academic question is why some patients do not require dose escalation but continue to maintain good relief on the same dose over many months.

2. Addiction

Clinical pain management has emphasised a difference between the clinical and the laboratory pharmacology of opioids. It is as though there were one opioid pharmacology when the opioid is used to counteract pain and another when it is not.

The respiratory depression which haunts prescribers in acute pain management is seen readily in studies of volunteers who are not in pain. Respiratory depression is minimal in patients with opioid-sensitive pain, given appropriate doses of opioid. The balance between pain and opioid respiratory effects is seen clearly in chronic pain. Patients maintained on oral morphine, with no clinical respiratory depression, and who then receive successful nerve blocks, must have their morphine dose reduced. Failure to reduce the dose results in respiratory depression (Hanks et al. 1981; McQuay 1988). One explanation is that the respiratory centre receives nociceptive input (Arita et al. 1988). Presence of this input counterbalances any respiratory depressant effect of the opioid. Absence of this input, because of the successful nerve block, leaves the respiratory depressant effect of the opioid unopposed. This has been shown beautifully in volunteers (BORGBJERG et al. 1996).

The clinical message is that opioids need to be titrated against pain. Doses higher than necessary for the relief of pain run the risk of respiratory depression. Prophylactic use of opioids, infusion without regard to pain experienced, doses greater than those required for analgesia (as in deliberate intensive therapy unit use to facilitate ventilation of a patient), use for purposes other than analgesia (e.g. sedation), or use in non-nociceptive pain all therefore carry potential risk. Concern about respiratory depression should not inhibit the appropriate use of opioids to provide analgesia when the pain may reasonably be thought to be opioid sensitive. A postoperative patient still complaining of pain when the previous dose can be assumed to have been absorbed needs more drug.

Similarly the drug-seeking behaviour synonymous with street addiction is not found in patients after pain relief with opioids, in childbirth, after operations or after myocardial infarction (PORTER and JICK 1980). Street addicts are not in pain. The political message is that medical use of opioids does not create street addicts. Medical use may indirectly increase availability to those who are already addicts, but restricting medical use hurts patients.

B. Morphine and Metabolites

I. What Are They?

1. Chemistry

To make sense of morphine metabolism the structure-activity relationships must be understood. Alterations to the structure change the pharmacological activity and may have important clinical consequences. The basic principles have been known for some time and were well summarised in a WHO Bulletin published as long ago as 1955 (BRAENDEN et al. 1955).

The most important positions on the morphine molecule, because of their implications for both activity and morphine metabolism, are the phenolic hydroxyl at position 3, the alcoholic hydroxyl at position 6, and at the nitrogen atom (Fig. 1). Both hydroxyl groups can be converted to ethers or esters (e.g. heroin, diacetylmorphine), and these changes alter clinical effect. Changes on the hydroxyl groups are opposite in direction; additions at the phenolic 3-hydroxyl group reduce pharmacological activity considerably, by perhaps more than 90%. By contrast, modification at the alcoholic 6-hydroxyl position results in an activation of the molecule, with the resulting compound being two to four times more potent as an analgesic than morphine after parenteral dosing in standard tests. These rules are not absolute, however, and some substitutions at the 6-hydroxyl (e.g. conjugation with long aliphatic acids) reduce activity because of steric and other considerations. Short-chain fatty

diamorphine　　　　　6-monoacetylmorphine　　　　　morphine

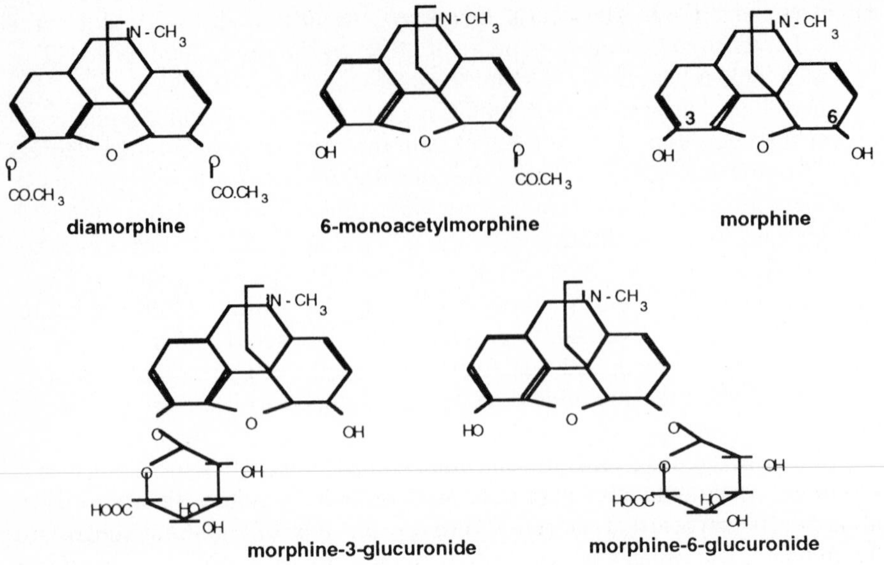

morphine-3-glucuronide　　　　morphine-6-glucuronide

Fig. 1. Structural formulae for morphine, diamorphine and metabolites

acid substitutions (such as 3,6-dibutanoylmorphine) have been used to increase the lipophilicity and potency of morphine (OWEN and NAKATSU 1984; TASKER and NAKATSU 1984).

The tertiary character of the nitrogen atom is crucial for morphine's analgesic activity. Chemical modifications which make the nitrogen quaternary (as with N-oxide) greatly diminish analgesic potency because of reduced penetration into the CNS. Changes to the methyl substituent on the nitrogen are also important; replacement of the methyl group with 3-carbon alkyl groups not only reduces the analgesic action but actually produces compounds which antagonise the actions of morphine, such as nalorphine.

2. Analysis

Studies of morphine kinetics and metabolism require adequate methods of analysis. Results from inadequate analytical methods should be interpreted with caution. The kinetic and dynamic differences demonstrated between different species increase the difficulties. SVENSSON et al. (1982) developed a high-performance chromatographic procedure (HPLC) which measured morphine and its 3- and 6-glucuronides simultaneously. These analyses were facilitated by the high concentrations found in plasma when patients take large oral morphine doses. Similar results have also been described using differential radioimmunoassay (HAND et al. 1987a) in which samples were measured with morphine antisera of different specificities. A specific radioimmunoassay for the determination of morphine-6-glucuronide in human plasma has been reported (CHAPMAN et al. 1995).

II. How Are They Made? Enzymology

Morphine glucuronides are formed by enzyme-catalysed transfer of glucuronic acid from uridine diphosphoglucuronic acid (UDP); the enzymes responsible are microsomal UDP glucuronyl transferases. This is a series of functionally distinct enzymes found in liver, kidney, intestines and other organs. The products of glucuronidation are excreted by the urine and bile. Whether the glucuronide is excreted by urine or bile depends upon the molecular weight and polarity of the conjugate. Compounds with larger molecular weight (higher than 300 Da) and low water solubility are more often excreted in the bile. Morphine glucuronides, being very water soluble, are expected to be excreted in the urine.

1. Liver

It is generally assumed that morphine conjugation occurs primarily in the liver, although the evidence is not compelling. For instance, the Michaelis constant for hepatic glucuronidation in human and animal tissue is in the order of 2 mmol/l (SAWE et al. 1982), which is some tens of thousands of times greater than the usual plasma concentrations of morphine. The implication of this high Michaelis constant is that, at therapeutic concentrations of around 200 nmol/l, the liver microsomal glucuronidation systems would work far too slowly to account for the rates of morphine glucuronidation. As an example of this, rat hepatocytes are able to glucuronidate nalorphine but not morphine, even at high intracellular concentrations (IWAMOTO and KLAASEN 1978).

Different morphine conjugates may arise from the actions of different enzymes. When the natural (−) and the synthesised (+) morphine enantiomers were tested for glucuronidation, the (+) enantiomer was conjugated preferentially at the 6-position of the conjugate rather than the 3-position (RANE et al. 1985). This work serves to emphasise the complexity of morphine metabolism at the sub-cellular (rather than the whole-body) level.

COUGHTRIE et al. (1989) showed that morphine glucuronide formation was influenced by both enantiomer and body "region". In rat liver microsomes natural (−)-morphine formed only the 3-O-glucuronide, whereas the unnatural (+)-morphine formed glucuronides at both the 3-OH and 6-OH positions, with the 6-O-glucuronide being the principal product. In human liver microsomes both the 3-OH-and 6-OH positions were glucuronidated by each of the enantiomers, the 3-O-glucuronide being the major product with (−)-morphine, and the 6-OH position preferred by the (+)-enantiomer. Two UDP-glucuronosyltransferase isoenzymes were responsible for the glucuronidation of morphine in rat liver. Morphine UDP-glucuronosyltransferase produced glucuronides at both the (−)-3-OH and (+)-6-OH positions, the other formed only the (+)-morphine-3-glucuronide (M3G). In human kidney there was glucuronidation ability at the 3-OH but not the 6-OH position (morphine-6-glucuronide, M6G).

Dechelotte et al. (1993) compared morphine uptake and biotransformation to M3G and M6G in isolated cells from guinea pig stomach, intestine, colon and liver. Morphine was glucuronidated to M3G by gastric, intestinal, colonic and liver cells, and to M6G by all except gastric cells. They found that small and large intestine epithelium, such as liver, formed M6G, and that gastric, intestinal and colonic epithelia inactivated morphine to M3G.

Knodell et al. (1982) ligated the inferior vena cava above the entrance to the hepatic veins and reduced the hepatic blood flow to less than 50% of controls; morphine clearance was unaltered, and the conclusion was that there were extrahepatic sites for morphine metabolism. Similar conclusions have been made in humans, in whom the disposition and elimination of indocyanin green and morphine were studied in healthy controls and cirrhotic patients (Patwardhan et al. 1981). There was a significant decrease in indocyanin green clearance but no alteration in morphine kinetics, again with the suggestion of some extrahepatic site of glucuronidation. This is unlikely to be the intestine, as drugs (e.g. morphine) with low lipophilicity are not subject to extensive gut wall glucuronidation (Rance and Shillingford 1977). The inability of the gut to metabolise morphine is supported by in vivo data (Knodell et al. 1982).

2. Kidney

There is unfortunately no clear evidence for an alternative organ of metabolism. Rabbit kidney tubules are able to metabolise morphine to glucuronides at the same sort of concentrations found in plasma in vivo (Schali and Roch-Ramel 1982), and the perfused rat kidney can actively excrete morphine (Ratcliffe et al. 1985). These data, however, do not substantiate the idea of significant renal glucuronidation in man.

Milne et al. (1993) used sheep to study the regional formation and extraction of M3G and M6G. There was significant extraction of morphine by the liver and kidney, net extraction of M3G and M6G by the kidney, and net formation of M3G by the gut. In a subsequent paper (Milne et al. 1995) they infused morphine or M3G into sheep and calculated regional net extraction ratios and total and regional clearances. They found prolonged elimination of M3G formed in situ from morphine compared with after M3G infusion. M3G was not converted back into morphine or M6G.

Mazoit et al. (1990) measured the hepatic extraction ratio of morphine directly in six patients having radiological procedures. The hepatic extraction ratio was 0.65 ± 0.11. No concentration gradient was observed between the artery and the superior mesenteric vein, showing that no gut wall metabolism of morphine occurred. Total body clearance was 38% greater than the hepatic clearance, and they concluded that the extrahepatic extraintestinal clearance of morphine probably occurred through the kidney.

Van Crugten et al. (1991) studied the renal handling of morphine, M3G and M6G in an isolated perfused rat kidney. They found renal handling of morphine to be a complex combination of glomerular filtration, active tubular secretion, and possibly active reabsorption, with the glucuronide metabolites, larger and less lipophilic than morphine, undergoing net tubular reabsorption.

3. Central Nervous System

The ability of M6G to penetrate the blood-brain barrier unchanged was confirmed using radioactively labelled M6G (YOSHIMURA et al. 1973). The analgesic activity of M6G did not appear to be due to hydrolysis of the conjugate in the brain or elsewhere; only conjugated morphine was found in rat brain after intraperitoneal M6G injections (SHIMOMURA et al. 1971). Evidence of transformation of M6G to morphine in brain tissue has been conflicting. WAHLSTROM et al. (1988) showed ability of CNS to metabolise M6G to morphine. SANDOUK et al. (1991) found after intracerebroventricular administration of morphine in four cancer patients that brain is able to metabolise morphine to M3G and M6G.

III. Where Are They Found?

1. Urine Studies

In humans more than 90% of an administered dose of morphine is excreted in the urine. Only about 10% is unchanged morphine, and M3G is the major metabolite (Table 1). M6G was formerly thought to be a minor metabolite, with less than 1% of the dose being in this form in post-addict males on high doses; more recent studies, using plasma samples, suggest that this figure is much too low (HAND et al. 1987a). Using differential radioimmunoassay, the amounts of morphine and 3- and 6-glucuronide found in the urine of patients on oral morphine therapy were in the mean ratio of 1:20:1.5 (Hand, McQuay, Moore, unpublished observations). The diglucuronide (morphine-3,6-diglucuronide) has also been found in urine to a small extent (YEH et al. 1979).

Morphine-3-ethereal sulphate (the major metabolite of morphine in the cat and chicken; MORI et al. 1972) accounts for perhaps 5% of a dose of morphine in humans (YEH et al. 1977). Ethereal sulphates are formed through the action of hepatic microsomal sulphokinases (BOERNER et al. 1975). Morphine-6-sulphate, although sought, has not been identified in any species.

Normorphine and normorphine-6-glucuronide have also been found in human urine (YEH et al. 1977). Normorphine is formed by hepatic microsomal oxidation and can account for about 5% of urinary excretion products of morphine in man (BOERNER et al. 1975).

Minor metabolites of morphine, such as codeine (3-O-methyl morphine) and morphine N-oxide have been identified in the urine of humans taking large doses of morphine chronically (YEH et al. 1977). They account for minor proportions (less than 1%) of an administered dose of morphine in man.

2. Plasma

In plasma only morphine, M3G and M6G have been identified. M6G was not thought to be present until recent years. Studies using HPLC demonstrated appreciable levels of M6G in the plasma of cancer-pain patients on high oral doses of morphine. The M6G levels were higher than those of morphine itself and about 10% of the concentration of M3G (SVENSSON et al. 1982).

One study which encapsulates the plasma data (HASSELSTRÖM and SÄWE 1993) administered single intravenous 5-mg and oral 20-mg doses of morphine to seven healthy volunteers and found that clearance of morphine to form M3G and M6G was 57.3% and 10.4%, respectively, and that renal clearance was 10.9% of total systemic plasma clearance. Twenty percent of a dose remained as unidentified residual clearance. The proportions of the dose found as M6G and M3G were the same by either route. A major finding was a slowly declining phase of morphine and metabolites that was evident both in both plasma and urine. The terminal half-lives were long, morphine 15 ± 16.5h, M3G 11.2 ± 2.7h and M6G 12.9 ± 4.5h. A greater proportion of morphine and metabolites was excreted during the slowly declining phase after the oral dose than the intravenous dose, which they suggested was due to enterohepatic recycling. The renal clearance of M6G and morphine exceeded creatinine clearance, which they attributed to an active secretion process. The time course for the plasma concentrations (measured by using differential radioimmunoassay) of morphine, M3G and M6G after a single oral dose of 10mg morphine is shown in Fig. 2.

3. Central Nervous System

BARJAVEL et al. (1994) used transcortical microdialysis after subcutaneous morphine, M3G and M6G in rats. Maximum brain opioid concentrations were

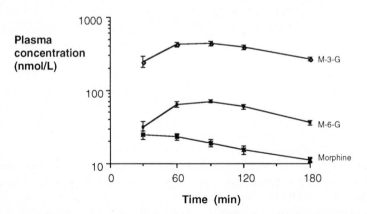

Fig. 2. Plasma concentrations of morphine, morphine-3-glucuronide and morphine-6-glucuronide. Plasma concentrations of morphine, morphine-3-glucuronide and morphine-6-glucuronide after a single oral dose of 10mg morphine sulphate pentahydrate in 12 volunteers (mean ± sem). Redrawn from JONES et al. (1988)

reached at the same time, 0.75 h. Penetration and elimination rates in the extracellular space of the rat brain cortex for the hydrophilic metabolites were similar to those of morphine. They concluded that in spite of their structural differences the glucuronide metabolites are capable of crossing the blood-brain-barrier at the same rate as morphine, but in greater quantity.

STAIN et al. (1995) found that subcutaneous M6G at the same doses as morphine produced a greater degree of analgesia with longer duration of action on behavioural tests. Concentrations of morphine and M6G in brain extracellular fluid were measured using microdialysis. They concluded that M6G is much more potent than morphine in the rat and attributed the difference to the higher levels of M6G in plasma and brain extracellular fluid.

IV. What Do They Do? Pharmacology

The analgesic activity of morphine conjugates remains intriguing despite many years' investigation. Whereas diamorphine (INTURRISI et al. 1984) and M3G do not bind to opioid receptors, 6-monoacetylmorphine, morphine, morphine-6-glucuronide (M6G) and normorphine do (CHRISTENSEN and JORGENSEN 1987).

There is also the prospect of M6G working at a different receptor. ROSSI et al. (1995) used antisense oligodeoxynucleotides directed against distinct Giα subunits of the morphine receptor to distinguish between morphine and M6G analgesia. The insensitivity of M6G towards the MOR-1 antisense probe and differential sensitivity towards G protein α subunit antisense oligodeoxynucleotides led them to believe that M6G acts through a different opioid receptor than morphine.

1. Morphine-3-Glucuronide

M3G has no analgesic activity (SCHULZ and GOLDSTEIN 1972), but it does have CNS stimulatory effects not mediated through opioid receptors (WOOLF 1981; YAKSH et al. 1986; YAKSH and HARTY 1988). Reports of antagonism of morphine analgesia by M3G (SMITH et al. 1990; GONG et al. 1992) are best interpreted as functional because there is good evidence that there is no direct pharmacological antagonism (HEWETT et al. 1993; SUZUKI et al. 1993). This is not surprising given the fact that M3G does not bind to opioid receptors.

2. Morphine-6-Glucuronide

The more recent evidence of M6G action on opioid receptors was anticipated by the observations that it is antagonised by nalorphine and demonstrates cross-tolerance with morphine (SHIMOMURA et al. 1971). M6G, unlike M3G, proved three to four times more potent than morphine as an analgesic after subcutaneous injection in mice and 45 times more potent after intracerebroventricular injection (SHIMOMURA et al. 1971). The difference in the potency ratio was attributed to slower entry of the glucuronide into the CNS compared with morphine (SHIMOMURA et al. 1971), and nalorphine-6-

sulphate had been shown to be a more potent antagonist than nalorphine itself (Oguri 1980). This greater analgesic potency has been confirmed, with 10–20 times greater intrathecal potency of M6G in the rat than morphine (Pasternak et al. 1987; Sullivan et al. 1989).

3. Morphine and Metabolites: Plasma and CSF Ratios

The greater potency of M6G than morphine has important clinical implications (Osborne et al. 1990; McQuay et al. 1990). It has long been known quantitatively to be an important metabolite (Boerner et al. 1975; Shimomura et al. 1971). Many studies have now investigated the ratios of parent to metabolite plasma concentrations (Table 2).

Table 2 and Figs. 3 and 4 show the ratios of metabolites to morphine in plasma after single doses of morphine, and the ratios of CSF:plasma concentrations for the two metabolites. Despite a variety of assays used and disparate study designs, a pattern does emerge. After single oral doses the median M6G:morphine plasma concentration ratio is 5.4 (range 0.96–11, $n = 11$) and that for M3G:morphine 25.0 (range 9.9–56, $n = 11$; Table 4). The corresponding ratios after single intravenous doses are about six times lower at 0.6 (range 0.29–2.0) for M6G:morphine plasma concentration ratio and 6.1 (2.8–11.1) for M3G:morphine (Tables 2, 4). The difference reflects the first-pass metabolism, which applies to the oral route but not the intravenous. The median plasma concentration ratios for multiple oral doses (Tables 3, 4) are 5.1 (1.9–17) for M6G:morphine and 31.4 (22.1–121) for M3G:morphine.

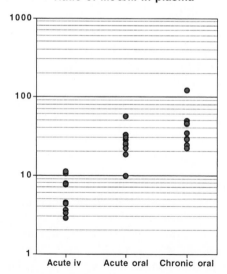

Fig. 3. Ratio of M3G to morphine in plasma for single intravenous and oral doses, and for multiple oral doses

Table 2. Morphine and metabolites in plasma and CSF after single morphine doses

Reference	Patient group	Route	n	Dose (mg)	Time	Origin of ratio	Metabolite: morphine		CSF: plasma	
							M6G	M3G	M6G	M3G
Babul and Darke 1993	Volunteers	Oral	6	10	24h	AUC	2.7	18.3		
		Rectal	6	10	24h	AUC	1.3	9.3		
D'Honneur et al. 1994	Elective surgery, normal renal function	Oral	8	30	4h	Single sample	5.4	22	0.07	0.1
	Elective surgery, impaired renal function	Oral	6	30	4h	Single sample	9.9	25	0.018	0.014
Hasselstrom and Säwe 1993	Volunteers	Oral	7	20	72h	AUC	3.6	29.9		
Hand et al. 1987b	Elective surgery	IV	15	5	72h	AUC	0.7	7.7		
		IM	15	10	95 min	Single sample	0.37	4.3	0.023	0.005
		Oral	11	30 CR	140 min	Single sample	0.96	9.9	0.008	0.004
Hoskin et al. 1989	Volunteers	Oral/buccal	6	10	12h	AUC	11			
		IV	6	5	12h	AUC	2			
Osborne et al. 1990	Volunteers	Oral	10	11.7	12h	AUC	9.7	55.8		
		IV	10	5	12h	AUC	1.4	7.9		
Poulain et al. 1990	Patients	Oral	2	10	12h	AUC	10			
Säwe et al. 1985	Patients	Oral	6	20/25	24h	AUC	2.5	24.4	0.27	
		IV	6	4	24h	AUC		11.1		
Sear et al. 1989a	Anasthetised	IV	5	10	24h	AUC	0.43	3.3		
	Anasthetised renal transplant	IV	9	10	24h	AUC	1.78	10.6		
Sear et al. 1989b	Anasthetised middle aged	IV	10	10	180 min	AUC	0.58	4.5		
	Anasthetised elderly	IV	10	10	180 min	AUC	0.37	3.6		
Sear et al. 1989c	Anasthetised	IV	10	10	180 min	AUC	0.54	4.3		
	Awake	IV	9	10	180 min	AUC	0.29	2.8		
Westerling et al. 1995	Volunteers	IV	14	10	72h	AUC	1.4	7.6		
		Oral	14	30	72h	AUC	6.4	32.4		
		Oral CR	14	30	72h	AUC	5.4	28.1		

IM, Intramuscular; IV, intravenous; CR, controlled release; AUC = area under the curve.

Table 3. Morphine and metabolites in plasma and CSF after multiple morphine doses

Reference	Route	n	Time	Origin of ratio	Metabolite: morphine		CSF:plasma	
					M6G	M3G	M6G	M3G
Bigler et al. 1990	Intrathecal	1	5h	AUC	0.75	4.6	0.8	0.25
Faura et al. 1996	Oral	39	60 min normal, 12 min CR	Single sample	5.8	46		
Goucke et al. 1994	Oral	9	4h after last dose, CR	Single sample	3.8	22.1	0.14	0.16
	Subcutaneous	2						
McQuay et al. 1990	Oral	151	Random	Single sample	5.1	28.4		
Peterson et al. 1990	Oral	21	Trough	Single sample	4	28.8		
	Subcutaneous							
Portenoy et al. 1991b	Oral (2)/IV (1)	3	Random	Single sample	1.9		0.08 (ventric)	
	Oral (3)/IV (5)	8	Random	Single sample			0.12 (lumbar)	
Portenoy et al. 1991a	IV Infusion	8	Random	Single sample	1.2			
Portenoy et al. 1992	3-h IV infusion	14	7h	AUC	0.54			
Poulain et al. 1988	Oral	10	12h	AUC	8.1	45		
Samuelsson et al. 1993	Epidural	14–35	Trough	Single sample	2	8.4	0.33	0.27
Säwe et al. 1983	Oral solution	2	4–6h	AUC	4	34		
Säwe 1986	Oral	15	4h	AUC	2.7	24.2		
Tiseo et al. 1995	Oral	71	Random/trough	Single sample	6.1			
	Parenteral	38	Random/trough	Single sample	2.7			
Wilkinson et al. 1992	Oral	10	12h	AUC	6.2	49		
	Rectal	10	12h	AUC	4.2	29		
Wolff et al. 1995	Oral	34	Trough	Single sample	17	121	0.09	0.14

Blank cells indicate where no information was given or found. Dosing was variable for these patients with chronic cancer pain. Median values were taken where available. CR, Controlled release.

These are similar to those found after single oral doses. This implies that there is little difference in metabolism between the single and multiple dosing contexts. It also means that studies of this phenomenon carried out after either single or multiple doses can with equal validity be extrapolated to the other situation. The M6G:morphine plasma ratios of 3.6 and 5 lead straight back into the argument about how much M6G contributes to the total analgesic effect of a dose of morphine (Table 6; HAND et al. 1987b; McQUAY et al. 1987; OSBORNE et al. 1988).

The crucial observation for morphine in man is whether the active metabolite morphine-6-glucuronide appears in the CNS to interact with opioid receptors and thus produce analgesia. Table 2 shows the CSF:plasma ratios of M6G and M3G after single doses and Table 3 those after multiple doses. Summmarised (Table 5), there is clear evidence that M6G does indeed penetrate into CSF from plasma. There is some hint that M6G penetrates to a

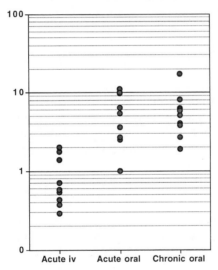

Fig. 4. Ratio of M6G to morphine in plasma for single intravenous and oral doses, and for multiple oral doses

Table 4. Summary of plasma morphine/metabolite ratios

Status	Route	Studies	Morphine-6-glucuronide			Morphine-3-glucuronide		
			Mean	Median	Range	Mean	Median	Range
Single	IV	11	0.9	0.6	0.29–2	6.3	6.1	2.8–11.1
Single	oral	11	6.1	5.4	0.96–11	27.3	25.0	9.9–55.8
Multiple	oral	11	5.9	5.1	1.9–17	43.7	31.4	22.1–121

Table 5. Summary of CSF/plasma ratios of morphine metabolites

Status	Route	Studies	Morphine-6-glucuronide			Morphine-3-glucuronide		
			Mean	Median	Range	Mean	Median	Range
Single	IM	1	0.023			0.005		
Single	Oral	4	0.0915	0.044	0.008–0.27	0.0393	0.014	0.004–0.1
Multiple	Oral	2	0.115		0.09–0.14	0.15		0.14/0.16
Multiple	Epidural	1	0.33			0.27		
Multiple	Intrathecal	1	0.8			0.25		

Table 6. CSF concentrations of morphine and morphine-6-glucuronide

	Morphine	M6G
CSF concentration relative to morphine	1	0.12
CSF potency relative to morphine[a]	1	13
Contribution to analgesia[b]	1	1.56
Percent of total analgesia	39	61

Values for CSF concentrations are from multiple oral dosing (Table 5).
[a] Intrathecal potency relative to morphine for M6G from (SULLIVAN et al. 1989).
[b] The contribution to analgesia is calculated by multiplying the CSF concentration relative to morphine by the relative potencies.

greater extent than M3G, perhaps by a multiple of 2–4. Looking at the difference in CSF:plasma ratios between single and multiple doses, the small amount of data shows higher values for both M6G and M3G in CSF after multiple doses. The values for multiple epidural and intrathecal dosing are, not surprisingly, much higher.

4. Clinical Effects

Given the greater potency the puzzle then is over how much M6G contributes to the total analgesia resulting from a dose of morphine. Simple calculation suggests that M6G contributes substantially (Table 6). If the relative potency of M6G to morphine in the CSF of humans is similar to that after intrathecal injection in rodents, i.e. about 10- to 20-fold greater potency (SULLIVAN et al. 1989), it may be argued that about 60% of the analgesia from multiple doses of morphine may be due to M6G (Table 6).

Against this, several clinical studies have failed to show any relationship between M6G plasma concentrations and analgesia or other opioid effects (SOMOGYI et al. 1993; VAN DONGEN et al. 1994) or indeed between M6G:morphine plasma concentration ratio and effect, although others have been more successful (PORTENOY et al. 1992; FAURA et al. 1996), and some have approached this through modelling techniques (WESTERLING et al. 1995). There are still no adequate randomised double-blind studies of the analgesic and other effects of M6G given on its own.

HANNA et al. (1990) compared the analgesic efficacy of intrathecal M6G 500 µg with morphine 500 µg in a single-blind cross-over study of three patients with chronic cancer pain. The mean requirement for patient-controlled analgesia with pethidine was 393.3(227.4) mg/24 h during the morphine part of the trial and 226.7(113.6) mg/24 h with M6G.

PEAT et al. (1991) studied the respiratory responses to intravenous morphine (0.12 mg/kg), M6G (0.03 mg/kg) and placebo in six volunteers using a single-blind randomised crossover design. Five volunteers also had M6G 0.06 mg/kg. After placebo or M6G (at both doses) there was no change in end-tidal CO_2 whilst the subjects were breathing air. After morphine there was a significant rise. Morphine reduced the ventilatory response to 5.5% CO_2 significantly at all times tested. M6G (at both doses) reduced the response to CO_2 at 20 and 40 min after administration, but to a significantly lower extent than morphine.

THOMPSON et al. (1995) compared analgesia (ischaemic limb) and respiratory function after 10 mg of intravenous morphine or M6G (1, 3.3 and 5 mg) in a double-blind, randomised study of ten volunteers. Morphine produced significant increase in arterial PCO_2 at 45 min, and in transcutaneous PCO_2 from 15 min to 4 h. Blood gas and transcutaneous PCO_2 were unchanged after M6G at all three doses.

OSBORNE et al. (1992) compared the cardiorespiratory and analgesic effects of four different dose levels (0.5, 1, 2, and 4 mg/70 kg) of intravenous M6G in an open study of 20 cancer patients with pain. M6G exerted a 'useful' analgesic effect in 17/19 patients for periods ranging between 2 and 24 h. No correlation was observed between dose or plasma M6G concentrations and duration or degree of analgesia. No clinically significant changes in cardiorespiratory parameters were observed. No patients reported sedation or euphoria. Nausea and vomiting were 'notably absent' in all cases.

These preliminary studies do suggest an analgesic effect of M6G, but the claim that M6G has less respiratory depressant potential than morphine will have to be addressed at equianalgesic dosing, and it is not clear that this has been achieved.

V. Pathophysiology

1. Liver Disease

The traditional view has been that use of morphine in patients with liver disease may result in excessive sedation and precipitate hepatic encephalopathy (LAIDLAW et al. 1961; TWYCROSS and LACK 1983). Two studies of morphine kinetics in patients with cirrhosis (PATWARDHAN et al. 1981; HASSELSTROM et al. 1986) have shown only very minor alterations of morphine kinetics in cirrhotic patients. Subsequent work, however, has shown kinetic change with liver disease. HASSELSTROM et al. (1990) studied oral and intravenous kinetics of morphine in seven cirrhotic patients with a history of encephalopathy. Morphine plasma clearance was significantly lower, its terminal elimination half-life longer and its oral bioavailability greater in the cirrhotic patients than in those with normal liver function. Plasma M3G:morphine ratios were significantly lower in the cirrhotic patients after oral, but not after intravenous, doses. MAZOIT et al. (1987) compared plasma morphine concentrations in six volunteers with those in eight cirrhotic patients. Cirrhotics had significantly longer morphine terminal half-life, attributed to lower total body clearance.

2. Kidney Disease

Morphine clearance is decreased and its analgesic effects increased in elderly patients (KAIKO et al. 1982), who have decreased renal function. In renal failure morphine produced effects and side effects of unexpected degree and duration (MOSTERT et al. 1971; DON et al. 1975; McQUAY and MOORE 1984; REGNARD and TWYCROSS 1984). The evidence suggests that this is because of the accumulation in plasma of morphine glucuronides, especially M6G (SÄWE et al. 1986; OSBORNE et al. 1986; BODD et al. 1990).

D'HONNEUR et al. (1994) compared plasma and CSF concentrations of morphine glucuronides in patients with normal renal function and those with renal failure. Plasma concentrations of glucuronides were significantly higher. CSF concentrations of M6G and M3G continued to rise over at least 24 h. At 24 h CSF M6G concentrations were 15 times greater in patients with renal failure than in those with normal renal function.

HANNA et al. (1993) gave 30 μg/kg M6G to 12 patients with chronic renal failure (dialysis-dependent) and 6 with good renal function after renal transplantation. The M6G elimination half-life was significantly shorter, and the clearance greater, in the transplanted group than in the dialysed and non-dialysed groups.

McQUAY et al. (1990) studied 151 patients with chronic cancer pain during chronic treatment with oral morphine. Dose of morphine, age, sex, renal and hepatic dysfunction, and other drugs accounted for 70% of the variance in plasma concentrations of morphine, M3G and M6G. Plasma creatinine greater than 150 μmol/l was associated with significant increase in M3G and M6G plasma concentrations (Fig. 5).

MILNE et al. (1992) gave morphine by constant intravenous infusion to 15 intensive-care patients with diverse renal function. There were significant linear relationships between measured renal creatinine clearance and the renal clearances of morphine, M3G and M6G.

OSBORNE et al. (1993) compared the pharmacokinetics of morphine and its glucuronide metabolites in three groups of patients with kidney failure (nondialyzed, receiving dialysis, and transplantation) with a group of normal healthy volunteers. Patients with kidney failure had a significantly higher morphine area under the curve than control subjects. There was also an increase in M3G and M6G that was several times greater than the increase in morphine area under the curve. This metabolite accumulation was reversed by kidney transplantation.

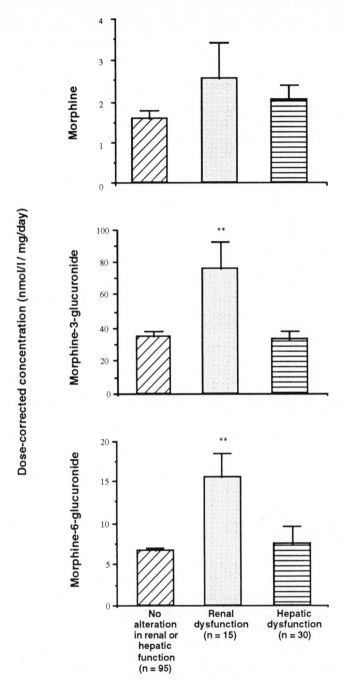

Fig. 5. Dose-corrected plasma concentrations (nmol/l per mg/day) for morphine, M3G and M6G for patients with normal renal and hepatic function ($n = 95$), renal dysfunction ($n = 15$) and hepatic dysfunction ($n = 30$). Redrawn from (McQUAY et al. 1990). Significantly higher plasma concentrations of M3G and M6G in renal dysfunction (** $p < 0.01$, Newman-Keuls test)

Peterson et al. (1990) found in 21 patients on oral or subcutaneous morphine that plasma concentrations of M3G and M6G, when divided by the morphine concentration, were significantly related to the calculated creatinine clearance of the patient.

Sear et al. (1989a) compared the kinetics of 10 mg intravenous morphine in nine patients with end-stage renal failure and five healthy anaesthetised patients. There were no differences between the two groups regarding morphine elimination half-life or clearance. Peak concentrations of M3G and M6G were significantly greater in the renal transplant patients, as were the area under the curve values (0–24h).

Somogyi et al. (1993) studied 11 cancer patients on long-term oral morphine. They detected no relationship between the renal clearance of morphine, M3G and M6G and that of creatinine. Renal tubular handling of all three opioids varied widely between patients, and there was evidence of either net renal tubular secretion or reabsorption.

This renal work highlights the role of the kidney in removing the major morphine metabolites. The evidence suggests that once renal function declines to a creatinine clearance of 50 ml/min or below, the accumulation of morphine metabolites, especially that of M6G (Bodd et al. 1990) becomes significant. Clinical problems should arise only if fixed dose schedules are used with an initial dose level that is too high.

3. Drug Interactions

Earlier reports of interactions between cimetidine and morphine have been rebutted (Mojaverian et al. 1982). Wahlstrom et al. (1994) studied the interactions of tricyclic antidepressants with morphine glucuronidation. All tricylics studied inhibited morphine glucuronidation, nortriptyline in non-competitive and amitriptyline and clomipramine in competitive or mixed manner. Inhibition occurred at a concentration ratio of tricyclic to morphine close to that seen in patients on treatment.

C. Conclusions

Much of the detail of morphine metabolism and excretion is still to be worked out. The clinical implication thus far is that the accumulation of the active metabolite M6G in renal dysfunction may produce both analgesia and unwanted effects. Fixed dose schedules with high initial doses should be avoided if renal problems are suspected. The precise contribution of M6G to the 'total' effect of a dose of morphine remains a puzzle.

References

Arita H, Kogo N, Ichikawa K (1988) Locations of medullary neurons with non-phasic discharges excited by stimulation of central and/or peripheral chemoreceptors and by activation of nociceptors in cat. Brain Res 442:1–10

Arner S, Meyerson BA (1988) Lack of analgesic effect of opioids on neuropathic and idiopathic forms of pain. Pain 33:11–23

Babul N, Darke AC (1993) Disposition of morphine and its glucuronide metabolites after oral and rectal administration: evidence of route specificity. Clin Pharmacol Ther 54:286–92

Barjavel M, Sandouk P, Plotkine M, Scherrmann JM (1994) Morphine and morphine metabolite kinetics in the rat brain as assessed by transcortical microdialysis. Life Sci 55:1301–1308

Bigler D, Christensen CB, Eriksen J, Jensen N-H (1990) Morphine, morphine-6-glucuronide and morphine-3-glucuronide concentrations in plasma and cerebrospinal fluid during long-term high-dose intrathecal morphine administration. Pain 41:15–18

Bodd E, Jacobsen D, Lund E, Ripel A, Mørland J, Wiik-Larsen E (1990) Morphine-6-glucuronide might mediate the prolonged opioid effect of morphine in acute renal failure. Hum Exp Toxicol 9:317–321

Boerner U, Abbott S, Roe RL (1975) The metabolism of morphine and heroin in man. Drug Metab Rev 4:39–73

Borgbjerg FM, Nielsen K, Franks J (1996) Experimental pain stimulates respiration and attenuates morphine induced respiratory depression. A controlled study in human volunteers. Pain 64:123

Braenden OJ, Eddy NB, Halbach H (1955) Synthetic substances with morphine-like effect. Bull World Health Organ 13:937–998

Chapman DJ, Cross MJ, Joel SP, Aherne GW (1995) A specific radioimmunoassay for the determination of morphine-6-glucuronide in human plasma. Ann Clin Biochem 32:297–302

Christensen CB, Jorgensen LN (1987) Morphine-6-glucuronide has high affinity for the opioid receptor. Pharmacol Toxicol 60:75–76

Colpaert FC, Niemegeers CJE, Janssen PAJ, Maroli AN (1980) The effects of prior fentanyl administration and of pain on fentanyl analgesia: tolerance to and enhancement of narcotic analgesia. J Pharmacol Exp Ther 213:418–426

Coughtrie MWH, Ask B, Rane A, Burchell B, Hume R (1989) The enantioselective glucuronidation of morphine in rats and humans. Biochem Pharmacol 38:3273–3280

Dechelotte P, Sabouraud A, Sandouk P, Hackbarth I, Schwenk M (1993) Uptake, 3-, and 6-glucuronidation of morphine in isolated cells from stomach, intestine, colon, and liver of the guinea pig. Drug Metab Dispos 21:13–17

D'Honneur G, Gilton A, Sandouk P, Scherrmann JM, Duvaldestin P (1994) Plasma and cerebrospinal fluid concentrations of morphine and morphine glucuronides after oral morphine. The influence of renal failure. Anesthesiology 81:87–93

Don HF, Dieppa RA, Taylor P (1975) Narcotic analgesics in anuric patients. Anesthesiology 42:745–747

Faura CC, Moore RA, Horga JF, Hand CW, McQuay HJ (1996) Morphine and morphine-6-glucuronide plasma concentrations and effect in cancer pain. J Pain Sympt Manage 11:95–102

Gong Q-L, Hedner T, Hedner J, Björkman R, Hedner T (1992) Morphine-3-glucuronide may functionally antagonise morphine-6-glucuronide induced antinociception and ventilatory depression in the rat. Pain 48:249–255

Goucke CR, Hackett LP, Ilett KF (1994) Concentrations of morphine, morphine-6-glucuronide and morphine-3-glucuronide in serum and cerebrospinal fluid following morphine administration to patients with morphine-resistant pain. Pain 56:145–149

Hand CW, Moore RA, McQuay HJ, Allen MC, Sear JW (1987a) Analysis of morphine and its major metabolites by differential radioimmunoassay. Ann Clin Biochem 24:153–60

Hand CW, Blunnie WP, Claffey LP, McShane AJ, McQuay HJ, Moore RA (1987b) Potential analgesic contribution from morphine-6-glucuronide in CSF (letter). Lancet 2:1207–1208

Hanks GW, Twycross RG, Lloyd JW (1981) Unexpected complication of successful nerve block. Anaesthesia 36:37–39

Hanna MH, Peat SJ, Woodham M, Knibb A, Fung C (1990) Analgesic efficacy and csf pharmacokinetics of intrathecal morphine-6-glucuronide: comparison with morphine. Br J Anaesth 64:547–550

Hanna MH, D'Costa F, Peat SJ, Fung C, Venkat N, Zilkha TR, Davies S (1993) Morphine-6-glucuronide disposition in renal impairment. Br J Anaesth 70:511–514

Hasselström J, Säwe J (1993) Morphine pharmacokinetics and metabolism in humans. Enterohepatic recycling and relative contribution of metabolites to active opioid concentrations. Clin Pharmacokinet 24:344–354

Hasselstrom J, Eriksson LS, Persson A, Rane A, Svensson JO, Sawe J (1986) Morphine metabolism in patients with liver cirrhosis. Acta Pharmacol Toxicol [Suppl] V:101

Hasselstrom J, Eriksson S, Persson A, Rane A, Svensson JO, Sawe J (1990) The metabolism and bioavailability of morphine in patients with severe liver cirrhosis. Br J Clin Pharmacol 29:289–297

Hewett K, Dickenson AH, McQuay HJ (1993) Lack of effect of morphine-3-glucuronide on the spinal antinociceptive actions of morphine in the rat: an electrophysiological study. Pain 53:59–63

Hoskin PJ, Hanks GW, Aherne GW, Chapman D, Littleton P, Filshie J (1989) The bioavailability and pharmacokinetics of morphine after intravenous, oral and buccal administration in healthy volunteers. Br J Clin Pharmacol 27:499–505

Houde RW (1985) The analgesic connection: the Nathan B. Eddy memorial lecture, vol 55. In: Harris LS (ed) Problems of drug dependence. NIDA Research Monograph, pp 4–13

Houde RW, Wallenstein SL, Beaver WT (1966) Evaluation of analgesics in patients with cancer pain. In: Lasagna L (ed) International encyclopedia of pharmacology and therapeutics. Pergamon, Oxford, pp 59–98

Inturrisi CE, Max M, Umans J, Schultz M, Shin S, Foley KM, Houde R (1984) The pharmacokinetics of heroin in patients with chronic pain. N Engl J Med 310:1213–1217

Iwamoto K, Klaasen CD (1978) Uptake of morphine and nalorphine by isolated rat hepatocytes. J Pharmacol Exp Ther 206:181–189

Jadad AR, Carroll D, Glynn CJ, Moore RA, McQuay HJ (1992) Morphine responsiveness of chronic pain: double-blind randomised crossover study with patient-controlled analgesia. Lancet 339:1367–1371

Jones SF, McQuay HJ, Moore RA, Hand CW (1988) Morphine and ibuprofen compared using the cold pressor test. Pain 34:117–122

Kaiko RF, Wallenstein SL, Rogers AG, Grabinski PY, Houde RW (1982) Narcotics in the elderly. Med Clin North Am 66:1079–1089

Knodell RG, Farleigh RM, Steele NM, Bond JH (1982) Effects of liver congestion on hepatic drug metabolism in the rat. J Pharmacol Exp Ther 221:52–57

Kupers RC, Konings H, Adriaensen H, Gybels JM (1991) Morphine differentially affects the sensory and affective pain ratings in neurogenic and idiopathic forms of pain. Pain 47:5–12

Laidlaw J, Read AE, Sherlock S (1961) Morphine tolerance in hepatic cirrhosis. Gastroenterology 40:389–396

Mazoit JX, Sandouk P, Zetlaoui P, Scherrmann JM (1987) Pharmacokinetics of unchanged morphine in normal and cirrhotic subjects. Anesth Analg 66:293–298

Mazoit JX, Sandouk P, Scherrmann JM, Roche A (1990) Extrahepatic metabolism of morphine occurs in humans. Clin Pharmacol Ther 48:613–618

McQuay HJ (1988) Potential problems of using both opioids and local anaesthetic (letter). Br J Anaesth 61:121

McQuay HJ (1989) Opioids in chronic pain. Br J Anaesth 63:213–226

McQuay HJ (1990) The logic of alternative routes. J Pain Sympt Manage 5:75–77

McQuay HJ (1991) Opioid clinical pharmacology and routes of administration. Br Med Bull 47:703–717

McQuay H, Moore A (1984) Metabolism of narcotics (letter). BMJ 288:237

McQuay H, Moore A (1994) Need for rigorous assessment of palliative care. BMJ 309:1315–1316

McQuay HJ, Moore RA, Hand CW, Sear JW (1987) Potency of oral morphine (letter). Lancet 2:1458–1459

McQuay HJ, Carroll D, Faura CC, Gavaghan DJ, Hand CW, Moore RA (1990) Oral morphine in cancer pain: influences on morphine and metabolite concentration. Clin Pharmacol Ther 48:236–244

Milne RW, Nation RL, Somogyi AA, Bochner F, Griggs WM (1992) The influence of renal function on the renal clearance of morphine and its glucuronide metabolites in intensive-care patients. Br J Clin Pharmacol 34:53–59

Milne RW, Sloan PA, McLean CF, Mather LE, Nation RL, Runciman WB, Rutten AJ, Somogyi AA (1993) Disposition of morphine and its 3- and 6-glucuronide metabolites during morphine infusion in the sheep. Drug Metab Dispos 21:1151–1156

Milne RW, McLean CF, Mather LE, Nation RL, Runciman WB, Rutten AJ, Somogyi AA (1995) Comparative disposition of morphine-3-glucuronide during separate intravenous infusions of morphine and morphine-3-glucuronide in sheep. Importance of the kidney. Drug Metab Dispos 23:334–342

Mojaverian P, Fedder IL, Vlasses PH, Rotmensch HH, Rocci ML, Swanson BN, Ferguson RK (1982) Cimetidine does not alter morphine disposition in man. Br J Clin Pharmacol 14:809–813

Moore RA, Hand CW, McQuay HJ (1987) Opioid metabolism and excretion. In: Budd K (ed) Update in opioids. Clinical anaesthesiology. Baillere Tindall, London, pp 829–858

Mori M, Oguri K, Yoshimura H, Shimomura K, Kamata O, Ueki S (1972) Chemical synthesis and analgesic effect of morphine ethereal sulfates. Life Sci 11:525–533

Mostert J, Evers JL, Hobika JH, Moore RH, Ambrus JL (1971) Cardiorespiratory effects of anaesthesia with morphine or fentanyl in chronic renal failure and cerebral toxicity after morphine. Br J Anaesth 43:1053–1060

Nagle CJ, McQuay HJ (1990) Opiate receptors; their role in effect and side-effect. Curr Anaesth Crit Care 1:247–252

Oguri K (1980) Conjugated metabolites of morphine and their pharmacological activity. Yakugaku Zasshi 117–25

Osborne R, Joel S, Trew D, Slevin M (1988) Analgesic activity of morphine-6-glucuronide. Lancet 1:828

Osborne R, Joel S, Trew D, Slevin M (1990) Morphine and metabolite behavior after different routes of morphine administration: demonstration of the importance of the active metabolite morphine-6-glucuronide. Clin Pharmacol Ther 47:12–19

Osborne R, Thompson P, Joel S, Trew D, Patel N, Slevin M (1992) The analgesic activity of morphine-6-glucuronide. Br J Clin Pharmacol 34:130–138

Osborne R, Joel S, Grebenik K, Trew D, Slevin M (1993) The pharmacokinetics of morphine and morphine glucuronides in kidney failure. Clin Pharmacol Ther 54:158

Osborne RJ, Joel SP, Slevin ML (1986) Morphine intoxication in renal failure: the role of morphine-6-glucuronide. BMJ 292:1548–1549

Owen JA, Nakatsu K (1984) Morphine diesters. II. Blood metabolism and analgesic activity in the rat. Can J Physiol Pharmacol 62:452–456

Pasternak GW, Bodnar RJ, Clark JA, Inturrisi CE (1987) Morphine-6-glucuronide, a potent mu agonist. Life Sci 41:2845–2849

Patwardhan RV, Johnson RF, Hoyumpa A, Sheehan JJ, Desmond PV, Wilkinson GR, Branch RA, Schenker S (1981) Normal metabolism of morphine in cirrhosis. Gastroenterology 81:1006–1011

Peat SJ, Hanna MH, Woodham M, Knibb AA, Ponte J (1991) Morphine-6-glucuronide effects on ventilation in normal volunteers. Pain 45:101

Peterson GM, Randall CT, Paterson J (1990) Plasma levels of morphine and morphine glucuronides in the treatment of cancer pain: relationship to renal function and route of administration. Eur J Clin Pharmacol 38:121–124

Portenoy RK, Foley KM, Inturrisi CE (1990) The nature of opioid responsiveness and its implications for neuropathic pain: new hypotheses derived from studies of opioid infusions. Pain 43:273–286

Portenoy RK, Foley KM, Stulman J, Khan E, Adelhardt J, Layman M, Cerbone DF, Inturrisi CE (1991a) Plasma morphine and morphine-6-glucuronide during chronic morphine therapy for cancer pain: plasma profiles, steady-state concentrations and the consequences of renal failure. Pain 47:13–19

Portenoy RK, Khan E, Layman M et al (1991b) Chronic morphine therapy for cancer pain: plasma and cerebrospinal fluid morphine and morphine-6-glucuronide concentrations. Neurology 41:1457

Portenoy RK, Thaler HT, Inturrisi CE, Friedlander-Klar H, Foley KM (1992) The metabolite morphine-6-glucuronide contributes to the analgesia produced by morphine infusion in patients with pain and normal renal function. Clin Pharmacol Ther 51:422–431

Porter J, Jick H (1980) Addiction rate in patients treated with narcotics. N Engl J Med 302:123

Poulain P, Hoskin PJ, Hanks GW, A-Omar O, Walker VA, Johnston A et al (1988) Relative bioavailability of controlled release morphine tablets (MST Continus) in cancer patients. Br J Anaesth 61:569–574

Poulain P, Ribon AM, Hanks GW, Hoskin PJ, Aherne GW, Chapman DJ (1990) CSF concentrations of morphine-6-glucuronide after oral administration of morphine. Pain 41:115–116

Rance MJ, Shillingford JS (1977) The metabolism of phenolic opioids by rat intestine. Xenobiotica 7:529–536

Rane A, Gawronska-Szlarz B, Svensson J (1985) Natural (−) and unnatural (+) enantiomers of morphine: comparative metabolism and effect of morphine and phenobarbital treatment. J Pharmacol Exp Ther 234:761–765

Ratcliffe PJ, Sear JW, Hand CW, Moore RA (1985) Morphine transport in the isolated perfused rat kidney. Proc EDTA ERA 22:1109–1114

Regnard CFB, Twycross RG (1984) Metabolism of narcotics. BMJ 288:860–860

Rossi GC, Standifer KM, Pasternak GW (1995) Differential blockade of morphine and morphine-6 beta-glucuronide analgesia by antisense oligodeoxynucleotides directed against MOR-1 and G-protein alpha subunits in rats. Neurosci Lett 198:99–102

Rowbotham MC, Reisner-Keller LA, Fields HL (1991) Both intravenous lidocaine and morphine reduce the pain of postherpetic neurlagia. Neurology 41:1024–1028

Samuelsson H, Hedner T, Venn R, Michalkiewicz A (1993) CSF and plasma concentrations of morphine and morphine glucuronides in cancer patients receiving epidural morphine. Pain 52:179–185

Sandouk P, Serrie A, Scherrmann JM, Langlade A, Bourre JM (1991) Presence of morphine metabolites in human cerebrospinal fluid after intracerebroventricular administration of morphine. Eur J Drug Metab Pharmacokinet 3:166–171

Säwe J (1986) Morphine and its 3- and 6-glucuronides in plasma and urine during chronic oral administration in cancer patients. In: Foley KM, Inturrisi CE (eds) Advances in pain research and therapy, vol 8. Opioid analgesics in the management of clinical pain. Raven, New York, pp 45–55

Säwe J, Pacifici GM, Kager L, von Bahr C, Rane A (1982) Glucuronidation of morphine in human liver and interaction with oxazepam. Acta Anaesthesiol Scand S74:47–51

Säwe J, Dahlstrom B, Rane A, Svensson J-O (1983) Steady state kinetics and analgesic efect of oral morphine in cancer patients. Eur J Clin Pharmacol 24:537–542

Säwe J, Kager L, Svensson J, Rane A (1985) Oral morphine in concer patients: in vivo kinetics and in vitro hepatic glucuronidation. Br J Clin Pharmacol 19:495–501

Säwe J, Odar-Cederlof I, Svensson JO, Arner B (1986) Kinetics of morphine in patients with renal failure. Acta Pharmacol Toxicol [Suppl] V:102

Säwe J, Kager L, Svensson J-O, Rane A (1995) Oral morphine in cancer patients: in vivo kinetics and in vitro hepatic glucuronidation. Br J Clin Pharmacol 19:495–501

Schali C, Roch-Ramel F (1982) Transport and metabolism of (3H)morphine in isolated, nonperfused proximal tubular segments of the rabbit kidney. J Pharmacol Exp Ther 223:811–815

Schulz R, Goldstein A (1972) Inactivity of narcotic glucuronides as analgesics and on guinea-pig ileum. J Pharmacol Exp Ther 183:404–410

Sear JW, Hand CW, Moore RA, McQuay HJ (1989a) Studies on morphine disposition: influence of renal failure on the kinetics of morphine and its metabolites. Br J Anaesth 62:28–32

Sear JW, Hand CW, Moore RA (1989b) Studies on morphine disposition: plasma concentrations of morphine and its metabolites in anesthetized middle-aged and elderly surgical patients. J Clin Anesth 1:164–169

Sear JW, Hand CW, Moore RA, McQuay HJ (1989c) Studies on morphine disposition: influence of general anaesthesia on plasma concentrations of morphine and its metabolites. Br J Anaesth 62:22–27

Shimomura K, Kamata O, Ueki S, Ida S, Oguri K, Yoshimura H, Tsukamoto H (1971) Analgesic effect of morphine glucuronides. Tohoku J Exp Med 105:45–52

Smith MT, Watt JA, Cramond T (1990) Morphine-3-glucuronide – a potent antagonist of morphine analgesia. Life Sci 47:579–585

Somogyi AA, Nation RL, Olweny C, Tsirgiotis P, van Crugten J, Milne RW, Cleary JF, Danz C, Bochner F (1993) Plasma concentrations and renal clearances of morphine, morphine-3-glucuronide and morphine-6-glucuronide in cancer patients receiving morphine. Clin Pharmacokinet 24:413–420

Stain F, Barjavel MJ, Sandouk P, Plotkine M, Scherrmann JM, Bhargava HN (1995) Analgesic response and plasma and brain extracellular fluid pharmacokinetics of morphine and morphine-6-beta-d-glucuronide in the rat. J Pharmacol Exp Ther 274:852–857

Sullivan AF, McQuay HJ, Bailey D, Dickenson AH (1989) The spinal antinociceptive actions of morphine metabolites morphine-6-glucuronide and normorphine in the rat. Brain Res 482:219–224

Suzuki N, Kalso E, Rosenberg PH (1993) Intrathecal morphine-3-glucuronide does not antagonize spinal antinociception by morphine or morphine-6-glucuronide in rats. Eur J Pharmacol 249:27–250

Svensson J-O, Rane A, Sawe J, Sjoquist F (1982) Determination of morphine, morphine-3-glucuronide and (tentatively) morphine-6-glucuronide in plasma and urine using ion-pair high performance liquid chromatography. J Chromatogr 230:427–432

Tasker RAR, Nakatsu K (1984) Evaluation of 3, 6-dibutanoylmorphine as an analgesic in vivo: comparison with morphine and 3, 6-diacetylmorphine. Life Sciences 34:1659–1667

Tasker RR, Tsuda T, Hawrylyshyn P (1983) Clinical neurophysiological investigation of deafferentation pain. In: Bonica JJ, Lindblom U, Iggo A (eds) Advances in pain research and therapy, vol 5. Proceedings of the 3rd World Congress on Pain. Raven, New York, pp 713–738

Thompson PI, Joel SP, John L, Wedzicha JA, Maclean M, Slevin ML (1995) Respiratory depression following morphine and morphine-6-glucuronide in normal subjects. Br J Clin Pharmacol 40:145–152

Tiseo PJ, Thaler HT, Lapin J, Inturrisi CE, Portenoy RK, Foley KM (1995) Morphine-6-glucuronide concentrations and opioid-related side effects: a survey in cancer patients. Pain 61:47–54

Twycross RG, Lack S (1983) Symptom control in far advanced cancer; pain relief. Pitman, London

Van Crugten JT, Sallustio BC, Nation RL, Somogyi AA (1991) Renal tubular transport of morphine, morphine-6-glucuronide, and morphine-3-glucuronide in the isolated perfused rat kidney. Drug Metab Dispos 19:1087–1092

van Dongen RT, Crul BJ, Koopman-Kimenai PM, Vree TB (1994) Morphine and morphine-glucuronide concentrations in plasma and CSF during long-term administration of oral morphine. Br J Clin Pharmacol 38:271–273

Wahlstrom A, Winblad B, Bixo M, Rane A (1988) Human brain metabolism of morphine and naloxone. Pain 35:121–127

Wahlstrom A, Lenhammar L, Ask B, Rane A (1994) Tricyclic antidepressants inhibit opioid receptor binding in human brain and hepatic morphine glucuronidation. Pharmacol Toxicol 75:23–27

Westerling D, Persson C, Hoglund P (1995) Plasma concentrations of morphine, morphine-3-glucuronide, and morphine-6-glucuronide after intravenous and oral administration to healthy volunteers: relationship to nonanalgesic actions. Ther Drug Monit 17:287–301

Wilkinson TJ, Robinson BA, Begg EJ, Duffull SB, Ravenscroft PJ, Schneider JJ (1992) Pharmacokinetics and efficacy of rectal versus oral sustained-release morphine in cancer patients. Cancer Chemother Pharmacol 31:251–254

Wolff T, Samuelsson H, Hedner T (1995 Aug) Morphine and morphine metabolite concentrations in cerebrospinal fluid and plasma in cancer pain patients after slow-release oral morphine administration. Pain 62:147–154

Woolf CJ (1981) Intrathecal high dose morphine produces hyperalgesia in the rat. Brain Res 29:491–495

Yaksh TL, Harty GJ (1988) Pharmacology of the allodynia in rats evoked by high dose intrathecal morphine. J Pharmacol Exp Ther 244:501–507

Yaksh TL, Harty GJ, Onofrio BM (1986) High doses of spinal morphine produce a nonopiate receptor mediated hyperesthesia; clinical and theoretic implications. Anesthesiology 64:590–597

Yeh SY, Gorodetzky CW, Krebs HA (1977) Isolation and identification of morphine 3- and 6-glucuronide, morphine 3,6-diglucuronide, morphine 3-ethereal sulfate, normorphine, and normorphine 6-glucuronide as morphine metabolites in humans. J Pharm Sci 66:1288–1293

Yeh SY, Krebs HA, Gorodetzky CW (1979) Isolation and identification of morphine. N-oxide α- and β-dihydromorphines, β- or γ-isomorphine, and hyroxylated morphine as morphine metabolites in several mammalian species. J Pharm Sci 68:133–140

Yoshimura H, Ida S, Oguri K, Tsukamoto H (1973) Biochemical basis for analgesic activity of morphine-6-glucuronide. I. Penetration of morphine-6-glucuronide in the brain of rats. Biochem Pharmacol 22:1423–1430

CHAPTER 14

Inhibitory Neurotransmitters and Nociception: Role of GABA and Glycine

D.L. HAMMOND

A. Introduction

As the two most important inhibitory amino acid neurotransmitters in the central nervous system, γ-aminobutyric acid (GABA) and glycine play important roles in the processing of nociceptive information. At present three receptors for GABA receptors are recognized – $GABA_A$, $GABA_B$, and $GABA_C$ – and two for glycine – Gly_A and Gly_B. This chapter reviews briefly the pharmacology, anatomy, and molecular biology of these two neurotransmitters and their receptors and then examine their roles in acute and persistent nociception.

B. GABA

I. Molecular Biology, Pharmacology, and Distribution

1. Molecular Biology

The $GABA_A$ receptor is comprised of four different subunits (α, β, γ, and δ) that are arranged as a pentamer and form the wall of a ligand-gated ion channel permeable to Cl^-. Activation of this receptor increases Cl^- conductance and results in hyperpolarization. Multiple isoforms or splice variants exist for three of the subunits (α_{1-6}, β_{1-4}, γ_{1-4}, and δ) with the consequence that there are at least 15 different subunits from which the $GABA_A$ receptor can be assembled. If all the possible homo- and hetero-oligomeric combinations of these 15 subunits are considered, more than 150000 different types of $GABA_A$ receptor could exist. Fortunately, the results of immunoprecipitation and immunocytochemical studies suggest that only 12 different combinations of these subunits exist in appreciable quantities in the central nervous system. The principal stoichiometric arrangement is ($2\alpha_x$, $1\beta_x$, and $2\gamma_x$); one γ may be replaced by a δ. In addition to binding sites for GABA, the $GABA_A$ receptor has allosteric binding sites for a wide variety of agents that can positively or negatively modulate the actions of GABA (see below). These modulatory agents include benzodiazepines, ethanol, barbiturates, inhalational anesthetics, and neurosteroids. Considerable effort has been expended to identify the subunits that correspond to the allosteric binding sites for GABA and its many modulatory agents. These studies indicate that each different subunit (and their different pentameric combinations) endows the $GABA_A$ receptor with distinctive pharmacological properties. For example, a γ subunit is required for binding of benzodiazepine ligands, but it is the isoform of the α subunit that dictates the affinity of this receptor for various benzodiazepine receptor agonists, antagonists and inverse agonists. These studies predict a significant, if not daunting, heterogeneity of $GABA_A$ receptors in the central nervous system (BURT and KAMATCHI 1991; MacDONALD and OLSEN 1994; RABOW et al. 1995; SIEGHART 1995; STEPHENSON 1995).

The $GABA_B$ receptor is a G protein coupled receptor and, unlike the $GABA_A$ receptor, it has yet to be cloned. Activation of this receptor decreases Ca^{2+} conductance, increases K^+ conductance, and inhibits adenyl cyclase. The inhibition of Ca^{2+} conductance occurs predominantly at presynaptic loci and results in a decrease in neurotransmitter release. The increase in K^+ conductance occurs predominantly at postsynaptic loci and results in hyperpolarization. Multiple subtypes of the $GABA_B$ receptor are proposed to exist on the basis of differential sensitivity to $GABA_B$ receptor agonists and antagonists, differential sensitivity of pre- vs. postsynaptic receptors to inhibition by pertussis toxin, and differential sensitivity of the presynaptic receptors on terminals of excitatory vs. inhibitory neurons to inhibition by pertussis toxin (BONANNO and RAITERI 1993; BORMANN 1988; BOWERY 1989, 1993; KERR and ONG 1995; MOTT and LEWIS 1994).

The $GABA_C$ receptor is the most recent of the GAB_A receptors to be identified. Like the $GABA_A$ receptor, the $GABA_C$ receptor is a ligand-gated ion channel that is permeable to Cl^-, and its activation causes hyperpolarization. However, unlike the $GABA_A$ receptor, it is a homo-oligomeric arrangement of ρ_1 or ρ_2 subunits. Moreover, its affinity for GABA is tenfold greater than that of the $GABA_A$ receptor, and the mean open time of its channel is five times longer than that of the $GABA_A$ receptor (BORMANN and FEIGENSPAN 1995).

2. Pharmacology

Table 1 summarizes prototypic agonists and antagonists for the $GABA_A$, $GABA_B$, and $GABA_C$ receptors. The $GABA_A$ receptor is often referred to as the bicuculline-sensitive, baclofen-insensitive GABA receptor. Agonists for the $GABA_A$ receptor include isoguvacine, muscimol, and 4,5,6,7-tetrahydroisoxazolo[4, 5-c]pyridin-2-ol (THIP). Antagonists for the $GABA_A$ receptor include bicuculline and SR 95531. Although picrotoxin is often referred to as a $GABA_A$ receptor antagonist, it actually blocks the Cl^- channel noncompetitively and does not compete for the site at which GABA binds. The actions of GABA at the $GABA_A$ receptor are enhanced by neurosteroids such as the progesterone metabolite 5α-pregnan-3α-ol-20-one, inhalational anesthetics such as halothane and isoflurane, and barbiturates such as pentobarbital and phenobarbital. At low concentrations these agents increase the duration that the Cl^- channel is open in the presence of GABA. However, at higher concentrations they are able to directly activate the Cl^- channel in the

Table 1. Characteristics of Three Types of GABA Receptor

	Bicuculline	Baclofen	Agonist	Antagonist	Modulators
GABA$_A$	Sensitive	Insensitive	Isoguvacine Muscimol THIP	Bicuculline Picrotoxin	Benzodiazepines Anesthetics Neurosteroids
GABA$_B$	Insensitive	Sensitive	Baclofen 3-APPA	Phaclofen 2-OH-saclofen CGP35348 CGP55845A	None
GABA$_C$	Insensitive	Insensitive	TACA CACA	Picrotoxin	None

THIP, 4,5,6,7-tetrahydroisoxazolo-[4,5-c]pyridin-3-ol; 3-APPA, 3-amino-propylphosphinic acid; CGP35348, 3-amino-propyl(diethoxymethyl)phosphinic acid; CGP55845,A 3-N[1-(S)(3,4-dichlorophenyl)ethyl]amino-2-(S)-hydroxypropyl-P-benzyl-phosphinic acid; TACA, *trans*-4-aminocrotonic acid; CACA, *cis*-4-aminocrotonic acid.

absence of GABA. Benzodiazepine receptor agonists such as diazepam and zolpidem also potentiate the effects of GABA at the GABA$_A$ receptor, but do so by increasing the frequency with which the Cl⁻ channel opens in the presence of GABA. Conversely, inverse agonists at the benzodiazepine receptor such as methyl, 6,7, dimethoxy-4-ethyl-β-carboline-3-carboxylate attenuate the effects of GABA by decreasing the frequency with which the channel opens (KERR and ONG 1992; MACDONALD and OLSEN 1994; RABOW et al. 1995; SIEGHART 1995).

The GABA$_B$ receptor is classically described as the baclofen-sensitive, bicuculline-insensitive GABA receptor. Agonists for the GABA$_B$ receptor include baclofen and 3-aminopropyl phosphinic acid, although the latter may be a partial agonist at some types of GABA$_B$ receptors. Antagonists for this receptor include phaclofen, CGP 35348, CGP 55845 and SCH 50911. There are no known modulators of the action of GABA at the GABA$_B$ receptor (BOLSER et al. 1995; KERR and ONG 1995).

The GABA$_C$ receptor is referred to as the baclofen-insensitive, bicuculline-insensitive GABA receptor. Prototypic agonists for this receptor include GABA, and *trans*- and *cis*-4-aminocrotonic acid. As expected of a Cl⁻ channel, the GABA$_C$ receptor is antagonized by picrotoxin, although to a lesser extent than the GABA$_A$ receptor. Importantly, the GABA$_C$ receptor is not antagonized by bicuculline (BORMANN and FEIGENSPAN 1995).

3. Distribution in the Central Nervous System

The distribution of GABA, its synthetic enzyme glutamic acid decarboxylase, and its catabolic enzyme GABA transaminase, as well as the localization of its receptors in the central nervous system have been extensively examined using autoradiographic, immunocytochemical, and in situ hybridization techniques (BOWERY et al. 1987; FRITSCHY and MOHLER 1995; NAGAI et al. 1983, 1985;

OLSEN et al. 1990; OTTERSEN and STORM-MATHIESEN 1984; PALACIOS et al. 1981; RICHARDS et al. 1987; WISDEN et al. 1992). Of greatest interest in the present context are the high concentrations of GABA, $GABA_A$, or $GABA_B$ receptors in regions of the central nervous system that are implicated in either the afferent transmission of nociceptive information or the production of antinociception. These regions include the (a) superficial laminae of the spinal and medullary dorsal horns (BOWERY et al. 1987; MA et al. 1993; PATRICK et al. 1983; TODD and SULLIVAN 1990; WALDVOGEL et al. 1990); (b) medullary and pontine nuclei such as the nucleus raphe magnus (NRM), nucleus reticularis gigantocellularis pars α (NGCpα), the A5 catecholamine nucleus and the periaqueductal gray matter (PAG; BOWERY et al. 1987; FRITSCHY and MOHLER 1995; JONES et al. 1991; KIHARA and KUBO 1989; KWIAT et al. 1993; REICHLING and BASBAUM 1990a; WILLIAMS and BEITZ 1990); and (c) various subnuclei of the thalamus (OLSEN et al. 1990; OTTERSEN and STORM-MATHIESEN 1984; PALACIOS et al. 1981). The $GABA_C$ receptor is located predominantly in the retina. It is not considered further here, although the ρ_2 subunit does occur in discrete locations of the central nervous system, including the spinal cord (BORMANN and FEIGENSPAN 1995).

II. Role of GABA in Nociceptive Processing at the Level of the Spinal Cord

GABA in the spinal cord is derived principally from interneurons (MIYATA and OTSUKA 1975; TODD and MCKENZIE 1989). However, there is a small contribution from the spinal projections of GABAergic neurons in the medulla (BLESSING 1990; FUJI et al. 1985; JONES et al. 1991; MILLHORN et al. 1987; REICHLING and BASBAUM 1990a). The highest concentrations of GABA, and $GABA_A$ and $GABA_B$ receptors, occur in the superficial laminae of the dorsal horn (BOWERY et al. 1987; MIYATA and OTSUKA 1975; WALDVOGEL et al. 1990).

Several lines of evidence suggest that GABA is well situated to modulate the afferent transmission of nociceptive information by presynaptic mechanisms. First, it is estimated that 20%–40% of $GABA_A$ and $GABA_B$ receptors are located on the terminals of small-diameter primary afferent neurons because the numbers of these receptors are significantly reduced in rats treated neonatally with capsaicin (PRICE et al. 1984; SINGER and PLACHETA 1980). Second, intracellular recordings from dorsal root ganglion neurons indicate that $GABA_A$ and $GABA_B$ receptors are present on the terminals of Aδ and C primary afferent fibers (DÉSARMENIEN et al. 1984). The $GABA_B$ receptor agonist baclofen inhibits spontaneous and evoked excitatory postsynaptic potentials recorded from dorsal horn neurons in slices of rat spinal cord (KANGRGA et al. 1991) and inhibits the C fiber-evoked activation of dorsal horn neurons in vivo (DICKENSON et al. 1985; HENRY 1982). The effects of $GABA_A$ receptor agonists have not been directly examined. However, intravenous injection of midazolam to spinalized rats or the intrathecal administration of diazepam suppresses the activation of dorsal horn neurons by Aδ or C fiber stimulation (CLAVIER et al. 1992; JURNA 1984). As benzodiazepine receptor agonists, midazolam and diazepam would be expected to enhance the actions of GABA at the GABA$_A$ receptor.

Third, GABA-immunoreactive axons and vesicle-containing dendrites in the substantia gelatinosa of the rat are situated presynaptic to the central axons of type I synaptic glomeruli, which arise from unmyelinated primary afferent neurons (TODD and LOCHHEAD 1990). GABA-immunoreactive axons and vesicle-containing dendrites are also situated presynaptic to the terminals of high-threshold Aδ mechanonociceptors in laminae I–III of the cat and monkey (ALVAREZ et al. 1992). Other investigators, however, only rarely observe vesicle-containing GABA-immunoreactive dendrites or axons to be situated presynaptic to the central axons of synaptic glomeruli (CARLTON and HAYES 1990). In these studies GABA-immunoreactive vesicle-containing dendrites are more frequently situated postsynaptic to primary afferent terminals, sometimes in a reciprocal synaptic arrangement with the terminals or as a member of a synaptic triad in which the GABA-immunoreactive vesicle-containing dendrite is postsynaptic to the primary afferent terminal and presynaptic to another, unlabeled profile (CARLTON and HAYES 1990; HAYES and CARLTON 1992; TODD and LOCHHEAD 1990). The latter synaptic arrangements do not exclude a presynaptic mechanism of action but do suggest alternate mechanisms for the modulation of nociceptive transmission by GABA in the dorsal horn (see CARLTON and HAYES 1990; HAYES and CARLTON 1992 for discussion).

Fourth, GABA$_A$ or GABA$_B$ receptor agonists inhibit the evoked release of neurotransmitters from the dorsal horn, although these findings are by no means consistent. For example, the GABA$_A$ receptor agonist muscimol modestly inhibits the release of substance P from in vivo superfusates of the cat spinal cord evoked by high-intensity stimulation of the sciatic nerve (GO and YAKSH 1987) but does not inhibit the release of substance P evoked either by addition of K$^+$ (BOURGOIN et al. 1992) or stimulation of the attached dorsal roots (MALCANGIO and BOWERY 1993) in slices of spinal cord. However, GABA$_A$ receptor agonists do inhibit the K$^+$-evoked release of calcitonin gene-related peptide, a selective marker of primary afferent neurons, from minced slices of spinal cord (BOURGOIN et al. 1992). The GABA$_B$ receptor agonist baclofen inhibits the release of glutamate (KANGRGA et al. 1991) and substance P (MALCANGIO and BOWERY 1993) that is evoked by stimulation of the attached dorsal roots in slices of rat spinal cord. However, baclofen does not inhibit the release of substance P or calcitonin gene-related peptide evoked by addition of K$^+$ to minced slices of spinal cord (BOURGOIN et al. 1992; SAWYNOK et al. 1982), nor does it inhibit the in vivo release of substance P into superfusates of the cat spinal cord evoked by high-intensity stimulation of the sciatic nerve (GO and YAKSH 1987). The differences among these studies may reflect the use of different experimental paradigms and means of release, as well as the fact that several of the neurotransmitters (e.g., substance P and glutamate) originate from intrinsic neurons, as well as from primary afferent neurons.

GABA is also well situated in the dorsal horn to regulate afferent transmission by a postsynaptic mechanism. Iontophoretic administration of GABA or the $GABA_A$ receptor agonist muscimol inhibits the excitation of spinothalamic tract neurons or nociceptive specific laminae I or II neurons by excitatory amino acids, an effect that is consistent with a postsynaptic site of action (JONES et al. 1990; LIN et al. 1996; WILLCOCKSON et al. 1984). In addition, baclofen hyperpolarizes dorsal horn neurons in slices of spinal cord by increasing K^+ conductance (KANGRGA et al. 1991). Administration of baclofen to the dorsal horn by dialysis also inhibits the excitation of spinothalamic tract neurons by iontophoretic administration of glutamate, although the magnitude of the effect is small (LIN et al. 1996). Finally, the soma and dendrites of spinothalamic tract neurons possess GABAergic synapses (CARLTON et al. 1992).

1. Studies of Acute Nociception

The collective results of these anatomical, neurochemical, and electrophysiological studies of the actions of GABA in the spinal cord lead to the prediction that GABA receptor agonists should modulate the afferent transmission of nociceptive information and produce antinociception. This postulate is supported by the results of behavioral studies. In the rat, intrathecal administration of $GABA_A$ receptor agonists such as muscimol or isoguvacine produces a modest increase in response latencies in the tail-flick or hot-plate tests (HAMMOND and DROWER 1984; McGOWAN and HAMMOND 1993a; ROBERTS et al. 1986), increases the vocalization threshold to noxious electrical stimulation of the tail (ROBERTS et al. 1986), and suppresses formalin-induced pain behaviors (DIRIG and YAKSH 1995). In the mouse, intrathecally administered muscimol antagonizes the caudally directed biting and scratching behavior and the thermal hyperalgesia produced by intrathecal administration of excitatory amino acids (AANONSEN and WILCOX 1989). However, it does not suppress the biting and scratching behavior evoked by substance P (HWANG and WILCOX 1989). In the mouse intrathecally administered muscimol does not increase tail-flick latency (HWANG and WILCOX 1989), although intrathecally administered isoguvacine is effective in this test in this species (HOLMES and FUJIMOTO 1994). The antinociception produced by $GABA_A$ receptor agonists is antagonized by picrotoxin or bicuculline (AANONSEN and WILCOX 1989; DIRIG and YAKSH 1995; McGOWAN and HAMMOND 1993a; ROBERTS et al. 1986). An involvement of endogenously released GABA in the modulation of sensory transmission is further suggested by the results of studies with $GABA_A$ receptor antagonists. Intrathecal administration of high doses of picrotoxin ($>1\,\mu g$) or bicuculline ($>0.3\,\mu g$) decreases the threshold for tail shock-induced vocalization, induces mechanical allodynia, and produces spontaneous pain behaviors (McGOWAN and HAMMOND 1993a; ROBERTS et al. 1986; YAKSH 1989). $GABA_A$ receptor antagonists also enhance the response of dorsal horn neurons to touch and to activation of Aβ fibers and decrease the threshold for activation of these neurons by an innocuous mechanical stimulus (SIVILOTTI and WOOLF 1994).

Agents that enhance the actions of GABA at the GABA$_A$ receptor can also produce antinociception. For example, intrathecal administration of midazolam increases the escape threshold for transcutaneous electrical stimulation in the rat (SERRAO et al. 1989) or for noxious visceral distention in the rabbit (CRAWFORD et al. 1993) and suppresses the sympathetic response to high-intensity stimulation of the tibial nerve in the dog (NIV et al. 1983). Intrathecal administration of diazepam or midazolam also produces a very modest increase in tail-flick response latency (NIV et al. 1988; ZAMBOTTI et al. 1991), although this effect is not observed by all investigators (SERRAO et al. 1989). Similarly, intrathecal pretreatment with midazolam suppresses formalin-induced pain behaviors (AIGOUY et al. 1992), although, again, this effect is not observed by all investigators (DIRIG and YAKSH 1995). The ability of benzodiazepine agonists to produce antinociception is likely to be highly dependent on the concentration of endogenous GABA.

Intrathecal administration of GABA$_B$ receptor agonists also produces antinociception. In the rat, intrathecal administration of baclofen increases response latencies in the tail-flick and hot-plate tests in a dose-dependent and stereospecific manner (ARAN and HAMMOND 1991; HAMMOND and DROWER 1984; SAWYNOK and DICKSON 1985; WILSON and YAKSH 1978) and suppresses both phase 1 and phase 2 responses to injection of formalin in the hindpaw (DIRIG and YAKSH 1995). In the mouse, intrathecal administration of baclofen suppresses the caudally directed biting and scratching behavior induced by intrathecal injection of substance P but does not suppress that induced by intrathecal administration of excitatory amino acid antagonists (AANONSEN and WILCOX 1989; HWANG and WILCOX 1989). Finally, intrathecally administered baclofen also produces a dose-dependent increase in shock titration threshold in the primate (YAKSH and REDDY 1981). The antinociception produced by baclofen is antagonized by phaclofen and CGP 35348 (ARAN and HAMMOND 1991; DIRIG and YAKSH 1995; HAMMOND and WASHINGTON 1993; HWANG and WILCOX 1989). Although intrathecal administration of GABA$_B$ receptor antagonists does not alter tail-flick or hot-plate response latencies (HAMMOND and WASHINGTON 1993; HAO et al. 1994), very high doses of CGP 35348 cause mechanical allodynia (HAO et al. 1994).

The ability of GABA$_A$ and GABA$_B$ receptor agonists to produce antinociception after intrathecal administration supports a role of spinal GABA$_A$ and GABA$_B$ receptors in the modulation of nociceptive sensitivity. However, these findings provide little information about the role of endogenous GABA in the modulation of nociceptive sensitivity by neuronal pathways. This deficit has been addressed by recent studies that examined the effects of intrathecally administered GABA$_A$ or GABA$_B$ receptor antagonists on the antinociception elicited by activation of bulbospinal pain modulatory pathways. For example, the antinociception produced by microinjection of L-glutamate in the ventromedial medulla (McGOWAN and HAMMOND 1993a,b) and intracerebroventricular administration of δ-opioid receptor agonists (HOLMES and FUJIMOTO 1994; KILLIAN et al. 1995; RADY and FUJIMOTO 1995) is attenuated by intrathecal administration of GABA$_A$ or GABA$_B$ receptor antagonists. Intrathecal administration of GABA$_A$ receptor antagonists also reduces the inhibition of dorsal horn neurons produced by stimulation of the PAG in the monkey (LIN et al. 1994, 1996), although GABA$_B$ receptor antagonists are ineffective (LIN et al. 1996). These results suggest that (a) a release of GABA in the spinal cord mediates in part the antinociception produced by activation of endogenous pathways, and (b) that the afferent transmission of nociceptive information in the spinal cord is subject to modulation by endogenously released GABA acting at either GABA$_A$ or GABA$_B$ receptors.

2. Studies of Persistent or Neuropathic Pain

With the recent development of several rodent models of persistent inflammatory pain or neuropathic pain, investigators have examined the role of GABA in the hyperalgesia, allodynia, inflammation, and spontaneous pain that occur in response to tissue or nerve injury. It was initially proposed that these sequelae result from an enhancement of excitatory inputs and a loss of inhibitory tone in the dorsal horn. However, a close examination of the data suggests that the response of the GABAergic system is dependent on the type of injury. Moreover, if a loss of inhibition does occur, it may be as obvious as a decrease in the number of GABA-immunoreactive neurons or as subtle as a downregulation of the receptor. Clearly more studies are needed for a better understanding of the response of the GABAergic system and its role in the development and the maintenance of the behavioral sequelae to injury.

The hypothesis that a loss of inhibition in the spinal cord dorsal horn mediates the allodynia and hyperalgesia induced after tissue or nerve injury is based on the observations that the levels of GABA and the number of GABA-immunoreactive neurons in the dorsal horn decrease after transection of the sciatic nerve (CASTRO-LOPES et al. 1993), chronic constriction of the sciatic nerve (IBUKI et al. 1996), or ischemia of the spinal cord (ZHANG et al. 1994). In the case of spinal cord ischemia the decrease in number of GABA-immunoreactive neurons is transient and is temporally correlated with the onset and resolution of mechanical allodynia (ZHANG et al. 1994). The loss of these neurons is of much longer duration after chronic constriction injury with a near complete loss observed 3 weeks after injury. However, this "loss" is also not permanent as GABA-immunoreactive neurons reappear by 7 weeks, although in fewer numbers than in control animals (IBUKI et al. 1996). A long term "loss" of GABA-immunoreactive neurons also occurs after transection of the sciatic nerve (CASTRO-LOPES et al. 1993). The binding of GABA to its receptors may also be altered. For example, 2–4 weeks after transection of the sciatic nerve binding to GABA$_B$ receptors in lamina II is decreased. This decrease is attributed to a loss of $GABA_B$ receptors situated on the terminals of primary afferents (CASTRO-LOPES et al. 1995). By comparison, binding to $GABA_A$ receptors in lamina II of the dorsal horn increases after sciatic nerve transection, an effect that is attributed to an upregulation of these receptors in response to a decrease in the levels of GABA or the aberrant innervation of lamina II by large-diameter myelinated primary afferents that possess $GABA_A$ receptors (CASTRO-LOPES et al. 1995). Surprisingly, there is no significant change in the density of $GABA_B$ binding sites in the spinal cord 2–3 weeks after chronic constriction injury (SMITH et al. 1994); the effect on $GABA_A$ receptors has not been examined.

Several investigators have examined the effects of $GABA_A$ and $GABA_B$ receptor agonists on the behavioral sequelae to injury. In rats with ischemia-induced injury of the spinal cord, systemic administration of low doses of baclofen alleviates the mechanical allodynia (HAO et al. 1991) and normalizes the response of dorsal horn neurons to innocuous mechanical stimuli in spinalized rats (HAO et al. 1992). The $GABA_A$ receptor agonists muscimol and THIP are without effect in these animals (HAO et al. 1991, 1992; Wiesenfeld-Hallin, personal communication). Similarly, intrathecal administration of either muscimol or baclofen or systemic administration of baclofen alleviates the thermal hyperalgesia and mechanical allodynia produced by chronic constriction injury of the sciatic nerve in the rat (SMITH et al. 1994; YAMAMOTO and YAKSH 1991).

The ability of $GABA_A$ or $GABA_B$ receptor agonists to suppress the mechanical allodynia or thermal hyperalgesia produced by injury has been interpreted as evidence that a loss of GABA-mediated inhibition in the dorsal horn mediates these behavioral sequelae. However, the simple ability of a receptor agonist to suppress hyperalgesia or allodynia is not sufficient evidence to implicate this receptor or neurotransmitter in the mechanism of action. Rather, studies with receptor antagonists provide a more direct examination of the involvement of the endogenous neurotransmitter. The study by YAMAMOTO and YAKSH (1993) is particularly enlightening in this respect. Intrathecal administration of 1–3 µg bicuculline on the day of surgery and for 2 days after loose ligation of the sciatic nerve causes a dose-dependent enhancement of the thermal hyperalgesia that develops in this model. This finding suggests that GABA serves a protective function after injury, and that its antagonism results in enhanced excitation of the spinal cord. Although this finding clearly implicates GABA in the development of these behavioral sequelae, even more interesting would be an analysis of the effects of these antagonists at *later* times. If a "permanent" loss of GABA-mediated inhibition has occurred, the antagonists should be relatively ineffective when administered at this later time. A finding that they continue to enhance the allodynia and hyperalgesia would call into question the hypothesis that these behavioral sequelae result from a loss of GABA-mediated inhibition in the spinal cord.

By comparison, the response of the GABAergic system to inflammatory pain, such as that induced by injection of carrageenan or complete Freund's adjuvant in one hindpaw, is quite different from that induced by nerve injury. The number of neurons immunoreactive for glutamic acid decarboxylase or its messenger RNA increases in the dorsal horn within 4 days of the injection of complete Freund's adjuvant in one hindpaw of the rat (CASTRO-LOPES et al. 1994b; NAHIN and HYLDEN 1991). The increase in messenger RNA for glutamic acid decarboxylase persists for nearly 3 weeks (CASTRO-LOPES et al. 1994b). The levels of GABA itself and the number of GABA-immunoreactive neurons in the spinal cord dorsal horn also increase shortly after the injection of either complete Freund's adjuvant or carrageenan (CASTRO-LOPES et al. 1992, 1994a). These increases are abolished by transection of the sciatic nerve or by the destruction of C fibers by neonatal administration of capsaicin (CASTRO-LOPES et al. 1994a). The latter finding suggests that the levels of GABA are increased as a compensatory response to increased afferent input. Furthermore, binding to $GABA_B$ receptors in the spinal cord is modestly decreased 3–4 weeks after injection of complete Freund's adjuvant (CASTRO-LOPES et al. 1995), an effect attributed to downregulation of this receptor in response to elevated levels of GABA (MALCANGIO et al. 1993). No significant changes in $GABA_A$ receptor binding occur after the induction of inflammation (CASTRO-LOPES et al. 1995). Interestingly, the stimulus-evoked release of substance P from slices of the spinal cord from monoarthritic rats is significantly greater than in control animals (MALCANGIO and BOWERY 1994). This evoked release is greatly increased in the presence of a $GABA_B$ but not a $GABA_A$ receptor antagonist (MALCANGIO and BOWERY 1994). As antagonists lack intrinsic activity, the enhanced action of the antagonist can be ascribed only to an increased release of GABA and activation of $GABA_B$ receptors. Systemic administration of a $GABA_B$ receptor antagonist also enhances the thermal hyperalgesia induced by injection of complete Freund's adjuvant. Although systemically administered baclofen is able to modestly suppress the thermal hyperalgesia, a relatively high dose is required (MALCANGIO and BOWERY 1994). This latter finding is consistent with a downregulation of the $GABA_B$ receptor. However, there appears to be no change in the potency of baclofen to suppress mechanical hyperalgesia induced by complete Freund's adjuvant (SMITH et al. 1994). On a final note, recent studies suggest that spinal $GABA_A$ but not $GABA_B$ receptors, may modulate the development of inflammation and thermal hyperalgesia associated with inflammation. Specifically, intraspinal administration of $GABA_A$ receptor antagonists, but not a $GABA_B$ receptor antagonist, alleviates the hyperalgesia induced by injection of kaolin in the knee joint (SLUKA et al. 1993) and prevents the release of excitatory amino acids in the spinal cord (SLUKA et al. 1994). Primary afferent depolarization and antidromic dorsal root reflexes are mediated by an action of GABA at $GABA_A$ receptors situated presynaptically on the terminals of primary afferent neurons. Antagonism of this receptor is thought to prevent the generation of these antidromic volleys and the accompanying reflex release of inflammatory and algogenic substances in the periphery.

III. GABAergic Modulation of Supraspinal Nuclei

A discussion of the role of GABA at each of the many supraspinal nuclei involved in the processing of nociceptive information is beyond the scope of this chapter. This section reviews the role of GABA in modulating the activity of neurons in the NRM and NGCpα of the ventromedial medulla and the PAG in the pons. Chemical or electrical stimulation of these nuclei produces antinociception that is mediated in part by activation of neurons that project to the spinal cord and the release of a variety of neurotransmitters including enkephalins, serotonin, norepinephrine, and GABA in the spinal cord (HAMMOND 1986; JONES 1992). Although these three nuclei are strongly implicated in the regulation of nociceptive sensitivity, GABA is also likely to be an important inhibitory influence on the activity of other nuclei involved in descending modulation of spinal afferent transmission such as the nucleus paragigantocellularis lateralis (LOVICK 1987), pontine catecholamine nuclei (KWIAT et al. 1993), and other nuclei involved in the ascending transmission of nociceptive information such as the thalamus, amygdala, or somatosensory cortex (OLIVÉRAS and MONTAGNE-CLAVEL 1994; OLIVÉRAS 1995; POORE and HELMSTETTER 1994; ROBERTS et al. 1992).

1. GABA$_A$ Receptors

The existence of GABA$_A$ receptors in the PAG, NRM, and NGCpα has been demonstrated by autoradiographic (BOWERY et al. 1987) and immunocytochemical methods (FRITSCHY and MOHLER 1995; GAO et al. 1993; WILLIAMS and BEITZ 1990). It is estimated that between 37.5% and 50% of the synapses on the soma and dendrites of PAG neurons that project to the NRM are GABAergic (REICHLING and BASBAUM 1990b; WILLIAMS and BEITZ 1990). Moreover, more than 50% of the dendrites of NRM neurons that project to the spinal cord are situated postsynaptic to GABA-immunoreactive terminals (CHO and BASBAUM 1991). (A small portion of this input may derive from GABAergic neurons of the PAG that project to the NRM; WILLIAMS and BEITZ 1990). Recent immunocytochemical studies using antibodies to the α_1 or α_3 subunits of the GABA$_A$ receptor indicate that both serotonergic and nonserotonergic neurons of the NRM and NGCpα possess GABA$_A$ receptors (GAO et al. 1993; HAMA et al. 1995) and that a portion of these neurons project to the spinal cord (HAMA et al. 1995). These anatomical findings indicate that neurons in the PAG that project to the NRM or NGCpα, as well as neurons in the NRM and NGCpα that project to the spinal cord receive substantial input from GABAergic afferents. The results of electrophysiological and pharmacological investigations indicate that this input is inhibitory and tonically active. For example, iontophoretic administration of GABA inhibits the spontaneous discharge of neurons in the PAG, whereas the GABA$_A$ receptor antagonist bicuculline significantly increases the activity of these neurons (BEHBEHANI et al. 1990). Microinjection of bicuculline in the PAG selectively decreases the response of dorsal horn neurons to noxious thermal stimuli without affecting their response to innocuous brush (SANDKÜHLER et al. 1989), a mechanism consistent with the production of antinociception. Indeed, microinjection of the $GABA_A$ receptor antagonists picrotoxin or bicuculline in the PAG increases tail-flick response latency (MOREAU and FIELDS 1986), and concurrently increases the spontaneous activity of "off-cells" while decreasing the spontaneous activity of "on-cells" in the NRM (MOREAU and FIELDS 1986). Conversely, microinjection of THIP, a $GABA_A$ receptor agonist, in the PAG produces a modest hyperalgesia (DEPAULIS et al. 1987). These findings suggest that an excitatory projection from the PAG to the NRM is under tonic, inhibitory control by GABAergic processes mediated by $GABA_A$ receptors. Similar observations have been made in the NRM and NGCpα. For example, microinjection of $GABA_A$ receptor antagonists such as bicuculline or picrotoxin in the NRM or the NGCpα increases tail-flick response latency and decreases responses to noxious pinch (DROWER and HAMMOND 1988; HEINRICHER and KAPLAN 1991), whereas microinjection of $GABA_A$ receptor agonists in these same nuclei decreases tail-flick latency and enhances responses to noxious pinch (DROWER and HAMMOND 1988; HEINRICHER and KAPLAN 1991). The increase in tail-flick latency is accompanied by an increase in the discharge of "off-cells" in the NRM (HEINRICHER and TORTORICI 1994). Thus, as is the PAG, the NRM and NGCpα are subject to a tonic, inhibitory input mediated by GABA at presumably postsynaptic $GABA_A$ receptors (GAO et al. 1993; HAMA et al. 1995).

2. $GABA_B$ Receptors

$GABA_B$ receptors are also present in the PAG, NRM, and NGCpα (BOWERY et al. 1987). However, the action of GABA at these receptors is less well understood. An early study indicated that microinjection of $0.8–1.5\,\mu g$ racemic baclofen at sites in the PAG produces a modest increase in tail-flick response latency but is relatively ineffective at sites in the NRM and NGCpα (LEVY and PROUDFIT 1979). However, a recent reexamination of the effects of a wide dose range of the active isomer of baclofen indicates that its actions are more complex than originally thought. For example, microinjection of very low doses (0.1–1.0 ng) of baclofen in the NRM and NGCpα produces a modest increase in tail-flick latency that is ascribed to activation of presynaptic $GABA_B$ receptors on inhibitory noradrenergic or GABAergic inputs to this nucleus. Inhibition of the tonic release of norepinephrine or GABA results in disinhibition (activation) of neurons in the NRM and NGCpα and the production of antinociception (THOMAS et al. 1995). Intermediate doses of baclofen (5–30 ng) are without effect. However, microinjection of still higher doses of baclofen (50–150 ng) produces a significant decrease in tail-flick latency, an effect that is ascribed to activation of postsynaptic $GABA_B$ receptors causing hyperpolarization and an inhibition of NRM neurons (THOMAS et al. 1995). This interpretation is consistent with electrophysiological findings that low concentrations of baclofen preferentially activate presynaptic $GABA_B$ receptors (see THOMAS et al. 1995 for discussion). Microinjection of the $GABA_B$ receptor antagonist CGP 35348 in the NRM or NGCpα does not alter thermal nociceptive threshold (THOMAS et al. 1996) suggesting that, unlike $GABA_A$ receptors, $GABA_B$ receptors in the NRM and NGCpα are not tonically activated.

3. Role of GABA in the Antinociceptive Effects of Morphine

For a time, the universal inhibitory effect of opioids appeared to be at odds with their ability to produce antinociception, presumably by activation of neurons in the PAG, NRM, and NGCpα. However, as our understanding of the role of GABA at supraspinal sites increased, it was proposed that the antinociceptive effects of locally or systemically administered opioids result from an inhibition of inhibitory GABAergic inputs to the PAG, NRM, or NGCpα. This postulate now has substantial support. For example, intracellular recordings from neurons of the NRM in slices of brainstem indicate that the μ-opioid receptor agonists morphine or [D-Ala^2, NMePhe^4, Gly^{5}ol]enkephalin decrease the amplitude of evoked GABA-mediated synaptic potentials with little effect on either the resting membrane potential or the amplitude of the evoked excitatory synaptic potentials (PAN et al. 1990). These findings are consistent with a presynaptic inhibition of GABA-mediated inhibitory inputs to the NRM. Additional support is provided by the observation that the antinociception produced by microinjection of morphine in the PAG is antagonized by microinjection of $GABA_A$ recetor agonists such as muscimol and THIP at the same site (DE PAULIS et al. 1987; MOREAU and FIELDS 1986; ROMANDINI and SAMANIN 1984; ZAMBOTTI et al. 1982). Finally, morphine inhibits the veratridine-induced release of GABA into microdialysates of the lateral PAG, although it has no effect on the basal release of GABA (RENNO et al. 1992).

C. Glycine

Glycine is closely related to GABA in its structure and mechanism of action. This section focuses on the role of glycine at the strychnine-sensitive receptor (Gly_A) in the modulation of nociception. The role of glycine at the strychnine-insensitive modulatory binding site associated with the N-methyl-D-aspartate receptor (Gly_B) is reviewed by Dickenson (this volume).

I. Molecular Biology and Pharmacology

The glycine receptor is comprised of two subunits, α and β, that are arranged as a pentamer and form the wall of an ion channel permeable to Cl^-. Activation of the receptor results in an increase in Cl^- conductance and hyperpolarization of the neuron. The stoichiometry of the Gly_A receptor is $(3\alpha_x, 2\beta)$. As with the $GABA_A$ receptor, multiple isoforms ($\alpha_{1-4)}$ and several splice variants of the α subunit exist. Isoforms of the β have yet to be identified. These multiple isoforms and splice variants of the α subunit endow the glycine receptor with unique pharmacological characteristics. For example, the glycine receptor is comprised of α_1 and, to a lesser extent, α_3 subunits in the adult. However, during the first 2 weeks of life the receptor is composed predominantly of α_2 subunits. The presence of this neonatal isoform substantially diminishes the receptor's affinity for strychnine and is thought to be the reason why neonatal rats are insensitive to the convulsant action of strychnine. This developmental change in sensitivity to strychnine was the first indication that subtypes of the glycine receptor might exist. Although the molecular biology of the glycine receptor predicts that multiple subtypes are likely to exist, functional characterization of these different subtypes is currently hampered by the limited number of available ligands. At present glycine is the sole prototypic agonist for the glycine receptor. Other amino acids also bind to this receptor but with diminished potency in the rank order of β-alanine > taurine > L-alanine > L-serine. There is also only one prototypic antagonist for this receptor, strychnine. The identification and functional characterization of the predicted subtypes of the glycine receptor will depend on the future development of additional potent agonists and antagonists (BÉCHADE et al. 1994; BETZ et al. 1994; VANDENBERG and SCHOFIELD 1994).

II. Role of Glycine in Nociceptive Processing at the Level of the Spinal Cord

The dorsal horn of the spinal cord contains high concentrations of glycine, although the levels are less than in the ventral horn (DALY 1990; PATRICK et al. 1983). Glycine-immunoreactive neurons are localized predominantly in deeper laminae of the dorsal horn, with fewer numbers in lamina I (VAN DEN POL and GORCS 1988). Glycine-immunoreactive neurons are estimated to represent 9%, 14%, and 46% of the neurons in laminae I, II, and III, respectively (TODD and SULLIVAN 1990). Interestingly, immunocytochemical studies indicate that GABA and glycine colocalize in many neurons in the dorsal horn. In fact, nearly every glycine-immunoreactive neuron in laminae I–III also contains GABA. A significant proportion of GABA-immunoreactive neurons also contain glycine, with estimates ranging from 30% in lamina I to 64% in lamina III (TODD and SULLIVAN 1990). High densities of the strychnine-sensitive glycine receptor (BASBAUM 1988; BOHLHALTER et al. 1994; VAN DEN POL and GORCS 1988; ZARBIN et al. 1981) and its messenger RNA (MALOSIO et al. 1991) are present in laminae II (inner), III, IV, and V of the dorsal horn.

The mechanism by which glycine modulates afferent transmission in the dorsal horn is one of postsynaptic inhibition. Immunocytochemical analyses at the electron microscopic level indicate that glycine receptors are predominantly postsynaptic in the dorsal horn (MITCHELL et al. 1993; VAN DEN POL and GORCS 1988). Furthermore, the density of glycine receptors in the spinal cord is not diminished by neonatal administration of capsaicin, which destroys small-diameter unmyelinated primary afferents (SINGER and PLACHETA 1980). Finally, intraspinal or iontophoretic administration of glycine inhibits the excitation of spinothalamic tract neurons by glutamate, an effect consistent with a postsynaptic site of action (WILLCOCKSON et al. 1984). Intraspinal administration of glycine also inhibits the pinch-evoked excitation of spinothalamic tract neurons; this effect is antagonized by strychnine (LIN et al. 1994). In contrast, intraspinal administration of strychnine increases the spontaneous activity of spinothalamic tract neurons and enhances their response to innocuous mechanical stimuli and to a lesser extent to noxious pinch (LIN et al. 1994). Intrathecal administration of strychnine also increases the response of unidentified dorsal horn neurons to innocuous touch, decreases their threshold for mechanical stimulation and enhances responses to stimulation of $A\beta$ fibers (SIVILOTTI and WOOLF 1994). Given the large proportions of neurons that colocalize GABA and glycine in the dorsal horn, it is perhaps expected that many neurons in the deeper laminae of the dorsal horn colocalize both $GABA_A$ and glycine receptors in close apposition on the soma and dendrites (BOHLHALTER et al. 1994).

Intrathecal administration of high doses of strychnine ($>1\,\mu g$) in unanesthetized rats induces caudally directed biting and scratching behaviors and touch-evoked allodynia and decreases vocalization threshold to electrical shock of the tail (BEYER et al. 1985; FRENK et al. 1988; YAKSH 1989). In anesthetized rats injected intrathecally with strychnine, hair deflection elicits a vigorous increase in heart rate and blood pressure and a prolonged withdrawal response of the hindlimb of a magnitude similar to that produced by a noxious stimulus (SHERMAN and LOOMIS 1994; YAKSH 1989). Strychnine does not alter response latency in the tail-flick test (BEYER et al. 1985). The initial finding that intrathecally administered glycine by itself does not produce antinociception in the tail-flick test or tail-shock test (BEYER et al. 1985) but rather produces a syndrome reminiscent of nociception (BEYER et al. 1985; LARSON 1989) appeared to be at odds with an inhibitory role of this amino acid in the dorsal horn. However, this lack of effect has since been attributed to concomitant activation of the Gly_B receptor, at which glycine acts to potentiate the effect of glutamate at the N-methyl-D-aspartate receptor (LARSON 1989). Thus, glycine does significantly increase the vocalization threshold for tail shock and increases response latency in the tail-flick test when administered in the presence of an antagonist of the N-methyl-D-aspartate receptor (BEYER et al. 1992). Although these findings with exogenously administered glycine receptor agonists and antagonists implicate glycine in the modulation of nociceptive threshold, they provide little insight into the role of endogenous glycine. The results of more recent studies indicate that glycine may play an important role in the antinociception produced by activation of bulbospinal pain modulatory pathways. For example, electrical stimulation of the NRM using stimulus intensities that are able to suppress the responses of dorsal horn neurons to noxious stimuli results in a release of glycine into microdialysates of the spinal cord (SORKIN et al. 1993). Furthermore, intraspinal administration of strychnine partially attenuates the suppression of spinothalamic tract neurona responses to brush, noxious pinch, and noxious heat that is produced by stimulation of the PAG (LIN et al. 1994) or the NRM (SORKIN et al. 1993). Additional insight is provided by two studies of neuropathic pain. Specifically, intrathecal administration of strychnine on the day of surgery and the 2 days after loose ligation of the sciatic nerve significantly enhances the thermal hyperalgesia that develops in this model (YAMAMOTO and YAKSH 1993). Systemic administration of strychnine also increases the number of "dark" neurons that occur in the dorsal horn after chronic constriction injury (SUGIMOTO et al. 1990). These data suggest that glycine plays an important protective role in the spinal cord, and that its removal augments the response of dorsal horn neurons to injury.

III. Role of Glycine at Supraspinal Nuclei

The concentration of glycine and the density of glycine receptors are much lower in the brainstem than in the spinal cord and are lower still at more rostral levels of the neuraxis (DALY 1990; PROBST et al. 1986; VAN DEN POL and GORCS 1988; ZARBIN et al. 1981). Although the PAG, NRM, and nucleus reticularis gigantocellularis do contain small numbers of strychnine-sensitive glycine receptors (PROBST et al. 1986; ZARBIN et al. 1981), the actions of glycine or strychnine in these and other supraspinal nuclei have not been extensively examined. The observation that microinjection of strychnine in the NRM does not increase tail-flick response latency suggests that these neurons are not subject to a tonic, inhibitory glycinergic input (HEINRICHER and KAPLAN 1991).

D. Summary

Whether the mechanism of action is an increase in Cl^- conductance, a decrease in Ca^{2+} conductance, or an increase in K^+ conductance, the predominant action of GABA in the central nervous system is one of inhibition. In the spinal cord GABA is well-situated to effect profound inhibition of the afferent transmission of nociceptive information by either pre- or postsynaptic mechanisms. Supraspinally the activity of bulbospinal pain modulatory pathways appears to be powerfully and tonically suppressed by GABA acting at $GABA_A$ receptors. The removal of this inhibitory tone may be an important means by which antinociception is produced. Despite its close structural and mechanistic relationship to GABA, the role of glycine in modulating nociceptive transmission is less well understood. The fact that glycine colocalizes with GABA in many spinal neurons and that $GABA_A$ and glycine receptors are found in close apposition on dorsal horn neurons suggests that glycine and GABA may interact to afford enhanced inhibition under certain conditions. This possibility clearly warrants further investigation.

Note added in Proof. Expression cloning of the $GABA_B$ receptor was recently achieved by Kaupmann and colleagues [Nature (1997) 386:239–246].

Acknowledgement. This work was supported by Public Health Service Grant DE11423.

References

Aanonsen LM, Wilcox GL (1989) Muscimol, gamma-aminobutyric acid$_A$ receptors and excitatory amino acids in the mouse spinal cord. J Pharmacol Exp Ther 248:1034–1038

Aigouy L, Fondras JC, Pajot J, Schoeffler P, Woda A (1992) Intrathecal midazolam versus intrathecal morphine in orofacial nociception: an experimental study in rats. Neurosci Lett 139:97–99

Alvarez FJ, Kavookjian ZM, Light AR (1992) Synaptic interactions between GABA-immunoreactive profiles and the terminals of functionally defined myelinated nociceptors in the monkey and cat spinal cord. J Neurosci 12:2901–2917

Aran S, Hammond DL (1991) Antagonism of baclofen-induced antinociception by intrathecal administration of phaclofen or 2-hydroxy-saclofen, but not delta-aminovaleric acid in the rat. J Pharmacol Exp Ther 257:360–368

Basbaum AI (1988) Distribution of glycine receptor immunoreactivity in the spinal cord of the rat: cytochemical evidence for a differential glycinergic control of lamina I and V neurons. J Comp Neurol 278:330–336

Béchade C, Sur C, Triller A (1994) The inhibitory glycine receptor. Bioessays 16:735–744

Behbehani MM, Jiang M, Chandler SD, Ennis M (1990) The effect of GABA and its antagonists on midbrain periaqueductal gray neurons in the rat. Pain 40:195–204

Betz H, Kuhse J, Fischer M, Schmieden V, Laube B, Kuryatov A, Langosch D, Meyer G, Bormann J, Runström N, Matzenbach B, Kirsch J, Ramming M (1994) Structure, diversity and synaptic localization of inhibitory glycine receptors. J Physiol (Paris) 88:243–248

Beyer C, Roberts LA, Komisaruk BR (1985) Hyperalgesia induced by altered glycinergic activity at the spinal cord. Life Sci 37:875–882

Beyer C, Komisaruk BR, Lòpez-Colomè A, Caba M (1992) Administration of AP5, a glutamate antagonist, unmasks glycine analgesic action in the rat. Pharmacol Biochem Behav 42:229–232

Blessing WW (1990) Distribution of glutamate decarboxylase-containing neurons in rabbit medulla oblongata with attention to intramedullary and spinal projections. Neuroscience 37:171–185

Bohlhalter S, Mohler H, Fritschy J-M (1994) Inhibitory neurotransmission in rat spinal cord: co-localization of glycine- and $GABA_A$-receptors at GABAergic synaptic contacts demonstrated by triple immunofluorescence staining. Brain Res 642:59–69

Bolser DC, Blythin DJ, Chapman RW, Egan RW, Hey JA, Rizzo C, Kuo S-C, Kreutner W (1995) The pharmacology of SCH 50911: a novel, orally-active GABA-B receptor antagonist. J Pharmacol Exp Ther 274:1393–1398

Bonanno G, Raiteri M (1993) Multiple $GABA_B$ receptors. Trends Pharmacol Sci 14:259–261

Bormann J (1988) Electrophysiology of $GABA_A$ and $GABA_B$ receptor subtypes. Trends Neurosci 11:112–116

Bormann J, Feigenspan A (1995) $GABA_C$ receptors. Trends Neuroscience 18:515–519

Bourgoin S, Pohl M, Benoliel JJ, Maugorgne A, Collin E, Hamon M, Cesselin F (1992) γ-Aminobutyric acid, through $GABA_A$ receptors, inhibits the potassium-stimulated release of calcitonin gene-related peptide – but not that of substance P-like material from rat spinal cord slices. Brain Res 583:344–348

Bowery NG (1989) GABA$_B$ receptors and their significance in mammalian pharmacology. Trends Pharmacol Sci 10:401–407

Bowery NG (1993) GABA$_B$ receptor pharmacology. Annu Rev Pharmacol Toxicol 33:109–147

Bowery NG, Hudson AL, Price GW (1987) GABA$_A$ and GABA$_B$ receptor site distribution in the rat central nervous system. Neuroscience 20:365–383

Burt DR, Kamatchi GL (1991) GABA$_A$ receptor subtypes: from pharmacology to molecular biology. FASEB J 5:2916–2923

Carlton SM, Hayes ES (1990) Light microscopic and ultrastructural analysis of GABA-immunoreactive profiles in the monkey spinal cord. J Comp Neurol 300:162–182

Carlton SM, Westlund KN, Zhang D, Willis WD (1992) GABA-immunoreactive terminals synapse on primate spinothalamic tract cells. J Comp Neurol 322:528–537

Castro-Lopes JM, Tavares I, Tölle TR, Coito A, Coimbra A (1992) Increase in GABAergic cells and GABA levels in the spinal cord in unilateral inflammation of the hindlimb in the rat. Eur J Neurosci 4:296–301

Castro-Lopes JM, Tavares I, Coimbra A (1993) GABA decreases in the spinal cord dorsal horn after peripheral neurectomy. Brain Res 620:287–291

Castro-Lopes JM, Tavares I, Tölle TR, Coimbra A (1994a) Carrageenan-induced inflammation of the hind foot provokes a rise of GABA-immunoreactive cells in the rat spinal cord that is prevented by peripheral neurectomy or neonatal capsaicin treatment. Pain 56:193–201

Castro-Lopes JM, Tölle TR, Pan B, Zieglgänsberger W (1994b) Expression of GAD mRNA in spinal cord neurons of normal and monoarthritic rats. Mol Brain Res 26:169–176

Castro-Lopes JM, Malcangio M, Pan B, Bowery NG (1995) Complex changes of GABA$_A$ and GABA$_B$ receptor binding in the spinal cord dorsal horn following peripheral inflammation or neurectomy. Brain Res 679:289–297

Cho HJ, Basbaum AI (1991) GABAergic circuitry in the rostral ventral medulla of the rat and its relationship to descending antinociceptive controls. J Comp Neurol 303:316–328

Clavier N, Lombard M-C, Besson J-M (1992) Benzodiazepines and pain: effects of midazolam on the activities of nociceptive non-specific dorsal horn neurons in the rat spinal cord. Pain 48:61–71

Crawford ME, Jensen FM, Toftdahl DB, Madsen JB (1993) Direct spinal effect of intrathecal and extradural midazolam on visceral noxious stimulation in rabbits. Br J Anaesth 70:642–646

Daly EC (1990) The biochemistry of glycinergic neurons. In: Ottersen OP, Storm-Mathiesen J (eds) Glycine neurotransmission. Wiley, Chicester, pp 25–66

Depaulis A, Morgan MM, Liebeskind JC (1987) GABAergic modulation of the analgesic effect of morphine microinjected in the ventral periaqueductal grey matter of the rat. Brain Res 436:223–228

Désarmenien M, Feltz P, Occhipinti G, Santangelo F, Schlicter R (1984) Coexistence of GABA$_A$ and GABA$_B$ receptors on Aδ and C primary afferents. Br J Pharmacol 81:327–333

Dickenson AH, Brewer CM, Hayes NA (1985) Effects of topical baclofen on C fibre-evoked neuronal activity in the rat dorsal horn. Neuroscience 14:557–562

Dirig DM, Yaksh TL (1995) Intrathecal baclofen and muscimol, but not midazolam are antinociceptive in the rat-formalin model. J Pharmacol Exp Ther 275:219–227

Drower EJ, Hammond DL (1988) GABAergic modulation of nociceptive threshold: effects of THIP and bicuculline microinjected in the ventral medulla of the rat. Brain Res 450:316–324

Frenk H, Bossut D, Urca G, Mayer DJ (1988) Is substance P a primary afferent neurotransmitter for nociceptive input? I. Analysis of pain-related behaviors resulting from intrathecal administration of substance P and 6 excitatory compounds. Brain Res 455:223–231

Fritschy JM, Mohler H (1995) $GABA_A$-receptor heterogeneity in the adult rat brain: differential regional and cellular distribution of seven major subunits. J Comp Neurol 359:154–194

Fuji K, Senba E, Fuji S, Nomura I, Wu J-Y, Ueda Y, Tohyama M (1985) Distribution, ontogeny and projections of cholecystokinin-8, vasoactive intestinal polypeptide and γ-aminobutyrate-containing neuron systems in the rat spinal cord: an immuno-histochemical study. Neuroscience 14:881–894

Gao B, Fritschy JM, Benke D, Mohler H (1993) Neuron-specific expression of $GABA_A$-receptor subtypes: differential association of the α_1- and α_3-subunits with serotonergic and GABAergic neurons. Neuroscience 54:881–892

Go VLW, Yaksh TL (1987) Release of substance P from the cat spinal cord. J Physiol (Lond) 391:141–167

Hama AT, Fritschy J-M, Seighart W, Hammond DL (1995) $GABA_A$ recetpor subunits on bulbospinal neurons of the rat. Soc Neurosci Abstr 21:1639

Hammond DL (1986) Control systems for nociceptive afferent processing: the descending inhibitory pathways. In: Yaksh TL (ed) Spinal afferent processing. Plenum, New York, pp 363–390

Hammond DL, Drower EJ (1984) Effects of intrathecally administered THIP, baclofen and muscimol on nociceptive threshold. Eur J Pharmacol 103:121–125

Hammond DL, Washington JD (1993) Antagonism of L-baclofen-induced antino-ciception by CGP 35,348 in the spinal cord of the rat. Eur J Pharmacol 234:255–262

Hao J-X, Xu X-J, Aldskogius H, Seiger Å, Wiesenfeld-Hallin Z (1991) Allodynia-like effect in rat after ischaemic spinal cord injury photochemically induced by laser irradiation. Pain 45:175–185

Hao J-X, Xu X-J, Yu Y-X, Seiger Å, Wiesenfeld-Hallin Z (1992) Baclofen reverses the hypersensitivity of dorsal horn wide dynamic range neurons to mechanical stimu-lation after transient spinal cord ischemia: implications for a tonic GABAergic inhibitory control of myelinated fiber input. J Neurophysiol 68:392–396

Hao J-X, Xu X-J, Wiesenfeld-Hallin Z (1994) Intrathecal γ-aminobutyric acid$_B$ ($GABA_B$) receptor antagonist CGP 35348 induces hypersensitivity to mechanical stimuli in the rat. Neurosci Lett 182:299–302

Hayes ES, Carlton SM (1992) Primary afferent interactions: analysis of calcitonin gene-related peptide-immunoreactive terminals in contact with unlabeled and GABA-immunoreactive profiles in the monkey dorsal horn. Neuroscience 47:873–896

Heinricher MM, Kaplan HJ (1991) GABA-mediated inhibition in rostral ventromedial medulla: role in nociceptive modulation in the lightly anesthetized rat. Pain 47:105–113

Heinricher MM, Tortorici V (1994) Interference with GABA transmission in the rostral ventromedial medulla: disinhibition of off-cells as a central mechanism in nociceptive modulation. Neuroscience 63:533–546

Henry JL (1982) Effects of intravenously administered enantiomers of baclofen on functionally identified units in lumbar dorsal horn of the spinal cat. Neuropharmacology 21:1073–1083

Holmes BB, Fujimoto JM (1994) [D-Pen^2-D-Pen^5]enkephalin, a delta opioid agonist, given intracerebroventricularly in the mouse produces antinociception through mediation of spinal GABA receptors. Pharmacol Biochem Behav 49:675–682

Hwang AS, Wilcox GL (1989) Baclofen, γ-aminobutyric acid$_B$ receptors and substance P in the mouse spinal cord. J Pharmacol Exp Ther 248:1026–1033

Ibuki T, Hama AT, Wang X-T, Pappas GD, Sagen J (1996) Loss of GABA-immunore-activity in the spinal dorsal horn of rats with peripheral nerve injury and promo-tion of recovery by adrenal medullary grafts. Neuroscience (in press)

Jones BE, Holmes CJ, Rodriguez-Veiga E, Mainville L (1991) GABA-synthesizing neurons in the medulla: their relationship to serotonin-containing and spinally projecting neurons in the rat. J Comp Neurol 313:349–367

Jones SL (1992) Descending control of nociception. In: Light AR (ed) The initial processing of pain and its descending control: spinal and trigeminal systems. Karger, Basel, pp 201–295

Jones SL, Sedivec MJ, Light AR (1990) Effects of iontophoresed opioids on physiologically characterized laminae I and II dorsal horn neurons in the cat spinal cord.
Brain Res 532:160–174

Jurna I (1984) Depression of nociceptive sensory activity in the rat spinal cord due to the
intrathecal administration of drugs: effects of diazepam. Neurosurgery 15:917–920

Kangrga I, Jiang M, Randic M (1991) Actions of (–) baclofen on rat dorsal horn
neurons. Brain Res 562:265–275

Kerr DIB, Ong J (1992) GABA agonists and antagonists. Med Res Rev 12:593–636

Kerr DIB, Ong J (1995) GABA$_B$ receptors. Pharmacol Ther 67:187–246

Kihara M, Kubo T (1989) Immunocytochemical localization of GABA containing
neurons in the ventrolateral medulla oblongata of the rat. Histochemistry 91:309–
314

Killian P, Holmes BB, Takemori AE, Portoghese PS, Fujimoto JM (1995) Cold water
swim stress- and delta-2 opioid-induced analgesia are modulated by spinal γ-
aminobutyric acid$_A$ receptors. J Pharmacol Exp Ther 274:730–734

Kwiat GC, Liu H, Williamson AM, Basbaum AI (1993) GABAergic regulation of
noradrenergic spinal projection neurons of the A5 cell group in the rat: an electron
microscopic analysis. J Comp Neurol 330:557–570

Larson AA (1989) Intrathecal GABA, glycine, taurine or beta-alanine elicits
dyskinetic movement in mice. Pharmacol Biochem Behav 32:505–509

Levy RA, Proudfit HK (1979) Analgesia produced by microinjection of baclofen and
morphine at brain stem sites. Eur J Pharmacol 57:43–55

Lin Q, Peng Y, Willis WD (1994) Glycine and GABA$_A$ antagonists reduce the inhibition of primate spinothalamic tract neurons produced by stimulation in
periaqueductal gray. Brain Res 654:286–302

Lin Q, Peng YB, Willis WD (1996) Role of GABA receptor subtypes in inhibition of
primate spinothalamic tract neurons: difference between spinal and periaqueductal gray inhibition. J Neurophysiol 75:109–122

Lovick TA (1987) Tonic GABAergic and cholinergic influences on pain control and
cardiovascular control neurones in nucleus paragigantocellularis lateralis in the
rat. Pain 31:401–409

Ma W, Saunders PA, Somogyi R, Poulter MO, Barker J (1993) Ontogeny of GABA$_A$
receptor subunit mRNAs in rat spinal cord and dorsal root ganglia. J Comp Neurol
338:337–359

MacDonald RL, Olsen RW (1994) GABA$_A$ receptor channels. Annu Rev Neurosci
17:569–602

Malcangio M, Bowery NG (1993) γ-aminobutyric acid$_B$, but not γ-aminobutyric acid$_A$
receptor activation, inhibits electrically evoked substance P-like immunoreactivity
release from the rat spinal cord in vitro. J Pharmacol Exp Ther 266:1490–1496

Malcangio M, Bowery NG (1994) Spinal cord SP release and hyperalgesia in
monoarthritic rats: involvement of the GABA$_B$ receptor system. Br J Pharmacol
113:1561–1566

Malcangio M, Da Silva H, Bowery NG (1993) Plasticity of GABA$_B$ receptor in rat
spinal cord detected by autoradiography. Eur J Pharmacol 250:153–156

Malosio M-L, Marquèze-Pouey B, Kuhse J, Betz H (1991) Widespread expression of
glycine receptor subunit mRNAs in the adult and developing rat brain. EMBO J
10:2401–2409

McGowan MK, Hammond DL (1993a) Antinociception produced by microinjection of
L-glutamate into the ventromedial medulla of the rat: mediation by spinal GABA$_A$
receptors. Brain Res 620:86–96

McGowan MK, Hammond DL (1993b) Intrathecal GABA$_B$ antagonists attenuate the
antinociception produced by microinjection of L-glutamate into the ventromedial
medulla of the rat. Brain Res 607:39–46

Millhorn DE, Hokfelt T, Seroogy K, Oertel W, Verhofstad AAJ, Wu JY (1987)
Immunohistochemical evidence for colocalization of gamma-aminobutyric acid
and serotonin in neurons of the ventral medulla oblongata projecting to the spinal
cord. Brain Res 410:179–185

Mitchell K, Spike RC, Todd AJ (1993) An immunocytochemical study of glycine receptor and GABA in laminae I-III of rat spinal dorsal horn. J Neurosci 13:2371–2381

Miyata Y, Otsuka M (1975) Quantitative histochemistry of gamma-aminobutyric acid in cat spinal cord with special reference to presynaptic inhibition. J Neurochem 25:239–244

Moreau JL, Fields HL (1986) Evidence for GABA involvement in midbrain control of medullary neurons that modulate nociceptive transmission. Brain Res 397:37–46

Mott DD, Lewis DV (1994) The pharmacology and function of central GABA$_B$ receptors. Int Rev Neurobiol 36:97–223

Nagai T, McGeer PL, McGeer EG (1983) Distribution of GABA-T-intensive neurons in the rat forebrain and midbrain. J Comp Neurol 218:220–238

Nagai T, Maeda T, Imai H, McGeer PL, McGeer EG (1985) Distribution of GABA-T-intensive neurons in the rat hindbrain. J Comp Neurol 231:260–269

Nahin RL, Hylden JLK (1991) Peripheral inflammation is associated with increased glutamic acid decarboxylase immunoreactivity in the rat spinal cord. Neurosci Lett 128:226–230

Niv D, Whitwam JG, Loh L (1983) Depression of nociceptive sympathetic reflexes by the intrathecal administration of midazolam. Br J Anaesth 55:541–547

Niv D, Davidovich S, Geller E, Urca G (1988) Analgesic and hyperalgesic effects of midazolam: dependence on route of administration. Anesth Analg 67:1169–1173

Olivéras JL (1995) Cortical application of picrotoxin as a model of central pain in the rat. Soc Neurosci Abstr 21:650

Olivéras J-L, Montagne-Clavel J (1994) The GABA$_A$ receptor antagonist picrotoxin induces a "pain-like" behavior when administered into the thalamic reticular nucleus of the behaving rat: a possible model for "central" pain? Neurosci Lett 179:21–24

Olsen RW, McCabe RT, Wamsley JK (1990) GABA$_A$ receptor subtypes: autoradiographic comparison of GABA, benzodiazepine and convulsant binding sites in the rat central nervous system. J Chem Neuroanat 3:59–76

Ottersen OP, Storm-Mathiesen J (1984) Glutamate-and GABA-containing neurons in the mouse and rat brain, as demonstrated with a new immunocytochemical technique. J Comp Neurol 229:374–392

Palacios JM, Wamsley JK, Kuhar MJ (1981) High affinity GABA receptors-autoradiographic localization. Brain Res 222:285–307

Pan ZZ, Williams JT, Osborne PB (1990) Opioid actions on single nucleus raphe magnus neurons from rat and guinea-pig in vitro. J Physiol (Lond) 427:519–532

Patrick JT, McBride WJ, Felten DL (1983) Distribution of glycine, GABA, aspartate, and glutamate in the rat spinal cord. Brain Res Bull 10:415–418

Poore LH, Helmstetter FJ (1994) Forebrain modulation of nociceptive reflexes: effects of GABA antagonists in the amygdala. Soc Neurosci Abstr 20:767

Price GW, Wilkin GP, Turnbull MJ, Bowery NG (1984) Are baclofen-sensitive GABA$_B$ receptors present on primary afferent terminals of the spinal cord? Nature 307:71–74

Probst A, Cortés R, Palacios JM (1986) The distribution of glycine receptors in the human brain. A light microscopic autoradiographic study using [3H]strychnine. Neuroscience 17:11–35

Rabow LE, Russek SJ, Farb DH (1995) From ion currents to genomic analysis: recent advances in GABA$_A$ receptor research. Synapse 21:189–274

Rady JJ, Fujimoto JM (1995) Spinal GABA receptors mediate brain delta opioid analgesia in Swiss Webster mice. Pharmacol Biochem Behav 51:655–659

Reichling DB, Basbaum AI (1990a) Contribution of brainstem GABAergic circuitry to descending antinociceptive controls. I. GABA-immunoreactive projection neurons in the periaqueductal gray and nucleus raphe magnus. J Comp Neurol 302:370–377

Reichling DB, Basbaum AI (1990b) Contribution of brainstem GABAergic circuitry to descending antinociceptive controls. II. Electron microscopic immunocytochemical evidence of GABAergic control over the projection from the periaqueductal gray to the nucleus raphe magnus in the rat. J Comp Neurol 302:378–393

Renno WM, Mullett MA, Beitz AJ (1992) Systemic morphine reduces GABA release in the lateral but not the medial portion of the midbrain periaqueductal gray of the rat. Brain Res 594:221–232

Richards JG, Schoch P, Haring P, Takacs B, Mohler H (1987) Resolving GABA$_A$/ benzodiazepine receptors: cellular and subcellular localization in the CNS with monoclonal antibodies. J Neurosci 7:1866–1886

Roberts LA, Beyer C, Komisaruk BR (1986) Nociceptive responses to altered GABAergic activity at the spinal cord. Life Sci 39:1667–1674

Roberts WA, Eaton SA, Salt TE (1992) Widely distributed GABA-mediate afferent inhibition processes within the ventrobasal thalamus of rat and their possible relevance to pathological pain states and somatotopic plasticity. Exp Brain Res 89:363–372

Romandini S, Samanin R (1984) Muscimol injection in the nucleus raphe dorsalis blocks the antinociceptive effect of morphine in rats: apparent lack of 5-hydroxytryptamine involvement in muscimol's effects. Br J Pharmacol 81:25–29

Sandkühler J, Willman E, Fu Q-G (1989) Blockade of GABA$_A$ receptors in the midbrain periaqueductal gray abolishes nociceptive spinal dorsal horn neuronal activity. Eur J Pharmacol 160:163–166

Sawynok J, Dickson C (1985) D-Baclofen is an antagonist at baclofen receptors mediating antinociception in the spinal cord. Pharmacology 31:248–259

Sawynok J, Kato N, Havlicek V, LaBella FS (1982) Lack of effect of baclofen on substance P and somatostatin release from the spinal cord in vitro. Naunyn Schmied Arch Pharmacol 319:78–81

Serrao JM, Stubbs SC, Goodchild CS, Gent JP (1989) Intrathecal midazolam and fentanyl in the rat: evidence for different spinal antinociceptive effects. Anesthesiology 70:780–786

Sherman SE, Loomis CW (1994) Morphine insensitive allodynia is produced by intrathecal strychnine in the lightly anesthetized rat. Pain 56:17–29

Sieghart W (1995) Structure and pharmacology of γ-aminobutyric acid$_A$ receptor subtypes. Pharmacol Rev 47:181–234

Singer E, Placheta P (1980) Reduction of [3H]muscimol binding sites in rat dorsal spinal cord after neonatal capsaicin. Brain Res 202:484–487

Sivilotti L, Woolf CJ (1994) The contribution of GABA$_A$ and glycine receptors to central sensitization: disinhibition and touch-evoked allodynia in the spinal cord. J Neurophysiol 72:169–179

Sluka KA, Willis WD, Westlund KN (1993) Joint inflammation and hyperalgesia are reduced by spinal bicuculline. Neuroreport 5:109–112

Sluka KA, Willis WD, Westlund KN (1994) Inflammation-induced release of excitatory amino acids is prevented by spinal administration of a GABA$_A$ but not by a GABA$_B$ receptor antagonist in rats. J Pharmacol Exp Ther 271:76–82

Smith GD, Harrison SM, Birch PJ, Elliott PJ, Malcangio M, Bowery NG (1994) Increased sensitivity to the antinociceptive activity of (±) baclofen in an animal model of chronic neuropathic, but not chronic inflammatory hyperalgesia. Neuropharmacology 33:1103–1108

Sorkin LS, McAdoo DJ, Willis WD (1993) Raphe magnus stimulation-induced antinociception in the cat is associated with release of amino acids as well as serotonin in the lumbar dorsal horn. Brain Res 618:95–108

Stephenson FA (1995) The GABA$_A$ receptors. Biochem J 310:1–9

Sugimoto T, Bennett GJ, Kajander KC (1990) Transsynaptic degeneration in the superficial dorsal horn after sciatic nerve injury: effects of a chronic constriction injury, transection, and strychnine. Pain 42:205–213

Thomas DA, McGowan MK, Hammond DL (1995) Microinjection of baclofen in the ventromedial medulla of the rat produces antinociception or hyperalgesia. J Pharmacol Exp Ther 275:274–284

Thomas DA, Naverette I, Graham BA, McGowan MK, Hammond DL (1996) Antinociception produced by systemic R(+)-baclofen hydrochloride is attenuated by CGP 35348 administered to the spinal cord or ventromedial medulla. Brain Res 718:129–137

Todd AJ, Lochhead V (1990) GABA-like immunoreactivity in type I glomeruli of rat substantia gelatinosa. Brain Res 514:171–174

Todd AJ, McKenzie J (1989) GABA-immunoreactive neurons in the dorsal horn of the rat spinal cord. Neuroscience 31:799–806

Todd AJ, Sullivan AC (1990) Light microscope study of the coexistence of GABA-like and glycine-like immunoreactivities in the spinal cord of the rat. J Comp Neurol 296:496–505

van den Pol AN, Gorcs T (1988) Glycine and glycine receptorimmunoreactivity in brain and spinal cord. J Neurosci 8:472–492

Vandenberg RJ, Schofield PR (1994) Inhibitory ligand-gated ion channel receptors: molecular biology and pharmacology of $GABA_A$ and glycine receptors. In: Peracchia C (ed) Handbook of membrane channels: molecular and cellular physiology. Academic, San Diego, pp 317–332

Waldvogel HJ, Faull RLM, Jansen KLR, Dragunow M, Richards JG, Mohler H, Street P (1990) GABA, GABA receptors and benzodiazepine receptors in the human spinal cord: an autoradiographic and immunohistochemical study at the light and electron microscopic levels. Neuroscience 39:361–385

Willcockson WS, Chung JM, Hori Y, Lee KH, Willis WD (1984) Effects of iontophoretically released amino acids and amines on primate spinothalamic tract cells. J Neurosci 4:732–740

Williams FG, Beitz AJ (1990) Ultrastructural morphometric analysis of GABA-immunoreactive terminals in the ventrocaudal periaqueductal grey: analysis of the relationship of GABA terminals and the $GABA_A$ receptor to periaqueductal grey-raphe magnus projection neurons. J Neurocytol 19:686–696

Wilson PR, Yaksh TL (1978) Baclofen is antinociceptive in the spinal intrathecal space of animals. Eur J Pharmacol 51:323–330

Wisden W, Laurie DJ, Monyer H, Seeburg PH (1992) The distribution of 13 $GABA_A$ receptor subunit mRNAs in the rat brain. I. Telencephalon, diencephalon, mesencephalon. J Neurosci 12:1040–1062

Yaksh TL (1989) Behavioral and autonomic correlates of the tactile-evoked allodynia produced by spinal glycine inhibition: effects of modulatory receptor systems and excitatory amino acid antagonists. Pain 37:111–123

Yaksh TL, Reddy SVR (1981) Studies in the primate on the analgetic effects associated with intrathecal actions of opiate, alpha-adrenergic agonists and baclofen. Anesthesiology 54:451–467

Yamamoto T, Yaksh TL (1991) Spinal pharmacology of thermal hyperesthesia induced by incomplete ligation of sciatic nerve. Anesthesiology 75:817–826

Yamamoto T, Yaksh TL (1993) Effects of intrathecal strychnine and bicuculline on nerve compression-induced thermal hyperalgesia and selective antagonism by MK-801. Pain 54:79–84

Zambotti F, Zonta N, Parenti M, Tommasi R, Vicentini L, Conci F, Mantegazza P (1982) Periaqueductal gray matter involvement in the muscimol-induced decrease of morphine antinociception. Naunyn Schmiedebergs Arch Pharmacol 318:368–369

Zambotti F, Zonta J, Tammiso R, Conci F, Hafner B, Zecca L, Ferrario P, Mantegazza P (1991) Effects of diazepam on nociception in rats. Naunyn Schmied Arch Pharmacol 344:84–89

Zarbin MA, Wamsley JK, Kuhar MJ (1981) Glycine receptor: light microscopic autoradiographic localization with [^{3}H]strychnine. J Neurosci 1:532–547

Zhang A-L, Hao J-X, Seiger Å, Xu X-J, Wiesenfeld-Hallin Z, Grant G, Aldskogius H (1994) Decreased GABA immunoreactivity in spinal cord dorsal horn neurons after transient spinal cord ischemia in the rat. Brain Res 656:187–190

CHAPTER 15

The Role of Descending Noradrenergic and Serotoninergic Pathways in the Modulation of Nociception: Focus on Receptor Multiplicity

M.J. Millan

A. General Introduction

Monoamines play a key role in the modulation of nociception at all levels of the neuroaxis; on cutaneous (and other) nocisponsive fibres in interaction with sympathetic terminals; in the dorsal horn (DH) of the spinal cord, the site of primary processing of afferent nociceptive information; in the thalamus and other targets of ascending nociceptive information wherein the integration of nociceptive input is pursued; and in those higher limbic and cortical structures responsible for the conscious (cognitive and emotional) appreciation of pain. Perhaps the most familiar of these roles is the ability of monoamines to modify the flow of nociceptive information to the brain via an action in the DH of the spinal cord. In this respect there is fragmentary evidence that dopamine, possibly by antinociceptive and pronociceptive actions at dopamine D_2 and D_1 receptors, respectively, may be implicated (BJÖRKLUND and SKAGERSBERG 1982; BOURGOIN et al. 1993; FLEETWOOD-WALKER et al. 1988; KIRITSKY-ROY et al. 1994; SCATTON et al. 1984). Further, the recent discovery of dopamine D_4 receptors in human spinal cord (MATSUMOTO et al. 1996) suggests that a role of other dopamine receptor types in spinal mechanisms for the modulation of nociception should not be ignored. However, the vast majority of available data concerning the integration of nociceptive information in the DH relates to the role of adrenergic and serotoninergic mechanisms. They thus comprise the principal focus of the present article. Evidence in favour of descending inhibition has been reviewed elsewhere (ADVOKAT 1988; BASBAUM and FIELDS 1984; LE BARS 1988; MILLAN 1995; PROUDFIT 1992; STAMFORD 1995). Here emphasis is afforded to the remarkable multiplicity of adrenergic (AR) and serotoninergic receptors which has emerged over the past 5 years, and which has yet to be fully assimilated into studies of pain and its modulation.

B. Control of Sympathetic and Motor Function at the Segmental Level: Relevance to Pain and Its Modulation

Before embarking on a detailed discussion of the role of noradrenaline (NAD) and serotonin (5-HT) in the DH in the modulation of nociception, it is important to point out that adrenergic and serotoninergic fibres provide an intense innervation of the sympathetic and parasympathetic nuclei of the thoraco-lumbar intermediolateral cell column (IML) and sacral intermediate zone, respectively (see COOTE 1988; MILLAN 1995; PROUDFIT 1992; WU and WESSENDORF 1993). Adrenergic and serotoninergic mechanisms play a key role therein the control of autonomic and cardiovascular function (COOTE 1988; EISENACH 1994; LOEWY 1990; MARKS et al. 1990; SOLOMON et al. 1989). This is of significance in several respects.

First, in algesiometric tests care should be taken that autonomic/cardio-vascular effects do not interfere with test results (LIN et al. 1993; LIGHTMAN et al. 1993). Further, in addition to the impact of drugs upon autonomic function at the level of the IML, the possibility of rostral drug distribution leading to cardiovascular side effects by actions in the brainstem should be recalled (EISENACH 1994; EISENACH et al. 1993; HAYASHI and MAZE 1993; HORVÁTH et al. 1994; MARWAHA et al. 1983; McCALL and CLEMENT 1994). Second, the sympathetic system may contribute to the maintenance of certain painful states, including reflex sympathetic dystrophy in humans (SCHOTT 1995). Con-sequently inhibition of sympathetic activity may alleviate such conditions (see CAMPBELL et al. 1992; DELLEMIJN et al. 1994; VERDUGO and OCHOA 1994). Indeed, in addition to peripheral (pro- and antinociceptive) actions at sympa-thetic terminals themselves (BYAS-SMITH 1995; KHASAR et al. 1995; OUSEPH and LEVINE 1995), a component of the antinociceptive actions of α_2-AR ago-nists (in particular, against neuropathic pain) may reflect inhibition of sympathetic outflow at the spinal level (RAUCK et al. 1993; YAKSH et al. 1995). Third, peripherally administered adrenergic drugs increase arterial pressure by vaso constriction and activation of high pressure baroceptors leads to a stimulation of vagal afferents and subsequently the engagement of descending adrenergic (and cholinergic) pathways mediating antinociception (REN et al. 1988, 1991; RANDICH and MAIXNER 1984; THURSTON and HELTON 1996; WATKINS et al. 1990). Thus, a modulation of sympathetic and/or para-sympathetic outflow at the segmental level leading to changes in arterial pressure may ultimately feedback onto the DH to modify nociceptive process-ing. Motoneurones (MNs) in the ventral horn (VH) are also subject to a pronounced and complex pattern of adrenergic and serotoninergic influence (CONNELL et al. 1989; GERIN et al. 1995; GUYENET et al. 1994; HOLSTEGE and KUYPERS 1987; HOWE et al. 1987; PALMERI and WIESENDENGER 1990; WALLIS 1994; WU and WESSENDORF 1993). Such actions are expressed behaviourally in a spectrum of motor effects (BERVOETS and MILLAN 1994; EIDE and HOLE 1991; FONE et al. 1991; XU et al. 1994b) and may potentially modify per-formance in algesiometric paradigms – although motor actions in the VH do *not* themselves account for the antinociceptive actions of α_2-AR agonists (HÄMÄLÄINEN et al. 1995). Rostral drug transfer to the brain may also be of significance in the induction of motor sedation (EISENACH 1994; HAYASHI and MAZE 1993).

C. Noradrenaline, Adrenaline and Adrenergic Receptors

I. Multiple Adrenergic Receptors

Multiple types of α_1-AR, α_2-AR and β-AR have been cloned (Table 1) the physiological significance of which is still under exploration. Spinal populations of α_2-ARs have long been implicated in the modulation of nociception, and their activation elicits robust antinociception under many conditions. They thus comprise the focus of the present discussion, in particular the potential significance of specific α_2-AR subtypes. As regards α_1-ARs, they are present at only low concentrations in the DH, and only fragmentary data for pro- and/or antinociceptive actions in the DH are available, while there is currently little information pertaining to the significance of α_{1A}-AR, α_{1B}-AR and α_{1D}-AR subtypes in the modulation of nociception (HAYES et al. 1986; HOWE et al. 1983; JONES 1992; PIERIBONE et al. 1994). There is evidence for a low level of mRNA encoding β_1-ARs in the spinal cord (NICHOLAS et al. 1993a), and β-ARs may be localized on capsaicin-sensitize primary afferents (PATTERSON and HARDEY 1987), but functional evidence for a role of spinal β-ARs in the modulation of nociception is as yet lacking (YAKSH 1985).

Table 1. Multiple adrenergic receptors (ARs) and pain: key characteristics

Receptor type	Transduction mechanisms	Selective agonist	Selective antagonist	DH	DRG	IML	SYMG	VH
α_{1A}	↑ g Ca²⁺	Oxymetazoline	(+)-Niguldipine	(++)	?	(++)	?	(++)
α_{1B}	↑ PLC	–	CEC	+	0	++	0	++
α_{1D}	↑ gCa²⁺	NAD	BMY 7378	0	0	0	0	++
rα_{2A}	⎰↓AC/	Guanabenz	BRL 44408	+++	+	+++	++	+/0
hα_{2A}	⎱↑ gK⁺/↓ gCa²⁺	Guanfacine		+++	?	++	?	++
rα_{2B}	⎰↓AC/		Prazosin	0	+	0	++	0
hα_{2B}	⎱↑ gK⁺/↓ gCa²⁺	–	ARC 239	++	?	+++	?	++
rα_{2C}	⎰↓ AC	–	Prazosin	+	+++	0	++	++
hα_{2C}	⎱↑ gK⁺/↓ gCa²⁺		ARC 239	+	?	+	?	+/0
β_1	↑ AC	Xamoterol	Betaxolol	+	0	0	0	0
β_2	↑ AC	Salbutamol	ICI 118551	0	0	0	0	0
β_3	↑ AC	CL 316243	SR 59396	?	?	?	?	?

NAD, Noradrenaline; AC, adenyl cyclase; PLC, phospholipase C; DH, dorsal horn; DRG, dorsal root ganglion; IML, intermediolateral cell column; SYMG, sympathetic ganglion; VH, ventral horn. The rα_{2A}-AR is the rat homologue of the human hα_{2A}-AR and is also known as the α_{2D} site. Many "selective" ligands have other activities but are useful for differentiating amongst adrenergic receptor subtypes, e.g. oxymetazoline (2A); (+)-nigulpidine (Ca²⁺ channels); BMY 7378 (5-HT$_{1A}$) and prazosin (α_1). CEC (chlorethylclonidine) irreversibly inactivates α_{1B} and to a lesser extent α_{1D} sites. Other preferential α_2-AR subtype ligands are discussed in the text. Only major transduction mechanisms, if possible for native populations, are given. Other transduction systems and cell-specific coupling mechanisms should not be ignored. The localization of α_{1A}-ARs is extrapolated from functional rather than neuroanatomical studies and requires direct demonstration. α_1-ARs are likely upregulated and/or "upmodulated" on primary afferents in some painful conditions.

II. Functional Organization of Noradrenergic and Adrenergic Input to the Dorsal Horn

1. Origins of Descending Noradrenergic and Adrenergic Pathways

Adrenergic pathways derived from medullary C1 and C2 nuclei and noradrenergic pathways derived from pontine A5, A6 (locus coeruleus (LC) and A7/ (subcoeruleus) clusters, provide a rich innervation of the spinal cord. The relative contribution of these noradrenergic cell groups is still under discussion, and not only inter-species differences may exist but even genetic differences within a single rat strain (CLARK et al 1991; KWIAT and BASBAUM 1992; PROUDFIT 1992). There is a dense plexus of terminals in structures involved in the reception, processing and rostrad transfer of nociceptive information: superficial laminae I and II, deeper laminae IV and V and the central grey matter surrounding the central canal, lamina X (CLARK and PROUDFIT 1991; FRITSCHY and GRZANNA 1990; KWIAT and BASBAUM 1992; LAMOTTE 1986; PROUDFIT 1992; WESTLUND 1992). Indeed, lamina I and II and, less markedly, lamina V receive an intense input from small-diameter, high-threshold, nocisponsive, primary afferent $A\delta$ and C fibres (BESSON and CHAOUCH 1987; FIELDS et al. 1991) which co-release calcitonin gene related peptide (CGRP), substance P and glutamate (GLU), the actions of which are mediated co-operatively by CGRP (1 or 2), neurokinin type 1/2 and α-amino-3-hydroxy-5-methyl-4-isoxazolepropionic acid (AMPA)/metabotropic/N-methyl-D-aspatate (NMDA) receptors, respectively (DICKENSON 1990; SEGUIN et al. 1995; URBAN et al. 1994; WILLIS 1994). Further, both superficial (I) and deeper (IV/V) laminae, as well as lamina X, are the origin of ascending pathways via which nociceptive information reaches the brain (BESSON and CHAOUCH 1987). There is a significant co-existence of NAD with other transmitters, such as GABA, in the LC (IJIMA et al. 1992). A question of current interest is the synaptic relationships between the terminals of noradrenergic projections and intrinsic DH neurones. In this regard, the possibility of volume transmission (possibly involving glia cells) has been evoked (see RIDET et al. 1993, 1994). Nevertheless, there is convincing anatomical (DOYLE and MAXWELL 1991a,b; SATOH et al. 1982; see WESTLUND 1992; WILLIS 1992) and functional evidence (see below) that NAD (and adrenaline) exert direct actions via α_2-ARs upon the activity of projection neurones (PNs), interneurones (INs) and, possibly, primary afferent terminals in the DH.

2. Influence on Projection Neurones and Interneurones in the Dorsal Horn

a) Inhibitory Actions

A major component of the antinociceptive actions of NAD and α_2-AR agonists in the DH is expressed postsynaptically to primary afferent fibres (PAFs), likely upon PNs. Of particular interest is the inhibitory influence of NAD and α_2-AR agonists upon the activity of those, "convergent", "multireceptorial" or "wide dynamic range" (WDR) neurones which are responsive to both noxious and innocuous input, and including spinocervical, spinomesencephalic and spinothalamic tract (STT) neurones: that is, the major routes for the rostrad transfer of nociceptive information to supraspinal centres (BESSON and CHAOUCH 1987). Inhibition of these neurones is exerted preferentially against noxious as compared to noxious-stimuli (however, see WILLIS 1988, 1992) and against stimulation of C and Aδ fibres versus Aβ fibre input upon the administration of α_2-AR agonists either locally by iontophoresis, by the intravenous route following disruption of descending pathways or topically by intrathecal administration onto the surface of the spinal cord (BELCHER et al. 1978; DAVIES and QUINLAN 1985; FLEETWOOD-WALKER 1992; FLEETWOOD-WALKER et al. 1985; HEADLEY et al. 1978; MURATA et al. 1989; SATOH et al. 1979; SULLIVAN et al. 1987, 1992b; WILLCOCKSON et al. 1984; ZHAO and DUGGAN 1987). NAD and α_2-AR agonists block the excitation of WDR neurones elicited by natural noxious stimuli and capsaisin as well as by GLU and substance P, indicative of actions *postsynaptic* to PAF terminals. Further, the ability of α_2-AR agonists to suppress the *spontaneous* firing of STT PNs is consistent with a direct action postsynaptic to primary afferents (BELCHER et al. 1978; MURATA et al. 1989; PERTOVAARA et al. 1993; WILLCOCKSON et al. 1984).

The above actions are pharmacologically well-defined; thus they are seen across a number of species with several α_2-AR agonists, with L-NAD but not its inactive isomer D-NAD, and they are blocked by selective α_2-AR antagonists (see above citations). Although this pattern of effects has been best documented in deeper (IV/V) laminae, clear-cut inhibitory actions of NAD and α_2-AR agonists against GLU and noxious stimuli have also been obtained in superficial (I/II) laminae, employing both iontophoretic and systemic administration and recordings from identified PNs – including STT units (DAVIES and QUINLAN 1985; FLEETWOOD-WALKER 1992; FLEETWOOD-WALKER et al. 1985; HEADLEY et al. 1978; WILLIS 1992). In line with these observations, a hyperpolarizing influence of NAD has been shown in intracellular recordings of substantia gelatinosa (laminae I) cells in vitro: this action is direct and is accompanied by a decrease in spontaneous firing rate reflecting an α_2-AR-mediated opening of K^+ channels (NORTH and YOSHIMURA 1984).

b) Excitatory Actions

Interestingly, NORTH and YOSHIMURA (1984) also provided in vitro evidence for an excitatory action of NAD or some neurones in superficial laminae, and there have also been reports of excitatory actions of NAD on lamina I/II cells in vivo (FLEETWOOD-WALKER 1992; HOWE and ZIEGLGÄNSBERGER 1987; MILLAR and WILLIAMS 1989; MILLER and PROUDFIT 1990; TODD and MILLAR 1983) while stimulation in the vicinity of the periaqueductal grey (PAG), LC and other brainstem structures excites certain neurones in the DH (LIGHT et al. 1986; McMAHON and WALL 1988; MILLAR and WILLIAMS 1989; MOKHA et al. 1983).

Such effects might be related to the "paradoxical" ability of a low dose of intrathecal clonidine to release substance P and neurokinin A in rat spinal cord and to facilitate flexor reflexes (LUO and WIESENFELD-HALIN 1993; SULLIVAN et al. 1987; XU et al. 1992). It could be argued that an action of NAD is involved at highly sensitive α_2-AR autoreceptors inhibiting NAD release, thereby mimicking the effects of postsynaptic α_2-AR blockade. An alternative hypothesis, likewise consistent with the globally antinociceptive role of NAD at postsynaptic α_2-ARs, is that the excitatory actions of NAD in the DH are exerted at *inhibitory* INs (ININs) to PNs (MILLAR and WILLIAMS 1989; WILLIS 1992). However, it is unclear at the ionic level as to how *native* α_2-ARs mediate neuronal excitation (ENKVIST et al. 1996; JANSSON et al. 1995a,b), and one intruiging possibility is that α_1-ARs mediate the excitatory actions of NAD in the DH (BERGLES et al. 1996; DAVIES et al. 1988; FLEETWOOD-WALKER 1992; NORTH and YOSHIMURA 1984).

If excitatory actions of NAD are indeed expressed on ININs, this could explain the above-mentioned preferential blockade of the response of PNs to noxious stimuli in two ways: first, these (GABAergic?) ININs may be exclusively responsive to noxious stimuli, and, second, they may presynaptically inhibit the activity of nocisponsive Aδ and C fibres in superficial laminae (MILLAR and WILLIAMS 1989; WILLIS 1992). By way of analogy to the second of these mechanisms, it is possible that NAD, via α_2-ARs, inhibits excitatory INs (EXINs) in the DH (FIELDS et al. 1991; WILLIS 1992) and, should these be selectively responsive to noxious input, the preferential actions of NAD α_2-ARs and brainstem adrenergic stimulation upon nociceptive versus non-nociceptive input could also be explained. In some studies excitatory actions of NAD have been preferentially seen against low-threshold, *non*-noxious stimuli in superficial laminae (HOWE and ZIEGLGÄNSBERGER 1987; MILLAR and WILLIAMS 1989; TODD and MILLAR 1983), and their significance as regard Aβ fibre mediated mechanical allodynia require further elucidation. Further, the identity of the α-AR subtype involved in the excitation of DH neurones remains of importance to definitively determine.

3. Influence on Primary Afferent Fibres

An action of NAD on PAFs transmitting nociceptive information to the DH would also afford selective inhibition of noxious versus non-noxious excitation of PNs. One piece of supporting evidence is provided by the influence of NAD upon the excitability of C fibre terminals: however (a) both inhibitory and excitatory actions have been seen; (b) the pharmacology of these effects is poorly established; (c) they may reflect a local anaesthetic-like, nerve block (BUTTERWORTH and STRICHARTZ 1993; GAUMANN et al. 1990) – possibly independent of α_2-ARs; (d) they may be mediated indirectly since they are attenuated by interruption of synaptic transmission with Mg^{2+} or tetrodotoxin; and (e) it is possible that these effects reflect indirect changes in extracellular conductivity due to glial uptake of NAD (CALVILLO and GHIGNONE 1986;

CALVILLO et al. 1988; CURTIS et al. 1983; JEFTNIJA et al. 1981, 1983) Thus this presumed mechanism of a primary afferent depolarization-induced reduction in the release of substance P and other transmitters mediating nociceptive information in the DH requires further evaluation. Other studies have attempted to show that the release of substance P in the spinal cord is reduced by NAD and α_2-AR agonists. Thus veratridine or high K^+-induced release of substance P is reduced by clonidine and NAD, and this action is attenuated by α_2-AR antagonists (Go and YAKSH 1987; ONO et al. 1991; PANG and VASKO 1986). Further, employing a push-pull cannula implanted into the upper dorsal horn, KURAISHI et al. (1985) showed that NAD yohimbine-reversibly inhibits the release of substance P provoked by a noxious, mechanical stimulus.

These approaches do not clearly differentiate PAFs from other pools of substance P, that is, INs and bulbospinal pathways. To resolve this difficulty several types of study have been undertaken. First, employing an antibody microprobe implanted into the DH, LANG et al. (1994) showed that both NAD and α_2-AR agonists fail to modify the release of substance P provoked by C fibre stimulation in lamina II. Since this approach allows for some spatial resolution – and supraspinal sources of substance P had been surgically eliminated – the authors concluded that presynaptic inhibition does *not* occur. Second, CGRP is co-localized with substance P in PAFs (see CODERRE 1993); thus, although CGRP and substance P release may not invariably be correlated (COLLIN et al. 1994), co-modulation of their release would be consistent with the involvement of PAF pools of the latter. In a superfused preparation of the lumbar enlargement of rat spinal cord, BOURGOIN et al. (1993) reported that, in contrast to the decrease in substance P, the K^+-stimulated outflow of CGRP is *not* modified by NAD. Third, capsaicin selectively depolarizes fine-calibre substance P containing PAFs, such that it may isolate peripheral from spinal pools of substance P. In this regard there are contradictory findings since FRANCO-CERECEDA et al. (1992) reported that NAD does not modify capsaicin-induced release of CGRP from guinea pig spinal ganglia in culture whereas TAKANO and YAKSH (1992c) found that α_2-AR agonists reduce capsaisin-evoked release of substance P and CGRP in parallel from an in vitro preparation of rat spinal cord, an action reversed by atipamezole. Further, GLU is also present in PAFs wherein it is partially co-localized and co-modulated with substance P (see SEGUIN et al. 1995): α_2-AR agonists inhibit both the release of GLU from rat spinal cord synaptosomes (KAMISAKI et al. 1993) and the capsaicin-evoked release of GLU from the rat DH (UEDA et al. 1995), actions reversed by α_2-AR antagonists. Finally, NAD does not inhibit the capsaicin-evoked release of somatostatin, a putative nociceptive transmitter of PAFs (KURAISHI et al. 1991).

Nevertheless, the balance of evidence – underpinned by the neuroanatomical studies discussed below – suggests that there may indeed be a presynaptic component of α_2-AR-mediated antinociception which reflects an inhibition of the release of PAF nociceptive neurotransmitters. However, the possibility that GABAergic or other types of ININ intervene in the influence of NAD upon PAF terminals should not be neglected (SAKATANI et al. 1993), and *direct* presynaptic inhibition is unlikely to be more than a minor contribution to the global, spinal antinociceptive actions of α_2-AR agonists. First, based on the findings of binding studies performed in animals deprived neurochemically or surgically of PAF input, only a small percentage of α_2-ARs (≤20%) are localized on PAFs (HOWE et al. 1987; WIKBERG and HAJÓS 1987). Second, although the possibility of volume inhibition of PAFs should be born in mind (see above), ultrastructural evidence for axo-axonic synapses of NAD-synthetisizing neurones in the superficial DH is virtually lacking whereas there is evidence for both axo-dendritic and axo-somatic contacts (DOYLE and MAXWELL 1991a,b; SATOH et al. 1982; see PROUDFIT 1992; RIDET et al. 1993; WESTLUND 1992). Third, α_2-AR agonists elicit (see below) robust and generalized analgesia in many models employing *intense*, phasic stimuli, and it may be questioned whether an action restricted to a reduction in the release of substance P and/or GLU could reproduce this profile of activity (see SEGUIN et al. 1995). Fourth, the discharge of PNs in response to noxious stimulation is inhibited upon iotophoretic administration of NAD directly in laminae IV and V (see above), whereas PAF terminals project primarily in more superficial (I/II) laminae of the DH.

III. Descending Noradrenergic Inhibition

1. Involvement of Several Medullary Noradrenergic Nuclei

The above observations suggest that the DH is a major locus of the antinociceptive actions of α_2-AR agonists. Complementary to these observations, studies employing the intracellular marker of sustained nociceptive input, c-*fos*, have demonstrated that the induction of this immediate-early gene by noxious stimuli is inhibited by α_2-AR agonists (HONORÉ et al. 1996; PERTOVAARA et al. 1993) and the results of behavioural studies showing that spinal administration of α_2-AR agonists elicits antinociception are discussed below. These data provide the basis of the concept of descending inhibition whereby activation by opioids, noxious stimulation or stress of centripetal adrenergic fibres running from the pons to the DH plays a key role in antinociceptive mechanisms by limiting the flow of nociceptive information to supraspinal structures (see ADVOKAT 1988; BASBAUM and FIELDS 1984; JONES 1991; LE BARS 1988; PROUDFIT 1992; STAMFORD 1995).

Direct evidence has been obtained from studies of the effects of electrical and chemical (to avoid effects on fibres of passage) stimulation of the A5 adrenergic cell group. Such studies have shown that the antinociception induced can be primarily attributed to α_2-ARs. Further, although this A5 group provides a major input to the IML, a dissociation between the antinociceptive and cardiovascular effects of stimulation can be shown (BURNETT and GEBHART 1991; CLARK and PROUDFIT 1993; GUINAN et al. 1989). In analogy, many studies (see JONES and GEBHART 1986; PROUDFIT 1992) have indicated that electrical or chemical stimulation of the LC (and subcoeruleus) can elicit a behavioural antinociception and inhibit the response of deep laminae DH neurones to noxious stimulation independently of an influence upon arterial blood pressure. Further, stimulation of the LC is accompanied by changes in spinal levels of NAD (CRAWLEY et al. 1979) and most studies suggest that α_2-ARs in the DH play a major role in mediating the antinociception evoked by LC stimulation, although a contribution of cerebral opioidergic and serotoninergic mechanisms cannot be discounted (GIRADA et al. 1987; JONES and GEBHART 1986; MARGALIT and SEGAL 1979; MOKHA and IGGO 1987). Interestingly, it has been suggested that a co-release of neuropeptides may also be involved in the inhibition of DH neurones elicited by stimulation of the Kolliker fuse–LC cell group (ZHAO and DUGGAN 1988). The A7 cluster also yields antinociception upon its electrical or chemical (substance P) stimulation, and intrathecal administration of α_2-AR antagonists blocks this action without affecting the accompanying increase in blood pressure (YEOMANS and PROUDFIT 1992; YEOMANS et al. 1992). However, since this projection is predominantly ipsilateral, it is surprising that antinociception is evoked bilaterally. Further, although stimulation of the A7 nucleus inhibits the response of DH neurones to both noxious and non-noxious stimuli, data concerning the involvement of descending adrenergic pathways in this action remain contradictory (HODGE et al. 1986; ZHAO and DUGGAN 1988).

Overall, however, it is clear that activation of descending adrenergic pathways to the DH elicits antinociception. In line with these observations, many studies have found that the electrical or chemical stimulation of either the PAG of ventromedial medulla (VMM) provokes an antinociception attenuated by the spinal administration of α_2-AR antagonists or by depletion of spinal pools of NAD (AIMONE et al. 1987; BARBARO et al. 1985; JENSEN and YAKSH 1986; SATOH et al. 1982). It has been suggested that the actions of electrical stimulation are partly due to the antidromic activation of adrenergic collaterals from the A5 and A7 groups projecting both to the PAG and the DH (KWIAT and BASBAUM 1990). However, this is unlikely to account for the actions of chemical stimuli (such as GLU) in the PAG, and an alternative network has been proposed by PROUDFIT (1992), involving a PAG-VMM connection (of uncertain neurochemistry) and a VMM pathway to the A7 and, possibly A5, groups which involves substance P, the introduction of which into the A7 cluster elicits an antinociception mediated by spinal α_2-ARs (YEOMANS and PROUDFIT 1992; YEOMANS et al. 1992). Further, a direct PAG projection to noradrenergic nuclei likely exists (BEITZ et al. 1988).

Finally, although the nucleus raphe magnus (NRM) is rich in serotonergic neurones (see below), its stimulation increases NAD release in the DH, probably by activation of NRM afferents to the A5 nucleus and the subsequent engagement of descending antinociceptive adrenergic pathways to the DH: correspondingly, spinal α_2-ARs are involved in mediating antinociception elicited by NRM stimulation (BARBARO et al. 1985; BOWKER and ABHOLD 1990; GEBHART and RANDICH 1990; HAMMOND and YAKSH 1984; HAMMOND et al.

1985; IWAMOTO and MARION 1993; JENSEN and YAKSH 1984; SAGEN et al. 1983). Further, the NRM may also be involved in the induction of antinociception by stimulation of the A11 nucleus, the adrenergic neurones of which do not themselves project to the spinal cord (PROUDFIT 1992).

In parallel to such studies, the role of segmental adrenergic mechanisms in the antinociceptive actions of morphine at the cerebral level has been extensively examined. Overall, there is compelling evidence that DH-localized α_2-ARs are involved, although NAD may fulfil a synergistic role with 5-HT inas much as the the antinociception elicited by introduction of morphine into the PAG or VMM is only partially blocked by α_2-AR antagonists and often best reduced by the spinal co-administration of both α_2-AR and serotoninergic antagonists (AIMONE et al. 1987; ARVIDSSON et al. 1995; FANG and PROUDFIT 1996; GEBHART and RANDICH 1990; JENSEN and YAKSH 1986; SAWYNOK 1989; TSENG and TANG 1989; ZHUO and GEBHART 1990). Further, a role of other descending neurotransmitters, such as acetylcholine, glycine, GABA and enkephalin in descending inhibition should not be discounted (ANTAL et al. 1996; BLOMQVIST et al. 1994; SORKIN et al. 1993; ZHUO and GEBHART 1990, 1991).

2. Functional Modulation

Noxious stimulation (or exposure to stress) induces antinociception and suppresses the response of DH neurones to noxious stimuli. Several lines of evidence suggest that activation of descending adrenergic pathways (possibly via an opioidergic link in the PAG) is involved in this phenomenon. First, in both superfusate and dialysis studies the high-intensity somatic stimuli activation of $A\delta$ and C fibre afferent increases the synthesis and release of NAD in the DH (HAMMOND et al. 1985; MEN and MATSUI 1994a; TAKAGI et al. 1979; YAKSH 1985). Second, blockade of spinal adrenergic transmission and/or α_2-ARs inhibits certain models of stress-induced antinociception (ROCHFORD et al. 1992). Third, under conditions of both phasic and long-term noxious inflammatory stimulation, an induction of the rate-limiting enzyme for NAD synthesis, tyrosine-hydroxylase, has been detected in A5, A6 and A7 pontine adrenergic cell groups (CHO et al. 1995; GRANT and BENNO 1992). Fourth, changes in the spinal turnover of NAD and in the density of α_2-ARs have been seen in models of prolonged noxious input (WEIL-FUGAZZA et al. 1986; WILLIAMS et al. 1991). A role of adrenergic pathways from the LC in the modulation of nociception under these conditions has been proposed (CODERRE et al. 1993) and, indicative of the antinociceptive actions of endogenous adrenergic systems, STANFA and DICKENSON (1994) showed that idazoxan facilitates the C fibres response of DH neurones in inflamed but not normal rats. KAYSER et al. (1995) have recently documented antinociceptive action of clonidine in rats with inflammation. Finally, adrenergic mechanisms in the DH are involved in the induction of antinociception by the cerebral actions of neurotensin (NARANJO et al. 1989) and cannabinoids (LICHTMAN and MARTIN 1991).

IV. Pharmacology of Spinal Adrenergic Mechanisms Modulating Nociception

1. Experimental Data

There is substantial evidence for dose-dependent and robust antinociceptive properties of spinal administration of clonidine and other α_2-AR agonists by an action in the DH; early studies focused primarily on classic algesiometric models (see YAKSH 1985). Studies with more selective and efficacious α_2-AR agonists such as dex-medetomidine (DMT), S 18616 and UK 14304 have amply confirmed such findings (DANZEBRINK and GEBHART 1990; CAHUSAC et al. 1995; MILLAN et al. 1994, 1995; PERTOVAARA 1993; SAEKI and YAKSH 1991; SULLIVAN et al. 1992b; TAKANO and YAKSH 1993; WILD et al. 1994; Fig. 1) and extended these observations to "hyperalgesic" models employing tonic, subchronic or chronic exposure to inflammatory stimuli. Under these conditions, in analogy to μ-opioids, the spinal (or systemic) administration of α_2-AR agonists normalizes abnormally low nociceptive thresholds and more potently elicits antinociception than in untreated animals, and this in the absence of pronounced motor disruption (AULT and HILDEBRAND 1993; HYLDEN et al. 1991; IDÄNPÄÄN-HEIKKILÄ et al. 1994; KAYSER et al. 1992; MANSIKKA and PERTOVAARA 1995; MANSIKKA et al. 1996; PERTOVAARA and HÄMÄLLÄININ 1994; STANFA and DICKENSON 1994).

Of particular interest are paradigms of neuropathic pain, involving the perturbation, damage or destruction of peripheral nerves by, for example,

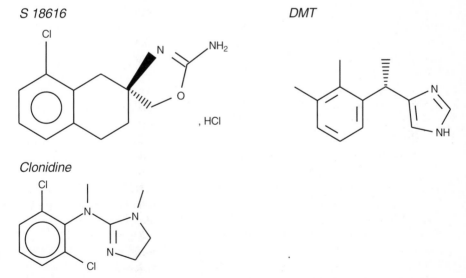

Fig. 1. Chemical structures of S 18616, DMT, and clonidine. S 18616 is a novel spiroimidazoline displaying high affinity, efficacy and selectivity for α_2-ARs: as well as antinociceptive properties in rodents

sciatic ligation. Under such conditions, the systemic or spinal administration of clonidine, DMT and other α_2-AR agonists generally normalizes the associated hyperalgesia and allodynia to mechanical stimuli and their potency may actually be enhanced relative to normal animals, although results appear to depend upon the injury type, the degree of sympathetic-dependence of the model and the quality of the noxious stimulus employed (HUNTER et al. 1996; KAYSER et al. 1995; LEIPHART et al. 1995; LUO et al. 1994; PUKE et al. 1994; XU et al. 1992; YAMAMOTO and YAKSH 1991; YAKSH et al. 1995).

The mechanisms underlying these apparent changes in sensitivity to α_2-AR agonists in models of nociceptive and neuropathic pain remain to be elucidated, although they may be related both to the above-mentioned neurochemical changes in NAD release and α_2-AR density. In fact, under conditions of long-term inflammatory and neuropathic pain, there occurs a complex series of changes involving (a) peripheral sequelae such as C fibre afferent barrage from inflamed tissue, ectopic (spontaneous and stimulated) neuroma and dorsal root ganglion (DRG) discharge, and sympathetic sprouting into the DRG, (b) central adaptive changes including sensitization (wind-up and heterotropic facilitation) triggered and maintained by GLU/NMDA receptors and facilitated by substance P/neurokinin receptors, and (c) central reorganization including loss of GABAergic ININ function and sprouting of Aβ fibres into superficial laminae (BURITOVA et al. 1996; CASTRO-LOPES et al. 1993; CODERRE et al. 1993; HAO et al. 1991, 1994; NACHEMSON and BENNETT 1993; SUGIMOTO et al. 1990; WILSON and KITCHENER 1996; WOOLF and DOUBELL 1994). Consequently, nociceptive information (mediated by Aδ/C fibres and NMDA receptors) is perceived as more intense (hyperalgesia) and non-nociceptive innocuous information (mediated by Aβ fibres via, possibly, AMPA receptors) is perceived as noxious (allodynia). Within this framework there are several possible sites of action at which α_2-AR agonists might act to not only reverse but even *prevent* the induction of chronic pain status. Possibilities include an influence of α_2-AR agonists upon peripheral inflammatory processes via induction of corticosterone secretion, direct vascular actions and the modulation of the activity of sympathetic or primary afferent terminals (CODERRE et al. 1993; HONORÉ et al. 1996; KHASER et al. 1995; LEE and YAKSH 1995; NAKAMURA and FERREIRA 1988; YAKSH et al. 1995).

Centrally, the presynaptic inhibition of GLU release from Aδ/C fibres in the DH and the postsynaptic inhibition of WDR PNs might be implicated. However, although such actions are likely involved in the control of painful states once established, the balance of evidence suggests that *pre*-emptive treatment with α_2-AR agonists does *not* markedly modify the generation or expression of nociceptive and neuropathic states, nor does it evoke a more pronounced antinociception than administration of α_2-ARs following onset of the states (LUO et al. 1994, 1995; MANSIKKA and PERTOVAARA 1995; PUKE and WIESENFELD-HALLIN 1993; SMITH et al. 1993; SULLIVAN et al. 1992a). Further, although clonidine reduces inflammation-induced induction of c-*fos* (HONORÉ et al. 1996; PERTOVAARA et al. 1993) – which may be involved in triggering central alterations in the processing of sensory information (CODERRE et al. 1993; GOGAS et al. 1996; HUNTER et al. 1995) – it does *not* attenuate the induction provoked by sciatic section (BASBAUM et al. 1991; LUO et al. 1994). In contrast, c-*fos* induction by nerve injury can be prevented by opioids (LUO et al. 1994, 1995). Indeed overall, there is a global tendency for morphine to be more effective than α_2-AR agonists in *preventing* the onset of such states whereas α_2-AR agonists are more effective in their *reversal* once established (LUO et al. 1994, 1995; McCARSON and KRAUSE 1995; WOOLF and CHANG 1993).

It is also likely that the actions of α_2-AR agonists reflect the degree to which an afferent barrage contributes to the onset and/or maintenance of painful states. For example, this is high for inflammatory hyperalgesia (e.g. MANSIKKA and PERTOVAARA 1995) yet relatively low (brief and intense) for injury-triggered central changes (e.g., PUKE and WIESENFELD-HALLIN 1993) and the former state is more sensitize to α_2-AR agonists. More generally, a possible explanation for the limited preventive activity of α_2-AR agonists against injury-induced painful states is that they involve excitotoxic, degenerative actions of GLU (via excessive stimulation of NMDA receptors) on ININs in the DH (CASTRO-LOPEZ et al. 1993; SUGIMOTO et al. 1990). α_2-AR agonists express only limited presynaptic release-inhibiting actions on fine-calibre primary afferents (BOURGOIN et al. 1993; see above) and are unlikely to inhibit the neuronal activity (protect) of most small ININs. As such they would not be expected to be as effective in preventing the hyperexcitability due to ININ loss as NMDA receptors antagonists (CODERRE 1993; HAO et al. 1991; PERSSON et al. 1995; SEGUIN et al. 1995; SMITH et al. 1994; WOOLF and DOUBELL 1994; XU et al. 1993, 1995). The painful state (especially allodynia), once established, however, might be moderated by the postsynaptic inhibitory actions of α_2-AR agonists versus Aβ-induced excitation of sensitized WDR and NS PNs and by presynaptic inhibitory actions of α_2-ARs on Aβ fibres (expressed directly or via GABAergic ININs; BERNARDI et al. 1995; MARCHAND et al. 1993; TEOH et al. 1996). An alternative hypothesis suggests that α_2-AR agonists may relieve allodynia by inhibiting sympathetic outflow via actions on preganglionic neurones in the IML (YAKSH et al. 1995). However, this would *not* be relevant to pain independent of sympathetic activity.

2. Clinical Data

The above-mentioned data with animal models of neuropathic pain are of special interest in the light of clinical data indicating that the chronic neuropathic pain due to cancer, back problems, diabetes or reflex sympathetic dystrophy is significantly relieved by epidural administration of clonidine (CARROLL et al. 1993; EISENACH 1994; EISENACH et al. 1995; HUNTOON et al. 1992; McQUAY 1992; RAUCK et al. 1993; see GLYNN 1992). As the efficacy of opioids in the management of neuropathic pain is still under dispute (ARNÉR and MEYERSON 1988), α_2-AR agonists would offer an attractive alternative.

Further, α_2-AR agonists may be effective in patients irresponsive or tolerant to opioids (COOMBS et al. 1985), although this remains to be rigorously confirmed, and the utility of α_2-AR agonists in suppressing the somatic symptoms of opioid withdrawal may be of significance in this context (BUCCAFUSCO 1990). Moreover, the issue of whether tolerance exists between opioids and α_2-AR agonists remains controversial (KANETO and INOUE 1990; LOOMIS et al. 1987; POST et al. 1988; SOLOMON and GEBHART 1988a; STEVENS et al. 1988; YAKSH 1985). On balance this seems likely to be the case, at least under certain conditions, since although μ-opioid receptors do not play a major role in mediating spinal α_2-AR antinociception (SULLIVAN et al. 1992a,b), α_2-AR and μ-opioid receptors share common cellular mechanisms of action on PNs (cy-clase inhibition, reduced gCa^{2+}, increased gK^+, etc.).

In addition to the pain accompanying the above-mentioned chronic disease states, clonidine elicits analgesia upon the epidural or intrathecal route under conditions of acute pain, including post-operative and labour pain. At modest doses this analgesia is expressed in the relative (though *not* absolute) absence of sedation and cardiovascular perturbation (BERNHARD et al. 1995; BERNARDI et al. 1995; BONNET et al. 1990a; EISENACH et al. 1993; FILOS et al. 1992, 1994; GLYNN 1992; HUNTOON et al. 1992; LUND et al. 1989). However, epidural clonidine can provoke both hypotension and bradycardia. Further, this may occur even at a magnitude comparable to the systemic routes, suggesting leakage to supraspinal sites, an assumption supported by the occurrence of (LC-mediated) sedation in some studies (BONNET et al. 1990a; BOUAZIZ et al. 1996; CARROLL et al. 1993; DE KOCK et al. 1993, 1995; EISENACH et al. 1993; KIRNO et al. 1993). Pretreatment with a bolus injection of clonidine or computerized control of injection rates may be advantageous in reducing such side effects (MENDEZ et al. 1990). The above clinical data were obtained with clonidine, which is a partial agonist. Further, it shows only modest selectivity to α_1-ARs, an action at which may modify sedative and other functional properties (GUO et al. 1991; SCHWINN et al. 1991). The availability of DMT, a ligand of greater selectivity and efficacy is thus of significance. However, although systemic DMT is active against the affective component of ischaemic and post-operative pain (AHO et al. 1991, 1992; JAAKOLA et al. 1991; KAUPPILA et al. 1991), its potential antinociceptive profile is disappointing, and the development of this drug has been reoriented towards cardioprotection, an action reflecting a reduction of stress-induced sympathetic activation (AANTAA and SCHEININ 1993; AHO et al. 1992; HAYASHI and MAZE 1993; JAAKOLA et al. 1992; LUND et al. 1989; WANG et al. 1994). Further, notwithstanding its improved selectivity and efficacy relative to clonidine, DMT is more lipophilic, a disadvantage for spinal administration since its redistribution by spinal vasculature and rostral migration in the cerebrospinal fluid may limit the intensity and duration of analgesia and worsen extraspinal side effects (EISENACH et al. 1994; PERTOVAARA et al. 1993).

There is thus a need for a modestly lipophilic drug of marked α_2-AR selectivity and efficacy which would allow for a more rigorous evaluation of the utility of spinal administration of α_2-AR agonists as analgesics. Such a drug should be less markedly redistributed and attain targets in the DH more easily than the deeper IML and VH, structures at the origin of cardiovascular and motor side effects, respectively. The polar clonidine derivative ST 91 and oxymetazoline are examples of lipophobic drugs which yield antinociception upon intrathecal administration to rats (SHERMAN et al. 1987; TAKANO and YAKSH 1992a,b), but they have not been evaluated epidurally in humans. It should be mentioned that the degree and rapidity of tolerance to the antinociceptive α_2-ARs *themselves* is an important consideration and likely depends on several factors, including drug efficacy (EISENACH et al. 1994; HAYASHI et al. 1995; MAZE et al. 1995). Although there are indications that the sedative and sympatholytic properties of α_2-AR agonists develop tolerance more rapidly than their antinociceptive actions, this is *not* the case for their hypotensive actions (HAYASHI et al. 1995; LOOMIS et al. 1987, 1988; REID et al. 1994; STEVENS and YAKSH 1989; Millan et al., unpublished observations). In summary, although spinal clonidine evokes neither pruritus, urinary retention, nausea nor marked respiratory depression (opioidergic side effects), there remains a need for further studies to establish whether the spinal administration of α_2-AR agonists alone can assume a broader role in the management of painful state in the absence of pronounced side effects.

3. Facilitation of the Actions of Local Anaesthetics and Opioids

α_2-AR agonists may be of use in association with other anaesthetic and analgesic drug classes. Local anaesthetics are broadly used drugs epidurally, for example, in obstectrics, and spinal clonidine or DMT is even more effective than opioids in increasing their duration of analgesic action and improving their efficacy (BONNET et al. 1990b; CARABINE et al. 1992; CIGARINI et al. 1992; EISENBACH 1994; GLYNN 1988; GLYNN and O'SULLIVAN 1996; HUNTOON et al. 1992; NISHIKAWA and DOHI 1990; O'MEARA and GIN 1993; SINGELYN et al. 1992). α_2-ARs agonists also markedly reduce anaesthetic requirements during surgery irrespective of the route of anaesthetic administration (AANTAA and SCHEININ 1993; HAYASHI and MAZE 1993). This action is seen upon utilization of the μ-opioid agonists, fentanyl and sufentanil as anaesthetics (AANTAA and SCHEININ 1993; ERKOLA et al. 1994; FLACKE et al. 1987; GHINGONE et al. 1986; JAVIS et al. 1992;) and the question arises as to whether the *analgesic* effects of μ-opioids may likewise be reinforced.

Indeed, there is extensive experimental evidence demonstrating that the spinal (or systemic) administration of α_2-AR agonists (clonidine or DMT) and μ-opioids synergistically evokes antinociception – while reducing respiratory depression – likely without an increase in tolerance development (GURTU et al. 1994; KNOWLES et al. 1994; MONASKI et al. 1990; OSSIPOV et al. 1990a,b; PLUMMER et al. 1992; VONHOF and SIRÉN 1991; YAMAGUCHI et al. 1994). This mutual analgesic action is possibly due to joint inhibition of WDR PNs upon which α_2-ARs and μ-opioid receptors may be co-localized (McFADZEAN and

DOCHERTY 1989), and, at least in the LC, α_2-AR and μ-opioid agonists enhance a common K^+ current (NORTH 1989). Such mutual facilitatory analgesic effects are seen for both inflammatory-nociceptive (HONORÉ et al. 1996) and neuropathic pain states (OSSIPOV et al. 1996b), in both behavioural (above citations) and electrophysiological studies (GINZBURG and SELZTER 1990; KALSO et al. 1993; OMOTE et al. 1991; OSSIPOV et al. 1990a; SULLIVAN et al. 1987, 1992a). Potentiation is consistently seen between α_2-AR agonists and μ-opioid agonists (above citations) and may also occur between α_2-AR agonists and κ agonists, at least for cutaneous stimuli in rats (GORDON et al. 1992; HARADA et al. 1995; MALMBERG and YAKSH 1993; OSSIPOV et al. 1990b) and dental pain in humans (GORDON et al. 1992). However, results with α_2-AR and δ-agonists are contradictory, and several studies suggest independence of δ-opioid and α_2-AR antinociception at the spinal level (HARADA et al. 1995; KALSO et al. 1993; OMOTE et al. 1991; ROERIG et al. 1992; STEVENS and YAKSH 1992; SULLIVAN et al. 1992a).

Clinical data with systemic administration of clonidine and DMT suggest that there does indeed exist a mutual facilitation of α_2-AR and μ-opioid evoked antinociception without deterioration of respiratory depression (AHO et al. 1991; BENHAMOU et al. 1994; DE KOCK et al. 1993; SEGAL et al. 1991). Such observations of an increased intensity and duration of opioid-analgesia (in the absence of increased side effects) by co-administration of clonidine have been extended to the spinal route (CAPOGNA et al. 1995; DE KOCK et al. 1993, 1995; EISENACH et al. 1994a; FOGARTY et al. 1993; GRACE et al. 1995; JAVIS et al. 1992; MOGENSEN et al. 1992; MOTSCH et al. 1990; VAN ESSEN et al. 1991).

Although clinical studies remain to be performed, there is evidence for synergistic interactions between α_2-AR and muscarinic (M_1) mechanisms of antinociception in the DH – in the absence of worsened hypotension (ABRAM and WINE 1995; EISENBACH and GEBHART 1995). Further, spinal α_2-AR agonists and NMDA antagonists yield synergistic blockade of neuropathic pain in the absence of increased side effects (LEE and YAKSH 1995) while adenosinergic and adrenergic mechanisms of antinociception may also interact in the DH (SAWYNOK and REID 1996).

V. α_2-AR Subtypes and Antinociception

1. Localization of α_2-AR Subtypes in the Dorsal Horn

a) Radioligand Binding and Antibody Studies

α_2-ARs are present in a high density in the superficial laminae of the DH and at a somewhat lower density in deeper laminae; further, their concentration is relatively low in the VH, while they are abundant in the IML (DASHWOOD et al. 1985; SEYBOLD 1986; SIMMONS and JONES 1988). The density of α_2-ARs appears to be maximal in the lumbar region of the rat, whereas in humans the greatest density is encountered in sacral segments (SIMMONS and JONES 1988; LAWHEAD et al. 1992). UHLÉN and WIKBERG (1991) showed that [^{3}H]RX 821002, which does not discriminate betwen multiple α_2-AR subtypes

(RENOUARD et al. 1994), labels a homogeneous population of sites in rat spinal cord with characteristics almost identical to α_{2A}-AR in rat cortex and to α_{2A}-AR, but not α_{2B}-AR, sites in rat kidney. In an analogous study LAWHEAD et al. (1992) reported that the pattern of displacement of [^{3}H]RX 821002 and of a further α_2-AR antagonist, [^{3}H]rauwolscine, in human spinal cord is powerfully correlated to affinities at several preparations of pure α_{2A}-ARs but poorly correlated to tissues expressing exclusively α_{2B}-ARs or α_{2C}-ARs. These authors concluded that α_{2A}-ARs receptors comprise at least 80%–90% of α_2-ARs in human spinal cord. This interpretation has been underpinned by a study (UHLÉN et al. 1992, 1994) in the rat utilizing a novel radioligand [^{3}H]-MK 912 which possesses a modest (ca. 15-fold) preference for α_{2C}- versus α_{2A}-ARs. The majority of sites identified (ca. 95%) were α_{2A}-ARs and the remainder – undetectable by non-subtype-selective radioligands – presented a profile corresponding to α_{2C}-ARs. In a complementary approach ROSIN et al. (1993) generated antibodies against α_{2A}-ARs and histochemically localized these sites in rat spinal cord, affording an insight into their topographical organization. In thoracic cord numerous labelled cells were localized in the superficial laminae I and II. A markedly lower density of cells was observed in deeper laminae (IV/V). At the cervical and lumbar levels, further, labelled cells were virtually restricted to superficial layers and lamine IV–VI. Throughout the spinal cord, α_{2A}-ARs have also been detected by selective antibodies in lamina X. As mentioned above, although this region is not traditionally associated with the reception and integration of nociceptive information, cells therein receive both cutaneous and visceral nociceptive input, and laminae X provides an input to the STT and several other ascending tracts (CARLTON et al. 1991; LA MOTTE 1988).

b) mRNA Studies of α_2-AR Subtypes in the Dorsal Horn: Intrinsic Neurones

These binding and antibody studies converge in showing that α_{2A}-ARs are present in significant quantities in rat and human DH and indicate the presence of a minor population of α_{2C}-ARs, an issue which has been further addressed employing comparative studies of the mRNA encoding α_2-AR subtypes. In a northern blot analysis ZENG and LYNCH (1991) found that mRNA encoding α_{2A}-ARs predominates in rat spinal cord, with α_{2C} ARs present at a markedly lower density and α_{2B}-ARs non-detectable. Subsequently NICHOLAS et al. 1993b, employing an in situ hybridization approach, likewise detected cells expressing α_{2A}-ARs in lamina I/II whereas α_{2C}-AR labelled cells showed only a diffuse labelling in the DH, and α_{2B}-AR-labelled cells were absent. These data reinforce the impression that α_{2A}-ARs predominate in the DH (BERKOWITZ et al. 1994). Collectively this organization also supports the notion that α_{2A}-ARs are concentrated in superficial versus deeper laminae. Thus, although there is evidence for direct inhibition of PNs in deeper laminae by α_2-AR agonists, and some deeper laminae send dendrites into superficial regions, this organization is consistent with the notion that superficially localized INs play a role in the mediation of the influence of descending noradrenergic pathways upon PNs in deeper laminae.

c) mRNA Studies of α_2-AR Subtypes in Dorsal Root Ganglion and Sympathetic Ganglia

Interestingly, in a study of α_2-AR expression in DRG, NICHOLAS et al. (1993b) found a pattern of data *opposite* to that in the DH, with a preponderance of α_{2C}-AR over α_{2A}-AR labelled neurones, together with an absence of α_{2B}-ARs. This observation was confirmed by MARCHAND et al. (1993) who found little or no evidence for α_{2A}-ARs whereas 75% of medium/large and 25% of small cells were labelled by a probe recognizing both α_{2C}-ARs and α_B-ARs. The presence of α_{2B}/α_{2C}-ARs in small neurones provides an anatomical basis for a role of $\alpha_{2(C)}$-ARs in the presynaptic modulation of afferent nociceptive information transmitted by small-calibre fibres. Further, the presence of α_{2C}-ARs on *large* neurones suggests that they may also modulate information relayed by *large*-diameter Aβ fibres transmitting normally non-nociceptive information, and which may be related to the above ability of NAD to modulate the response of PNs to not only nociceptive but also non-nociceptive information. Importantly, further, in neuropathic and other painful states, Aβ fibres transmit mechanical information underlying allodynic states (WOOLF and DOUBELL 1994).

These observations also thus provide a substrate for a putative presynaptic – in addition to postsynaptic – modulation of the allodynia of neuropathic pain states (see above). In addition, they raise the possibility of actions of α_2-AR agonists on the *peripheral* terminals of small and large calibre fibres (KHASAR et al. 1995, see below). Finally, certain neuropathic states are dependent upon the integrity of sympathetic transmission and the presence of $\alpha_{2B/C}$-ARs but not α_{2A}-ARs in paravertebral sympathetic ganglia suggests that an action of $\alpha_{2B/C}$-AR ligands on sympathetic terminals also influences neuropathic pain states (KHASAR et al. 1995, see below). It would be important to determine whether α_2-AR subtypes exist in *human* DRG and sympathetic ganglia.

d) α_2-AR Subtype Localization in Relation to Sympathetic and Motor Function

There is extensive neuroanatomical, electrophysiological and behavioural evidence (ASTON-JONES et al. 1991; GUYENET et al. 1994; MILLAN et al. 1994; NICHOLAS et al. 1993b; ROSIN et al. 1993; AANTAA and SCHEININ 1993) that the LC (A6), subcoeruleus, A5 and A7 adrenergic projections to the DH synthesize α_{2A}-ARs but neither α_{2B}-ARs nor α_{2C}-ARs. In addition to their dendritic localization, these are transported to the terminals in the DH, where they operate as inhibitory autoreceptors (REIMANN and SCHNEIDER 1989). In analogy, descending adrenergic pathways originating in the C1 and C3 regions of the medulla, as well as descending raphe-derived serotoninergic pathways, bear α_{2A}-ARs, although not α_{2B}-ARs or α_{2C}-ARs (ROSIN et al. 1993; GUYENET et al. 1994; SCHEININ et al. 1994). Thus, even though α_{2A}-AR agonists elicit antinociception postsynaptically to adrenergic pathways in the DH, at low doses they might counteract this action in simultaneously activating α_{2A}-AR autoreceptors and inhibiting the antinociceptive actions of adrenergic pathways. In analogy, α_{2A}-AR agonists may suppress the anti- (and pro-) nociceptive influence of descending serotoninergic transmission to the DH.

As concerns sympathetic outflow, further, an inhibition of excitatory noradrenergic, adrenergic and serotoninergic inputs to the IML by inhibitory α_2-auto and heteroceptors contributes to the sympatholytic properties of clonidine and other α_{2A}-AR agonists (LOEWY 1990; GUYENET et al. 1994). Further, the presence of a high density of mRNA encoding α_{2A}-ARs (but not α_{2AB}-ARs or α_{2C}-ARs) in the IML of the rat, and of a high density of α_{2A}-ARs, α_{2B}-ARs and, to a lesser degree α_{2C}-ARs, in the IML of human spinal cord, suggests that α_{2A}-ARs also locally inhibit sympathetic outflow. As concerns the rat VH, antibody studies failed to detect α_{2A}-ARs (ROSIN et al. 1993), while only occasional cells displaying mRNA were found in the dorsal aspect of the VH by NICHOLAS et al. (1993b). These data suggest that the motor-inhibitory actions of α_2-AR agonists in rat are expressed predominantly at the level of the LC, although a minor pre- or postsynaptic influence of α_2-AR agonists upon MNs themselves should not be excluded (AANTAA and SCHEININ 1993; BERVOETS and MILLAN 1994; MILLAN et al. 1994). Interestingly, although mRNA for α_{2B}-ARs is likewise absent from the rat VH, this region displays a significant amount of mRNA for α_{2C}-ARs (NICHOLAS et al. 1993a), suggesting that α_{2C}-ARs are involved in the regulation of motor function at the spinal level.

e) mRNA Studies of α_2-AR Subtypes in Human Spinal Cord

Inasmuch as species (rat, human) differences in α_2-AR subtype distribution may exist (BERKOVITZ and MILLAN 1994), a recent study of the distribution of mRNA encoding multiple α_2-ARs in human spinal cord is of importance (STAFFORD-SMITH et al. 1995). This confirmed the presence of α_{2A}-ARs in superficial (I/II) and deeper (IV/V) laminae of the DH throughout the length of the spinal cord, consistent with a role in the modulation of nociception. Further, α_{2A}-AR mRNA was present in the IML of thoracic and rostral lumbar segments, and in the parasympathetic IML of the sacral cord. α_{2C}-ARs were seen in only a modest density in superficial and deeper laminae of the DH, in the IML and (more weakly) in the VH of only the lumbar zone. However, in marked distinction to the rat, α_{2B}-ARs were present throughout the cord in both superficial and deeper laminae, and in a particularly high concentration in the sacral region. Further, they were also found in a high density in the sympathetic IML, the parasympathetic intermediate zone and the VH.

2. Functional Evidence for Multiple α_2-AR Subtypes Modulating Nociception

a) Early Results and Pharmacological Tools

An early indication that multiple α_2-AR subtypes may modulate nociception at the segmental level was provided by UHLÉN et al. (1990) who reported that the antinociceptive actions of two α_2-ARs agonists, UK 14304 (non-subtype-selective) and guanfacine (a preferential α_{2A}-AR agonist), were differentially modified by the elimination of spinal pools of NAD. These results are consistent with a role of an α_{2A}-AR and a non-α_{2A}-AR in the modulation of nociception in the rat. The lack of highly selective α_2-AR agonists and antagonists has complicated the further characterization of the role of putative α_2-AR subtypes. Nevertheless, whereas guanfacine, guanabenz and oxymetazoline are preferential α_{2A}-AR agonists, ST 91 appears to exert its actions via a non-α_{2A}-AR (although this is *not* synonymous with α_{2B}-/α_{2C}-AR selectivity, see below); BRL 44408 behaves as a preferential antagonist at α_{2A}-ARs versus $\alpha_{2B/2C}$-ARs while yohimbine, rauwolscine, imiloxan and WB 4101 show a mild, and ARC 239 and prazosin, a marked, preference for $\alpha_{2B/2C}$-ARs versus rat α_{2A}-ARs (RENOUARD et al. 1994). The judicious use of these ligands in conjunction with a consideration of the localization of α_2-AR subtypes allows for the formulation of reasonable hypotheses concerning their respective implication in the modulation of nociception.

b) Modulation of the Release of Primary Afferent Transmitters in the Dorsal Horn: A Role for α_{2C}-ARs

In this light we may recall evidence (above) for a preponderance of α_{2C}-AR mRNA in small DRG neurones. The transport of α_{2C}-ARs to the central terminals of these neurones which release substance P, CGRP and GLU in the DH would provide a potential substrate for a presynaptic antinociceptive action of NAD at α_{2C}-ARs. Indeed, in line with this possibility there is a striking homogeneity amongst results obtained in several species and employing diverse techniques as concerns the ability of prazosin, yohimbine and rauwolscine to moderate the inhibitory influence of NAD, clonidine, ST 91 and other α_2-AR agonists upon the release of substance P, CGRP and/or GLU in the DH (BOURGOIN et al. 1993; KURAISHI et al. 1985; ONO et al. 1991; TAKANO and YAKSH 1992c; UEDA et al. 1995). Although prazosin is a potent antagonist at α_1-ARs, selective α_1-AR agonists do not modify the release of substance P, CGRP or GLU in the DH (see YAKSH 1985 and above citations). Further, although prazosin blocks α_{2B}-ARs, these do not exist in DRG and are present in only a low level in the rat DH, tending to exclude an indirect implication of α_{2B}-ARs via INs. Thus the antagonist properties of prazosin at α_{2C}-ARs likely underlie its actions. Interestingly, prazosin also reduces the inhibitory influence of systemic administration of morphine upon noxious stimulus-evoked release of substance P in the DH in vivo consistent with the possibility that α_{2C}-ARs might contributes to the influence of descending noradrenergic inhibition upon PAF activity (KURAISHI et al. 1983b). Functional evidence along these lines was also presented by CAMARATA and YAKSH (1985). KURAISHI et al. (1985) also showed that prazosin alone potentiates the influence of noxious stimuli upon substance P release, indicative of a *tonic* activity of these noradrenergic pathways at α_{2C}-ARs (see STANFA and DICKENSON 1994). This action was specific inasmuch as resting substance P release (likely from an intrinsic source) was not modified. A further indirect argument in favour of a primary role of α_{2C}-ARs is the report that the preferential α_{2A}-AR agonist, oxymetazoline, does not modify capsaicin-evoked GLU release in rat DH, whereas this was inhibited by ST 91 (UEDA et al. 1995). Indeed, TAKANO and YAKSH (1992c) showed that ST 91 prazosin-reversibly inhibits substance P releases in rat DH, although in this study CGRP release curiously was not affected.

The above observations argue for a role of α_{2C}-ARs in the inhibition of primary afferent transmission in the DH. However, in certain studies prazosin only submaximally interferes with the actions of α_2-AR agonists. Further, there is a minor population of cells expressing α_{2A}-ARs in the DRG while the ability of DMT block capsaicin-induced substance P and CGRP release in rat DH is prevented by atipamezole (RENOUARD et al. 1994) yet *resistant* to prazosin (TAKANO and YAKSH 1992c). This suggests that α_{2A}-ARs *also* play a minor role in presynaptic inhibition, although it cannot be excluded that these are located on INs rather than afferent terminals themselves.

To summarize, these data suggest that the release of PAF pools of substance P, CGRP and GLU in the DH is inhibited presynaptically by α_{2C}-ARs in the rat; in addition, a modest contribution of α_{2A}-ARs cannot be discounted. Nevertheless, as discussed above, presynaptic α_2-ARs on PAF neurones likely play a comparatively minor role in the global antinociceptive actions of α_2-AR agonists. Indeed, there is an abundance of evidence indicating that the antinociceptive actions of NAD and other α_2-AR agonists in behavioural and electrophysiological models are *insensitive* to prazosin – this remaining a major exclusion criteria of α_1-AR involvement.

c) Behavioural Studies: A Key Role for α_{2A}-ARs

The preferential α_{2A}-AR agonist oxymetazoline was shown by SHERMAN et al. (1987) to elicit phentolamine-reversible antinociception upon intrathecal administration to rats, providing an early indication that α_{2A}-ARs play a role in the induction of antinociception. Several lines of evidence have subsequently corroborated the notion that α_{2A}-ARs play the major role in the induction of antinociception.

First, α_{2A}-ARs predominate over other α_2-AR subtypes in the DH of both rat and humans, and they are strategically localized postsynaptically to PAFs for the modulation of nociception (see above). Second, α_{2A}-ARs couple positively to (inwardly rectifying) K^+ conductances; this provides a transduction mechanism for the direct hyperpolarization and inhibition of both PNs and

EXINs feeding forward onto these (see ENKVIST et al. 1996; JANSSON et al. 1995; NORTH 1989). Further, the ability of α_{2A}-AR activation to close Ca^{2+}-channels offers a mechanism both for inhibition of PNs and for an inhibitory influence upon primary afferent transmitter release (AANTAA and SCHEININ 1993; ENKVIST et al. 1996; HORVÁTH et al. 1992; JANSSON et al. 1995; LIPSCOMBE et al. 1989; NACIF-COELHO et al. 1994). Third, the antinociception elicited by intrathecal DMT is insensitive to prazosin, imiloxan and WB 4101 and is only weakly inhibited by yohimbine yet potently blocked by both atipamazole and idazoxan, two potent α_{2A}-AR antagonists with no subtype selectivity (TAKANO and YAKSH 1992b, 1993). Further, the vast majority of studies with spinal administration of α_2-AR agonists have observed resistance to prazosin in contrast to potent blockade by mixed $\alpha_{2A/B/C}$-AR antagonists (see MILLAN et al. 1994; TAKANO and YAKSH 1993; YAKSH 1985). Fourth, systemic and epidural administration of guanfacine and guanabenz, preferential α_{2A}-AR agonists, evokes antinociception across several tests in rats (MILLAN et al. 1994; SMITH et al. 1992). Fifth, the antinociceptive actions of guanfacine, guanabenz and several further α_2-AR agonists are abolished by idazoxan, atipamazole and BRL 44408, only weakly inhibited by yohombine, rauwolscine, and insensitive to prazosin, WB 4101 and ARC 239 (MILLAN et al. 1994). Sixth, across a total of 17 antagonists, blockade of the antinociceptive actions of α_2-AR agonist, UK 14304, was correlated more powerfully with affinity at α_{2A}-ARs (0.81) than α_{2B} (0.61) or α_{2C}-ARs – (0.59; MILLAN et al. 1994). Seventh, in recent studies of knock-out mice with null mutations of α_{2A}-AR – but not α_{2B} or α_{2C}-ARs – the antinociceptive actions of α_2-AR agonists were modified (K. Limbird, unpublished observation, quoted in LANIER et al. 1996; HUNTER, J.C., pers. Comm.).

d) Behavioural Studies: A Possible Role of Other α_2-AR Subtypes?

Although the above data offer unequivocal evidence for a principal antinociceptive role of α_{2A}-ARs, they leave open the possibility that additional α_2-ARs are implicated. It might be argued that α_{2C}-ARs are involved inasmuch as they are present in rat and human DH and may possess similar, if not identical, intracellular transduction mechanisms as α_{2A}-ARs, although this remains to be confirmed in CNS tissue (see ENKVIST et al. 1996; JANSSON et al. 1995; RENOUARD et al. 1994). Similar arguments could also be advanced for α_{2B}-ARs in human DH, should their existence be corroborated. XU et al. (1993), further, suggested that activation of α_{2C}-ARs underlies the amplification of antinociceptive actions of clonidine in rats with sciatic damage, although they later withdrew this proposition (PUKE et al. 1994). In addition, comparative studies of the antinociception elicited by intrathecal injection of DMT, clonidine and ST 91 in the rat have led to the suggestion that a second, non-α_{2A}-AR mediates antinociception in the hot-plate test (TAKANO and YAKSH 1992a,b, 1993). Thus, DMT- and clonidine-induced antinociception was potently blocked by atipamezole and idazoxan, less potently blocked by yohimbine and resistant to prazosin whereas the action of ST 91 was blocked by prazosin, yohimbine, imiloxan and WB 4101 (TAKANO et al. 1992a). Further, in the electrophysiological study of HOWE et al. (1983), the effect of ST 91 was also inhibited by prazosin. TASKER et al. (1992) also reported that prazosin is more effective than idazoxan in blocking ST 91-induced antinociception in the formalin test.

These data are consistent with a role of α_{2C}-ARs (see above data on presynaptic inhibition). Further evidence that DMT and clonidine but not ST 91 act at α_{2A}-ARs has been provided by two lines of evidence. First, in distinction to DMT and clonidine, ST 91 provokes neither sedation nor hypotension, actions mediated by α_{2A}-ARs (LIN et al. 1993; MILLAN et al. 1994; PALMARI and WIESENDANGER 1990; ROSIN et al. 1993; VAYSSETTES-COURSAY et al. 1996). Second, animals tolerant to DMT do not display tolerance to ST 91 and vice versa (TAKANO and YAKSH 1993). Thus ST 91 likely acts at a different population of receptors than DMT. However, ST 91 is a weak ligand at *all* α_2-AR subtypes and has very little if any α_{2C}-AR preference (PUKE et al. 1994; RENOUARD et al. 1994, V. Audinot and M.J. Millan, unpublished observation). Further, idazoxan and atipamezole *failed* to block its antinociceptive actions (TAKANO and YAKSH 1992a,b) despite their potent affinity at *all* α_2-AR subtypes (RENOUARD et al. 1994). These points question the role of α_{2C}-ARs and perhaps those of α_2-ARs in general in the actions of ST 91 although the possible existence of a novel α_2-AR subtype *cannot* formally be excluded. In fact, a role of antinociceptive α_1-ARs cannot be convincingly discounted in the actions of ST 91 inasmuch as WB 4101 is, as prazosin, a potent α_1-AR antagonist while yohimbine and imiloxan have only modest α_2-AR versus α_1-AR selectivity. A role of α_1-ARs is, moreover, consistent with the notion (TAKANO and YAKSH 1993) that for induction of antinociception clonidine shares a common receptor with both DMT (α_{2A}-AR) and ST 91 (α_1-AR?).

Further questioning the putative implication of α_{2C}-ARs (or α_{2B})-ARs in the actions of ST 91 are recent studies of knock-out α_{2B}-AR and α_{2C}-AR mice which appear to show little disruption of adrenergic mechanisms of antinociception (Maze, unpublished observation, cited in LANIER et al. 1996; HUNTER, J.C., pers. Comm.). Thus further work is required to identify the mechanism of action of ST 91. More generally there is a need for careful studies of the potential role of multiple α_2-AR (*and* α_1-AR) subtypes in the modulation of nociception in the DH employing appropriate pharmacological tools in combination with behavioural studies and, where possible, recordings from identified DH neurones. Finally, the above discussion reveals that α_{2A}-ARs mediate not only antinociception but also sedation in the LC and hypotension (via inhibition of sympathetic outflow at sites in the VMM, in the IML and on sympathetic terminals) exploding the simplistic concept that α_{2A}-AR subtype targetting may allow for the dissociation of analgesia from motor and cardiovascular side effects.

D. Serotonin and Serotonin Receptors

I. Multiple Serotonin Receptors

Multiple 5-HT receptors display contrasting patterns of coupling to ionic and soluble cellular transduction systems (BOESS and MARTIN 1994; MILLAN 1995; see Table 2). Such differences support the hypothesis that various 5-HT receptor types, where co-localized on individual neurones – or on separate neurones of a homogeneous functional unit – differentially modify neuronal activity and correspondingly fulfil contrasting functional roles, for example, in the control of mood (MILLAN 1995; MILLAN et al. 1992). Electrophysiological and neuroanatomical support for this concept has been acquired in several tissues including the cortex, septum and most pertinently the spinal cord (ASHBY et al. 1994; BOBKER 1994; MILLAN 1995; MURASE et al. 1990). The latter observation has been assimilated into a theoretical framework whereby individual 5-HT receptor types play differential roles in the control of nociception at the level of the DH. This hypothesis (MILLAN 1995) can accommodate many confusing and contradictory data concerning ostensible pronociceptive versus antinociceptive actions of 5-HT. Selective actions of novel drugs at individual 5-HT receptor types may, further, permit the separation of antinociceptive actions from undesired cardiovascular, motor and endocrine side effects. The multiplicity of functionally contrasting 5-HT receptors offers the opportunity for more effective exploitation of serotoninergic mechanisms of analgesia.

Table 2. Multiple serotoninergic receptors and pain: key characteristics

Receptor type	Transduction mechanisms	Selective agonist	Selective antagonist	DH	DRG	IML	SYMG	VH
5-HT_{1A}	$\downarrow$ AC/$\uparrow$ gK$^+$/$\downarrow$ gCa^{2+}	8-OH-DPAT	WAY 100635	+++	(+)?	+/0	++	0/+
5-HT_{1B}/(5-HT_{1D})	$\downarrow$ AC	GR 46611	SB 224289	+++	++	+	++	+
5-HT_{1E}	$\downarrow$ AC	–	–	?	?	?	?	?
5-HT_{1F}	$\downarrow$ AC	Ly 334370	–	?	–	?	–	?
5-HT_{2A}	$\uparrow$ PLC/$\downarrow$ gK$^+$	α-CH3-5-HT	MDL 100907	+	++	+	++	+
5-HT_{2B}	$\uparrow$ PLC/$\downarrow$ gK$^+$	BW 723C86	SB 204741	0/+	–	?	–	0/+
5-HT_{2C}	$\uparrow$ PLC/$\downarrow$ gK$^+$	RO 60175	SB 242084	+	+	+	–	++
5-HT_3	$\uparrow$ gCa^{2+}/gNa^{2+}$\uparrow$PLC	2-CH3-5-HT	Granisetron	+++	+++	+/0	++	+/0
5-HT_4	$\uparrow$ AC	SC 53116	GR 125487	?	?	?	?	?
5-HT_{5A}	$\downarrow$ AC?	–	–	?	–	–	–	?
5-HT_{5B}	?	–	–	?	–	–	–	?
5-HT_6	$\uparrow$ AC	–	–	+?	–	?	+	?
5-HT_7	$\uparrow$ AC	–	–	+?	++	?	++	?

AC, Adenyl cyclase; PLC, phospholipase C; DH, dorsal horn; DRG, dorsal root ganglion; IML, intermediolateral cell column; SYMG, sympathetic ganglion; VH, ventral horn. The 5-HT_{1B} (rodent) and $5\text{-HT}_{1D\beta}$ (man and guinea pig) are species homologues. Only major transduction mechanisms, if possible for native populations, are given. Other transduction systems and cell-specific coupling mechanisms should not be ignored. 5-HT_6 sites are found in superior cervical but not in lumbar sympathetic ganglia.

II. Functional Organization of Serotoninergic Input to the Dorsal Horn

1. Origin of Descending Serotoninergic Pathways

The principal source of the serotoninergic innervation of the DH is the NRM of the VMM (BOWKER and ABBOTT 1990; KWIAT and BASBAUM 1990, 1992). The NRM contains a substantial population of *non*-serotoninergic cells (JONES and LIGHT 1992) and certain neurotransmitters there are co-localized with 5-HT in a subset of neurones, for example, glycine, GABA, substance P and enkephalin, of which descending pools at least of GABA, glycine and enkephalin may elicit antinociception in the DH (ANTAL et al. 1996; ARDVISSON et al. 1992; JONES et al. 1991; NICHOLAS et al. 1992; SORKIN et al. 1993; WU and WESSENDORF 1992). Nevertheless, in distinction to the IML and VH, most serotoninergic fibres projecting to the DH probably do *not* contain co-transmitters (ANTAL et al. 1996; ARDVISSON et al. 1992; BOWKER and ABBOTT 1990; JONES and LIGHT 1992; SORKIN et al. 1993; YANG and HELKE 1995; WU and WESSENDORF 1992, 1993).

2. Influence on Projection Neurones in the Dorsal Horn

The entire rostro-caudal length of the DH receives a largely ipsilateral innervation via the dorsolateral funiculus, although contralateral collaterization occurs in the DH itself; all laminae are richly innervated (BULLITT and LIGHT 1989), and varicosities and fibres are most numerous in superficial laminae 1 and II. Classically, PNs – especially those in the superficial laminae – present extensive serotonergic synaptic contacts, although recent studies have claimed the comparative scarcity of these profiles in the DH (in contrast to the VH) and suggested that "volume transmission" occurs whereby 5-HT expresses its actions at loci well removed from its site of release, possible involving interactions with glia cells (LIGHT et al. 1983; MARLIER et al. 1991a; MAXWELL and JANKOWSKA 1996; MAXWELL et al. 1983; MILETIC et al. 1984; RIDET et al. 1993; RUDA 1990; RUDA et al. 1986). In the light of complementary electrophysiological findings, direct, monosynaptic (or indirect volume) actions of 5-HT at STT and other PNs likely modulates the flow of nociceptive information to the brain (BELCHER et al. 1978; HEADLEY et al. 1978; JORDAN et al. 1979; WILLIS 1992; WILLCOCKSON et al. 1984; YEZIERSKI et al. 1982).

3. Influence on Interneurones in the Dorsal Horn

Serotoninergic pathways may also modulate the activity of PNs via inhibitory actions on relay, laminae-II localized EXINs which project to superficial and deeper laminae inasmuch as inhibitory action of iontophoretic 5-HT in deep PNs are *scarce* (FIELDS et al. 1991; LIGHT and KAVOOKJIAN 1988; WILLIS 1992). Of significance is also the involvement of ININs targetted by serotoninergic fibres. Although there is anatomical evidence that some of these are enkephalinergic (or dynorphinergi, GLAZER and BASBAUM 1984; MILETIC et al.

1984; RUDA 1990), functional evidence that opioidergic mechanisms are involved in the actions of 5-HT at the spinal level is controversial, and this mechanism is unlikely to play major role (CRISP and SMITH 1989; HO and TAKEMORI 1989; KELLSTEIN et al. 1988; MONROE et al. 1995; PAUL and HORNBY 1995; SPANOS et al. 1989; VASKO et al. 1984).

Of likely greater importance are GABAergic and possibly glycinergic ININs, a subpopulation of which may be co-localized (ALHAIDER et al. 1991; GLAZER and BASBAUM 1984; HAYES and CARLTON 1992; TODD et al. 1996; XU et al. 1993; YOSHIMURA and NISHI 1995). Indeed, the differential modulation of GABAergic ININ activity by excitatory 5-HT$_3$ (and 5-HT$_2$) as compared to inhibitory 5-HT$_{1A}$ receptors, may underlie their anti- and pro-nociceptive actions, respectively (ALHAIDER et al. 1991; MILLAN 1995; SUGIYAMA and HUANG 1995; see below). GABAergic ININs are also important because their functional hypoactivity (and possibly degeneration due to excitotoxic actions of NMDA receptors) contributes to chronic neuropathic pain states, together with other changes such as rewiring and alterations in DH neuronal sensitivity (see above and WOOLF and DOUBELL 1994).

Although the direct role of 5-HT in the induction of and response to such states remains surprisingly little explored, a role of DH pools of 5-HT seems probable inasmuch as DH-localized serotoninergic neurones are affected by both acute and long-term noxious stimulation and by manipulations modifying the activity of primary afferent nociponsive fibres (GODEFROY et al. 1987; MARLIER et al. 1992; MEN and MATSUI 1994a,b; TAGUCHI and SUZUKI 1992; WEIL-FUGAZZA 1990). Further, sprouting of serotoninergic neurones has been seen following nerve damage (WANG et al. 1991). There are also indications for alterations in serotoninergic turnover in chronic pain patients (see VON KNORRING 1990). Indeed, activation of DH-localized 5-HT$_{1A}$-receptors on ININs may provide an empirical model of the allodynia-like, mechanosensitivity of neuropathic pain states (MILLAN 1995; see below). In this light, it is also of interest that descending serotoninergic fibres modulate the transmission of (normally) non-nociceptive sensory information to the brain via an influence upon postsynaptic dorsal column neurones (BESSON and CHAOUCH 1987; WU and WESSENDORF 1992).

4. Influence on Primary Afferent Fibres

Despite indications for the existence of 5-HT receptors on PAF terminals (see below) there is little anatomical evidence for axo-axonic serotoninergic synapses in the DH (LIGHT et al. 1983; MAXWELL et al. 1983; MILETIC et al. 1984; RUDA 1990). Further, no clear data for the specific modulation of C and Aδ fibre excitability by serotoninergic mechanisms has been forthcoming (CARSTENS et al. 1981; HOLZIV et al. 1985). In addition, in vitro attempts to demonstrate that 5-HT modulates release of substance P in the DH of the rat have met with little success (see CESSELIN et al. 1994) and, although YONEHARA et al. (1991) showed that 5-HT inhibits noxious stimulus-elicited release of 5-HT in the trigeminal nucleus, a role of intervening GABAergic or other ININs could not be excluded. Nevertheless, 5-HT inhibits the DH capsaicin-evoked release of somastostatin, which may be implicated in inflammatory hyperalgesia (Kuraishi et al. 1991). Further, the marked influence of 5-HT on the peripheral terminals of PAFs, the occurrence of the mRNA for several 5-HT receptor types in the DRG and the possible role of "volume" actions on primary afferent terminals suggest that this question deserves further analysis (see Millan 1995; Pierce et al. 1996; Ridet et al. 1993).

III. Descending Serotoninergic Inhibition

The concept that descending serotoninergic fibres exert an inhibitory influence upon the flow of nociceptive information to the supraspinal level has dominated thinking for more than a decade (Basbaum and Fields 1984). However, the generality of this role has been challenged (Millan 1995). It is thus appropriate to briefly review this concept, which has its roots in both neuroanatomical studies (see above) and in observations of the antinociceptive actions of brainstem stimulation and of spinal administration of 5-HT (Advokat 1988; Antal et al. 1996; Basbaum and Fields 1984; Besson and Chaouch 1987; Le Bars 1988; Sawynok 1989). According to this theory, activation of descending serotoninergic pathways contributes to the analgesic properties of both morphine as well as of endogenous opioids released by electrical stimulation of the NRM, PAG and other VMM structures. However, it now seems unlikely that descending serotoninergic pathways fulfil a universal or generalized antinociceptive role.

First, stimulation of NRM more consistently increases extracellular levels of NAD than of 5-HT in the DH while spinal α_2-ARs are involved in the associated antinociception (Barbaro et al. 1985; Bowker and Abhold 1990; Gebhart and Randich 1990; Hammond and Yaksh 1984; Hammond et al. 1985; Iwamoto and Marion 1993; Jensen and Yaksh 1984). Second, activation of descending enkephalinergic, glycinergic and/or GABAergic neurones may contribute to stimulation-induced antinociception from the NRM and other structures (Antal et al. 1996; Blomqvist et al. 1994; Lin et al. 1994, 1996; Sorkin et al. 1993; Yezierski et al. 1982). Third, centripetal serotoninergic neurones do *not* invariably respond to noxious stimuli (Auerbach et al. 1985; Chaing and Xiang 1987; Matos et al. 1992). Fourth, *none* of the "on or off" cells implicated in the modulation of spinal nociception contains 5-HT. Although half of the "neutral" cells are serotoninergic, their role is unclear and they are unresponsive to morphine (Fields et al. 1991; Potrebic et al. 1994). Fifth, conduction velocities of antinociception-mediating and on/off cells are in the myelinated range, whereas serotoninergic axons from the NRM are unmyelinated (Basbaum et al. 1988). Sixth, pharmacological and chemical interruption of spinal serotoninergic transmission only variably affects basal nociceptive thresholds, opioid- and stimulation-induced antinociception (JOHANNESSEN et al. 1982; KURAISHI et al. 1983a,b; MILNE and GAMBLE 1990; VONVOIGTLANDER et al. 1984; YEZIERSKI et al. 1982; see LE BARS 1988; SAWYNOK 1989): further, it facilitates the antinociceptive effects of clonidine, the GABA$_B$ agonist, baclofen, and stress, and reduces the hyperalgesia elicited by intraplantar formalin (DUAN and SAWYNOK 1987; HUTSON et al. 1982, 1983; SAWYNOK 1989; TJØLSEN et al. 1991). Seventh, administration of spinal 5-HT itself can elicit behavioural hyperalgesia and antagonize the antinociceptive action of intrathecal NAD and morphine (ADVOKAT 1993; CLATWORTHY et al. 1988; CRISP et al. 1991; CRISP and SMITH 1989; SOLOMON et al. 1989). Eighth, 5-HT and descending serotoninergic pathways exert not only inhibition but also excitation of superficial and deep laminae neurones in the DH and direct inhibition of the latter is remarkably rare (BELCHER et al. 1978; EKBLOM et al. 1991; FIELDS et al. 1991; JORDAN et al. 1979; MURASE et al. 1990; REN et al. 1988, 1991; TODD and MILLAR 1983; YEZIERSKI et al. 1982; ZEMLAN et al. 1994; ZHUO and GEBHART 1991). These observations support the argument (MILLAN 1995) of several contrasting (pro- and antinociceptive) actions of 5-HT in the DH, probably mediated by different receptor types.

IV. Pharmacology of Spinal Serotoninergic Mechanisms Modulating Nociception

1. 5-HT$_{1A}$ Receptors

a) Localization and Neuronal Mechanisms of Action

5-HT$_{1A}$ receptors are prominent in rat and human DH, where they appear to display an incremental rostro-caudal gradient from cervical to lumbo-sacral regions, although this has recently been contested (LAPORTE et al. 1995, in press; MARLIER et al. 1991b; POMPEIANO et al. 1992; THOR et al. 1993). As shown by radioligand, mRNA and antibody studies, they are particularly concentrated in superficial I/II laminae. In contrast, they are almost undetectable in the rat VH and the IML – with the exception of the dorsomedial nucleus of the pedundal nerve which controls urinary function (KIA et al. 1996; MARLIER et al. 1991b; POMPANEIO et al. 1992; RIAD et al. 1991; THOR et al. 1993; but see KHECK et al. 1995). The human VH *does*, however, contains 5-HT$_{1A}$ receptors, albeit at a density ten-fold lower than in the DH. Lesion studies in the rat indicate that 5-HT$_{1A}$ receptors are localized postsynaptically to serotoninergic neurones (BERVOETS et al. 1993; LAPORTE et al. 1995), and they are likewise not found on descending adrenergic pathways consistent with their hypothesized presence on intrinsic neurones (LAPORTE et al. 1995; see below). Nevertheless, destruction of PAFs is associated with a minor reduction in the density of 5-HT$_{1A}$ in the superficial DH, suggesting that a fraction may be localized on these (LAPORTE et al. 1995). This suggestion is supported by the discovery of mRNA encoding 5-HT$_{1A}$ sites in the dorsal ganglion (POMPEIANO et al. 1992). Furthermore, 5-HT$_{1A}$ receptors have been claimed to reduce the activity of capsaicin-sensitive primary afferents by closing Ca^{2+} channels (DEL MAR et al. 1994). However, the high concentration of the 5-HT$_{1A}$ receptor agonist 8-OH-DPAT utilized questions this interpretation and 8-OH-DPAT fails to modify the release of substance P from primary afferents in dorsal horn slices (BOURGOIN et al. 1993). Further, it is difficult to exclude the occurrence of transsynaptic degeneration in denervation studies (SUGIMOTO et al. 1990), and a recent study failed to detect mRNA encoding 5-HT$_{1A}$ receptors in lumbar DRG (PIERCE et al. 1996). They did, however, detect 5-HT$_7$ receptors, for which 8-OH-DPAT has significant affinity. A of 5-HT$_7$ receptors might thus be responsible for certain peripheral (pronociceptive) actions previously attributed to 5-HT$_{1A}$ receptors (PIERCE et al. 1996).

b) Functional Actions

In an early study of WDR neurones, iontophoretic administration of 8-OH-DPAT non-selectively suppressed their response to both noxious and non-noxious stimuli (EL-YASSIR et al. 1988), suggesting that activation of 5-HT$_{1A}$ receptors does not elicit a selective antinociceptive action against Aδ/C fibre stimulation – although the significance of actions against normally innocuous (Aβ) mediated stimuli in neuropathic painful states should be recalled (see above). In a fraction (20%) of cells spontaneous activity is increased by 8-OH-DPAT, an observation which has been linked to an increase in receptive field size and an enhancement of nociceptive withdrawal reflexes (MURPHY and ZEMLAN 1990; MURPHY et al. 1992; ZEMLAN et al. 1983). This interpretation has been supported by Ali et al. (1994) who, employing intrathecal injection of 8-OH-DPAT, observed both an increase in the response of DH neurones to noxious stimulation and a reduced tail-flick latency to a noxious stimulus. These findings corroborate previous studies reporting pronociceptive actions of 5-HT$_{1A}$ agonists in both tail-flick and other algesiometric paradigms (CRISP et al. 1991; FASMER et al. 1986; SOLOMON and GEBHART 1988a,b; see MILLAN 1994). Further, 5-HT$_{1A}$ agonists increase scratching elicited by intrathecal NMDA or substance P in mice (ALHAIDER and WILCOX 1993 but see EIDE and HOLE 1991) and specifically inhibit the induction of antinociception by both nicotine (DAMAJ et al. 1994) and μ-opioid agonists (ARTS et al. 1991; MILLAN and COLPAERT 1991a,b; MILLAN et al. 1991, 1996). In analogy, stress and defeat induces analgesia is attenuated by spinal actions of 5-HT$_{1A}$ receptor agonists (HUTSON et al. 1983; RODGERS et al. 1991). Bearing in mind evidence that 5-HT (possibly via 5-HT$_{1A}$) receptors inhibit the antinociceptive effects of the GABA$_B$ agonist baclofen and of the α_2-AR agonist clonidine (see above), this counteraction of antinociceptive mechanisms by 5-HT$_{1A}$ receptors in the DH appears to be quite broadly expressed. In analogy, 5-HT$_{1A}$ receptors may mediate descending facilitation of DH neurones by stimulation of vagal afferents or of the nucleus reticularis gigantocellularis (ZHUO and GEBHART 1991).

One further "pronociceptive" effect mediated by 5-HT$_{1A}$ receptors is that of "spontaneous tail-flicks" (STFs) – tail-flicks in the "absence" of noxious stimulation (MILLAN et al. 1991) a response reflecting activation of 5-HT$_{1A}$ receptors in the DH (BERVOETS et al. 1993). The induction and modulation of STFs may be dissociated from tail-flicks elicited by phasic noxious stimuli and from a generalized perturbation of motor function (MILLAN et al. 1996). Indeed, STFs represent a *sensory* rather than motor phenomenon integrated in the DH (BERVOETS et al. 1993) and display striking similarities to certain experimental models of the mechanical allodynia seen in neuropathic pain. Thus STFs are little affected by opioids, bradykinin type1 and 2 antagonists, neurokinin type 1 and 2 antagonists and aspirin (MILLAN et al. 1996). In contrast, STFs are potently blocked by systemic or spinal administration of antagonists at NMDA (and coupled glycine$_B$) receptors, which are implicated in sensitization processes underlying chronic pain, as well as antagonists at AMPA receptors, which are implicated in Aβ fibre-mediated mechanical allodynia (MELLER et al. 1993; URBAN et al. 1994; WOOLF and DOUBELL 1994; XU et al. 1993, 1995). α_2-AR agonists as well as muscimol and baclofen, agonists at GABA$_A$ and GABA$_B$ receptors, respectively, also block STFs. As with α_2-AR agonists (see above), GABAergic agonists are active in both experimental and clinical neuropathic pain states (ANGHINAH et al. 1994; XU et al. 1993). As suggested above, GABAergic ININs may bear inhibitory 5-HT$_{1A}$ receptors such that the blockade of STFs by GABAergic agonists would be equivalent to the restoration of 5-HT$_{1A}$ receptor-interrupted – like GABAergic transmission inhibitory to WDR PNs. Thus 5-HT$_{1A}$ receptor activation in the DH, possibly via inhibition of GABAergic and other types of IN, may relieve inhibition of WDR neurones and enhance nociception. This would enhance their sensitivity in a manner similar to that confronted in some neuropathic painful states where GABAergic IN activity is compromized.

However, several caveats must be noted. First, this is an empirical model which mimics only one component of such painful states. Second, the relationship of STFs to spinally integrated processes involved in the modulation of non-noxious information and of motor response still requires further evaluation (FARKAS and ONO 1995). Indeed, in electrophysiologial and behavioural studies of spinal responses it is not a priori possible to be certain that changes are associated with an increase in access of nociceptive information into the brain (MURPHY and ZEMLAN 1990; ZEMLAN et al. 1994), that is, accompanied by a consequent sensation of "pain" rather than just in the motor reflex arc. Third, there is currently no evidence that administration of 5-HT$_{1A}$ receptor agonists to man elicits pain and the clinical relevance of these effects requires clarification (KISHORE-KUMAR 1989). In fact, some studies have suggested antinociceptive actions of 5-HT$_{1A}$ agonists (BRAS et al. 1990; DANZEBRINK and GEBHART 1991a; EIDE and HOLE 1991; MJELLEM et al. 1993; MURPHY et al. 1992; XU et al. 1994a,b). A rigorous pharmacological demonstration that 5-HT$_{1A}$ receptors in the DH elicit antinociception in these studies was not, however, presented, and antinociceptive actions of 8-OH-DPAT, buspirone and other

5-HT$_{1A}$ receptor agonists have generally proven resistant to serotonergic antagonists (DANZEBRINK and GEBHART 1991a; MILLAN 1994). Indeed, both α_2-adrenergic and dopamine D$_2$ receptors have been implicated in their antinociceptive actions (MILLAN and COLPAERT 1991a,b; POST and ARCHER 1990; GIORDANO 1991). Moreover, even where 5-HT$_{1A}$ receptors appear to be involved in the putative antinociceptive actions of 5-HT$_{1A}$ receptor agonists, their marked cardiovascular, endocrine and other actions may modify behaviour in algesiometric tests and underlie an apparent antinociception (MILLAN et al. 1994; GIORDANO and LaVERNE 1992).

Notwithstanding these arguments, several recent papers have reopened the possibility that DH-localized 5-HT$_{1A}$ receptors can specifically inhibit ascending nociceptive transmission, for example, in response to cerebral administration of μ-opioids and to NRM stimulation, as well as in a model of sciatic ligation and in an algesiometric paradigm reflecting the affective component of pain (CERVO et al. 1994; LIN et al. 1996; MILLAN 1995; MILLAN et al. 1996; POWELL and DYKSTRA 1995; ROBLES et al. 1996; SÁNCHEZ et al. 1995; XU et al. 1994a,b; ZEMLAN et al. 1994). Such actions would presumably be mediated at PNs, EXINs or terminals of PAFs

2. 5-HT$_{1B}$/5-HT$_{1D}$ Receptors

a) Localization and Neuronal Mechanisms of Action

In the rat 5-HT$_{1B}$ receptors manifest a similar distribution to 5-HT$_{1A}$ receptors inasmuch as they are found preferentially in the DH (laminae I followed by III/IV) rather than the VH and IML. However, their overall density is lower than that of 5-HT$_{1A}$ sites, and they are found in relatively low amounts in laminae II, while they are also present in the corticospinal tract. A further distinction is provided by their presence as inhibitory autoreceptors on the terminals of serotoninergic neurones (MARLIER et al. 1991a,b; THOR et al. 1993). Nevertheless, the major population is localized postsynaptically to serotoninergic neurones (LAPORTE et al. 1995), likely on PNs themselves – or INs. In addition, 5-HT$_{1B}$ receptors may be present on fine-calibre PAFs since a 20% loss of sites is seen upon capsaicin treatment. In line with studies of homologous rodent 5-HT$_{1B}$ sites a recent study of human spinal cord employing [^{3}H]GTI, a radioligand which does not distinguish between 5-HT$_{1D\alpha}$ and 5-HT$_{1D\beta}$ receptors, revealed 5-HT$_{1D}$ receptors predominantly in the superficial laminae and present only at ten-fold lower levels in the VH (LAPORTE et al. 1996). mRNA encoding 5-HT$_{1B}$ sites has been detected in the rat trigeminal ganglia and DRG, while mRNA encoding 5-HT$_{1D\alpha}$ sites has been detected in guinea pig trigeminal ganglia. Further, mRNA encoding 5-HT$_{1D\beta}$ and 5-HT$_{1D\alpha}$ receptors is present in ganglia of the Vth cranial (trigeminal) nerve in man (BRUINVELS et al. 1992; DOUCET et al. 1995; LAPORTE et al. 1996; MILLS and MARTIN 1995; PIERCE et al. 1996; REBECK et al. 1994). The absence of receptor protein itself (BRUINVELS et al. 1992) suggests that receptors may be transported to peripheral terminals of these afferent *sensory* neurones and activation of $5\text{-}HT_{1B}/5\text{-}HT_{1D}$ receptors inhibits the peripheral release of neuropeptides from C fibres: this putative action would reduce neurogenic inflammation, a process implicated in the genesis of migraine headaches (see MILLAN 1995; MOSKOVITZ 1992; ZOCHODNE and Ho 1994). However, as regards central terminals of these primary afferents, despite the above-cited evidence for mRNA encoding $5\text{-}HT_{1B}$ sites in ganglia and for a loss of $5\text{-}HT_{1B}$ sites in the DH upon degeneration of primary afferents, the $5\text{-}HT_{1B/D}$ agonist, sumatriptan did not modify the release of CGRP or substance P in rat spinal cord (BOURGOIN et al. 1993). Antinociceptive actions at DH-localized $5\text{-}HT_{1B}$ receptors may thus predominantly be expressed postsynaptically to primary afferents in the DH.

b) Functional Actions

Activation of DH-localized $5\text{-}HT_{1B}$ sites in rodents mediates antinociception – and a decrease in receptive field size – against diverse modalities of noxious stimulation (ALHAIDER and WILCOX 1993; DANZEBRINK and GEBHART 1991a; McKEARNEY 1989; MURPHY and ZEMLAN 1990; MURPHY et al. 1992; SAWYNOK and REID 1994; SCHLICKER et al. 1992). Such actions are specific inasmuch as inhibition of the activity of WDR neurones is expressed against noxious but not non-noxious input (EL YASSIR et al. 1988). EL YASSIR et al. (1988) also provided evidence that activation of $5\text{-}HT_{1B}$ receptors contributes to the antinociceptive actions of NRM stimulation, that is, $5\text{-}HT_{1B}$ receptors may be involved in processes of descending inhibition. Biochemical evidence for a presynaptic action of $5\text{-}HT_{1B}$ agonists on PAFs is lacking (see above) and the ability of $5\text{-}HT_{1B}$ agonists to block GLU-induced firing of DH neurones supports the possibility of a postsynaptic locus of action (EL YASSIR and FLEETWOOD-WALKER 1990). Although serotoninergic terminals in the DH bear inhibitory $5\text{-}HT_{1B}$ autoreceptors, an inhibition of 5-HT release is unlikely to be involved in the antinociceptive actions of $5\text{-}HT_{1B}$ ligands inasmuch as their actions are not reduced in rats sustaining lesions of serotoninergic pathways (SAWYNOK and REID 1994). In line with evidence that spinal serotoninergic and adrenergic mechanisms may interact in the control of nociception, synergistic antinociceptive actions of $5\text{-}HT_{1B}$ and $\alpha_2\text{-}AR$ agonists have been documented (DANZEBRINK and GEBHART 1991b).

3. $5\text{-}HT_{2A/2C}$ Receptors

a) Localization and Neuronal Mechanisms of Action

The overall density of $5\text{-}HT_{2A}$ receptors in the spinal cord is very low, and they are diffusely distributed therein; indeed, despite the presence of mRNA encoding $5\text{-}HT_{2A}$ sites certain studies have failed to detect $5\text{-}HT_{2A}$ sites at all. The density of $5\text{-}HT_{2A}$ sites is, further, particularly low in the DH, although a minor population does probably exist here as well as, more densely, in the VH and

IML (HELTON et al. 1994; LAPORTE et al. 1995, 1996; MARLIER et al. 1991a,b; POMPEIANO et al. 1994; PRANZATELLI et al. 1992; THOR et al. 1993). The closely related 5-HT$_{2C}$ site appears to be present at higher concentrations although still at levels far below those of 5-HT$_{1A}$ sites; further, it is absent from cat spinal cord (CESSELIN et al. 1994; LAPORTE et al. 1996; MOLINEAUX et al. 1989; PRANZATELLI et al. 1992). Intriguingly, mRNA encoding both 5-HT$_{2C}$ and 5-HT$_{2A}$ receptors was recently reported in rat DRG (PIERCE et al. 1996). The presence of 5-HT$_{2A}$ sites in the DRG is consistent with evidence that they directly sensitize PAFs in the periphery, and these data raise the possibility of an analogous role for 5-HT$_{2C}$ sites (see MILLAN 1995). 5-HT$_{2B}$ mRNA has been found in the spinal cord of all species as yet examined, including rat and human (HELTON et al. 1994).

b) Functional Actions

In the light of the above-mentioned anatomical studies the interpretation of some early work (BANK et al. 1988; SOLOMON and GEBHART 1988b; see CESSELIN et al. 1994) that the blockade of 5-HT-induced antinociception by poorly selective 5-HT$_2$ antagonists reflects antagonism of 5-HT$_2$ sites must be taken with some caution. Indeed, comparatively little concrete evidence in favour of antinociceptive actions of spinal 5-HT$_{2A}$ sites has been forthcoming (CHOJNACKA-WAJCIK et al. 1994; CRISP et al. 1991; SAWYNOK and REID 1994; TAKESHITA and YAMEGUSHI 1995; XU et al. 1994a,b). Nevertheless, there are data suggesting that 5-HT$_{2A}$ sites may contribute to the antinociceptive effects elicited by PAG stimulation, stress, vagal stimulation, naloxone, cerebral μ-opioids and the benzamide, tiapride (EVANS et al. 1994; KIEFEL et al. 1989; LIN and WILLIS 1993; PAUL and PHILIPS 1986; PAUL et al. 1989; TAKESHITA et al. 1995; XU et al. 1994a). These findings require rigorous pharmacological corroboration. SUGIYAMA and HUANG (1995) have recently provided evidence that 5-HT$_{2A}$ receptors mediate inhibitory potentials in rat trigeminal neurones via the activation of GABAergic/glycinergic INs. This observation supports the concept (MILLAN 1995) that GABAergic INs may play a key role in mediating serotoninergic actions on PNs in the DH.

A clinical report that the 5-HT$_2$ antagonist, ritanserin, exerts antinociceptive properties has appeared and requires confirmation (SANDRINI et al. 1986). In fact, certain studies have suggested that spinal 5-HT$_{2A}$ or 5-HT$_{2C}$ receptors *potentiate* nociception (EIDE and HOLE 1991; Ho and TAKEMORI 1989; KJØSVIK et al. 1990; POWELL and DYKSTRA 1995; SÁNCHEZ et al. 1995; SAWYNOCK and REID 1994; XU et al. 1994a,b). This action may involve a facilatory action on PAF terminals reflecting the induction of phospholipase C and subsequently protein kinase C (HORI et al. 1996). On the other hand, an inhibition of DH release of NAD may also be implicated (CELUCH et al. 1992). The above observations suggest that a further clarification of the roles of 5-HT$_{2A}$, 5-HT$_{2B}$ and 5-HT$_{2C}$ receptors in the modulation of nociception at the spinal level would be of interest.

4. 5-HT₃ Receptors

a) Localization and Neuronal Mechanisms of Action

Radiolabelling and antibody studies have revealed that 5-HT$_3$ sites are highly concentrated in superficial laminae (particularly lamina I) in both rat and human spinal cord, whereas the VH and IML are virtually devoid of 5-HT$_3$ receptors (KIA et al. 1995; LAPORTE et al. 1992; WAEBER et al. 1989). They are localized neither on serotoninergic neurones themselves nor on descending adrenergic neurones (LAPORTE et al. 1995). The pronounced magnitude (>50%) of the decrease in the density of superficial 5-HT$_3$ sites provoked by destruction of unmyelinated PAFs suggests that a substantial proportion are localized on these, consistent with the presence of mRNA encoding 5-HT$_3$ sites in rat and mouse DRG (KIA et al. 1995; KIDD et al. 1993; LAPORTE et al. 1995, 1996; TECOTT et al. 1993; WAEBER et al. 1989). In line with their localization on PAFs, 5-HT$_3$ receptor antagonists inhibited CGRP release in rat spinal cord (SARIA et al. 1990), while there is electrophysiological evidence both for functional actions of 5-HT$_3$ receptors on DRG neurones (PHILIPPI et al. 1995; ROBERTSON and BEVAN 1991) and for direct depolarizing action of 5-HT$_3$ receptors on the peripheral terminals of PAFs (see MILLAN 1995). On the other hand, the 5-HT$_3$ agonist 2-methyl-5-HT failed to modify the release of substance P or CGRP in rat spinal cord (BOURGOIN et al. 1993). Thus a possible role of 5-HT$_3$ sites on PAFs in modulating nociceptive information remains to be further explored.

b) Functional Actions

Studies employing the preferential agonists at 5-HT$_3$ sites, 2-methyl-5-HT and metachloro-phenylbiguanide, as well as selective antagonists in interaction with 5-HT, suggest that activation of 5-HT$_3$ receptors in the DH evokes antinociception under some although not all conditions (CRISP et al. 1991; DANZEBRINK and GEBHART 1991a; GIORDANO 1991; GLAUM et al. 1990; XU et al. 1994). Further, 5-HT$_3$ antagonists block defeat-induced antinociception (RODGERS et al. 1991). In addition, inhibition of WDR neurones in the DH by 5-HT$_3$ receptor agonists or PAG stimulation is reduced by local (microdialysis) administration of antagonists at 5-HT$_3$ receptors: interestingly, responses to noxious as well as non-noxious mechanical stimulation are equally affected (PENG et al. 1995b). The excitatory influence of ondansetron alone suggests a degree of tonic activity at 5-HT$_3$ receptors. The central antinociceptive action of paracetamol was recently found to be inhibited by spinal administration of a 5-HT$_3$ antagonist (PELISSIER et al. 1995). As mentioned above, the role of 5-HT$_3$ sites on the central terminals of PAFs remains to be defined, and the reduction by 5-HT$_3$ agonists in the scratching provoked by spinal administration of substance P and NMDA suggests that their antinociceptive actions are expressed postsynaptically (ALHAIDER et al. 1991). Inasmuch as 5-HT$_3$ receptors are excitatory, such antinociceptive actions are unlikely to be exerted directly at PNs but rather via the engagement of GABAergic (and other) ININs (ALHAIDER et al. 1991; GIORDANO 1991; GLAZER and BASBAUM 1984; LIN et al. 1994; PENG et al. 1995b), possibly the same population as inhibited by pronociceptive 5-HT$_{1A}$ receptors (MILLAN 1995). Thus, both the behavioural antinociceptive actions of 5-HT$_3$ agonists and their ability to inhibit the excitation of WDR and high-threshold neurones by noxious stimulation and NMDA is blocked by the GABA$_A$ antagonists bicuculline and picrotoxin and (less completely) the GABA$_B$ antagonist phaclofen. One population of these GABA receptors may be localized on PAFs, but the major population likely targets PNs (ALHAIDER et al. 1991; ILIAKIS et al. 1996; LIN et al. 1994; PENG et al. 1995a; TEOH et al. 1996).

Finally, certain WDR neurones in the DH may be excited by 5-HT$_3$ receptors, an effect accompanied by increased nociception. This action is likely expressed on PNs directly, although EXINs or terminals of PAFs could be involved (ALI et al. 1996; SARIA et al. 1990).

5. Other 5-HT Receptor Types

It has been suggested that a substantial proportion (50%) of 5-HT$_1$ binding sites in superficial laminae of the rat spinal cord comprises a putative 5-HT$_{1S}$ site (ZEMLAN and SCHWAB 1991; ZEMLAN et al. 1990). There is some evidence for the occurrence of 5-HT$_6$ sites in rat spinal cord (WARD et al. 1995). The apparent existence of 5-HT$_7$ sites in the DH (GUSTAFSON et al. 1996) would be of particular interest in view of the presence of the corresponding mRNA in DRG and of their significant affinity for 8-OH-DPAT (ca. 25-fold lower than at 5-HT$_{1A}$ receptors; BOESS and MARTIN 1994; RUAT et al. 1994). Further, whereas 5-HT$_{1A}$ receptors inhibit adenyl cyclase, 5-HT$_7$ sites are positively coupled, and a paradoxical stimulation of adenyl cyclase activity with high (10–100 nM) concentrations of 8-OH-DPAT has been reported in cultures of spinal neurones (LUCAS et al. 1993). This is accompanied by a cAMP and c-*fos* dependent induction in the gene expression of dynorphin, a major component of endogenous mechanisms of pain control (MILLAN 1993; OSSIPOV et al. 1996; RILEY et al. 1996; STILLER et al. 1993). This observation, together with the modest potency (50 nM) of 8-OH-DPAT in reducing NMDA receptor-mediated excitation of DH neurones (MURASE et al. 1990), has led to the suggestion that the apparent spinal, antinociceptive actions of 8-OH-DPAT (generally seen at high doses and little characterized pharmacologically) may reflect the activation of putative 5-HT$_7$ receptors (MILLAN 1995). Interestingly, GUSTAFSON et al. (1996) suggested that 5-HT$_7$ sites, but not mRNA encoding 5-HT$_7$ receptors, exist in superficial laminae of the rat DH. This would be consistent with their presence of PAF terminals and the observation that DRG express mRNA encoding 5-HT$_7$ receptors (PIERCE et al. 1996). A possible role of 5-HT$_7$ sites in the inhibition of VH-localized MNs should also be considered (HASEGAWA and ONO 1996). Finally, 5-HT$_4$ agonists have been shown to elicit antinociception by a cholinergic mechanism (GHELARDINI et al. 1996).

E. General Discussion and Conclusions

In conclusion, there is extensive anatomical, electrophysiological and functional evidence that adrenergic and serotoninergic pathways descending from the brainstem to the spinal cord play a key role in the modulation of nociception. The potential importance of actions in the VH and IML should not be forgotten; in particular, the control of sympathetic outflow at the level of preganglionic neurones in the IML may markedly modify nociception in both inflammatory and neuropathic painful states. Nevertheless, it is the DH which is the principal site of action for the modulation of nociceptive information by adrenergic and serotoninergic mechanisms. In this regard there are clear differences amongst individual adrenergic and serotoninergic subtypes as concerns their influence upon nociception. Moreover, even one individual subtype may exert a complex pattern of affects reflecting multiple sites of interactions sites. For example, $5\text{-}HT_{1A}$, $5\text{-}HT_{2A}$ and $5\text{-}HT_3$ receptors may all mediate both pro- *and* antinociceptive actions in the DH. One simple explanation for this phenomenon could be that their actions are expressed both directly at PNs themselves and indirectly via ININs (MILLAN 1995). Receptor types decreasing cellular excitability (such as $5\text{-}HT_{1A}$) would elicit antinociception directly at PNs yet increase nociception via actions at ININs – the latter action predominating. The opposite would be anticipated for excitatory receptors such as $5\text{-}HT_3$ receptors – where direct excitation of PNs leading to antinociception appears to prevail.

Clearly, at the behavioural level the overall impact upon nociception depends upon the precise balance of such actions as well as any influence on primary afferent terminals etc. and sympathetic transmissions. In this regard the often neglected importance of observations following *systemic* drug administration should be mentioned. The availability of improved pharmacological tools, more precise information concerning the localization of various adrenergic and serotoninergic receptor subtypes, the application of more refined electrophysiological and behavioural techniques and the use of experimental models of both nociceptive and neuropathic pain should allow for additional progress in defining the pathophysiological significance and therapeutic potential of spinal adrenergic and serotoninergic mechanisms for the modulation of nociception.

Monoaminergic antidepressant drugs have found use in the treatment of neuropathic pain. Their principal action is likely the release of NAD onto α_2-ARs in the DH, although a facilatory role of 5-HT should not be discounted and other non-monoaminergic and cerebral mechanisms may also be involved. Analgesia is exerted independently of their antidepressant properties – as indicated by the lower dose range, more rapid action and dissociation of analgesic versus mood-elevating properties (DIRKSEN et al. 1994; ESCHALIER et al. 1994; HWANG and WILCOX 1987; MAX et al. 1991; ONGHENA and VAN HOUDENHOVE 1992). Further, clonidine and other α_2-AR agonists are attracting increasing interest as potential analgesic (and adjunct analgesic) agents (see above).

On the other hand, despite the success of the antimigraine 5-HT$_{1D}$ (or 5-HT$_1$-like) agonist sumatriptan (ZOCHODNE and HO 1994) therapeutically useful drugs with a predominantly *spinal, serotoninergic* mode of pain relief are still awaited. Indeed, the enormous research effort devoted to descending serotoninergic controls of nociceptive information over the past 15 years has generated to date little in terms of improved pain relief. This likely reflects the fact that the segmental modulation of nociceptive information is far more complicated than originally realized concerning the role of descending pathways, mechanisms underlying the induction and maintenance of painful states and, above all, the diverse role of multiple serotoninergic receptor types. It is this remarkable diversity of serotoninergic and ARs which offers the hope for the development of novel, effective and well-tolerated strategies for the relief of pain.

References

Aantaa R, Scheinin M (1993) Alpha$_2$-adrenergic agents in anaesthesia. Acta Anasthesiol Scand 37:433–448

Abram SE, Winne RP (1995) Intrathecal acetylcholinesterase inhibitors produce analgesia that is synergistic with morphine and clonidine in rats. Anesth Analg 81:501–507

Advokat C (1988) The role of descending inhibition in morphine-induced analgesia. Trends Pharmacol Sci 9:330–334

Advokat C (1993) Intrathecal coadministration of serotonin and morphine differentially modulates the tail-flick reflex of intact and spinal rats. Pharmacol Biochem Behav 45:871–879

Aho MS, Erkola OA, Scheinin M, Lehtinen AM, Kortila KT (1991) Effect of intravenously administered dexmedetomidine on pain after laparoscopic tubal ligation. Anesth Analg 73:112–118

Aho MS, Scheinin H, Lehtinen AM, Erkola OA, Vuorinen J, Korttila KT (1992) Intramuscularly administered dexmedetomidine attenuates hemodynamic and stress hormone responses to gynecologic laparoscopy. Anesth Analg 75:932–939

Aimone LD, Jones SL, Gebhart G (1987) Stimulation-produced descending inhibition from the periaqueductal gray and nucleus raphe magnus in the rat: mediation by spinal monoamines but not opioids. Pain 31:123–136

Alhaider AA, Wilcox GL (1993) Differential roles of 5-hydroxytryptamine1A and 5-hydroxytryptamine1B receptor subtypes in modulating spinal nociceptive transmission in mice. J Pharmacol Exp Ther 265:378–385

Alhaider AA, Lei SZ, Wilcox GL (1991) Spinal 5-HT3 receptor-mediated antinociception: possible release of GABA. J Neurosci 11:1881–1888

Ali Z, Wu G, Kozlov A, Barasi S (1994) The actions of 5-HT1 agonists and antagonists on nociceptive processing in the rat spinal cord: results from behavioural and electrophysiological studies. Brain Res 661:83–90

Ali Z, Wu G, Kozlov A, Barasi S (1996) The role of 5-HT$_3$ receptors in nociceptive processing in the rat spinal cord: results from behavioural and electrophysiological studies. Neurosci Lett 208:203–207

Anghinah R, Oliveira ASB, Gabbai AA (1994) Effect of baclofen on pain in diabetic neuropathy. Muscle Nerve 17:958–959

Antal M, Petkó M, Polgár E, Heizmann CW, Storm-Mathisen J (1996) Direct evidence of an extensive gabaergic innervation of the spinal dorsal horn by fibres descending from the rostral ventromedial medulla. Neuroscience 73:509–518

Arnér S, Meyerson BA (1988) Opioids in neuropathic pain. Pain Dig 3:15–22

Arts KS, Holmes BB, Fujimoto JM (1991) Differential contribution of descending serotonergic and noradrenergic systems to central Tyr-D-Ala-Gly-NMePhe-Gly-ol (DAMGO) and morphine-induced antinociception in mice. J Pharmacol Exp Ther 256:890–896

Arvidsson U, Cullheim S, Ulfhake B, Dagerlind A, Luppi P, Kitahama K, Jouvet M, Terenius L, Hokfelt T (1992) Distribution of enkephalin and its relation to serotonin in cat and monkey spinal cord and brain stem. Synapse 11:85–104

Arvidsson U, Dado RJ, Riedl M, Lee JH, Law PY, Loh HH, Elde, R, Wessendorf MW (1995) Delta-opioid receptor immunoreactivity. Distribution in brainstem and spinal cord, and relationship to biogenic amines and enkephalin. J Neurosci 15:1215–1235

Ashby CR, Edwards E, Wang RY (1994) Electrophysiological evidence for a functional interaction between 5-HT$_{1A}$ and 5-HT$_2$ receptors in the rat medial prefrontal cortex: an iontophoretic study. Synapse 17:173–181

Aston-Jones G, Shipley MT, Chouvet G, Ennis M, van Bockstaele E, Pieribone V, Shiekhattar R, Akaola H, Drtolet G, Astier B, Charléty P, Valentino RJ, Williams JT (1991) Afferent regulation of locus coeruleus neurones: anatomy, physiology and pharmacology. Prog Brain Res 88:47–75

Auerbach SB, Fornal C, Jacobs BL (1985) Response of serotonin-containing neurones in nucleus raphe magnus to morphine, noxious stimuli and PAG stimulation in freely moving cats. Exp Neurol 88:609–628

Ault B, Hildebrand LM (1993) Effects of excitatory amino acid receptor antagonists on a capsaicin-evoked nociceptive reflex: a comparison with morphine, clonidine and baclofen. Pain 52:341–349

Bank WA, Kastin AJ, Trentman TL, Hayes HS, Johnson BG, Galina ZH (1988) Mediation of serotonin-induced analgesia by the 5-HT2 receptor in the pentobarbital anesthetized mouse model. Brain Res Bull 21:887–891

Barbaro NM, Hammond DL, Fields HL (1985) Effects of intrathecally administered methysergide and yohimbine on microstimulation-produced antinociception in the rat. Brain Res 343:223–229

Basbaum AI, Fields HL (1984) Endogenous pain control systems: brainstem spinal pathways and endorphin circuitry. Annu Rev Neurosci 7:309–338

Basbaum AI, Zahs K, Lord B, Lakos S (1988) The fiber caliber of 5-HT immunoreactive axons in the dorsolateral funiculus of the spinal cord of the rat and cat. Somatosens Res 5:177–185

Basbaum AI, Chi SI, Levine JD (1991) Factors that contribute to peripheral nerve injury-evoked persistent expression of the C-fos proto-oncogene in the spinal cord of the rat. In: Besson JM, Guilbaud G (eds) Lesions of the primary afferents fibres as a tool for the study of clinical pain. Elsevier, Amsterdam, pp 205–218

Beitz AJ, Mullett MA, Brandt N (1988) The relationship of periaqueductal gray projections to bulbospinal neurons: a combined fluorogold-PHAL analysis. Soc Neurosci Abstr 14:856

Belcher G, Ryall RW, Schaffner B (1978) The differential effects of 5-hydroxytryptamine, noradrenaline and raphe stimulation on nociceptive and non-nociceptive dorsal horn interneurones in the cat. Brain Res 151:307–321

Benhamou D, Narchi P, Hamza J, Marx M, Peyrol MT, Sembeil F (1994) Addition of oral clonidine to postoperative patient-controlled analgesia with i.v. morphine. Br J Anaesth 72:537–540

Bergles DE, Doze VA, Madison DV, Smith SJ (1996) Excitatory actions of norepinephrine on multiple classes of hippocampal CA1 interneurones. J Neurosci 16:572–585

Berkowitz DE, Price DT, Bello EA, Page SO, Schwinn DA (1994) Localization of messenger RNA for three distinct α_2-adrenergic receptor subtypes in human tissues. Anesthesiology 81:1235–1244

Bernard JM, Kick O, Bonnet F (1995) Comparison of intravenous and epidural clonidine for postoperative patient-controlled analgesia. Anesth Analg 81:706–712

Bernardi PS, Valtschanoff JG, Weinberg RJ, Schmidt HHHW, Rustioni A (1995) Synaptic interactions between primary afferent terminals and GABA and nitric oxide-synthesizing neurons in superficial laminae of the rat spinal cord. J Neurosci 15:1363–1371

Bervoets K, Millan MJ (1994) 5-HT1A receptors and the tail-flick response. V. Opposite modulation of 5-HT1A receptor-induced spontaneous tail-flicks by α-1A – as compared to α-2D – adrenoceptors in rat lumbar spinal cord. J Pharmacol Exp Ther 269:110–120

Bervoets K, Rivet JM, Millan MJ (1993) 5-HT1A receptors and the tail-flick response. IV: Spinally-localized 5-HT1A receptors postsynaptic to serotoninergic ne-urones mediate spontaneous tail-flicks in the rat. J Pharmacol Exp Ther 264:95–104

Besson JM, Chaouch A (1987) Peripheral and spinal mechanisms of nociception. Physiol Rev 67:67–186

Björklund A, Skagerberg G (1982) Descending monoaminergic projections to the spinal cord. In: Sjölund B, Björklund A (eds) Brain stem control of spinal mechanisms. Elsevier Biochemical, Amsterdam, pp 55–88

Blomqvist A, Hermanson O, Ericson H, Larhammar D (1994) Activation of a bulbospinal opioidergic projection by pain stimuli in the awake rat. Neuroreport 5:461–464

Bobker DH (1994) A slow excitatory postsynaptic potential mediated by 5-HT$_2$ receptors in nucleus prepositus hypoglossi. J Neurosci 14:2428–2434

Boess FG, Martin IL (1994) Molecular biology of 5-HT receptors. Neuropharmacology 33:275–317

Bonnet F, Boico O, Rostaing S, Loriferne JF, Saada M (1990a) Clonidine-induced analgesia in postoperative patients: epidural versus intramuscular administration. Anesthesiology 72:423–427

Bonnet F, Buisson VB, Franÿois Y, Catoire P, Saada M (1990b) Effects of oral and subarachnoid clonidine on spinal anesthesia with bupivacaine. Reg Anesth 15:211–214

Bouaziz H, Tong C, Yoon Y, Hood DD, Eisenach JC (1996) Intravenous opioids stimulate norepinephrine and acetylcholine release in spinal cord dorsal horn. Systematic studies in sheep and an observation in a human. Anesthesiology 84:143–154

Bourgoin S, Pohl M, Mauborgne A, Benoliel JJ, Collin E, Hamon M, Cesselin, F (1993) Monoaminergic control of the release of calcitonin gene-related peptide- and substance P-like materials from rat spinal cord slices. Neuropharmacology 32:633–640

Bowker RM, Abbott LC (1990) Quantitative re-evaluation of descending serotonergic and non-serotonergic projections from the medulla of the rodent: evidence for extensive co-existence of serotonin and peptides in the same spinally projecting neurones, but not from the nucleus raphe magnus. Brain Res 512:15–25

Bowker RM, Abhold RH (1990) Evoked chages in 5-hydroxytryptamine and norepinephrine release: in vivo dialysis of the rat dorsal horn. Eur J Pharmacol 175:101–106

Bras H, Jankowska E, Noga B, Skoog B (1990) Comparison of effects of various types of NA and 5-HT agonists on transmission from group II muscle afferents in the cat. Eur J Neurosci 2:1029–1039

Bruinvels AT, Landwehrmeyer B, Moskowitz MA, Hoyer D (1992) Evidence for the presence of 5-HT1B receptor messenger RNA in neurones of the rat trigeminal ganglia. Eur J Pharmacol 227:357–359

Buccafusco JJ (1990) Participation of different brain regions in the anti-narcotic withdrawal action of clonidine in the dependent rat. Brain Res 513:8–14

Bullitt E (1989) Induction of c-fos-like protein within the lumbar spinal cord and thalamus of the rat following peripheral stimulation. Brain Res 493:391–397

Bullitt E, Light AR (1989) Intraspinal course of descending serotoninergic pathways innervating the rodent dorsal horn and lamina X. J Comp Neurol 286:231–242

Buritova J, Chapman V, Honoré P, Besson JM (1996) The contribution of GABA$_B$ receptor-mediated events to inflammatory pain processing: carrageenan oedema and associated c-Fos expression in the rat. Neuroscience 73:487–496

Burnett A Gebhart GF (1991) Characterization of descending modulation of nociception from the A5 cell group. Brain Res 546:271–281

Butterworth JF, Strichartz GR (1993) The α_2-adrenergic agonists clonidine and guanfacine produce tonic and phasic block of conduction in rat sciatic nerve fibers. Anesth Analg 76:295–301

Byas-Smith MG, Max MB, Muir, J, Kingman A (1995) Transdermal clonidine compared to placebo on painful diabetic neuropathy using a two-stage "enriched-enrollment" design. Pain 60:267–274

Cahusac, PMB, Morris R, Hill RG (1995) A pharmacological study of the modulation of neuronal and behavioural nociceptive responses in the rat trigeminal region. Brain Res 700:70–82

Calvillo O, Ghignone M (1986) Presynaptic effect of clonidine on unmyelinated afferent fibers in the spinal cord of the cat. Neurosci Lett 64:335–339

Calvillo O, Ghignone M, Madrid J (1988) Effects of α_1 adrenoceptor activation on the excitability of primary afferent terminals of the sural nerve in the spinal cord of the cat. Synapse 2:326–328

Camarata PJ, Yaksh TL (1985) Characterization of the spinal adrenergic receptors mediating the spinal effects produced by the microinjection of morphine into the periaqueductal gray. Brain Res 336:133–142

Campbell JN, Meyer RA, Davis KD (1992) Sympathetically maintained pain: a unifying hypothesis. In: Willis WD (ed) Hyperalgesia. Raven, New York, pp 141–149

Capogna G, Celleno D, Zangrillo A, Costantino P, Foresta S (1995) Addition of clonidine to epidural morphine enhances postoperative analgesia after cesarean delivery. Reg Anesth 20:57–61

Carabine UA, Milligan KR, Moore J (1992) Extradural clonidine and bupivacaine for postoperative analgesia. Br J Anaesth 68:132–135

Carroll D, Jahad A, King V, Wiffen P, Glynn C, McQuay H (1993) Single dose randomised double-blind double-dummy crossover comparison of epidural and intravenous clonidine in chronic pain. Br J Anaesth 71:665–669

Carstens E, Klumpp D, Randic M, Zimmerman M (1981) Effects of iontophoretically applied 5-hydroxytryptamine on the excitability of single primary afferent C- and A-fibers in the cat spinal cord. Brain Res 220:151–158

Castro-Lopes JM, Tavares I, Coimbra A (1993) GABA decreases in the spinal cord dorsal horn after peripheral neurectomy. Brain Res 620:287–291

Celuch, SM, Ramirez AJ, Enero MA (1992) Activation of 5-HT$_2$ receptors inhibits the evoked release of [^{3}H]-noradrenaline in the rat spinal cord. Gen Pharmacol 23:1063–1065

Cervo L, Rossi C, Tatarczynska E, Samanin R (1994) Role of 5-HT1A receptors in the antinociceptive action of 8-hydroxy-2-(di-n-propylamino)tetralin in the rat. Eur J Pharmacol 263:187–191

Cesselin F, Laporte AM, Miquel MC, Bourgoin S, Hamon M (1994) Serotonergic mechanisms of pain control. In: Gebhart GF, Hammond DL, Jensen TS (eds) Proceedings of the 7th World Congress on Pain, vol 2. International Association for the Study of Pain, Seattle, pp 669–695

Chiang CY, Xiang XK (1987) Does morphine enhance the release of 5-hydroxytryptamine in the rat spinal cord? An in vivo differential pulse voltammetry study. Brain Res 411:259–266

Cho HJ, Lee HS, Bae MA, Joo K (1995) Chronic arthritis increases tyrosine hydroxylase mRNA levels in the pontine noradrenergic cell groups. Brain Res 695:96–99

Chojnacka-Wójcik E, Klodzinska A, Deren-Wesolek A (1994) Involvement of 5-HT$_{2C}$ receptors in the m-CPP-induced antinociception in mice. Pol J Pharmacol 46:423–428

Cigarini I, Kaba A, Brohon E, Brichant JF, Damas F, Hans P, Dutz F, Albert A, Lamy M (1992) Epidural clonidine in labor analgesia: a comparative study. Anesthesiology 77:A989

Clarke PBS, Proudfit HK (1991) The projection of locus coeruleus neurones to the spinal cord in the rat determined by anterograde tracing combined with immunocytochemistry. Brain Res 538:231–245

Clark FM, Proudfit HK (1993) The projections of noradrenergic neurones in the A5 catecholamine cell group to the spinal cord in rat: anatomical evidence that A5 neurones modulate nociception. Brain Res 616:200–210

Clark FM, Yoemans DC, Proudfit HK (1991) The noradrenergic innervation of the spinal cord: differences between two substrains of Sprague-Dawley rats determined using retrograde tracers combined with immunocytochemistry. Neurosci Lett 125:155–158

Clatworthy A, Williams JH, Barasi S (1988) Intrathecal 5-hydroxytryptamine and electrical stimulation of the nucleus raphe magnus in rats both reduce the antinociceptive potency of intrathecally administered noradrenaline. Brain Res 455:300–306

Coderre TJ (1993) The role of excitatory amino acid receptors and intracellular messengers in persistent nociception after tissue injury in rats. Mol Biol 7:119–146

Coderre TJ, Katz J, Vaccarino AL, Melzack R (1993) Contribution of central neuroplasticity to pathological pain: review of clinical experimental evidence. Pain 52:259–285

Collin E, Frechilla D, Pohl M, Bourgoin S, Mauborgne A, Hamon, M, Cesselin F (1994) Differential effects of the novel analgesic, S 12813–4, on the spinal release of substance P- and calcitonin gene-related peptide-like materials in the rat. Naunyn Schmiedebergs Arch Pharmacol 349:387–393

Connell LA, Majid A, Wallis DJ (1989) Involvement of α_1-adrenoceptors in the depolarizing but not the hyperpolarizing responses of motoneurones in the neonate rat to noradrenaline. Neuropharmacology 28:1399–1409

Coombs DW, Saunders RL, Lachance D, Savage S, Ragnarsson TS, Jensen LE (1985) Intrathecal morphine tolerance: use of intrathecal clonidine, DADLE, and intraventricular morphine. Anesthesiology 62:357–363

Coote JH (1988) The organisation of cardiovascular neurones in the spinal cord. Rev Physiol Biochem Pharmacol 110:147–285

Coyle DE (1996) Efficacy of animal models for neuropathic pain. Pain Dig 6:7–20

Crawley JN, Roth RH, Mass JW (1979) Locus coeruleus stimulation increases noradrenergic metabolite levels in rat spinal cord. Brain Res 166:180–184

Crisp T, Smith DJ (1989) A local serotonergic component involved in the spinal antinociceptive action of morphine. Neuropharmacology 28:1047–1053

Crisp T, Stafinsky, JL, Spanos, LJ, Uram M, Perni VC, Donepudi HB (1991) Analgesic effects of serotonin and receptor-selective serotonin agonists in the rat spinal cord. Gen Pharmacol 22:247–251

Curtis DR, Leah JD, Peet MJ (1983) Effects of noradrenaline and 5-hydroxytryptamine on spinal Ia afferent terminations. Brain Res 258:328–332

Damaj MI, Glennon RA, Martin BR (1994) Involvement of the serotonergic system in the hypoactive and antinociceptive effects of nicotine in mice. Brain Res Bull 33:199–203

Danzebrink RM, Gebhart GF (1990) Antinociceptive effects of intrathecal adrenoceptor agonists in a rat model of visceral nociception. J Pharmacol Exp Ther 253:698–705

Danzebrink RM, Gebhart GF (1991a) Evidence that spinal 5-HT1, 5-HT2 and 5-HT3 receptor subtypes modulate responses to noxious colorectal distension in the rat. Brain Res 538:64–75

Danzebrink, RM, Gebhart GF (1991b) Intrathecal administration of clonidine with serotonin receptor agonists produces supra-additive visceral antinociception in the rat. Brain Res 555:35–42

Dashwood MR, Gilbey MP, Spyer KM (1985) The localization of adrenoceptors and opiate receptors in regions of the cat central nervous system involved in cardiovascular control. Neuroscience 15:537–551

Davies J, Quinlan JE (1985) Selective inhibition of responses of feline dorsal horn neurones to noxious cutaneous stimuli by tizanidine (DS103-282) and noradrenaline: involvement of α_2-adrenoceptors. Neuroscience 16:673–682

Davies M, Wilkinson LS, Roberts MHT (1988) Evidence for excitatory 5-HT$_2$ receptors on rat brainstem neurones. Br J Pharmacol 94:483–491

De Kock M, Crochet B, Morimont C, Scholtes JL (1993) Intravenous or epidural clonidine for intra- and postoperative analgesia. Anesthesiology 79:525–531

De Kock M, Famenne F, Deckers G, Scholtes JL (1995) Epidural clonidine or sufentanil for intraoperative and postoperative analgesia. Anesth Analg 81:1154–1162

Del Mar LP, Cardenas CG, Scroggs RS (1994) Serotonin inhibits high-threshold Ca2+ channel currents in capsaicin-sensitive acutely isolated adult rat DRG neurones. J Neurophysiol 72:2551–2554

Dellemijn HL, Fields RR, Allen WR, McKay WR, Rowbotham MC (1994) The interpretation of pain relief and sensory changes following sympathetic blockade. Brain 117:1475–1487

Dickenson AH (1990) A cure for wind up: NMDA receptor antagonists as potential analgesics. Trends Pharmacol Sci 11:307–309

Dirksen R, Van Diejen D, Van Luijtelaar EJJM, Booij LHDJ (1994) Site- and test-dependent antinociceptive efficacy of amitriptyline in rats. Pharmacol Biochem Behav 47:21–26

Doucet E, Pohl M, Fattaccini CM, Adrien J, El Mestikawy S, Hamon M (1995) In situ hybridiztion evidence for the synthesis of 5-HT$_{1B}$ receptor in serotoninergic neurones of anterior raphe nuclei in the rat brain. Synapse 19:18–28

Doyle CA, Maxwell DJ (1991a) Catecholaminergic innervation of the spinal dorsal horn: a correlated light and electron microscopic analysis of tyrosine hydroxylase-immunocytochemical study. Neuroscience 45:161–176

Doyle CA, Maxwell DJ (1991b) Ultrastructural analysis of noradrenergic nerve terminals in the cat lumbosacral spinal dorsal horn: a dopamine-beta-hydroxylase-immunocytochemical study. Brain Res 563:329–333

Duan J, Sawynok J (1987) Enhancement of clonidine-induced analgesia by lesions induced with spinal and intracerebroventricular administration of 5,7-dihydroxytryptamine. Neuropharmacology 26:323–329

Eide PK, Hole K (1991) Different role of 5-HT1A and 5-HT2 receptors in spinal cord in the control of nociceptive responsiveness. Neuropharmacology 30:727–731

Eisenach JC (1994) Alpha-2 agonists and analgesia. Exp Opin Invest Drugs 3:1005–1010

Eisenach JC, Detweiler D, Hood D (1993) Hemodynamic and analgesic actions of epidurally administered clonidine. Anesthesiology 78:277–287

Eisenach JC, D'Angelo R, Taylor C, Hood D (1994a) An isobolographic study of epidural clonidine and fentanyl after cesarean section. Anesth Analg 79:285–290

Eisenach JC, DuPen S, Dubois M, Miguel R, Allin D (1995) Epidural clonidine analgesia for intractable cancer pain. Pain 61:391–399

Eisenach JC, Shafer SL, Bucklin BA, Jackson C, Kallio A (1994b) Pharmacokinetics and pharmacodynamics of intraspinal dexmedetomidine in sheep. Anesthesiology 80:1349–1359

Eisenbach JC, Gebhart GF (1995) Intrathecal amitriptyline. Antinociceptive interactions with intravenous morphine and intrathecal clonidine, neostigmine and carbamylcholine in rats. Anesthesiology 83:1036–1045

Ekblom A, Hansson P, Thomsson M (1991) L-Tryptophan supplementation does not affect postoperative pain intensity or consumption of analgesics. Pain 44:249–254

El-Yassir N, Fleetwood-Walker SM (1990) A 5-HT1-type receptor mediates the antinociceptive effect of nucleus raphe magnus stimulation in the rat. Brain Res 523:92–99

El-Yassir N, Fleetwood-Walker SM, Mitchell R (1988) Heterogeneous effects of serotonin in the dorsal horn of the rat: the involvement of 5-HT1 receptor subtypes. Brain Res 456:147–158

Enkvist MOK, Hämäli̇nen H, Jansson CC, Kukkonen JP, Hautala R, Courtney MJ, Åkerman, KEO (1996) Coupling of astroglial α_2-adrenoreceptors to second messenger pathways. J Neurochem 66:2394–2401

Erkola O, Korttila K, Aho M, Haasio J, Aantaa A, Kallio A (1994) Comparison of intramuscular dexmedetomidine and midazolam premedication for elective abdominal hysterectomy. Anesth Analg 79:646–653

Eschalier A, Mestre C, Dubray C, Ardid D (1994) Why are antidepressants effective as pain relief? CNS Drugs 2:261–267

Evans AR, Jones SL, Blair RW (1994) Effects of vagal afferent nerve stimulation on noxious heat-eoked Fos-like immunoreactivity in the rat lumbar spinal cord. J Comp Neurol 346:490–498

Fang F, Proudfit HK (1996) Spinal cholinergic and monoamine receptors mediate the antinociceptive effect of morphine microinjected in the periaqueductal gray on the rat tail, but not the feet. Brain Res 722:95–108

Farkas S, Ono H (1995) Participation of NMDA and non-NMDA excitatory amino acid receptors in the mediation of spinal reflex potentials in rats: an in vivo study. Br J Pharmacol 114:1193–1205

Fasmer OB, Berge OG, Post C, Hole K (1986) Effects of the putative 5-HT1A agonist, 8-OH-2-(di-n-propylamino) amino tetralin, on nociceptive sensitivity in mice. Pharmacol Biochem Behav 25:883–888

Fields, HL, Heinricher MM, Mason P (1991) Neurotransmitters in nociceptive modulatory circuits. Annu Rev Neurosci 14:219–245

Filos KS, Goudas LC, Patroni O, Polyzou V (1992) Intrathecal clonidine as a sole analgesic for pain relief after cesarean section. Anesthesiology 77:267–274

Filos KS, Goudas LC, Patroni O, Polyzou V (1994) Hemodynamic and analgesic profile after intrathecal clonidine in humans. A dose-response study. Anesthesiology 81:591–601

Flacke JW, Bloor BC, Flake WE (1987) Reduced narcotic requirement by clonidine with improved hemodynamic and adrenergic stability in patients undergoing coronary bypass surgery. Anesthesiology 67:11–19

Fleetwood-Walker SM (1992) The antinociceptive effects of noradrenergic agonists on the activity of the spinal dorsal horn neurones. In: Besson JM, Guilbaud G (eds) Towards the use of noradrenergic agonists for the treatment of pain. Excerpta Medica/Elsevier Science, Amsterdam, pp 181–196

Fleetwood-Walker SM, Mitchell R, Hope PJ, Molony V, Iggo A (1985) An $\alpha 2$ receptor mediates the selective inhibition by noradrenaline of nociceptive responses of identified dorsal horn neurones. Brain Res 334:243–254

Fleetwood-Walker SM, Hope PJ, Mitchell R (1988) Antinociceptive actions of descending dopaminergic tracts on cat and rat dorsal horn somatosensory neurones. J Physiol (Lond) 399:335–348

Fogarty DJ, Carabine UA, Milligan KR (1993) Comparison of the analgesic effects of intrathecal clonidine and intrathecal morphine after spinal anaesthesia in patients undergoing total hip replacement. Br J Anaesth 71:661–664

Fone KCF, Robinson AJ, Marsden CA (1991) Characterization of the 5-HT receptor subtypes involved in the motor behaviours produced by intrathecal administration of 5-HT agonists in rats. Br J Pharmacol 103:1547–1555

Franco-Cereceda A, Rydh M, Dalsgaard C (1992) Nicotine- and capsaicin-, but not potassium-evoked, CGRP-release from cultured guinea-pig spinal ganglia is inhibited by Ruthenium red. Neurosci Lett 137:72–74

Fritschy JM, Grzanna R (1990) Demonstration of two separate descending noradrenergic pathways to the spinal cord: evidence for an intragriseal trajectory of locus coeruleus axons in the superficial layers of the dorsal horn. J Comp Neurol 291:553–582

Gaumann DM, Brunet PC, Jirounek P (1990) Clonidine enhances the effects of lidocaine on C-fiber action potential. Anesth Analg 74:719–725

Gebhart GF, Randich A (1990) Brainstem modulation of nociception. In: Klemm WR, Vertes RP (eds) Brainstem mechanisms of behavior. Wiley, New York, pp 315–352

Gerin C, Becquet D, Privat A (1995) Direct evidence for the link between mono-aminergic descending pathways and motor activity. I. A study with microdialysis probes implanted in the ventral funiculus of the spinal cord. Brain Res 704:191–201

Ghelardini C, Galeotti N, Casamenti F, Malmberg-Aiello P, Pepeu G, Gualtieri, F, Bartolini A (1996) Central cholinergic antinociception induced by 5-HT4 agonists: BIMU 1 and BIMU 8. Life Sci 58:2297–2309

Ghingone M, Quintin L, Duke PC, Kelher CH, Calvillo O (1986) Effects of clonidine on narcotic requorements and hemodynamic response during induction of fentanyl anesthesia and endotracheal intubation. Anesthesiology 64:36–42

Ginzburg R, Seltzer Z (1990) Subarachnoid spinal cord transplantation of adrenal medulla suppresses chronic neuropathic pain behavior in rats. Brain Res 523:147–150

Giordano J (1991) Analgesic profile of centrally administered 2- methylserotonin against acute pain in rats. Eur J Pharmacol 199:233–236

Giordano J, LaVerne R (1992) Putative mechanisms of buspirone-induced antinociception in the rat. Pain 50:365–372

Girada MN, Brennan JJ, Martindale ME, Foreman RD (1987) Effects of stimulating the subcoeruleus-parabrachial region on the non-noxious and noxious responses of T1-T5 spinathalamic tract neurones in the primate. Brain Res 409:19–30

Glaum SR, Proudfit HK, Anderson EG (1990) 5-HT3 receptors modulate spinal noci-ceptive reflexes. Brain Res 510:12–16

Glazer EJ, Basbaum AI (1984) Axons which take up [^{3}H]serotonin are presynaptic to enkephalin immunoreactive neurons in cat dorsal horn. Brain Res 298:386–391

Glynn CL (1992) The spinal noradrenergic systems in the transmission of pain in patients. In: Besson JM, Guilbaud G (eds) Towards the use of noradrenergic agonists for the treatment of pain. Excerpta Medica/Elsevier Science, Amsterdam, pp 197–210

Glynn C, O'Sullivan K (1996) A double-blind randomised comparison of the effects of epidural clonidine, lignocaine and the combination of clonidine and lignocaine in patients with chronic pain. Pain 64:337–343

Go VL, Yaksh TL (1987) Release of subtance P from the cat spinal cord. J Physiol (Lond) 391:141–167

Godefroy F, Weil-Fugazza J, Besson JM (1987) Complex temporal changes in 5-hydroxytryptamine synthesis in the central nervous system induced by experimen-tal polyarthritis in the rat. Pain 28:223–238

Gogas KR, Cho HJ, Botchkina GI, Levine JD, Basbaum AI (1996) Inhibition of noxious stimulus-evoked pain behaviors and neuronal fos-like immunoreactivity in the spinal cord of the rat by supraspinal morphine. Pain 65:9–15

Gordon NC, Heller PH, Levine JD (1992) Enhancement of pentazocine analgesia by clonidine. Pain 48:167–169

Grace D, Bunting H, Milligan KR, Fee JP (1995) Postoperative analgesia after co-administration of clonidine and morphine by the intrathecal route in patients undergoing hip replacement. Anesth Analg 80:86–91

Grant SJ, Benno RH (1992) Both phasic sensory stimulation and tonic pharmacologi-cal activation increase fos-like immunoreactivity in the rat locus coeruleus. Syn-apse 12:112–118

Guinan MJ, Rothfeld JM, Pretel S, Culhane ES, Carstens E, Watkins LR (1989) Electrical stimulation of the rat ventral midbrain elicits antinociception via the dorsolateral funiculus. Brain Res 485:333–348

Guo TZ, Tinklenberg J, Oliker R, Maze M (1991) Central α1-adrenoceptor stimulation functionally antagonizes the hypnotic response to dexmedetomidine, an α2-adrenoceptor agonist. Anesthesiology 75:252–256

Gurtu S, Shukla, S, Mukerjee D (1994) Morphine, clonidine coadministration in subanalgesic doses-effective control of tonic pain. Neuroreport 5:715–717

Gustafson EL, Durkin MM, Bard JA, Zgombick J, Branchek TA (1996) A receptor autoradiographic and in situ hybridization analysis of the distribution of the 5-HT$_7$ receptor in rat brain. Br J Pharmacol 117:657–666

Guyenet PG, Stornetta, RL, Riley T, Norton FR, Rosin, DL, Lynch, KR (1994) Alpha$_{2A}$-adrenergic receptors are present in lower brainstem catacholaminergic and serotoninergic innervating spinal cord. Brain Res 638:285–294

Hama AT, Sagen J (1993) Reduced pain-related behavior by adrenal medullary transplants in rats with experimental painful peripheral neuropathy. Pain 52:223–231

Hämäläinen MM, Jyväsjärvi E, Pertovaara A (1995) Can the α_2-adrenoceptor agonist-mediated suppression of nocifensive reflex responses be due to an action on motoneurones or peripheral nociceptors? Neurosci Lett 196:29–32

Hammond DL, Yaksh TL (1984) Antagonism of stimulation-produced antinociception by intrathecal administration of methylsergide or phentolamine. Brain Res 298:329–337

Hammond DL, Tyce GM, Yaksh TL (1985) Efflux of 5-hydroxytryptamine and nora-drenaline into spinal cord superfusates during stimulation of the rat medulla. J Physiol (Lond) 359:151–162

Hao JX, Xu XJ, Aldskogius H, Seiger Å, Wiesenfeld-Hallin Z (1991) The excitatory amino acid receptor antagonist MK-801 prevents the hypersensitivity induced by spinal cord ischemia in the rat. Exp Neurol 113:182–191

Hao JX, Xu XJ, Wiesenfeld-Hallin Z (1994) Intrathecal γ aminobutyric acidB (GABAB) receptor antagonist CGP 35348 induces hypersensitivity to mechanical stimuli in the rat. Neurosci Lett 182:299–302

Harada Y, Nishioka K, Kitahata LM, Kishikawa K, Collins JG (1995) Visceral antinociceptive effects of spinal clonidine combined with morphine, (D-Pen2, D-Pen5) enkephalin, or U50,488H. Anesthesiology 83:344–352

Hasegawa Y, Ono H (1996) Effect of ±-8-dihydroxy-2-(di-n-propylamino) tetralin hydrobromide on spinal motor systems in anesthetized intact and spinalized rats. Eur J Pharmacol 295:211–214

Hayashi, Y, Maze M (1993) Alpha$_2$ adrenoceptor agonists and anaesthesia. Br J Anaesth 71:108–118

Hayashi Y, Guo TZ, Maze M (1995) Desensitization to the behavioral effects of alpha$_2$-adrenergic agonists in rats. Anesthesiology 82:954–962

Hayes AG, Skingle M, Tyers MB (1986) Antagonism of alpha-adrenoceptor agonist-induced antinociception in the rat. Neuropharmacology 25:397–402

Hayes ES, Carlton SM (1992) Primary afferent interactions: analysis of calcitonin gene-related peptide-immunoreactive terminals in contact with unlabeled and GABA-immunoreactive profiles in the monkey dorsal horn. Neuroscience 47:873–896

Headley PM, Duggan AW, Griersmith BT (1978) Selective reduction of noradrenaline and 5-hydroxytryptamine of nociceptive responses of cat dorsal horn neurones. Brain Res 145:185–189

Helton LA, Thor KB, Baez M (1994) 5-Hydroxytryptamine$_{2A}$, 5-hydroxytryptamine$_{2B}$ and 5-hydroxytryptamine$_{2C}$ receptor mRNA expression in the spinal cord of rat, monkey and human. Neuroreport 5:2617–2620

Ho BY, Takemori AE (1989) Serotonergic involvement in the antinociceptive action of and the development of tolerance to the kappa-opioid receptor agonist, U-50,488H. J Pharmacol Exp Ther 250:508–514

Hodge CJ, Apkarian AV, Stevens, R (1986) Inhibition of dorsal horn cell responses by stimulation of the Kolliker-Fuse nucleus. J Neurosurg 65:825–833

Holstege JC, Kuypers HGJM (1987) Brainstem projections to spinal motoneurones: an update. Neuroscience 23:809–821

Holziv G, Shefner SA, Anderson EG (1985) Serotonin depolarizes type A and C primary afferents: an intracellular study in bullfrog dorsal root ganglion. Brain Res 327:71–79

Honoré P, Chapman V, Buritova J, Besson JM (1996) To what extent do spinal interactions between an alpha-2 adrenoceptor agonist and a μ opioid agonist influence noxiously evoked c-fos expression in the rat? A pharmacological study. J Pharmacol Exp Ther 278:303–403

Hori Y, Endo K, Takahashi T (1996) Long-lasting synaptic facilitation induced by serotonin in superficial dorsal horn neurones of the rat spinal cord. J Physiol (Lond) 492 (3):867–876

Horváth G, Szikszay M, Benedek G (1992) Calcium channels are involved in the hypnotic-anesthetic action of dexmedetomidine in rats. Anesth Analg 74:884–888

Horváth G, Kovács M, Szikszay M, Benedek G (1994) Mydriatic and antinociceptive effects of intrathecal dexmedetomidine in conscious rats. Eur J Pharmacol 253:61–66

Howe JR, Zieglgänsberger W (1987) Responses of rat dorsal horn neurones to natural stimulation and to iontophoretically applied norepinephrine. J Comp Neurol 255:1–17

Howe JR, Wang JY, Yaksh TL (1983) Selective antagonism of the antinociceptive effect of intrathecally applied alpha adrenergic agonists by intrathecal prazosin and intrathecal yohimbine. J Pharmacol Exp Ther 224:552–558

Howe JR, Yaksh TL, Go VLW (1987) The effect of unilateral dorsal root ganglionectomies or ventral rhizotomies on $\alpha2$-adrenoceptor binding to, and the substance P, enkephalin, and neurotensin content of, the cat lumbar spinal cord. Neuroscience 21:385–394

Hunter, JC, Woodburn VL, Durieux C, Pettersson EKE, Poat JA, Hughes J (1995) C-fos antisense oligodeoxynucleotide increases formalin-induced nociception and regulates preprodynorphin expression. Neuroscience 65:485–492

Hunter JC, Lewis R, Eglen RM, Fontana DJ (1996) The role of α and β adrenoceptors in a rodent model of neuropathic pain. Br J Pharmacol 117:237P

Huntoon M, Eisenach JC, Boese P (1992) Epidural clonidine after cesarean section: appropriate dose and effect of prior local anesthesic. Anesthesiology 76:187–183

Hutson PH, Tricklebank MD, Curzon G (1982) Enhancement of footshock-induced analgesia by spinal 5,7-dihydroxytryptamine lesions. Brain Res 237:367–372

Hutson PH, Tricklebank MD, Curzon, G (1983) Analgesia induced by brief footshock: blockade by fenfluramine and 5-methoxy-N,N-dimethyltryptamine and prevention of blockade by 5-HT antagonists. Brain Res 279:105–110

Hwang AS, Wilcox GL (1987) Analgesic properties of intrathecally administered heterocyclic antidepressants. Pain 28:343–355

Hylden JLK, Thomas DA, Iadarola MJ, Nahin RL, Dubner R (1991) Spinal opioid analgesic effects are enhanced in a model of unilateral inflammation/hyperalgesia: possible involvement of noradrenergic mechanisms. Eur J Pharmacol 194:135–143

Idänpään-Heikkilä J, Kalso EA, Seppälä T (1994) Antinociceptive actions of dexmedetomidine and the kappa-opioid agonist U-50,488H against noxious thermal, mechanical and inflammatory stimuli. J Pharmacol Exp Ther 271:1306–1313

Iijima K, Sato M, Kojima N, Ohtomo K (1992) Immunocytochemical and in situ hybridization evidence for the coexistence of GABA and tyrosine hydroxylase in the rat locus ceruleus. Anat Rec 234:593–604

Iliakis B, Anderson NL, Irish PS, Henry MA, Westrum LE (1996) Electron microscopy of immunoreactivity patterns for glutamate and gamma-aminobutyric acid in synaptic glomeruli of the feline spinal trigeminal nucleus (subnucleus caudalis). J Comp Neurol 366:465–477

Iwamoto ET, Marion L (1993) Adrenergic, serotonergic and cholinergic components of nicotinic antinociception in rats. J Pharmacol Exp Ther 265:777–789

Jaakola ML, Salonen M, Lehtinen R, Scheinin H (1991) The analgesic action of dexmedetomidine, a novel alpha-2-adrenoceptor agonist, in healthy volunteers. Pain 46:281–285

Jaakola ML, Melkkila AT, Kanto J, Kallio A, Scheinin H, Scheinin M (1992) Dexmedetomidine reduces intraocular pressure, intubation responses and anaesthetic requirements in patients undergoing ophthalmic surgery. Br J Anaesth 68:570–575

Jansson CC, Karp M, Oker-Blom C, Näsman J, Savola JM, Åkerman KEO (1995a) Two human α_2-adrenoceptor subtypes α_2A-C10 and α_2B-C2 expressed in Sf9 cells couple to transduction pathway resulting in opposite effects on cAMP production. Eur J Pharmacol 290:75–83

Jansson CC, Marjamäki A, Luomala K, Savola JM, Scheinin M, Åkerman KEO (1995b) Coupling of human 2-adrenoceptor subtypes to regulation of cAMP production in transfected S115 cells. Eur J Pharmacol 266:165–174

Javis DA, Duncan SR, Segal IS, Maze M (1992) Ventilatory effects of clonidine alone and in the presence of alfentanil, in human volunteers. Anesthesiology 76:899–905

Jeftinija S, Semba K, Randic M (1981) Norepinephrine reduces excitability of single cutaneous primary afferent C-fibers in the cat spinal cord. Brain Res 219:456–463

Jeftinija S, Semba K, Randic M (1983) Norepinephrine reduces excitability of single cutaneous primary afferent C and A fibers in the cat spinal cord. Adv Pain Res Ther 5:271–276

Jensen TS, Yaksh TL (1984) Spinal monoamine and opiate systems partly mediate the antinociceptive effects produced by glutamate at brainstem sites. Brain Res 321:287–298

Jensen TS, Yaksh TL (1986) Examination of spinal monoamine receptors through which brainstem opiate-sensitive systems act in the rat. Brain Res 363:114–127

Johannessen JN, Watkins LR, Carlton SM, Mayer DJ (1982) Failure of spinal cord serotonin depletion to alter analgesia elicited from the periaqueductal gray. Brain Res 237:373–386

Jones BE, Holmes CJ, Rodriguez-Veiga E, Mainville L (1991) GABA-synthesizing neurones in the medulla: their relationship to serotonin-containing and spinally projecting neurones in the rat. J Comp Neurol 313:349–367

Jones SL (1991) Descending noradrenergic influences on pain. Prog Brain Res 88:381–394

Jones SL (1992) Noradrenergic modulation of noxious heat-evoked fos-like immunoreactivity in the dorsal horn of the rat sacral spinal cord. J Comp Neurol 325:435–445

Jones SL, Gebhart GF (1986) Quantitative characterization of ceruleospinal inhibition of nociceptive transmission in the rat. J Physiol (Lond) 56:1397–1410

Jones SL, Light AR (1992) Serotoninergic medullary raphe-spinal projection to the lumbar spinal cord in the rat: a retrograde immunohistochemical study. J Comp Neurol 322:599–610

Jordan LM, Kenshalo DR, Martin RF, Haber LH, Willis WD (1979) Two populations of spinothalamic tract neurones with opposite responses to 5-hydroxytryptamine. Brain Res 164:342–346

Kalso EA, Sullivan AF, McQuay HJ, Dickenson AH, Roques BP (1993) Cross-tolerance between mu opioid and alpha-2 adrenergic receptors, but not between mu and delta opioid receptors in the spinal cord of the rat. J Pharmacol Exp Ther 265:551–558

Kamisaki Y, Hamada T, Maeda K, Ishimura M, Itoh T (1993) Presynaptic α_2 adrenoceptors inhibit glutamate release from rat spinal cord synaptosomes. J Neurochem 60:522–526

Kaneto H, Inoue M (1990) Active site of adrenergic blockers to suppress the development of tolerance to morphine analgesia. Brain Res 507:35–39

Kauppila T, Kemppainen P, Tanila H, Pertovaara A (1991) Effect of systemic dexmedetomidine, an alpha-2-adrenoceptor agonist, on experimental pain in humans. Anesthesiology 74:3–8

Kayser V, Guilbaud G, Besson JM (1992) Potent antinociceptive effects of clonidine systematically administered in an experimental model of clinical pain, the arthritic rat. Brain Res 593:7–13

Kayser V, Desmeules J, Guilbaud G (1995) Systemic clonidine differentially modulates the abnormal reactions to mechanical and thermal stimuli in rats with peripheral mononeuropathy. Pain 60:275–285

Kellstein DE, Malseed RT, Goldstein FJ (1988) Opioid monoamine interactions in spinal antinociception: evidence for serotonin but not norepinephrine reciprocity. Pain 34:85–92

Khasar SG, Green PG, Chou B, Levine JD (1995) Peripheral nociceptive effects of a2 adrenergic receptor agonists in the rat. Neuroscience 66:427–432

Kheck NM, Gannon PJ, Azmitia EC (1995) 5-HT$_{1A}$ receptor localization on the axon hillock of cervical spinal motoneurones in primates. J Comp Neurol 355:211–220

Kia HK, Miguel MC, Brisorgueil MJ, Daval G, Riad M, El Mestikawy S, Hamon M, Vergé D (1996) Immunocytochemical localization of serotonin(1A) receptors in the rat central nervous system. J Comp Neurol 365:289–305

Kia HK, Miguel MC, McKernan RM, Laporte AM, Lombard MC, Bourgoin S, Hamon M, Vergé D (1995) Localization of 5-HT$_3$ receptors in the rat spinal cord. Immunohistochemistry and in situ hybridization. Neuroreport 6:257–261

Kidd EJ, Laporte AM, Langlois X, Fattacini CM, Doyen C, Lombard MC, Gozlan H, Hamon M (1993) 5-HT3 receptors in the rat central nervous system are mainly located on nerve fibre terminals. Brain Res 612:289–298

Kiefel JM, Paul D, Bodnar RJ (1989) Reduction in opioid and non-opioid forms of swim analgesia by 5-HT2 receptor antagonists. Brain Res 500:231–240

Kiritsky-Roy KA, Shyu BC, Danneman PJ, Morrow TJ, Belczynski C, Casey KL (1994) Spinal antinociception mediated by a cocaine-sensitive dopaminergic supraspinal mechanism. Brain Res 644:109–116

Kirno K, Lundin, S, Elam M (1993) Epidural clonidine depresses sympathetic nerve activity in humans by a supraspinal mechanism. Anesthesiology 78:1021–1027

Kishore-Kumar R, Schafer SS, Lawlor BA, Murphy DL, Max MB (1989) Single doses of the serotonin agonists buspirone and m-chlorophenylpiperazine do not relieve neuropathic pain. Pain 37:223–227

Kjøsvik A, Størkson R, Tjølson A, Hole K (1990) Activation of spinal 5-HT$_2$ receptors increase nociception in rats. Soc Neurosci Abstr 20:553P

Knowles MG, Wang C, Chakrabarti MK, Whitman JG (1994) Comparison of clonidine with fentanyl on phrenic nerve activity and their interaction in anaesthetized rabbits. Br J Anaesth 73:517–521

Kuraishi Y, Harada Y, Aratani S, Satoh M, Takagi H (1983a) Separate involvement of the spinal noradrenergic and serotoninergic systems in morphine analgesia: the differences in mechanical and thermal algesic tests. Brain Res 273:245–252

Kuraishi Y, Hirota N, Sugimoto M, Satoh M, Takagi H (1983b) Effects of morphine on noxious stimuli-induced release of substance P from rabbit dorsal horn in vivo. Life Sci 33:693–696

Kuraishi Y, Hirota N, Sato Y, Kaneko S, Satoh M, Takagi H (1985) Noradrenergic inhibition of the release of substance P from the primary afferents in the rabbit spinal dorsal horn. Brain Res 359:177–182

Kuraishi Y, Minami M, Satoh M (1991) Serotonin, but neither noradrenaline nor GABA, inhibits capsaicin-evoked release of immunoreactive somatostatin slices of rat spinal cord. Neurosci Res 9:238–245

Kwiat GC, Basbaum AI (1990) Organization of tyrosine hydroxylase- and serotonin-immunoreactive brainstem neurons with axons collaterals to the periaqueductal gray and the spinal cord in the rat. Brain Res 528:83–94

Kwiat GC, Basbaum AI (1992) The origin of brainstem noradrenergic and serotonergic projections to the spinal cord dorsal horn of the rat. Somatosens Mot Res 9:157–173

LaMotte CC (1986) Organization of dorsal horn neurotransmitter systems. In: Yaksh TL (ed) Spinal afferent processing. Plenum, New York, pp 97–116

LaMotte CC (1988) Lamina X of primate spinal cord: distribution of five neuropeptides and serotonin. Neuroscience 25:639–658

Lang CW, Hope PJ, Grubb BD, Duggan AW (1994) Lack of effect of microinjection of noradrenaline or medetomidine on stimulus-evoked release of substance P in the spinal cord of the cat: a study with antibody microprobes. Br J Pharmacol 103:951–957

Lanier SM, Lafontan M, Limbird LE, Paris H (1996) Summary of the ASPET-sponsored colloquium: alpha-2 adrenergic receptors: structure, function, and therapeutic implications, 25–27 Oct 1995. J Pharmacol Exp Ther 277:10–16

Laporte AM, Koscielniak T, Ponchant M, Vergé D, Hamon M, Gozlan H (1992) Quantitative autoradiographic mapping of 5-HT3 receptors in the rat CNS using [125I]iodo-zacopride and [3H]zacopride as radioligands. Synapse 10:271–281

Laporte AM, Fattaccini CM, Lombard MC, Chauveau J, Hamon M (1995) Effects of dorsal rhizotomy and selective lesion of serotonergic and noradrenergic systems on 5-HT$_{1A}$, 5-HT$_{1B}$ and 5-HT$_3$ receptors in the rat spinal cord. J Neural Transm 100:207–223

Laporte AM, Doyen C, Nevo IT, Chauveau J, Hauw JJ, Hamon M (1996) Autoradiographic mapping of serotonin 5-HT$_{1A}$, 5-HT$_{1D}$, 5-HT$_{2A}$ and 5-HT$_3$ receptors in the aged human spinal cord. J Chem Neuroanat 11:67–75

Lawhead RG, Blaxall HS, Bylund DB (1992) α_{2A} is the predominant α_2 adrenergic receptor subtype in human spinal cord. Anesthesiology 77:983–991

Le Bars D (1988) Serotonin and pain. In: Osborne NN, Hamon M (eds) Neuronal serotonin. Wiley, London, pp 171–230

Lee YW, Yaksh TL (1995) Analysis of drug interaction between intrathecal clonidine and MK-801 in peripheral neuropathic pain rat model. Anesthesiology 82:741–748

Leiphart JW, Dills CV, Zikel OM, Kim DL, Levy RM (1995) A comparison of intrathecally adminstered narcotic and nonnarcotic analgesics for experimental chronic neuropathic pain. J Neurosurg 82:595–599

Lichtman AH, Martin BR (1991) Cannabinoid-induced antinociception is mediated by a spinal α_2-noradrenergic mechanism. Brain Res 559:309–314

Lichtman AH, Smith FL, Martin BR (1993) Evidence that the antinociceptive tail-flick response is produced independently from changes in either tail-skin temperature or core temperature. Pain 55:283–295

Light AR, Kavookjian AM, Petrusz P (1983) The ultrastructure and synptic connections of serotonin-immunoreactive terminals in spinal laminae I and II. Somat Res 1:33–50

Light AR, Casale EJ, Menetrey DM (1986) The effects of focal stimulation in nucleus raphe magnus and periaqueductal gray on intracellularly recorded neurones in spinal laminae I and II. J Neurophysiol 56:555–571

Light AR, Kavookjian AM (1988) Morphology and ultrastructure of physiologically identified subsantia gelatinosa (lamina II) neurons with axons that terminate in deeper dorsal horn laminae (III–V). J Comp Neurol 267:172–189

Lin JC, Tsao WL, Lee HK, Wang Y (1993) Dissociation of hypertension and enhanced clonidine-induced antinociception in spontaneously hypertensive rats. Pain 53:53–58

Lin Q, Willis WD (1993) Application of methylsergide by microdialysis attenuates the inhibition of primate nociceptive spinothalamic tract neurons produced by stimulation in periaqueductal gray. Soc Neurosci Abstr 19:523

Lin Q, Peng, YB, Willis WD (1994) Glycine and GABA$_A$ antagonists reduce the inhibition of primate spinothalamic tract neurons produced by stimulation in periaqueductal gray. Brain Res 654:286–302

Lin Q, Peng, YB, Willis WD (1996) Antinociception and inhibition from the periaqueductal gray are mediated in part by spinal 5-hydroxytryptamine$_{1A}$ receptors. J Pharmacol Exp Ther 276:958–967

Lipscombe D, Kongsamut S, Tsien RW (1989) α-Adrenergic inhibition of sympathetic neurotransmitter release mediated by modulation of N-type calcium-channel gating. Nature 340:639–642

Loewy AD (1990) Central autonomic pathways. In: Loewy AD, Spyer KM (eds) Central regulation of autonomic function. Oxford University Press, New York, pp 88–103

Loomis CW, Milne B, Cervenko FW (1987) Determination of cross-tolerance in rat spinal cord using intrathecal infusion via sequential mini-osmotic pumps. Pharmacol Biochem Behav 26:131–139

Loomis CW, Milne B, Cervenko FW (1988) A study of the interaction between clonidine and morphine on analgesia and blood pressure during continuous intrathecal infusion in the rat. Neuropharmacology 27:191–199

Lucas JJ, Mellström B, Colado MI, Naranjo JR (1993) Molecular mechanisms of pain: serotonin 1A receptor agonists trigger transactivation by c-fos of the prodynorphin gene in spinal cord neurones. Neuron 10:599–611

Lund C, Qvitzau S, Greulich A, Hjorts Ø, Kehlet H (1989) Comparison of the effects of extradural clonidine with those of morphine on postoperative pain, stress responses, cardiopulmonary function and motor and sensory block. Br J Anaesth 63:516–519

Luo L, Wiesenfeld-Hallin Z (1993) Low-dose intrathecal clonidine releases tachykinins in rat spinal cord. Eur J Pharmacol 235:157–159

Luo L, Puke MJC, Wiesenfeld-Hallin Z (1994) The effects of intrathecal morphine and clonidine on the prevention and reversal of spinal cord hyperexcitability following sciatic nerve section in the rat. Pain 58:245–252

Luo L, Ji RR, Zhang Q, Iadarola MJ, Hökfelt T, Wiesenfeld-Hallin Z (1995) Effect of administration of high dose intrathecal clonidine or morphine prior to sciatic nerve section on c-fos expression in rat lumbar spinal cord. Neuroscience 68:1219–1227

Malmberg AB, Yaksh TL (1993) Pharmacology of the spinal action of ketorolac, morphine, ST-91, U50488H and L-PIA on the formalin test and an isobolographic analysis of the NSAID interaction. Anesthesiology 79:270–281

Mansikka H, Pertovaara A (1995) Influence of selective α_2-adrenergic agents on mustard oil-induced central hyperalgesia in rats. Eur J Pharmacol 281:43–48

Mansikka H, Idänpään-Heikkilä JJ, Pertovaara A (1996) Different roles of α_2-adrenoceptors of the medulla versus the spinal cord in modulation of mustard oil-induced central hyperalgesia in rats. Eur J Pharmacol 297:19–26

Marchand JE, Zhang X, Wurm WH, Kream RM (1993) Differential expression of alpha-2 adrenergic receptor subtypes by sensory and sympathetic neurones. Anesthesiology 79:A894

Margalit D, Segal M (1979) A pharmacologic study of analgesia produced by stimulation of the nucleus locus coeruleus. Psychopharmacology 62:169–173

Marks SA, Stein RD, Dashwood MR, Gilbey MP (1990) [3H]Prazosin binding in the intermediolateral cell column and the effects of iontophoresed methoxamine on sympathethic preganglionic neuronal activity in the anaesthesized cat and rat. Brain Res 530:321–324

Marlier L, Sandillon F, Poulat P, Rajaofetra N, Geffard M, Privat A (1991a) Serotonergic innervation of the dorsal horn of rat spinal cord: light and electron microscope immunocytochemical study. J Neurocytol 20:310–322

Marlier L, Teilhac JR, Cerruti C, Privat A (1991b) Autoradiographic mapping of 5-HT1, 5-HT1A, 5-HT1B and 5-HT2 receptors in the rat spinal cord. Brain Res 550:15–23

Marlier L, Poulat P, Rajaofetra N, Sandillon F, Privat A (1992) Plasticity of serotonergic innervation of the dorsal horn of the rat spinal cord following neonatal capsaicin treatment. J Neurosci Res 31:346–358

Marwaha J, Kehne JH, Commissaris RL, Lakoski J, Shaw W, Davis M (1983) Spinal clonidine inhibits neural firing in locus coeruleus. Brain Res 276:379–382

Matos FF, Rollema H, Brown JL, Basbaum AI (1992) Do opioids evoke the release of serotonin in the spinal cord? An in vivo microdialysis study of the regulation of extracellular serotonin in the rat. Pain 48:439–447

Matsumoto M, Hidaka K, Tada S, Tasaki Y, Yamaguchi T (1996) Low levels of mRNA for dopamine D_4 receptor in human cerebral cortex and striatum. J Neurochem 66:915–919

Max MB, Kishore-Kumar R, Schafer SC, Meister B, Gracely RH, Smoller B, Dubner R (1991) Efficacy of desipramine in painful diabetic neuropathy: a placebo-controlled trial. Pain 45:3–9

Maxwell DJ, Jankowska E (1996) Synaptic relationships between serotonin-immunoreactive axons and dorsal horn spinocerebellar tract cells in the cat spinal cord. Neuroscience 70:247–253

Maxwell DJ, Leranth CS, Verhofstad AAJ (1983) Fine structure of serotonin-containing axons in the marginal zone of the rat spinal cord. Brain Res 266:253–259

Maze M, Poree L, Rabin BC (1995) Anesthetic and analgesic actions of α_2-adrenoceptor agonists. Pharmacol Comm 6:175–182

McCall RB, Clement ME (1994) Role of serotonin1A and serotonin2 receptors in the central regulation of the cardiovascular system. Pharmacol Rev 46:231–243

McCarson KE, Krause JE (1995) The formalin-induced expression of tachykinin peptide and neurokinin receptor messenger RNAs in rat sensory ganglia and spinal cord is modulated by opate preadministration. Neuroscience 64:729–739

McFadzean I, Docherty RJ (1989) Noradrenaline- and enkephalin-induced inhibition of voltage-sensitive calcium currents in NG108-15 hybrid cells. Eur J Neurosci 1:141–147

McKearney JW (1989) Apparent antinociceptive properties of piperazine-type serotinin agonists: trifluoromethylphenylpiperazine, chlorophenylpiperazine and MK-212. Pharmacol Biochem Behav 32:657–660

McMahon SB, Wall PD (1988) Descending excitation and inhibition of spinal cord lamina I projection neurones. J Neurophysiol 59:1204–1219

McQuay HJ (1992) Is there a place for alpha2 adrenergic agonists in the control of pain. In: Besson JM, Guilbaud G (eds) Towards the use of noradrenergic agonists for the treatment of pain. Excerpta Medica/ElsevierScience, Amsterdam, pp 219–232

Meller ST, Dykstra CL, Gebhart GF (1993) Acute mechanical hyperalgesia is produced by coactivation of AMPA and metabotropic glutamate receptors. Neuroreport 4:879–888

Men DS, Matsui Y (1994a) Activation of descending noradrenergic system by peripheral nerve stimulation. Brain Res Bull 34:177–182

Men DS, Matsui Y (1994b) Peripheral nerve stimulation increases serotonin and dopamine metabolites in rat spinal cord. Brain Res Bull 33:625–632

Mendez R, Eisenbach JC, Kashtan K (1990) Epidural clonidine analgesia after cesarean section. Analgesia 73:848–852

Miletic V, Hoffert MJ, Ruda MA, Dubner E, Shigenaga Y (1984) Serotonergic axonal contacts on identified spinal dorsal neurones and their correlation with nucleus raphe magnus stimulation. J Comp Neurol 228:129–141

Millan MJ (1993) Multiple opioid systems and chronic pain. In: Herz A, Akil H, Simon E (eds) The opioids. Springer, Berlin Heidelberg New York, pp 127–162 (Handbook of experimental pharmacology, vol 104)

Millan MJ (1994) Serotonin and pain: evidence that activation of 5-HT1A receptors does not elicit antinociception against noxious thermal, mechanical and chemical stimuli in mice. Pain 58:45–61

Millan MJ (1995) Serotonin and pain: a reappraisal of its role in the light of receptor multiplicity. Semin Neurosci 7:409–419

Millan MJ, Colpaert FC (1991a) 5-Hydroxytryptamine (5-HT)1A receptors and the tail-flick response. III. Structurally diverse 5-HT1A partial agonists attenuate mu-but not kappa-opioid antinociception in mice and rats. J Pharmacol Exp Ther 256:993–1001

Millan MJ, Colpaert FC (1991b) 5-Hydroxytryptamine (5-HT)1A receptors and the tail-flick response. II. High efficacy 5-HT1A agonists attenuate morphine-induced antinociception in mice in a competitive-like manner. J Pharmacol Exp Ther 256:983–992

Millan MJ, Bervoets K, Colpaert FC (1991) 5-HT1A receptors and the tail-flick response. I. 8-OH-DPAT-induced spontaneous tail-flicks in the rat as an in vivo model of 5-HT1A receptor-mediated activity. J Pharmacol Exp Ther 256:973–982

Millan MJ, Canton H, Lavielle G (1992) Targeting multiple serotonin receptors: mixed 5-HT1A agonists – 5-HT1C/2 antagonists as therapeutic agents. Drug News Perspect 5:397–406

Millan MJ, Bervoets K, Rivet JM, Widdowson P, Renouard A, Le Marouille-Girardon S, Gobert A (1994) Multiple alpha2-adrenergic receptor subtypes. II. Evidence for a role of rat Rα2A-ARs in the control of nociception, motor behaviour and hippocampal synthesis of noradrenaline. J Pharmacol Exp Ther 270:958–972

Millan MJ, Bervoets K, Girardon S, Gobert A, Newman-Tancredi A, Audinot V, Rivet JM, Lacoste A, Cordi A (1995) S 18616: a potent, high efficacy and selective spiroimidazoline agonist at α2-adrenergic receptors (ARs). Am Soc Neurosci Abstr 21:1416

Millan MJ, Seguin L, Honoré P, Girardon S, Bervoets K (1996) Pro- and antinociceptive actions of serotonin (5-HT)1A agonists and antagonists in rodents: relationship to algesiometric paradigm. Behav Brain Res 73:69–77

Millar J, Williams GV (1989) Effects of iontophoresis of noradrenaline and stimulation of the periaqueductal gray on single-unit activity in the rat superficial dorsal horn. J Comp Neurol 287:119–133

Miller JF, Proudfit HK (1990) Antagonism of stimulation-produced antinociception from ventrolateral pontine sites by intrathecal administration of α-adrenergic antagonists and naloxone. Brain Res 530:20–34

Mills A, Martin GR (1995) Autoradiographic mapping of [3H]sumatriptan binding in cat brain stem and spinal cord. Eur J Pharmacol 280:175–178

Milne RJ, Gamble GD (1990) Behavioural modification of bulbospinal serotonergic inhibition and morphine analgesia. Brain Res 521:167–174

Mjellem N, Lund A, Hole K (1993) Different functions of spinal 5-HT1A and 5-HT2A receptor subtypes in modulating behaviour induced by excitatory amino acid receptor agonists in mice. Brain Res 626:78–82

Mogensen T, Eliasen K, Ejlersen E, Vegger P, Nielsen, IK, Kehlet, H (1992) Epidural clonidine enhances postoperative analgesia from a combined low-dose epidural bupivacaine and morphine regimen. Anesth Analg 75:607–610

Mokha SS, Iggo A (1987) Mechanisms mediating the brain stem control of somatosensory transmission in the dorsal horn of the cat's spinal cord: an intracellular analysis. Exp Brain Res 69:93–106

Mokha SS, McMillan, JA, Iggo A (1983) Descending influences on spinal nociceptive neurons from locus coeruleus actions pathway neuro transmitter and mechanisms. Adv Pain Res Ther 5:387–392

Molineaux SM, Jessell TM, Axel R, Julius D (1989) 5-HT1C receptor is a prominent serotonin receptor subtype in the central nervous system. Proc Natl Acad Sci USA 86:6793–6797

Monaski MS, Zinsmeister AR, Stevens CW, Yaksh TL (1990) Interaction of intrathecal morphine and ST-91 on antinociception in the rat: dose-response analysis, antagonism and clearance. J Pharmacol Exp Ther 254:383–392

Monroe PJ, Kradel BK, Smith DL, Smith DJ (1995) Opioid effects on spinal [3H]5-hydroxytryptamine release are not related to their antinociceptive action. Eur J Pharmacol 272:51–56

Moskowitz M (1992) Neurogenic versus vascular mechanisms of sumatriptan and ergot alkaloids in migraine. Trends Pharmacol 13:307–311

Motsch J, Gräber E, Ludwig K (1990) Addition of clonidine enhances postoperative analgesia from epidural morphine: a double-blind study. Anesthesiology 73:1067–1073

Murase K, Randic M, Shirasaki T, Nagakawa T, Akaike N (1990) Serotonin suppresses N-methyl-D-aspartate responses in acutely isolated spinal dorsal horn neurones of the rat. Brain Res 525:84–93

Murata K, Nakagawa I, Kumeta, LM, Collins, JG (1989) Intrathecal clonidine suppresses noxiously evoked activity of spinal wide dynamic range neurones in cats. Anesth Analg 69:185–191

Murphy AZ, Murphy RM, Zemlan FP (1992) Role of spinal serotonin1 receptor subtypes in thermally and mechanically elicited nociceptive reflexes. Psychopharmacology 108:123–130

Murphy RM, Zemlan FP (1990) Selective serotonin1A/1B agonists differentially affect spinal nociceptive reflexes. Neuropharmacology 29:463–468

Nachemson AK, Bennett GJ (1993) Does pain damage spinal cord neurons? Transsynaptic degeneration in rat following a surgical incision. Neurosci Lett 162:78–80

Nacif-Coelho C, Correa-Sales C, Chang LL, Maze M (1994) Perturbation of ion channel conductance alters the hypnotic response to the alpha$_2$-adrenergic agonist dexmedetomidine in the locus coeruleus. Anesthesiology 81:1527–1534

Nakamura M, Ferreira SH (1988) Peripheral analgesic action of clonidine: mediation by release of endogenous enkephalin-like substances. Eur J Pharmacol 146:223–228

Naranjo JR, Arned A, Molinero MT, Del Rio J (1989) Involvement of spinal monaminergic pathways in antinociception produced by substance P and neurotensin in rodents. Neuropharmacology 28:291–298

Nicholas AP, Pieribone VA, Arvidsson U, Hökfelt T (1992) Serotonin-, substance P- and glutamate/aspartate immunoreactivities in medullo-spinal pathways in rat and primate. Neuroscience 48:545–559

Nicholas AP, Pieribone VA, Hökfelt T (1993a) Cellular localization of messenger RNA for beta-1 and beta2 adrenergic receptors in rat brain: an in situ hybridization study. Neuroscience 56:1023–1039

Nicholas AP, Pieribone VA, Hökfelt T (1993b) Distributions of mRNAs for alpha-2 adrenergic receptor subtypes in rat brain: an in situ hybridization study. J Comp Neurol 328:575–594

Nishikawa T, Dohi S (1990) Clinical evaluation of clonidine added to lidocaine solution for epidural anesthesia. Anesthesiology 73:853–859

North RA (1989) Drug receptors and the inhibition of nerve cells. Br J Pharmacol 98:13–28

North RA, Yoshimura MJ (1984) The actions of noradrenaline on neurones of the rat substantia gelatinosa in vitro. J Physiol (Lond) 349:43–55

O'Meara ME, Gin T (1993) Comparison of 0.125% bupivacaine with 0.125% bupivacaine and clonidine as extradural analgesia in the first stage of labour. Br J Anaesth 71:651–656

Omote K, Kitahata L, Collins JG, Nakatani K, Nakagawa I (1991) Interaction between opiate subtype and alpha$_2$ adrenergic agonists in suppression of noxiously evoked activity of WDR neurones in the spinal dorsal horn. Anesthesiology 74:737–743

Onghena P, Van Houdenhove B (1992) Antidepressant-induced analgesia in chronic-malignant pain: a meta-analysis of 39 placebo-controlled studies. Pain 49:205–219

Ono H, Mishima A, Fuduka H, Vasko MR (1991) Inhibitory effects of clonidine and tizanidine on release of substance P from slices of rat spinal cord and antagonism by α-adrenergic receptor antagonists. Neuropharmacology 30:585–589

Ossipov MH, Harris S, Lloyd P, Messineo E (1990a) An isobolographic analysic of the antinociceptive effect of systematically and intrathecally administered combinations of clonidine and opiates. J Pharmacol Exp Ther 255:1107–1116

Ossipov MH, Lozito R, Messineo E, Green J, Harris J, Lloyd P (1990b) Spinal antinociceptive synergy between clonidine and morphine, U69593 and DPDPE: isobolographic analysis. Life Sci 46:171–176

Ossipov MH, Kovelowski CJ, Wheeker-Aceto H, Cowan A, Hunter JC, Lai J, Malan TP, Porreca F (1996a) Opioid antagonists and antisera to endogenous opioids increase the nociceptive response to formalin: demonstration of an opioid kappa and delta inhibitory tone. J Pharmacol Exp Ther 277:784–788

Ossipov MH, Lopez Y, Bian D, Nichols ML, Porreca F (1996b) Synergistic antinociceptive interactions of morphine and clonidine in rats with nerve-ligation injury. Anesthesiology (in press)

Ouseph AK, Levine JD (1995) α_1-Adrenoceptor-mediated sympathetically dependent mechanical hyperalgesia in the rat. Eur J Pharmacol 273:107–112

Palmeri A, Wiesendanger M (1990) Concomitant depression of locus coeruleus neurones and of flexor reflexes by an alpha-2-adrenergic agonist in rats: a possible mechanism for an alpha-2-mediated muscle relaxation. Neuroscience 34:177–187

Pang IH, Vasko MR (1986) Morphine and norepinephrine but not 5-hydroxytryptamine and gamma-butyric acid inhibit potassium-stimulated release of substance P from rat spinal cord slices. Brain Res 376:268–279

Patterson SI, Hanley MR (1987) Autoradiographic evidence for β-adrenergic receptors on capsaicin-sensitive primary afferent terminals in rat spinal cord. Neurosci Lett 78:17–21

Paul D, Hornby PJ (1995) Potentiation of intrathecal DAMGO antinociception, but not gastrointestinal transit inhibition, by 5-hydroxytryptamine and norepinephrine uptake blockade. Life Sci 56:PL83–87

Paul D, Phillips AG (1986) Selective effects of pirenpirone on anagesia produced by morphine or electrical stimulation at sites in the nucleus raphe magnus and periaqueductal grey. Psychopharmacology 88:172–176

Paul D, Mana MJ, Pfaus JG, Pinel JPJ (1989) Attenuation of morphine analgesia by the S2 antagonists, pirenperone and ketanserin. Pharmacol Biochem Behav 31:641–647

Pelissier T, Alloui A, Paeile C, Eschalier A (1995) Evidence of a central antino-ciceptive effect of paracetamol involving spinal 5-HT$_3$ receptors. Neuroreport 6:1546–1548

Peng, YB, Lin Q, Willis WD (1995a) The role of 5-HT$_3$ receptors in periaqueductal gray-induced inhibition of nociceptive dorsal horn neurones in rats. J Pharmacol Exp Ther 276:116–124

Peng YB, Lin Q, Willis WD (1995b) Involvement of alpha-2 adrenoceptors in the periaqueductal gray-induced inhibition of dorsal horn cell activity in rats. Soc Neurosci Abstr 21:1172

Persson J, Axelsson G, Hallin RG, Gustafsson LL (1995) Beneficial effects of ketamine in a chronic pain state with allodynia, possibly due to central sensitization. Pain 60:217–222

Pertovaara A (1993) Antinociception induced by alpha-2-adrenoceptor agonists, with special emphasis on medetomidine studies. Prog Neurobiol 40:691–709

Pertovaara A, Hämäläinen MM (1994) Spinal potentiation and supraspinal additivity in the antinociceptive interaction between systematically administered α_2-adrenoceptor agonist and cocaine in the rat. Anesth Analg 79:261–266

Pertovaara A, Bravo R, Herdegen T (1993) Induction and suppression of immediate-early genes in the rat brain by a selective alpha-2-adrenoceptor agonist and antagonist following noxious peripheral stimulation. Neuroscience 54:117–126

Philippi M, Vyklicky L, Kuffler DP, Orkand RK (1995) Serotonin- and proton-induced and modified ionic currents in frog sensory neurones. J Neurosci Res 40:387–395

Pierce PA, Xie GX, Levine JD, Peroutka SJ (1996) 5-hydroxytryptamine receptor subtype messenger RNAs in rat peripheral sensory and sympathetic ganglia: a polymerase chain reaction study. Neuroscience 70:553–559

Pieribone VA, Nicholas AP, Dagerlind Å, Hökfelt T (1994) Distribution of $\alpha 1$-adrenoceptors in rat brain revealed by in situ hybridization experiments utilizing subtype-specific probes. J Neurosci 14:4252–4268

Plummer JL, Cmielewski PL, Gourlay GK, Owen H, Cousins MJ (1992) Antino-ciceptive and motor effects of intrathecal morphine combined with intrathecal clonidine, noradrenaline, carbachol or midazolam in rats. Pain 49:145–152

Pompeiano M, Palacios JM, Mengod G (1992) Distribution and cellular localization of mRNA coding for 5-HT1A receptor in the rat brain: correlation with receptor binding. J Neurosci 12:440–453

Pompeiano M, Palacios JM, Mengod G (1994) Distribution of the serotonin 5-HT$_2$ receptor family mRNAs: comparison between 5-HT$_{2A}$ and 5-HT$_{2C}$ receptors. Mol Brain Res 23:163–178

Post C, Archer T (1990) Interactions between 5-HT and noradrenaline in analgesia. In: Besson JM (ed) Serotonin and pain. Excerpta Medica, Amsterdam, pp 153–174

Post C, Archer T, Minor BG (1988) Evidence for cross-tolerance to the analgesic effects between morphine and selective α_2-adrenoceptor agonists. J Neural Transm 72:1–9

Potrebic SB, Fields HL, Mason P (1994) Serotonin immunoreactivity is contained in one physiological cell class in the rat rostral ventromedial medulla. J Neurosci 14:1655–1665

Powell KR, Dykstra LA (1995) The role of serotonin in the effects of opioids in squirrel monkeys responding under a titration procedure. I. Kappa opioids. J Pharmacol Exp Ther 274:1305–1316

Pranzatelli MR, Murthy JN, Pluchino RS (1992) Identification of spinal 5-HT1C binding sites in the rat: characterization of [3H]mesulergine binding. J Pharmacol Exp Ther 261:161–165

Proudfit HK (1992) The behavioural pharmacology of the noradrenergic descending system. In: Besson JM, Guilbaud G (eds) Towards the use of noradrenergic agonists for the treatment of pain. Excerpta Medica/Elsevier Science, Amsterdam, pp 119–137

Puke MJC, Wiesenfeld-Hallin Z (1993) The differential effects of morphine and the α_2-adrenoceptor agonists clonidine and dexmedetomidine on the prevention and treatment of experimental neuropathic pain. Anesth Analg 77:104–109

Puke MJC, Luo L, Wiesenfeld-Hallin Z (1994) The spinal analgesic role of α α_2-adrenergic receptor subtypes in rats after peripheral nerve section. Eur J Pharmacol 260:227–232

Randich A, Maixner W (1984) Interactions between cardiovascular and pain regulatory systems. Neurosci Biobehav Rev 8:343–367

Rauck RL, Eisenbach JC, Jackson KE, Young LD, Southern BSN (1993) Epidural clonidine treatment for refractory reflex sympathetic dystrophy. Anesthesiology 79:1163–1169

Rebeck GW, Maynard KI, Hyman BT, Moskowitz MA (1994) Selective 5-HT1D serotonin receptor gene expression in trigeminal ganglia: implications for anti-migraine drug development. Proc Natl Acad Sci USA 91:3666–3669

Reid K, Hayashi Y, Guo TZ, Correa-Sales C, Nacif-Coelho C, Maze M (1994) Chronic administration of an α_2 adrenergic agonist desensitizes rats to anesthetic effects of dexmedetomidine. Pharmacol Biochem Behav 47:171–175

Reimann W, Schneider F (1989) Presynaptic α2-adrenoceptors modulate the release of [3H]noradrenaline from rat spinal cord dorsal horn neurones. Eur J Pharmacol 167:161–166

Ren K, Randich A, Gebhart GF (1988) Vagal afferent modulation of a nociceptive reflex in rats: involvement of spinal opioid and monoamine receptors. Brain Res 446:285–294

Ren K, Randich A, Gebhart GF (1991) Spinal serotonergic and kappa opioid receptors mediate facilitation of the tail flick reflex produced by vagal afferent stimulation. Pain 45:321–329

Renouard A, Widdowson PS, Millan MJ (1994) Multiple alpha2-adrenergic receptor subtypes. I. Comparison of [^{3}H]RX821002-labelled rat Rα2A-adrenergic receptors in cerebral cortex to human Hα2A-adrenergic receptors and other populations of 2-adrenergic subtypes. J Pharmacol Exp Ther 270:946–957

Riad M, El Mestikawy S, Vergé D, Gozlan H, Hamon M (1991) Visualisation and quantification of central 5-HT1A receptors with specific antibodies. Neurochem Int 19:413–423

Ridet JL, Rajaofetra N, Teilhac JR, Geffard M, Privat A (1993) Evidence for non-synaptic serotonergic and noradrenergic innervation of the rat dorsal horn and possible involvement of neuron-glia interactions. Neuroscience 52:143–157

Ridet JL, Tamir H, Privat A (1994) Direct immunocytochemical localization of 5-hydroxytryptamine receptors in the adult rat spinal cord: a light and electron microscopic study using an anti-idiotypic antiserum. J Neurosci 38:109–121

Riley RC, Zhao ZQ, Duggan AW (1996) Spinal release of immunoreactive dynorphin A(1-8) with the development of peripheral inflammation in the rat. Brain Res 710:131–142

Robertson B, Bevan S (1991) Properties of 5-hydroxytryptamine3 receptor-gated currents in adult rat dorsal root ganglion neurones. Br J Pharmacol 102:272–276

Robles LI, Barrios M, Del Pozo E, Dordal A, Baeyens JM (1996) Effects of K^+ channel blockers and openers on antinociception induced by agonists of $5\text{-}HT_{1A}$ receptors. Eur J Pharmacol 295:181–188

Rochford J, Dubé B, Dawes P (1992) Spinal cord alpha-2 noradrenergic receptors mediate conditioned analgesia. Psychopharmacology 106:235–238

Rodgers RJ, Shepherd JK, Donát P (1991) Differential effects of novel ligands for 5-HT receptor subtypes on nonopioid defensive analgesia in male mice. Neurosci Behav Rev 15:489–495

Roerig SC, Lei S, Kitto K, Hylden JKL, Wilox GL (1992) Spinal interactions between opioid and noradrenergic agonists in mice: multiplicativity involves delta and alpha-2 receptors. J Pharmacol Exp Ther 262:365–374

Rosin DL, Zeng D, Stornetta RL, Norton FR, Riley T, Okusa MO, Guyenet PG, Lynch KR (1993) Immunohistochemical localization of α_{2A}-adrenergic receptors in catecholaminergic and other brainstem neurons in the rat. Neuroscience 56:139–155

Ruat M, Traiffort E, Leurs R, Tardivel-Lacombe J, Diaz J, Arrang JM, Schwartz JC (1994) Molecular cloning, characterization, and localization of a high-affinity serotonin receptor (5-HT7) activating cAMP formation. Proc Natl Acad Sci USA 90:8547–8551

Ruda MA (1990) Serotonin and spinal dorsal horn neuronal circuitry. In: Besson JM (ed) Serotonin and pain. Excerpta Medica/Elsevier Science, Amsterdam, pp 73–84

Ruda MA, Bennett GJ, Dubner R (1986) Neurochemistry and neural circuitry in the dorsal horn. Prog Brain Res 66:219–268

Saeki S, Yaksh TL (1991) Suppression by spinal alpha-2 agonists of motor and autonomic responses evoked by low- and high-intensity thermal stimuli. J Pharmacol Exp Ther 260:795–802

Sagen J, Winker MA, Proudfit HK (1983) Hypoalgesia induced by the local injection of phentolamine in the nucleus raphe magnus blockade by depletion of spinal cord monoamines. Pain 16:253–264

Sakatani K, Chesler M, Hassan AZ, Lee M, Young W (1993) Non-synaptic modulation of dorsal column conduction by endogenous GABA in neonatal rat spinal cord. Brain Res 622:43–50

Sánchez A, Niedbala B, Feria M (1995) Modulation of neuropathic pain in rats by intrathecally injected serotonergic agonists. Neuroreport 6:2585–2588

Sandrini G, Alfonsi E, de Rysky C, Marini S, Facchinetti F, Nappi G (1986) Evidence for Serotonin-S_2 receptor involvement in analgesia in humans. Eur J Pharmacol 130:311–314

Saria A, Javorsky F, Humpel C, Gamse R (1990) 5-HT3 receptor antagonists inhibit sensory neuropeptide release from the rat spinal cord. Neuroreport 1:104–106

Satoh M, Kawajiri SI, Ukai Y, Yamamoto M (1979) Selective and non-selective inhibition by enkephalins and noradrenaline of nociceptive response of lamina V type neurons in the spinal dorsal horn of the rabbit. Brain Res 177:384–387

Satoh M, Kashiba A, Kimura H, Maeda T (1982) Noradrenergic axon terminals in the substantia gelatinosa of the rat spinal cord. Cell Tissue Res 222:359–378

Sawynok J (1989) The role of ascending and descending noradrenergic and serotoninergic pathways in opioid and non-opioid antinociception as revealed by lesion studies. Can J Physiol Pharmacol 67:975–988

Sawynok J, Reid A (1994) Spinal supersensitivity to 5-HT$_1$, 5-HT$_2$- and 5-HT$_3$ receptor agonists following 5,7-dihydroxytryptamine. Eur J Pharmacol 264:249–257

Sawynok J, Reid A (1996) Neurotoxin-induced lesions to central serotonergic, noradrenergic and dopaminergic systems modify caffeine-induced antinociception in the formalin test and locomotor stimulation in rats. J Pharmacol Exp Ther 277:646–653

Scatton B, Dubois A, Cudennec A (1984) Autoradiographic localization of dopamine receptors in the spinal cord of the rat using H-N-propylnorapomorphine. J Neural Transm 59:251–256

Scheinin M, Lomasney JW, Hayden-Hixson DM, Schambra UB, Caron MG, Lefkowitz RJ, Fremeau RT (1994) Distribution of α_2-adrenergic receptor subtype gene expression in rat brain. Mol Brain Res 21:133–149

Schlicker E, Werner U, Hamon M, Gozlan H, Nickel B, Szelenyi, I, Göthert M (1992) Anpirtoline, a novel, highly potent 5-HT$_{1B}$ receptor agonist with antinociceptive/antidepressant-like actions in rodents. Br J Pharmacol 105:732–738

Schott GD (1995) An unsympathetic view of pain. Lancet 345:634–365

Schwinn DA, Correa-Sales C, Page SO, Maze M (1991) Functional effects of activation of alpha-1 adrenoceptors by dexmedetomidine: in vivo and in vitro studies. J Pharmacol Exp Ther 259:1147–1152

Segal IS, Javis DJ, Duncan SR, White PF, Maze M (1991) Clinical efficacy of oral-transdermal clonidine combinations during the perioperative period. Anesthesiology 74:220–225

Seguin L, Le Marouille-Girardon S, Millan MJ (1995) Antinociceptive profiles of non-peptidergic neurokinin 1 and neurokinin 2 receptor antagonists: a comparison to other classes of antinociceptive agent. Pain 61:325–343

Seybold VS (1986) Neurotransmitter receptor sites in the spinal cord. In: Yaksh TL (ed) Spinal afferent processing. Plenum, New York, pp 117–139

Sherman S, Lommis C, Milne B, Cervenko F (1987) Prolonged spinal analgesia in the rat with the α-adrenoceptor agonist oxymetazoline. Eur J Pharmacol 140:25–32

Simmons RMA, Jones DJ (1988) Binding of [^{3}H]prazosin and [^{3}H]p-aminoclondine to α-adrenoceptors in rat spinal cord. Brain Res 445:338–349

Singelyn FJ, Dangoisse M, Bartholomee S, Gouverneur JM (1992) Adding clonidine to mepivacaine prolongs the duration of anesthesia and analgesia after axillary brachial plexus block. Reg Anesth 17:148–150

Smith BD, Baudendistel LJ, Gibbons JJ, Schweiss JF (1992) A comparison of two epidural α2-agonists, guanfacine and clonidine, in regard to duration of antinociception, and ventilatory and hemodynamic effects in goats. Anesth Analg 74:712–718

Smith GD, Harrison SM, Wiseman J, Elliott PJ, Birch PJ (1993) Pre-emptive administration of clonidine prevents development of hyperalgesia to mechanical stimuli in a model of mononeuropathy in the rat. Brain Res 632:16–20

Smith GD, Wiseman J, Harrison SM, Elliott PJ, Birch PJ (1994) Pre-treatment with MK-801, a non-competitive NMDA antagonist, prevents development of mechanical hyperalgesia in a rat model of chronic neuropathy, but not in a model of chronic inflammation. Neurosci Lett 165 79–83

Solomon RE, Gebhart GF (1988a) Intrathecal morphine and clonidine: antinociceptive tolerance and cross-tolerance and effects on blood pressure. J Pharmacol Exp Ther 245:444–454

Solomon RE, Gebhart GF (1988b) Mechanisms of effects of intrathecal serotonin on nociception and blood pressure in rats. J Pharmacol Exp Ther 245:905–912

Solomon RE, Brody MJ, Gebhart GF (1989) Pharmacological characterization of alpha-adrenoceptors involved in the antinociceptive and cardiovascular effects of intrathecally administered clonidine. J Pharmacol Exp Ther 251:27–38

Sorkin LS, McAdoo DJ, Willis WD (1993) Raphe magnus stimulation-induced antinociception in the cat is associated with release of amino acids as well as serotonin in the lumbar dorsal horn. Brain Res 618:95–108

Spanos LJ, Stafinsky JL, Crisp T (1989) A comparative analysis of monoaminergic involvement in the spinal antinociceptive action of DAMPGO and DPDPE. Pain 39:329–335

Stafford-Smith M, Schambra UB, Wilson KH, Page SO, Hulette C, Light AR, Schwinn DA (1995) α_2-Adrenergic receptors in human spinal cord: specific localized expression of mRNA encoding α_2-adrenergic receptor subtypes at four distinct levels. Mol Brain Res 34:109–117

Stamford JA (1995) Descending control of pain. Br J Anaesth 75:217–227

Stanfa LC, Dickenson AH (1994) Enhanced alpha-2 adrenergic controls and spinal morphine potency in inflammation. Neuroreport 5:469–472

Stevens CW, Yaksh TL (1989) Time course characteristics of tolerance development to continuously infused antinociceptive agents in rat spinal cord. J Pharmacol Exp Ther 251:216–223

Stevens C, Yaksh TL (1992) Studies of morphine and D-Ala2-D-Leu5-enkephalin (DADLE) cross-tolerance after continuous intrathecal infusion in the rat. Anesthesiology 76:596–603

Stevens CW, Monasky MS, Yaksh TL (1988) Spinal infusion of opiate and alpha-2 agonists in rats: tolerance and cross-tolerance studies. J Pharmacol Exp Ther 244:63–70

Stiller RU, Grubb BD, Schaible HG (1993) Neurophysiological evidence for increased kappa opioidergic control of spinal cord neurons in rats with unilateral inflammation at the ankle. Eur J Neurosci 5:1520–1527

Sugimoto T, Bennet GJ, Kajander KC (1990) Transsynaptic degeneration in the superficial dorsal horn after sciatic nerve injury: effects of a chronic constriction injury, transsection, and strychnine. Pain 42:205–213

Sugiyama BH, Huang LYM (1995) Activation of 5-HT2 receptors potentiates the spontaneous inhibitory postsynaptic currents on (sIPSCs) intrigeminal neurones. Am Soc Neurosci Abstr 21:1415

Sullivan AF, Dashwood MR, Dickenson AH (1987) α_2-Adrenoceptor modulation of nociception in rat spinal cord: localisation, effects and interaction with morphine. Eur J Pharmacol 138:169–177

Sullivan AF, Kalso EA, McQuay HJ, Dickenson AH (1992a) Evidence for the involvement of the μ but not δ opioid receptor subtype in the synergistic interaction between opioid and α_2 adrenergic antinociception in the rat spinal cord. Neurosci Lett 139:65–68

Sullivan AF, Kalso EA, McQuay HJ, Dickenson AH (1992b) The antinociceptive actions of dexmedetomidine on dorsal horn neuronal responses in the anaesthetized rat. Eur J Pharmacol 215:127–133

Taguchi K, Suzuki Y (1992) The response of the 5-hydroxyindole oxidation current to noxious stimuli in the spinal cord of anesthesized rats: modification by morphine. Brain Res 583:150–154

Takagi H, Shiomi H, Kuraishi Y, Fukui K, Ueda H (1979) Pain and the bulbospinal noradrenergic system. pain-induced increase in normetanephrine content in the spinal cord and its modification by morphine. Eur J Pharmacol 54:94–107

Takano Y, Yaksh TL (1992a) The effect of intrathecally administered imiloxan and WB4101: possible role of α2-adrenoceptor subtypes in the spinal cord. Eur J Pharmacol 219:465–468

Takano Y, Yaksh TL (1992b) Characterization of the pharmacology of intrathecally administered alpha-2 agonists and antagonists in rats. J Pharmacol Exp Ther 261:764–772

Takano Y, Yaksh TL (1993) Chronic spinal infusion of dexmedetomidine, ST 91 and clonidine: spinal alpha$_2$ adrenoceptor subtypes and intrinsic activity. J Pharmacol Exp Ther 264:327–335

Takano Y, Yaksh TL (1992c) In vitro release of calcitonin gene related peptide (CGRP), substance P (SP) and vasoactive intestinal polypeptide (VIP): modulation by alpha-2 agonists. In: Inoki R, Shigenaga Y, Tohyama M (eds) Processing and inhibition of nociceptive information. Elsevier Science, Amsterdam, pp 249–252

Takeshita N, Okhubo Y, Yamaguchi I (1995) Tiapride attenuates pain transmission through an direct activation of central serotoninergic mechanism. J Pharmacol Exp Ther 275:23–30

Takeshita N, Yamaguchi I (1995) Meta-chlorophenylpiperazine attenuates formalin-induced nociceptive responses through 5-HT$_{1/2}$ receptors in both normal and diabetic mice. Br J Pharmacol 116:3133–3138

Tasker RAR, Connell BJ, Yole MJ (1992) Systemic injections of alpha-1 adrenergic agonists produce antinociception in the formalin test. Pain 49:383–391

Tecott LH, Maricq AV, Julius D (1993) Nervous system distribution of the serotonin 5-HT3 receptor mRNA. Proc Natl Acad Sci USA 90:1430–1434

Teoh H, Malcangio M, Bowery NG (1996) GABA, glutamate and substance P-like immunoreactivity release: effects of novel GABA$_B$ antagonists. Br J Pharmacol 118:1153–1160

Thor KB, Nickolaus S, Helke CJ (1993) Autoradiographic localization of 5-hydroxytryptamine1A, 5-hydroxytryptamine1B and 5-hydroxytryptamine1C/2 binding sites in the rat spinal cord. Neuroscience 55:235–252

Thurston CL, Helton ES (1996) Effects of intravenous phenylephrine on blood pressure, nociception, and neural activity in the rostral ventral medulla in rats. Brain Res 717:81–90

Tjølsen A, Berge OG, Hole K (1991) Lesions of bulbo-spinal serotonergic or noradrenergic pathways reduce nociception as measured by the formalin test. Acta Physiol Scand 142:229–236

Todd KA, Millar J (1983) Respective fields and responses to iontophoretically applied noradrenaline and 5-hydroxytryptamine of units recorded in laminae I–III of cat dorsal horn. Brain Res 288:159–167

Todd AJ, Watt C, Spike RC, Sieghart W (1996) Colocalization of GABA, glycine and their receptors at synapses in the rat spinal cord. J Neurosci 16:974–982

Tseng LLF, Tang R (1989) Differential actions of the blockade of spinal opioid, adrenergic and serotonergic receptors on the tail-flick inhibition induced by morphine microinjected into dorsal raphe and central gray in rats. Neuroscience 33:93–100

Uhlén S, Wikberg JES (1991) Rat-spinal cord α_{2A}-adrenoceptors are of the α_{2A}-subtype: comparison with α_{2A}- and α_{2B}-adrenoceptors in rat spleen, cerebral cortex and kidney using [^{3}H]RX82102 ligand binding. Pharmacol Toxicol 69:341–350

Ueda M, Oyama T, Kuraishi Y, Akaike A, Satoh M (1995) Alpha2-adrenoceptor-mediated inhibition of capsaicin-evoked release of glutamate from rat spinal dorsal horn slices. Neurosci Lett 188:137–139

Uhlén S, Persson I, Alari C, Post C, Axelsson KL, Wikberg JES (1990) Antinociceptive actions of α_2-adrenoceptor agonists in the rat spinal cord: evidence for antinociceptive α_2-adrenoceptor subtype and dissociation of antinociceptive α_2-adrenoceptors from cyclic AMP. J Neurochem 55:1905–1914

Uhlén S, Xia Y, Chhajlani V, Felder CC, Wikberg JES (1992) [^{3}H]-MK912 binding delineates two α_2-adrenoceptor subtypes in rat CNS one of which is identical with the cloned A2d α_2-adrenoceptor. Br J Pharmacol 106:986–995

Ulhén S, Porter AC, Neubig RR (1994) The novel alpha-2 adrenergic radioligand [3H]-MK912 is alpha-2C selective among human alpha-2A, alpha-2B and alpha-2C adrenoceptors. J Pharmacol Exp Ther 271:1558–1565

Urban L, Thompson SWN, Dray A (1994) Modulation of spinal excitability: cooperation between neurokinin and excitatory amino acid neurotransmitters. Trends Neurosci 17:432–438

Vasko MR, Pang IH, Vogt M (1984) Involvement of 5-hydroxytryptamine-containing neurones in antinociception produced by injection of morphine into nucleus raphe magnus or onto spinal cord. Brain Res 306:341–348

Vayssettes-Courchay C, Bouysset F, Cordi A, Laubie M, Verbeuren TJ (1996) A comparative study of the reversal by different α_2-adrenoceptor antagonists of the central sympatho-inhibitory effect of clonidine. Br J Pharmacol 117:587–593

Verdugo RJ, Ochoa JL (1994) Sympathetically maintained pain. Neurology 44:1003–1010

Von Knorring L (1990) Serotonin metabolites in the CSF of chronic pain patients. In: Besson JM (ed) Serotonin and pain. Excerpta Medica/Elsevier Science, Amsterdam, pp 285–304

Vonhof S, Sirén AL (1991) Reversal of μ-opioid-mediated respiratory depression by α_2-adrenoceptor antagonism. Life Sci 49:111–119

VonVoigtlander PF, Lewis RA, Neff GL (1984) Kappa opioid analgesia is dependent on serotonergic mechanisms. J Pharmacol Exp Ther 231:270–274

Waeber C, Hoyer D, Palacios JM (1989) 5-Hydroxytryptamine3 receptors in the human brain: autoradiographic visualisation using [3H]ICS 205–930. Neuroscience 31:393–400

Wallis DI (1994) 5-HT receptors involved in initiation or modulation of motor patterns: opportunities for drug development. Trends Pharmacol Sci 15:288–292

Wang C, Knowles MG, Chakrabarti MK, Whitwam JG (1994) Clonidine has comparable effects on spontaneous sympathetic activity and afferent A delta and C-fiber-mediated somatosympathetic reflexes in dogs. Anesthesiology 81:710–717

Wang SD, Goldenberg ME, Murray M (1991) Plasticity of spinal systems after unilateral lumbosacral dorsal rhizotomy in the adult rat. J Comp Neurol 304:555–568

Ward RP, Hamblin MW, Lachowicz JE, Hoffman BJ, Sibley DR, Dorsa DM (1995) Localization of serotonin subtype 6 receptor messenger RNA in the rat brain by in situ hybridization histochemistry. Neuroscience 64:1105–1111

Watkins LR, Thurston CL, Fleshner M (1990) Phenylephrine-induced antinociception: investigations of potential neural and endocrine bases. Brain Res 528:273–284

Weil-Fugazza J (1990) Central metabolism and release of serotonin in pain and analgesia. In: Besson JM (ed) Serotonin and pain. Excerpta Medica, Amsterdam, p 339

Weil-Fugazza J, Godefroy F, Manceau V, Besson JM (1986) Increased norepinephrine and uric acid levels in the spinal cord of arthritic rats. Brain Res 374:190–194

Westlund KN (1992) Anatomy of noradrenergic pathways modulating pain. In: Besson JM, Guilbaud G (eds) Towards the use of noradrenergic agonists for the treatment of pain. Excerpta Medica/ElsevierScience, Amsterdam, pp 91–118

Wikberg JES, Hajós M (1987) Spinal cord $\alpha2$-adrenoceptors may be located postsynaptically with respect to primary sensory neurones: destruction of primary C-afferents with neonatal capsaicin does not affect the number of [3H]clonidine binding sites in mice. Neurosci Lett 76:63–68

Wild KE, Press JB, Raffa RB (1994) Alpha$_2$-adrenoceptors: can subtypes mediate selective analgesia? Analgesia 1:15–25

Willcockson WS, Chung, JM, Hori Y, Lee KH, Willis WD (1984) Effects of iontophoretically released amino acids and amines on primate spinothalamic tract cells. J Neurosci 4:732–740

Williams F, Birnbaum A, Wilcox G, Beitz A (1991) Hybridization histochemical analysis of spinal neurones that express the $\alpha2$-adrenergic receptor in a rat model of peripheral mononeuropathy. Soc Neurosci Abstr 17:1370

Willis WD (1988) Anatomy and physiology of descending control of nociceptive responses of dorsal horn neurons: a comprehensive review. Prog Brain Res 77:1–29

Willis WD (1992) Descending control systems: Physiological aspects. In: Besson JM, Guilbaud G (eds) Towards the use of noradrenergic agonists for the treatment of pain. Excerpta Medica/Elsevier Science, Amsterdam, pp 47–64

Willis WD (1994) Central plastic responses to pain. In: Gebhart GF, Hammond DL, Jensen TS (eds) Proceeding of the 7th World Congress on Pain, vol 2. International Association for the Study of Pain, Seattle, pp 301–324

Wilson P, Kitchener PD (1996) Plasticity of cutaneous primary afferent projections to the spinal dorsal horn. Prog Neurobiol 48:105–129

Woolf CJ, Chong MS (1993) Preemptive analgesia-treating postoperative pain by preventing the establishment of central sensitization. Anesth Analg 77:362–379

Woolf CJ, Doubell TP (1994) The pathophysiology of chronic pain – increased sensitivity to low threshold Aβ-fibre inputs. Curr Opin Biol 4:525–534

Wu J, Wessendorf MW (1992) Organization of the serotonergic innervation of spinal neurones in rats. I. Neuropeptide coexistence in varicosities innervating some spinothalamic tract neurones but not in those innervating postsynaptic dorsal column neurones. Neuroscience 50:885–898

Wu J, Wessendorf MW (1993) Organization of the serotonergic innervation of spinal neurones in rats. III. Differential serotonergic innervation of somatic and parasympathetic preganglionic motoneurones as determined by patterns of co-existing peptides. Neuroscience 55:223–233

Xu XJ, Hao JX, Seiger A, Wiesenfeld-Hallin Z (1993) Systemic excitatory amino acid receptor antagonists of the α-amino-3-hydroxy-5-methyl-4-isoxazolepropionic acid (AMPA) receptor and of the N-methyl-D-aspartate (NMDA) receptor relieve mechanical hypersensitivity after transient spinal cord ischemia in rats. J Pharmacol Exp Ther 267:140–144

Xu W, Qui XC, Han JS (1994a) Spinal serotonin 1A and 1C/2 receptors mediate supraspinal μ opioid-induced analgesia. Neuroreport 5:2665–2668

Xu W, Qui XC, Han JS (1994b) Serotonin receptor subtypes in spinal antinociception in the rat. J Pharmacol Exp Ther 269:1182–1189

Xu XJ, Puke MJC, Wiesenfeld-Hallin Z (1992) The depression effect of intrathecal clonidine on the spinal flexor reflex is enhanced after sciatic nerve section in rats. Pain 51:145–53

Xu XJ, Zhang X, Hökfelt T, Wiesenfeld-Hallin Z (1995) Plasticity in spinal nociception after peripheral nerve section: reduced effectiveness of the NMDA receptor antagonist MK-801 in blocking wind-up and central sensitization of the flexor reflex. Brain Res 670:342–346

Yaksh TL (1985) Pharmacology of spinal adrenergic systems which modulate spinal nociceptive processing. Pharmacol Biochem Behav 22:845–858

Yaksh TL, Pogrel JW, Lee YW, Chaplan SR (1995) Reversal of nerve ligation-induced allodynia by spinal alpha2 adrenoceptor agonists. J Pharmacol Exp Ther 272:207–214

Yamaguchi H, Watanabe S, Dohi S, Naito H (1994) Effect of additional clonidine on dose-responses of morphine on antinociception and $PaCO_2$ in rats. Anesth Analg 78:S493

Yamamoto T, Yaksh TL (1991) Spinal pharmacology of thermal hyperesthesia induced by incomplete ligation of sciatic nerve. Anesthesiology 75:817–826

Yang L, Helke CJ (1995) Effects of coexisting neurochemicals on the release of serotonin from the intermediate area of rat thoracic spinal cord. Synapse 21:319–323

Yeomans DC, Proudfit HK (1992) Antinociception induced by microinjection of substance P into the A7 catecholamine cell group in the rat. Neuroscience 49:681–691

Yeomans DC, Clark FM, Paice JA, Proudfit HK (1992) Antinociception induced by electrical stimulation of spinally projecting noradrenergic neurones in the A7 catecholamine cell group of the rat. Pain 48:449–461

Yezierski RP, Wilcox TK, Willis WD (1982) The effects of serotonin antagonists on the inhibition of primate spinothalamic tract cells produced by stimulation in nucleus raphe magnus or periaqueductal gray. J Pharmacol Exp Ther 220:266–277

Yonehara N, Shibutani T, Imai Y, Sawada T, Inoki R (1991) Serotonin inhibits release of substance P evoked by tooth pulp stimulation in trigeminal nucleus caudalis in rabbits. Neuropharmacology 30:5–13

Yoshimura M, Nishi S (1995) Primary afferent-evoked glycine- and GABA-mediated IPSPs in substantia gelatinosa neurones in the rat spinal cord in vitro. J Physiol (Lond) 482 (1):29–38

Zemlan FP, Schwab EF (1991) Characterization of a novel serotonin receptor subtype (5-HT$_{1S}$) in rat CNS: interaction with a GTP binding protein. J Neurochem 57:2092–2099

Zemlan FP, Kow L, Pfaff DW (1983) Spinal serotonin (5-HT) receptor subtypes and nociception. J Pharmacol Exp Ther 226:477–485

Zemlan FP, Schwab EF, Murphy RM, Behbehani MM (1990) Identification of a novel 5-HT1S binding site in rat spinal cord. Neurochem Int 16:503–513

Zemlan FP, Murphy RM, Behbehani MM (1994) 5-HT1A receptors mediate the effect of bulbospinal serotonin system on spinal dorsal horn nociceptive neurons. Pharmacology 48:1–10

Zeng D, Lynch KR (1991) Distribution of α2-adrenergic receptor mRNAs in the rat CNS. Mol Brain Res 10:219–225

Zhao ZQ, Duggan AW (1987) Clonidine and the hyper-responsiveness of dorsal horn neurones following morphine withdrawal in the spinal cat. Neuropharmacology 26:1499–1502

Zhao ZQ, Duggan AW (1988) Idazoxan blocks the action of noradrenaline but not spinal inhibition from electrical stimulation of the locus coeruleus and nucleus kolliker-fuse of the cat. Neuroscience 25:997–1005

Zhuo M, Gebhart GF (1990) Spinal cholinergic and monoaminergic receptors mediate descending inhibition from the nuclei reticularis gigantocellularis and gigantocellularis pars alpha in the rat. Brain Res 535:67–78

Zhuo M, Gebhart GF (1991) Spinal serotonin receptors mediate descending facilitation of a nociceptive reflex from the nuclei reticularis gigantocellularis and gigantocellularis pars alpha in the rat. Brain Res 550:35–48

Zochodne DW, Ho LT (1994) Sumatriptan blocks neurogenic inflammation in the peripheral nerve trunk. Neurology 44:161–163

CHAPTER 16

Neonatal Pharmacology of Pain

M. FITZGERALD

A. Introduction

It is only a little over a decade since interest arose in the development of pain processing in the mammalian nervous system, and there is now widespread recognition that more basic knowledge is required in this field. Clinical management of paediatric pain has been largely empirical, and there is considerable ignorance about the ability of the infant nervous system to react to painful stimuli and the sensitivity of the developing nervous system to analgesic therapy.

This review discusses the current state of knowledge of the developmental pharmacology of pain and analgesia. Pain pathways within the spinal cord are emphasized because this region is known to be a major site of nociceptive processing and has been the most thoroughly studied region in this field. The important message of this review is that pain transmission in the neonate cannot be considered simply as an immature or less efficient form of that found in the adult but rather involves quite different transient functional signalling pathways that are not a feature of the mature nervous system. As a result neonatal analgesic sensitivity differs considerably from that in the adult. Furthermore, many agents that are simply neurotransmitters in the adult, also have trophic actions regulating neuronal growth and synaptogenesis in the developing nervous system.

Before considering the pharmacology of neonatal pain it is important to appreciate the background against which the actions of excitatory and inhibitory agents are set in the immature nervous system. Neonatal spinal sensory pathways undergo considerable postnatal reorganization, both anatomical and physiological. These have been reviewed in detail elsewhere (FITZGERALD 1995; FITZGERALD and ANAND 1993) but are briefly summarized below and illustrated in Fig. 1.

I. Anatomical Background

At birth the spinal cord is still immature. The spinal cord develops ventrodorsally, beginning in embryonic life with motoneurons, followed by intermediate neurons and deep dorsal horn projection neurons and ending with the neurons of lamina I and II, substantia gelatinosa (SG) (ALTMAN and

BAYER 1984). As a result axodendritic growth of SG neurons only begins postnatally in the rat (BICKNELL and BEAL 1984). Synaptogenesis peaks in the first 2 postnatal weeks and is concentrated in the deep dorsal horn at P (postnatal day) 4–5 and in laminae II at P7–9 (CABALKA et al. 1990). Some, although by no means all, of these synapses arise from the primary afferents whose terminals undergo considerable postnatal maturation. Large myelinated cutaneous afferents arising mainly from low-threshold mechanoreceptors enter the spinal cord well before birth (FITZGERALD et al. 1991), but their terminals grow up dorsally and proceed to occupy both deep dorsal horn laminae and more superficial laminae I and II. This situation is maintained for 3 postnatal weeks before they finally withdraw to terminate in the deep dorsal horn as found in the adult (FITZGERALD et al. 1995). During their occupation of SG, A fibre terminals can be seen to form synaptic connections at electron microscopic level (COGGESHALL et al. 1995). C fibre afferents, which are largely nociceptors and small-diameter Aδ fibres, grow into the spinal cord only a few days before birth, and the formation of C fibre synaptic connections is almost entirely a postnatal event (FITZGERALD 1987). C-type afferent terminals are not observed within synaptic glomeruli at electron microscopic level until P5 (PIGNATELLI et al. 1989). Their final terminal region is SG, but, as discussed above, they are forced to share this region with A fibres for a considerable postnatal period. Competitive interaction takes place between the two afferent groups which results finally in exclusively C fibres occupying the region. If C fibres are selectively destroyed at birth with the neurotoxin capsaicin, A fibres remain in SG until adulthood (SHORTLAND et al. 1990).

II. Physiological Background

The postnatal maturation of synaptic connections between afferent C fibres and SG cells takes place over a prolonged period. Unlike low-threshold A fibres, which rapidly form synaptic connections prenatally and evoke brisk mono- and polysynaptic responses that can be recorded in the dorsal horn and from the ventral root soon after they grow into the spinal cord (FITZGERALD 1991a,b), C fibre activation is unable to evoke spike activity in the spinal cord until the 2nd postnatal week (FITZGERALD and GIBSON 1984; FITZGERALD 1988; HORI and WATANABE 1987). Responses to noxious mechanical stimulation or non-specific chemical irritants, such as formalin, both of which have an A fibre component, produce clear reflex activity and c-*fos* induction from birth (FITZGERALD and GIBSON 1984; WILLIAMS et al. 1990; SOYGUDER et al. 1994), but responses to pure C fibre inputs remain subthreshold for a considerable period postnatally (FITZGERALD 1991b).

In contrast to the slow development of C fibre mediated excitatory responses, the input from A fibres is apparently enhanced. Cutaneous reflexes in the newborn rat, kitten and human are exaggerated compared to the adult (see FITZGERALD 1995 for review). The elicitation of a flexor reflex response in kittens, rat pups and human infants often does not require a painful stimulus as in the adult but only light touch (EKHOLM 1967; FITZGERALD et al. 1987). Thresholds are lower, and the reflex responses more synchronized and long-lasting. Repeated skin stimulation results in considerable hyperexcitability or sensitization with generalized movements of all limbs. Significantly shorter latencies to paw withdrawal from heat have also been observed in neonates (LEWIN et al. 1993), and pain behaviour following formalin injection into the hindpaw, measured as frequency of paw flexion and paw licking, is greatly augmented in the 1st postnatal week (GUY and ABBOTT 1992). This period of hyperexcitability begins to decline after the 1st postnatal week in the rat (and after 30 weeks gestation in humans) gradually falling to adult levels at P20–30 (HAMMOND and RUDA 1991).

The physiological properties of dorsal horn cells in the 1st postnatal week are consistent with increased excitability of spinal reflexes. The synaptic linkage between afferents and dorsal horn cells is weak, and electrical stimulation often evokes only a few spikes at long latencies, but natural stimulation of receptive fields can often evoke long-lasting excitation lasting minutes which may lower the threshold to subsequent stimuli (FITZGERALD 1985). Repeated stimuli can build up considerable background activity in the cells. Furthermore, the receptive fields of the dorsal horn cells are larger in the newborn and gradually diminish over the first 2 postnatal weeks (FITZGERALD 1985). One factor contributing to increased excitability is the delayed postnatal maturation of descending inhibitory pathways travelling from the brainstem via the dorsolateral funiculus of the spinal cord to the dorsal horn (FITZGERALD and

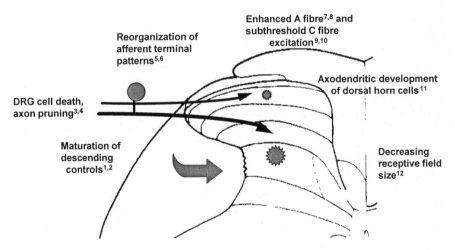

Fig. 1. Postnatal changes in the physiological and anatomical aspects of developing spinal pain pathways. References: *1*, FITZGERALD and KOLTZENBERG (1986); *2*, VAN PRAAG and FRENK (1992); *3*, COGGESHALL et al. (1994); *4*, HULSEBOSCH et al. (1986); *5*, PIGNATELLI et al. (1989); *6*, FITZGERALD et al. (1995); *7*, EKHOLM (1967); *8*, JENNINGS and FITZGERALD (1996); *9*, FITZGERALD (1988); *10*, HORI and WATANBE (1987); *11*, BICKNELL and BEAL (1984); *12*, FITZGERALD (1985)

Koltzenburg 1986). Although descending axons from brainstem projection neurons grow down the spinal cord early in fetal life, they do not extend collateral branches into the dorsal horn for some time and do not become functionally effective until postnatal day 10 in the rat. This lack of descending inhibition has important implications for the function of neonatal nociceptive pathways and explains why stimulus produced analgesia from the periacqueductal grey is not effective until P21 in rats (van Praag and Frenk 1991).

Figure 1 summarizes the points above and gives a brief overview of the anatomical and physiological situation in the developing spinal cord. The next sections consider the pharmacology of this system.

B. Neonatal Pharmacology of Excitatory Pathways Involved in Pain

I. Glutamate

1. NMDA Receptors

The neonatal spinal cord has a higher concentration of N-methyl-D-aspartate (NMDA) receptors in the grey matter than that observed in older animals (Gonzalez et al. 1993). All laminae in the dorsal horn are uniformly labelled with NMDA sensitive [^{3}H]glutamate until days 10–12, when higher densities begin to appear in substantia gelatinosa as in the adult. The differentiation progresses gradually, and P30 binding is similar to that in the adult. Furthermore, the affinity of the receptors for NMDA decreases with postnatal age (Hori and Kanda 1994). In the immature hippocampus, where similar high densities are found, NMDA-evoked excitatory postsynaptic potentials are much greater in amplitude and less sensitive to Mg^{2+} than in the adult (Morrisett et al. 1990). Furthermore, the antagonist activity of D-5-amino phosphonovaleric acid to the NMDA evoked response is two to three times greater during this period of NMDA hyperexcitability than in older animals (Brady et al. 1994). In the visual cortex and colliculus it has been shown that the NMDA channel open time is also developmentally regulated, resulting in NMDA currents that are several times longer in young animals than in adults (Hestrin 1992; Carmignoto and Vicini 1992) This situation is likely to be the same in the neonatal dorsal horn since NMDA-evoked calcium efflux in rat substantia gelatinosa is very high in the 1st postnatal week and then declines (Hori and Kanda 1994; see Fig. 2). Interestingly, neonatal capsaicin delays this developmental decline, suggesting that C fibre evoked NMDA-regulated Ca^{2+} may be related to postnatal maturation (Hori and Kanda 1994).

Molecular cloning and functional expression studies have revealed five members of NMDA receptor (NR) channel subunits. The NR2 subunits (A, B, C) are modulatory since their expression alters properties such as voltage-

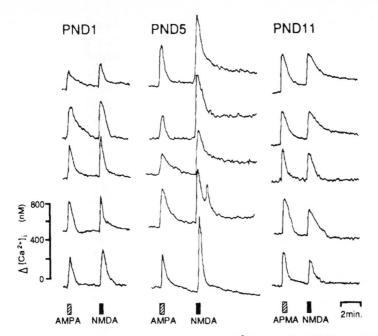

Fig. 2. Sample recordings of transient increases in Ca^{2+} induced by NMDA and AMPA at different ages. *Columns*, representative NMDA and AMPA responses of five individual neurons simultaneously recorded in each rat spinal cord slice from siblings at postnatal days (*PND*) 1, 5 and 11. (From Hori and Kanda 1994)

dependent Mg^{2+} block and deactivation kinetics of NMDA receptors. The NR2B subunit appears to predominate over the NR2A in developing cortex and cerebellum (Zhong et al. 1995) and may define NMDA properties in these areas in early life (Riva et al. 1994). There is also considerable rearrangement of the subunit composition of the NMDA channel complex during spinal cord development (Watanabe et al. 1994). The switch of receptor subunits appears to be activity dependent. In the rat cerebellum, where NR1 and NR2B predominate in the young rats and NR1, NR2A and NR2C in the adult, the switch from NR2B to NR2A is delayed if the cerebellum is chronically exposed to tetrodotoxin in culture (Audinat et al. 1994).

The change in NMDA receptor properties is thought to reflect its different roles during development from survival, migration and neurite growth which may require tonic activation by glutamate at extrasynaptic receptors to neurotransmission involving phasic activation of receptors at synapses. Chronic neonatal treatment with the NMDA anatagonist MK-801 leads to long-term effects on brain function and may lead to the development of a CNS with immature network properties. Important changes in the sharpening and fine tuning of synapses have been observed in the developing visual system following chronic NMDA blockade (see Hofer and Constantine-Paton 1994 for review), and administration of daily doses of MK-801 to embryonic chick disrupts the somatotopic organization of cutaneous nerve projections in the chick spinal cord (Mendelson 1994).

The role of the NMDA receptor in neonatal pain transmission has not been directly investigated. However, NMDA-dependent C fibre evoked depolarization of spinal cord cells and "wind-up" of cells to repeated C fibre stimulation has frequently been demonstrated in the young (8- to 14-day) spinal cord "in vitro" (Thompson et al. 1990; King and Lopez-Garcia 1993; Sivilotti et al. 1995). It can even been argued that these NMDA-dependent central changes in excitability are more pronounced in these preparations than in the adult, considering that (a) they are performed largely at room temperature, and (b) they are evoked by both $A\delta$ and C fibres whereas in the adult the effect is exclusively C fibre mediated (Woolf and King 1987).

2. AMPA Receptors

Receptor autoradiography of α-amino-3-hydroxy-5-methyl-isoxazole (AMPA) receptor expression in the neonatal spinal cord shows a wider distribution of R1, R2 and R3 than in the adult, which decrease over the first postnatal 3 weeks (Jacowec et al. 1995a). In situ hybridization studies to determine the distribution, temporal expression and potential subunit expression of AMPA receptors in the developing rat spinal cord have shown that there are considerable postnatal changes (Jacowec et al. 1995b; see Fig. 3). The GluR1, GluR2 and GluR4 subunits are more generally more abundant in the neonatal than in the adult cord although the ratio of Glu2 to Glu1, Glu3 and Glu4 is lower. Since Glu2 does not allow Ca^{2+} flux, there is relatively more non-NMDA dependent Ca^{2+} influx in neonates and therefore more downstream intracellular Ca^{2+} events. There are also changes in the distribution of the flip-flop variants with postnatal age. The functional importance of this lies in the fact that various combinations of subunits affect desensitization, ionic permeability and current/voltage relationships. The flip variants are generally more sensitive to agonists than the flop resulting in higher levels of depolarization from glutamate release. If the AMPA and NMDA receptors are co-localized, this could lead to enhanced NMDA receptor activation (Jacowec et al. 1995b).

Little is known about the functional role of immature AMPA receptors in neonatal pain but by postnatal days 10–14 in the rat the AMPA antagonist 6-cyano-7-nitroquinoxaline-2,3-dione abolishes dorsal horn cell firing to both low- and high-threshold inputs in vitro (King and Lopez-Garcia 1993). This is in contrast to the NMDA antagonist 5-amino phosphonovaleric acid, which selectively abolishes long latency C fibre evoked activity.

3. Metabotropic Receptors

Metabotropic glutamate receptors have recently been implicated in nociceptive transmission in adult spinal cord (Young et al. 1994), and they may also play a role in developing nociceptive mechanisms. There is evidence that

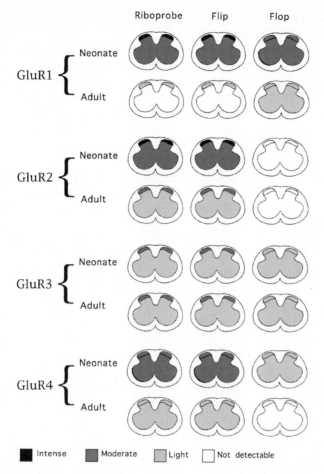

Fig. 3. Summary of in situ hybridization analysis of the developmental changes in expression of transcripts for AMPA receptor subunits in rat spinal cord. (From JACOWEC et al. 1995b)

metabotropic receptors are involved in long-term potentiation production in the neonatal but not the adult hippocampus (IZUMI and ZORUMSKI 1994). Certainly metabotropic glutamate receptors in the spinal cord are differentially regulated during development. Autoradiographical studies show that there are large numbers of low-affinity quisqualate binding sites at birth and fewer high affinity ones. In situ studies of the five subtypes mGluR1–mGluR5 show that mGluR, mGluR2 and mGluR4 are generally low at birth and increase to adult levels, whereas mGluR3 and mGluR5 are high at birth and decrease to adult levels (CATANIA et al. 1994). Signal transduction pathways mediated by mGluRs show opposing developmental patterns: phosphoinositide hydrolysis is very high in the 1st postnatal week and then decreases, whereas inhibition of cAMP formation is achieved only in the adult (Nicoletti et al. 1986; Casabona et al. 1992).

Functional studies of these changes in metabotropic receptors in the dorsal horn have not been undertaken, but the NMDA-dependent, long-duration, C fibre evoked slow ventral root potentials and their wind-up on repeated stimulation are unaffected by the metabotropic antagonist L-AP3 in 8–12 day cord (Thompson et al. 1992).

II. Neuropeptides

Somatostatin and substance P (SP) are present in the dorsal horn and dorsal root ganglia from well before birth, but levels increase considerably in the 2nd postnatal week (Senba et al. 1982). Immunostaining of neonatal lumbar cord shows that the adult pattern of distribution of SP and calcitonin gene related peptide are present by P4, but that adult staining intensities are not achieved until P10 (Reynolds and Fitzgerald 1992). This is also true of somatostatin and galanin (Marti et al. 1987). Levels of SP are regulated by nerve growth factor (NGF), and the administration of excess NGF to newborn rat pups upregulates SP in dorsal root ganglia (Goedert et al. 1981). It is interesting that the onset of NGF expression in the skin coincides with the onset of SP expression in cutaneous sensory neurons, and that a second postnatal surge in NGF production coincides with a substantial increase in SP levels (Constantinou et al. 1994). Administration of excess NGF to neonatal rats increases hypersensitivity to cutaneous stimulation and decreases nociceptive thresholds, which could be due to increased release of SP but is likely to involve several mechanisms (Lewin et al. 1993).

SP receptor density is maximal in the first 2 postnatal weeks; at P60 the cord has one-sixth of the binding sites present at P11. Furthermore, in the newborn there is the inverse receptor distribution of the adult. The superficial laminae have very few SP receptors, and the high density observed in the adult substantia gelatinosa is not apparent until the 2nd week of life (Charlton and Helke 1986; Kar and Quirion 1995; see Fig. 4). Recent analysis in 12–20 day rats shows that the neurokinin 1 (NK_1) receptors in SG are not on the neurons themselves but on lamina III and IV cell dendrites that run through lamina II and terminate in lamina I (Bleazard et al. 1994). Only 10% of the neurons in SG respond to a selective NK_1 receptor agonist, compared to 48% in deeper laminae. It seems likely therefore that the lack of these receptors in neonatal SG reflects the lack of dendritic growth of lamina III and IV cells at this age.

Other neuropeptide receptors, for vasoactive intestinal polypeptide, somatostatin, calcitonin gene related peptide, neurotensin, galanin and NK_3, are also overexpressed in the immature spinal cord but all to different extents, and some, such as galanin, show a clear concentration in SG from birth (Kar and Quirion 1995). Vasopressin receptors are transiently expressed in the immature cord, and physiological studies show them to be functionally active in the neonate (Tribollet et al. 1991) although they are lost in the adult.

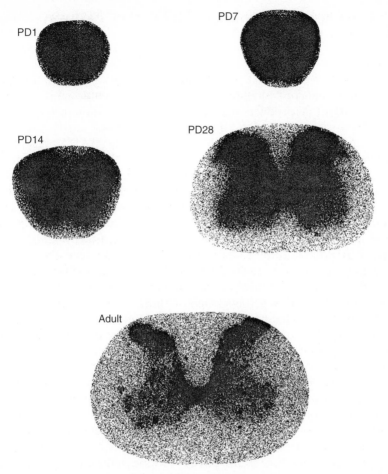

Fig. 4. Autoradiography study of SP/NK$_1$ binding in the developing rat lumbar spinal cord. Sections from postnatal days (*PD*) 1–28 and adult rats are shown. (From KAR and QUIRION 1995)

Despite low levels of SP in the 1st week of life it can be released from central terminals since stimulation of a newborn rat dorsal root at C fibre intensities produces a long-lasting ventral root potential that is blocked by SP antagonists (AKAGI et al. 1982). By P12 it can be shown that both NK$_1$ and NK$_2$ receptors are involved in C fibre evoked slow potentials (NAGY et al. 1994). On the other hand, SP it is not apparently released in sufficient quantities from peripheral C fibre terminals to produce neurogenic extravasation, which cannot be observed until P10 (FITZGERALD and GIBSON 1984) despite the fact that exogenously administered SP can produce extravasation before this age (GONZALEZ et al. 1991).

C. Neonatal Pharmacology of Inhibitory Pathways Involved in Pain

I. GABA

In the adult spinal cord γ-aminobutyric acid (GABA) is an inhibitory amino acid transmitter that produces membrane hyperpolarization through the activation of postsynaptic $GABA_A$ and $GABA_B$ receptors and in addition depresses transmitter release acting through presynaptic $GABA_B$ receptors. In the adult central nervous system GABAergic synaptic inhibition is known to play a crucial role in preventing the spread of excitatory glutamatergic activity. It has therefore been intriguing and exciting to find that GABA mediates most of the *excitatory* drive at early stages of development in the hippocampal CA3 region (STRATA and CHERUBINI 1994; BEN-ARI et al. 1994). Activation of $GABA_A$ receptors induces a depolarization and excitation of immature CA3 pyramidal neurons and increases intracellular Ca^{2+} during the 1st postnatal week of life. During the same developmental period the postsynaptic $GABA_B$-mediated inhibition is poorly developed. In contrast, the presynaptic $GABA_B$-mediated inhibition is well developed at birth and plays a crucial role in modulating the postsynaptic activity by depressing transmitter release at early postnatal stages (GAIARSA et al. 1995a,b). A similar situation occurs in the neonatal dorsal horn where, again, the function of GABA receptors is quite different from in the adult. In 90% of E15–16 dorsal horn neurons cultured for more than 1 week both GABA and glycine induced increased intracellular Ca^{2+} and depolarization (REICHLING et al. 1994). The depolarization and entry of Ca^{2+} through voltage-gated channels by bicuculline-sensitive GABA receptors and strychnine-sensitive glycine receptors decreased with age in culture, and by 30 days it was gone and these agents caused hyperpolarization (WANG et al. 1994). Whole-cell recording of E17–P3 motoneurons show that GABA currents are especially large at this age, and that GABA and glycine result in Cl^- efflux and membrane depolarization, in contrast to the adult where Cl^- influx and hyperpolarization occur. This is a Cl^- specific effect not involving HCO_3^- ions (GAO and ZISKIND-CONHAIM 1995), presumably arising from higher intracellular Cl^- in immature neurons perhaps due to immature co-transport mechanisms (BEN-ARI et al. 1994).

GABA is transiently overexpressed in developing spinal cord and during the first 2 postnatal weeks 50% of neurons are GABA-positive, compared to 20% in the 3rd postnatal week (SCHAFFNER et al. 1993). This is reflected in expression of the GABA-synthesizing enzyme glutamate decarboxylase (GAD) during development. At birth cells expressing two forms of GAD mRNA, GAD65 and GAD67, are widely distributed in all laminae, except in motoneurons of the spinal cord. There follows an overall decrease in the number of GAD mRNA-labelled cells in all layers, but a dramatic drop occurs in a subpopulation of cells within ventral portions of the spinal cord. There is a transient increase in expression between P7 and P14, after which there is a marked decline to adult (MA et al. 1994; SOMOGYI et al. 1995). The appearance of GAD-related mRNAs parallels expression of neuronal markers (light and heavy neurofilaments) and is also closely correlated with the expression of GABA, mRNAs encoding GABA$_A$ receptor subunits and depolarizing responses to GABA (SOMOGYI et al. 1995).

GABA is thought to be one of the classic neurotransmitters acting as a developmental signal. Transient increases in GAD mRNA expression during the early postnatal period coincide with, and may be linked to, synapse formation and synapse elimination of the developing spinal cord (MA et al. 1994). It has been shown that GABA plays a trophic role in the neuritic outgrowth of cultured hippocampal neurons (GAIARSA et al. 1995a).

There is evidence of a new biculline-baclofen insensitive type of GABA receptor which is evident during development (STRATA and CHERUBINI 1994).

II. Opiates

Opioids interact with the three opioid receptors μ, δ and κ and the endogenous opioid peptides – the enkephalins, dynorphins and endorphins – are not specific for any one receptor (DICKENSON 1994). Both μ and κ receptor binding sites appear in the rat spinal cord early in fetal life (E15) and δ sites do not appear until after birth (ATTALI et al. 1990). The density of μ and κ receptors at their peak are almost twice as great as in the adult whereas the density of δ sites is low. The κ sites predominate in the immature spinal cord, where they form 55%–80% of binding sites, peaking at day 7, but binding properties appear to be the same as in the adult. The μ sites represent 20%–38% of the population peaking at postnatal day 1 (ATTALI et al. 1990). Some caution is required in interpreting these percentages, however, since the adult values given in this study are not consistent with previous reports (see DICKENSON 1994). Autoradiography with radiolabelled specific μ receptor ligand FK 33–824 shows binding sites to be distributed widely across spinal cord laminae during early postnatal development, followed by selective modification to attain their adult distribution during the 3rd postnatal week. Unlike in the adult, where μ receptor binding is concentrated heavily in the superficial laminae of the dorsal horn, and only moderate amounts in laminae III–V, IX and X of the grey matter, the distribution in the first 2 postnatal weeks is marked by high densities in both superficial and deep dorsal and intermediate horn, with moderate amounts in the ventral horn (KAR and QUIRION 1995).

The reported effects of morphine in producing analgesia in infant rats has changed over the years. Early reports of higher susceptibility of newborn animals to the convulsive effect of systemic morphine have been shown to be unfounded through careful analysis of EEG and behaviour at 6–300mg/kg (VAN PRAAG and FRENK 1992). A number of studies have shown that in thermal and pressure tests of nociception the analgesic effects of morphine are weak until the 2nd postnatal week (ZHANG and PASTERNAK 1981; BARR et al. 1986; GIORDIANO and BARR 1987; FANSELOW and CRAMER 1988), but that the κ opiate ketocyclazocine is an effective analgesic in the 1st postnatal week, reaching adult potency by P10 (BARR et al. 1986). However, more recent studies emphasize the antinociceptive effects of morphine soon after birth. Morphine (0.5–4.0 mg/kg) produces a dose-related increase in hindlimb withdrawal latency to a hot plate from day 2, with maximum sensitivity at day 6 (BLASS et al. 1993), and the pain responses induced by the formalin inflammatory model is suppressed by 1–2 mg/kg morphine in 3 day old rats (MCLAUGHLIN et al. 1990). These discrepancies may arise from the central effects of opioids, especially those related to decreased respiration since brainstem μ receptors are also developmentally regulated postnatally (MURPHEY and OLSEN 1995). Another important point is the need to distinguish between the sedative and analgesic effects of morphine, a problem that has been recently addressed by ABBOT and GUY (1995) by comparing the suppression of specific and non-specific responses to intraplantar injection of formalin by morphine and by pentobarbital. This study shows that from the 1st postnatal day 1 mg/kg morphine produces behavioural analgesia that is qualitatively different from the sedative effects of pentobarbital.

In isolated spinal cords of 1- to 4-day-old rats β-endorphin, [D-Ala^2]Met-enkephalinamide and morphine depress the dorsal root potential in a naloxone reversible manner (SUZUE and JESSELL 1980). In 8- to 12-day-rats 0.1–20 μM morphine reduces the NMDA sensitive slow ventral root potential by 70% and shorter latency NMDA sensitive component by 30%, leaving the Aβ and early fibre C evoked components unaffected (SIVILOTTI et al. 1995).

Subcutaneous administration of Met^5-enkephalin in the neonate combined with peptidase inhibitors to prevent rapid degradation produces an inhibition of the tail-flick response and loss of the righting response, apparently mediated through the μ receptor. This effect is decreased at day 15 and lost by day 20, suggesting that the permeability of the blood-brain barrier against opioid peptides matures only after 2 postnatal weeks (OKA et al. 1992).

III. Monoamines

While 5-hydroxytryptamine 5-HT is clearly involved in spinal analgesia, the multiple receptor subtypes (14 mammalian 5-HT receptors now cloned) makes its mode of action obscure (see LUCAS and HEN 1995). 5-HT$_{1C}$ and 5-HT$_2$ receptors are distributed widely in the CNS in embryonic life (HELLENDALL et al. 1993; PRANZATELLI 1993; PRANZATELLI and GALVAN 1994). Transient expression of 5-HT$_{1B}$ receptors has been reported on thalmocortical axons (BENNETT-CLARKE et al. 1994) which are functionally active for the first 2 weeks of life, mediating presynaptic inhibition, but are gone after 2 weeks (RHOADES et al. 1994). However, the onset of expression of both 5-HT and its receptors precedes their specific functions in the spinal cord, suggesting that they, as with glutamate, play a trophic role during development (RAJAOFETRA et al. 1992; ZISKIND-CONHAIM et al. 1993).

5-HT projections grow into the ventral horn between embryonic days 16 and 18 (ZISKIND-CONHAIM et al. 1993) but are not present in the dorsal horn until birth. A laminar distribution is apparent at p 5, but the adult distribution and density is not achieved until the end of the 2nd week (MARTI et al. 1987; WANG et al. 1991). There also is evidence of a transient overexpression of 5-HT in the spinal cord at P14 (BREGMAN 1987). In motoneurons the responses to 5-HT are mediated by multiple receptor subtypes and increase significantly at the time that 5-HT projections first appear (ZISKIND-CONHAIM et al. 1993).

Noradrenergic axons invade the spinal cord at E16, beginning in the ventral cord and reaching the dorsal horn by P0. The pattern of innervation in the dorsal horn resembles that of the adult at P7 but adult density is not reached until P30 (RAJAOFETRA et al. 1992). Peak noradrenergic receptor development in rat spinal cord occurs at around P12, consistent with the analgesic effects of intrathecal noradrenaline and the α_2 agonist clonidine in P10 rat pups (HUGHES and BARR 1988). Noradrenaline containing terminals first appear in the dorsal horn at P4 and achieve the adult pattern by 14–21 days (COMMISSIONG 1983).

Levels of 5-HT are apparently not sufficient for effective function of descending inhibitory pathways to the spinal cord from the brainstem until the 2nd or 3rd postnatal week (FITZGERALD and KOLTZENBURG 1986; VAN PRAAG and FRENK 1991). D-Amphetamine (2 mg/kg) at doses that would enhance release of all three monoamines does not begin to affect pain behaviour before 10 days of age, suggesting that these monoamines are not fully functional in the pain pathways before that time (ABBOT and GUY 1995).

D. Concluding Comments

The study of the neonatal pharmacology of pain requires an understanding of the underlying developmental biology of the nervous system and of sensory neurons in particular. Many aspects of receptor distribution, density, ratio of subunits and functional properties undergo enormous changes in the pre- and postnatal periods. This has been interpreted in other systems, such as the hippocampus and the visual system, in terms of synaptogenesis and fine tuning of connections during development and no doubt is related to these events in the dorsal horn of the spinal cord also. However, spinal cord pain pathways are active from birth, and it is important to consider the effects of these develop-mental changes in transmitter/receptor systems on the functional properties of neonatal pain transmission and pain behaviour. This in turn influences the effectiveness of any analgesic therapy applied to the newborn. The introduc-tory section briefly discussed the differences in the physiological properties of neonatal pain pathways compared to those in the adult. It is tempting to suggest that the hyperexcitability of NMDA receptors and the depolarizing responses to GABA in immature sensory neurons are partly responsible for the exaggerated responses evoked by cutaneous stimulation in the neonate, but this has not been tested directly.

An enormous amount of research must still be carried out in this area. Increases in intracellular calcium may trigger a cascade of secondary events such as the activation of protein kinases and phosphatases, for example phospholipase A_2, leading to increases in intracellular arachidonic acid and the formation of cyclo-oygenase and lipoxygenase products and the synthesis of nitric oxide, all of which are implicated in nociceptive pathways. Recent evidence suggests that nitric oxide is not induced in the spinal cord by noxious stimulation until the 2nd postnatal week (SOYGUDER et al. 1994), but the developmental regulation of downstream events remains to be investigated.

References

Abbot FV, Guy ER (1995) Effects of morphine, pentobarbital and amphetamine on formalin-induced behaviours in infant rats: sedation versus specific suppression of pain. Pain 62:303–312

Akagi H, Konishi S, Yanagisawa M, Otsuka M (1983) Effects of capsaicin and a substance P antagonist on a slow reflex in isolated rat spinal cord. Neurochem Res 8:795–796

Altman J, Bayer S A (1984) The development of the rat spinal cord. Adv Anat Embryol Cell Biol 85:1–166

Attali B, Saya D, Vogel Z (1990) Pre- and postnatal development of opiate receptor subtypes in rat spinal cord. Dev Brain Res 53:97–102

Audinat E, Lambolez B, Rossier J, Crepel F (1994) Activity-dependent regulation of N-methyl-D-aspartate receptor subunit expression in rat cerebellar granule cells. Eur J Neurosci 6:1792–1800

Barr GA, Paredes W, Erickson KL, Zukin RS (1986) Kappa-opioid receptor mediated analgesia in the developing rat. Dev Brain Res 29:145–152

Ben-Ari Y, Tseeb V, Raggozzino D, Khazipov R, Gaiarsa JL (1994) Gamma-aminobutyric acid (GABA): a fast excitatory transmitter which may regulate the development of hippocampal neurones in early postnatal life. Prog Brain Res 102:261–73

Bennett-Clarke CA, Hankin MH, Leslie MJ, Chiaia NL, Rhoades RW (1994) Patterning of the neocortical projections from the raphe nuclei in perinatal rats: investigation of potential organizational mechanisms. J Comp Neurol 348:277–290

Bicknell HR, Beal JA (1984) Axonal and dendritic development of substantia gelatinosa neurons in the lumbosacral spinal cord of the rat. J Comp Neurol 226:508–522

Blass EM, Cramer CP, Fanselow MS (1993) The development of morphine induced antinociception in neonatal rats: a comparison of forpaw, hindpaw and tail retraction from a thermal stimulus. Pharm Biochem Behav 44:643–649

Bleazard L, Hill RG, Morris R (1994) The correlation between the distribution of the NK_1 receptor and the actions of tachykinin agonists in the dorsal horn of the rat indicates that substance P does not have a functional role on substantia gelatinosa (lamina II) neurons. J Neurosci 14:7655–7664

Brady RJ, Gorter JA, Monroe MT, Swann JW (1994) Developmental alterations in the sensitivity of hippocampal NMDA receptors to AP5. Dev Brain Res 83:190–196

Bregman BS (1987) Development of serotonin immunoreactivity in the rat spinal cord and its plasticity after neonatal spinal cord lesions. Dev Brain Res 34:245–263

Cabalka LM, Ritchie TC, Coulter JD (1990) Immunolocalization of a novel nerve terminal protein in spinal cord development. J Comp Neurol 295:83–91

Carmignoto G, Vicini S (1992) Activity dependent decrease in NMDA receptor re-
    'sponses during development of the visual cortex. Science 258:1007–1011
Casabona G, Genazzi AA, Di SM, Sortino MA, Nicoletti F (1992) Developmental
    changes in the modulation of cyclic AMP formation by the metabotropic
    glutamate receptor agonist 15,3R aminocyclopentane-1,3 dicarboxylicacid in brain
    slices. J Neurochem 89:1161–1163
Catania MV, Landwehrmeyer GB, Testa CM, Standaert DG, Penney JB Jr, Young AB
    (1994) Metabotropic glutamate receptors are differentially regulated during devel-
    opment. Neurosci 61:481–495
Charlton CG, Helke CJ (1986) Ontogeny of substance-P receptors in the rat spinal
    cord: quantitative changes in receptor number and differential expression in spe-
    cific loci. Dev Brain Res 29:81–91
Coggeshall RE, Pover CM, Fitzgerald M (1994) Dorsal root ganglion cell death and
    surviving cell numbers in relation to the development of sensory innervation in the
    rat hindlimb. Dev Brain Res 82:193–212
Coggeshall RE, Jennings E, Fitzgerald M (1995) Evidence that large myelinated pri-
    mary afferent fibres make synaptic contacts in lamina II of neonatal rats. Dev
    Brain Res 92:81–90
Commissiong JW (1983) The development of catecholaminergic nerves in the spinal
    cord of the rat. II. Regional development. Dev Brain Res 11:75–92
Constantinou J, Reynolds ML, Woolf CJ, Safieh-Garabedian B, Fitzgerald M (1994)
    Nerve growth factor levels in developing rat skin: upregulation following skin
    wounding. Neuroreport 5:2281–2284
Dickenson AH (1994) Where and how do opioids act? In: Gebhart GF, Hammond DL,
    Jensen TS (eds) Progress in pain research and management, vol 2. International
    Association for the Study of Pain, Seattle, pp 525–552
Ekholm J (1967) Postnatal changes in cutaneous reflexes and in the discharge pattern
    of cutaneous and articular sense organs. Acta Physiol Scand [Suppl] 297:1–
    130
Fanselow MS, Cramer CP (1988) The ontogeny of opiate tolerance and withdrawal in
    infant rats. Pharmacol Biochem Behav 31:431–438
Fitzgerald M (1985) The postnatal development of cutaneous afferent fibre input and
    receptive field organization in the rat dorsal horn. J Physiol (Lond) 364:1–18
Fitzgerald M (1987) The prenatal growth of fine diameter afferents into the rat spinal
    cord – a transganglionic study. J Comp Neurol 261:98–104
Fitzgerald M (1988) The development of activity evoked by fine diameter cutaneous
    fibres in the spinal cord of the newborn rat. Neurosci Lett 86:161–166
Fitzgerald M (1991a) A physiological study of the prenatal development of cutaneous
    sensory inputs to dorsal horn cells in the rat. J Physiol (Lond) 432:473–482
Fitzgerald M (1991b) The developmental neurobiology of pain. In: Bond M, Woolf CJ,
    Charlton M (eds) Proceedings of the 6th World Congress on Pain. Elsevier,
    Amsterdam, pp 253–261
Fitzgerald M (1995) Pain in infancy: some unanswered questions. Pain Rev 2:77–91
Fitzgerald M, Anand K (1993) The developmental neuroanatomy and neurophysiology
    of pain. In: Schechter NL, Berde CB, Yaster Y (eds) Pain in infants, children and
    adolescents. Williams and Wilkins, Baltimore, pp 11–31
Fitzgerald M, Gibson SJ (1984) The postnatal physiological and neurochemical devel-
    opment of peripheral sensory C fibres. Neuroscience 13:933–944
Fitzgerald M, Koltzenburg M (1986) The functional development of descending inhibi-
    tory pathways in the dorsolateral funiculus of the newborn rat spinal cord. Dev
    Brain Res 24:261–270
Fitzgerald M, Shaw A, Macintosh N (1987) The postnatal development of the cutane-
    ous flexor reflex: a comparative study in premature infants and newborn rat pups.
    Dev Med Child Neurol 30:520–526
Fitzgerald M, Reynolds ML, Benowitz LI (1991) GAP-43 expression in the developing
    rat lumbar spinal cord. Neurosci 41:187–199

Fitzgerald M, Butcher T, Shortland P (1995) Developmental changes in the laminar termination of A fibre cutaneous sensory afferents in the rat spinal cord dorsal horn. J Comp Neurol 348:225–233

Gaiarsa JL, McLean H, Congar P, Leinekugel X, Khazipov R, Tseeb V, Ben-Ari Y (1995a) Postnatal maturation of gamma-aminobutyric acidA and B-mediated inhibition in the CA3 hippocampal region of the rat. J Neurobiol 26:339–349

Gaiarsa JL, Tseeb V, Ben-Ari Y (1995b) Postnatal development of pre- and postsynaptic GABAB-mediated inhibitions in the CA3 hippocampal region of the rat. J Neurophysiol 73:246–255

Gao B-X, Ziskind-Conhaim L (1995) Development of glycine and GABA-gated currents in rat spinal motoneurons. J Neurophysiol 74:113–121

Giordano J, Barr GA (1987) Morphine and ketocyclazocine-induced analgesia in the developing rat: differences due to type of noxious stimulus and body topography. Dev Brain Res 32:247–253

Goedert M, Stoeckel K, Otten U (1981) Biological importance of the retrograde axonal transport of nerve growth factor in sensory neurons. Proc Natl Acad Sci USA 78:5895–5898

Gonzales R, Coderre TJ, Sherbourne CD, Levine JD (1991) Postnatal development of neurogenic in the rat. Neurosci Lett 127:25–27

Gonzalez DL, Fuchs JL, Droge MH (1993) Distribution of NMDA receptor binding in developing mouse spinal cord. Neurosci Lett 151:134–137

Guy ER, Abbott FV (1992) The behavioural response to formalin pain in preweanling rats. Pain 51:81–90

Hammond DL, Ruda MA (1991) Developmental alterations in nociceptive threshold, immunoreactive calcitonin-gene related peptide, substance P and fluoride resistant acid phosphatase in neonatally capsaicin treated rats. J Comp Neurol 312:436–450

Hellendall RP, Schambra UB, Liu JP, Lauder JM (1993) Prenatal expression of 5-HT_{1C} and 5-HT_2 receptors in the rat central nervous system. Exp Neurol 120:186–201

Hestrin S (1992) Developmental regulation of NMDA receptors-mediated synaptic at a central synapse. Nature 357:686–689

Hofer M, Constantine-Paton M (1994) Regulation of N-methyl-D-aspartate (NMDA) receptor function during the rearrangement of developing neuronal connections. Prog Brain Res 102:277–285

Hori Y, Kanda K (1994) Developmental alterations in NMDA receptor-mediated $[Ca^{2+}]i$ elevation in substantia gelatinosa neurons of neonatal rat spinal cord. Dev Brain Res 80:141–148

Hori Y, Watanabe S (1987) Morphine-sensitive late components of the flexion reflex in the neonatal rat. Neurosci Lett 78:91–96

Hughes HE, Barr GA (1988) Analgesic effects of intrathecally applied noradrenergic compounds in the developing rat: differences due to thermal vs mechanical nociception. Dev Brain Res 41:109–120

Hulsebosch CE, Coggeshall RE, Chung K (1986) Numbers of rat dorsal root axons and ganglion cells during postnatal development. Dev Brain Res 26:105–113

Izumi Y, Zorumski CF (1994) Developmental changes in the effects of metabotropic glutamate receptor antagonists on CA1 long-term potentiation in rat hippocampal slices. Neurosci Lett 176:89–92

Jacowec MW, Fox AJ, Martin CJ, Kalb RG (1995a) Quantitative and qualitative changes in AMPA receptor expression during spinal cord development. Neuroscience 67:893–907

Jacowec MW, Yen L, Kalb RG (1995b) In situ hybridization analysis of AMPA receptor subunit gene expression in the developing rat spinal cord. Neuroscience 67:909–920

Jennings E, Fitzgerald M (1996) C-fos can be induced in the neonatal rat spinal cord by both noxious and innocuous stimulation. Pain 68:301–306

Kar S, Quirion R (1995) Neuropeptide receptors in developing and adult rat spinal cord: an in vitro quantitative autoradiography study of calcitonin gene-related peptide, neurokinins, μ-opioid, galanin, somatostatin, neurotensin and vasoactive intestinal polypeptide receptors. J Comp Neurol 354:253–281

King AE, Lopez-Garcia JA (1993) Excitatory amino acid receptor mediated neurotransmission from cutaneous afferents in rat dorsal horn "in vitro". J Physiol (Lond) 472:443–457

Lewin GR, Ritter AM, Mendell LM (1993) Nerve growth factor-induced hyperalgesia in the neonatal and adult rat. J Neurosci 13:2136–2148

Lucas JJ, Hen R (1995) New players in the 5-HT receptor field: genes and knockouts. Trends Pharmocol Sci 16:217–252

Ma W, Behar T, Chang L, Barker JL (1994) Transient increase in expression of GAD65 and GAD67 mRNAs during postnatal development of rat spinal cord. J Comp Neurol 346:151–160

Marti E, Gibson SJ, Polak JM, Facer P, Springall DR, Van Aswegen G, Aitchison M, Koltzenburg M (1987) Ontogeny of peptide and amine-containing neurones in motor, sensory, and autonomic regions of rat and human spinal cord, dorsal root ganglia, and rat skin. J Comp Neurol 266:332–359

McLaughlin CR, Litchman AH, Fanselow MS, Cramer CP (1990) Tonic nociception in neonatal rats. Pharmacol Biochem Behav 36:859–862

Mendelson B (1994) Chronic embryonic MK-801 exposure disrupts the somatotopic organization of cutaneous nerve projections in the chick spinal cord Dev Brain Res 82:152–166

Morrisett RA, Mott DD, Lewis DV, Wilson WA, Swartzwelder HS (1990) Reduced sensitivity of the N-methyl-D-aspartate component of synaptic transmission to magnesium in hippocampal slices from immature rats. Dev Brain Res 56:257–262

Murphey LJ, Olsen GD (1995) Developmental change of mu receptors in neonatal guinea pig brain stem. Dev Brain Res 85:146–148

Nagy I, Miller BA, Woolf CJ (1994) NK$_1$ and NK$_2$ receptors contribute to C-fibre evoked slow potentials in the rat spinal cord. Neuroreport 5:2105–2108

Nicoletti F, Iadotola MJ, Wroblewski JT, Costa E (1986) Excitatory amino acid recognition sites coupled with inositol phospholipid metabolism: developmental changes and interaction with α_1-adrenoreceptors. Proc Natl Acad Sci USA 83:1931–1935

Oka T, Liu X-F, Kajita T, Ohgiya N, Ghoda K, Taniguchi T, Arai Y, Matsumiya T (1992) Effects of subcutaneous administration of enkephalins on tail-flick response and righting reflex of developing rats. Dev Brain Res 69:271–276

Pignatelli D, Ribeiro-da-Silva A, Coimbra A (1989) Postnatal maturation of primary afferent terminations in the substantia gelatinosa of the rat spinal cord. An electron microscope study. Brain Res 491:33–44

Pranzatelli MR (1993) Regional differences in the ontogeny of 5-hydroxytryptamine-1C binding sites in rat brain and spinal cord. Neurosci Lett 149:9–11

Pranzatelli MR, Galvan I (1994) Ontogeny of [^{125}I]iodocyanopindolol-labelled 5-hydroxytryptamine1B-binding sites in the rat CNS. Neurosci Lett 167:166–170

Rajaofetra N, Poulat P, Marlier L, Geffard M, Privat A (1992) Pre- and postnatal development of noradrenergic projections to the rat spinal cord: an immunocytochemical study. Dev Brain Res 67:237–246

Reichling DB, Kyrozis A, Wang J, McDermott AB (1994) Mechanisms of GABA and glycine depolarization-induced calcium transients in rat dorsal horn neurons. J Physiol (Lond) 476:411–421

Reynolds ML, Fitzgerald M (1992) Neonatal sciatic nerve section results in TMP but not SP or CGRP depletion from the terminal field in the dorsal horn of the rat: the role of collateral sprouting. Neuroscience 51:191–202

Rhoades RW, Bennett-Clarke CA, Shi MY, Mooney RD (1994) Effects of 5-HT on thalamocortical synaptic transmission in the developing rat. J Neurophysiol 72:2438–2450

Riva MA, Tascedda F, Molteni R, Racagni G (1994) Regulation of NMDA receptor subunit mRNA expression in the rat brain during postnatal development. Mol Brain Res 25:209–216

Schaffner AE, Behar T, Nadi S, Barker JL (1993) Quantitative analysis of transient GABA expression in embryonic and early postnatal rat spinal neurons. Dev Brain Res 72:265–276

Senba E, Hiosaka S, Hara Y, Inagaki S, Sakanaka M, Takatsuki K, Kawai Y, Tohyama M (1982) Ontogeny of the peptidergic system in the rat spinal cord. Immunohistochemical analysis. J Comp Neurol 208:54–66

Shortland P, Molander C, Fitzgerald M, Woolf CJ (1990) Neonatal capsaicin treatment induces invasion of the substantia gelatinosa by the arborizations of hair follicle afferents in the rat dorsal horn. J Comp Neurol 296:23–31

Sivilotti LG, Gerber G, Rawat B, Woolf CJ (1995) Morphine selectively depresses the slowest, NMDA-dependent component of C-fibre evoked synaptic activity in the rat spinal cord "in vitro". Eur J Neurosci 7:12–18

Somogyi R, Wen X, Ma W, Barker JL (1995) Developmental kinetics of GAD family mRNAs parallel neurogenesis in the rat spinal cord. J Neurosci 15:2575–2591

Soyguder Z, Schmidt HHHW, Morris R (1994) Postnatal development of nitric oxide synthase type I expression in the lumbar spinal cord of the rat: a comparison of c-fos in response to peripheral application of mustard oil. Neurosci Lett 180:188–192

Strata F, Cherubini E (1994) Transient expression of a novel type of GABA response in rat CA3 hippocampal neurones during development. J Physiol (Lond) 480:493–503

Suzue T, Jessell T (1980) Opiate analgesics and endorphins inhibit rat dorsal root potential in vitro. Neurosci Lett 16:161–166

Thompson SWN, King AE, Woolf CJ (1990) Activity dependent changes in rat ventral horn neurons "in vitro", summation of prolonged afferent evoked postsynaptic depolarizations produce a D-2-amino-5-phosphonovaleric acid sensitive wind-up. Eur J Neurosci 2:638–649

Thompson SWN, Gerber G, Sivilotti LG, Woolf CJ (1992) Long duration ventral root potentials in the neonatal rat spinal cord "in vitro", the effects of ionotropic and metabotropic excitatory amino acid receptor antagonists. Brain Res 595:87–97

Tribollet E, Goumaz M, Raggenbass M, Dubois-Dauphin M, Dreifuss JJ (1991) Early appearance and transient expression of vasopressin receptors in the brain of rat fetus and infant. An autoradiographical and electrophysiological study. Dev Brain Res 58:13–24

Van Praag H, Frenk H (1991) The development of stimulation-produced analgesia (SPA) in the rat. Dev Brain Res 64:71–76

Van Praag H, Frenk H (1992) The effects of systemic morphine on behaviour and EEG in newborn rats. Dev Brain Res 67:19–26

Wang J, Reichling DB, Kyrozis A, MacDermott AB (1994) Developmental loss of GABA- and glycine-induced depolarization and Ca^{2+} transients in embryonic rat dorsal horn neurons in culture. Eur J Neurosci 6:1275–1280

Wang SD, Goldberger ME, Murray M (1991) Normal development and the effects of early rhizotomy on spinal systems in the rat. Dev Brain Res 64:57–69

Watanabe M, Mishina M Inoue Y (1994) Distinct spatiotemporal distributions of the N-methyl-D-aspartate receptor channel subunit mRNAs in the mouse cervical cord. J Comp Neurol 345:314–319

Williams S, Evan G, Hunt SP (1990) Changing patterns of c-fos induction in spinal neurons following thermal cutaneous stimulation in the rat. Neuroscience 49:3673–3681

Woolf CJ, King AE (1987) Physiology and morphology of multireceptive neurons with C afferent fiber inputs in the deep dorsal horn of the rat lumbar spinal cord. J Neurophysiol 58:460–479

Young MR, Fleetwood-Walker SM, Mitchell R, Munroe FE (1994) Evidence for a role of metabotropic glutamate receptors in sustained nociceptive inputs to rat dorsal horn neurons. Neuropharmacology 33:141–144

Zhang AZ, Pasternak GW (1981) Ontogeny of opioid pharmacology and receptors: high and low affinity site differences. Eur J Pharmacol 73:29–40

Zhong J, Carrozza DP, Williams K, Pritchett DB, Molinoff PB (1995) Expression of mRNAs encoding subunits of the NMDA receptor in developing rat brain. J Neurochem 64:531–539

Ziskind-Conhaim L, Seebach BS, Gao BX (1993) Changes in serotonin-induced potentials during spinal cord development. J Neurophysiol 69:1338–1349

Subject Index

Subject Index

Springer
and the
environment

At Springer we firmly believe that an international science publisher has a special obligation to the environment, and our corporate policies consistently reflect this conviction.
We also expect our business partners – paper mills, printers, packaging manufacturers, etc. – to commit themselves to using materials and production processes that do not harm the environment. The paper in this book is made from low- or no-chlorine pulp and is acid free, in conformance with international standards for paper permanency.

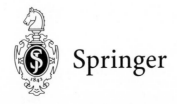

Springer

Printing: Saladruck, Berlin
Binding: Buchbinderei Lüderitz & Bauer, Berlin